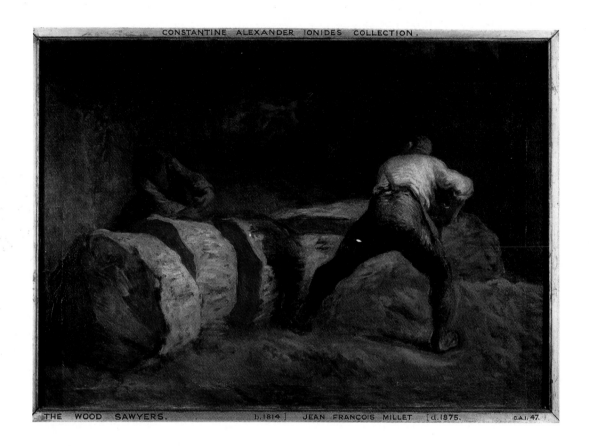

"Woodsawyers," by Jean Francois Millet (1850). (Reproduced with permission from the Victoria and Albert Museum, London.)

OCCUPATIONAL HAND & UPPER EXTREMITY INJURIES & DISEASES

EDITED BY **MORTON L. KASDAN** M.D., FACS

Associate Clinical Professor of Surgery (Plastic and Recon-
structive Surgery), University of Louisville School of Medicine;
Associate Clinical Professor, Occupational Medicine, University of
Kentucky Medical Center

HANLEY & BELFUS, INC./Philadelphia
MOSBY–YEAR BOOK/St. Louis • Baltimore • Boston • Chicago • London
Philadelphia • Sydney • Toronto

Publisher: HANLEY & BELFUS, INC.
                  210 S. 13th Street
                  Philadelphia, PA 19107
                  (215) 546-7293

North American and worldwide sales and distribution:

                  MOSBY-YEAR BOOK, INC.
                  11830 Westline Industrial Drive
                  St. Louis, MO 63146

In Canada: THE C.V. MOSBY COMPANY, LTD.
                  5240 Finch Avenue East
                  Unit 1
                  Scarborough, Ontario M1S 5A2
                  Canada

**Occupational Hand and Upper Extremity
  Injuries and Diseases**

ISBN 1-56053-002

Library of Congress Catalog Card Number 90-83166

Last digit is the print number: 9 8 7 6 5 4 3 2 1

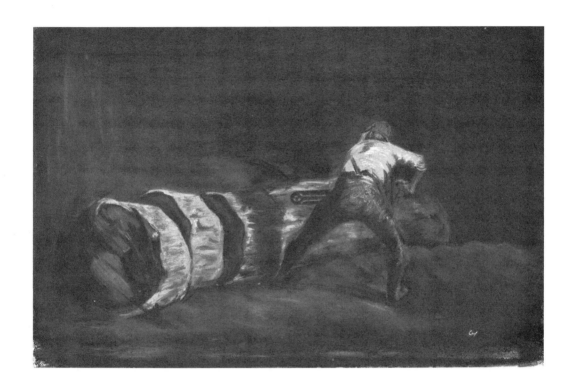

"Woodsawyer II," by Craig Wilkerson (1990).

DEDICATION

This book is dedicated to my teachers who helped me recognize the importance of education and hard work.

Morris and Sarah Kasdan
Harold E. Kleinert, M.D., F.A.C.S.
Richard A. Mladick, M.D., F.A.C.S.
Kenneth L. Pickrell, M.D., F.A.C.S.

CONTENTS

1. The Role of Motivation in the Recovery of the Hand 1
   Paul W. Brown, M.D.

2. Chronic Pain and the Injured Worker: A Sociobiological Problem........... 13
   Edward R. Chaplin, M.D.

3. Prevention of Occupational Hand Injuries 47
   Sidney J. Blair, M.D., F.A.C.S

4. Etiologies and Prevalence of Occupational Injuries to the Upper Extremity... 53
   Frank P. Vannier, M.D. and John F. Rose, M.D.

5. Anatomy of the Upper Extremity 61
   Joel B. Grad, M.D.

6. Psychological Evaluation of Hand Pain 75
   Richard K. Johnson, Ph.D.

7. How the Radiologist Can Help to Evaluate Injuries and Diseases of the
   Upper Extremity 89
   Jeri P. Irwin, M.D., William W. Joule, M.D.,
   Gary H. Peterson, M.D., Curt E. Liebman, M.D., and
   Jannice O. Aaron, M.D.

8. Neurologic Evaluation of the Upper Extremity........................... 115
   Michael R. Swenson, M.D. and David R. Villasana, M.D.

9. First Aid for Hand Injuries.. 131
   L. Scott Levin, M.D.

10. Local and Regional Block Anesthesia for the Upper Extremity.............. 143
    Donald M. Ditmars, Jr., M.D.

11. Preoperative Care of the Surgical Patient............................... 155
    Ann S. Kasdan, R.N.

12. Fingertip and Nail Bed Injuries 159
    Donald M. Ditmars, Jr., M.D.

13. Tendon Injuries of the Hand 171
    Mark R. Wilson, M.D. and Fred M. Hankin, M.D.

14. Occupational Hand Fractures and Dislocations. **181**
David P. Falconer, M.D., Paul J. Donahue, M.D.,
Melissa L. Barton, M.D., Charles J. MacDonald, M.D., and
Steven R. Sonkowsky, O.P.A.-C., R.P.A.

15. Replantations and Amputations of the Upper Extremity **215**
Luis R. Scheker, M.D. and David T. Netscher, M.D.

16. High-Pressure Injection Injuries: Preventable and Underestimated **233**
Morton L. Kasdan, M.D., F.A.C.S., and
Ramon O. Ryan, M.D., M.S.

17. Early Repair and Late Reconstruction of Crush Injuries. **239**
Ellen Beatty, M.D. and Robert J. Belsole, M.D.

18. Electrical Injuries **249**
Kevin P. Yakuboff, M.D. and Harold E. Kleinert, M.D.

19. Emergency Management of Thermal, Electrical, and Chemical Burns **259**
Leland R. Chick, M.D. and Graham D. Lister, M.B., Ch.B.

20. Peripheral Nerve Injuries and Their Management. **271**
R. Frederick Torstrick, M.D.

21. Diagnosis and Management of Occupational Disorders of the Shoulder **279**
Elin Barth, M.D. and Edward W. Berg, M.D.

22. Diagnosis and Management of Occupational Disorders of the Elbow **289**
Ronald C. Burgess, M.D.

23. Ligament Injuries of the Wrist **297**
Peter C. Amadio, M.D.

24. Ligament Injuries of the Hand. **311**
Raymond C. Noellert, M.D. and Fred M. Hankin, M.D.

25. Work-Related Vascular Injuries and Diseases. **319**
Anthony C. Berger, M.B.B.S., F.R.A.C.S. and
James M. Kleinert, M.D.

26. Management of Carpal Tunnel Syndrome **341**
Robert M. Szabo, M.D. and Michael Madison, Ph.D.

27. Cumulative Trauma Disorders and Compression Neuropathies of the
Upper Extremities. **353**
Linda H. Mosely, M.D., F.A.C.S., Roberta M. Kalafut, D.O.,
Paula D. Levinson, P.T., and Sue A. Mokris, O.T.R.

28. Tendinitis of the Upper Extremity. **403**
Janet R. Chipman, M.D., Morton L. Kasdan, M.D., F.A.C.S. and
Daniel G. Camacho, M.D., F.A.C.S.

29. Infections of the Hand **423**
Robert L. Reid, M.D., F.A.C.S.

30. Postoperative Care. **433**
Lois E. Thompson, R.N.

31. Occupational Contact Dermatitis of the Upper Extremity **443**
Chester L. Davidson, M.D.

32. Arthritis of the Hand and Upper Extremity in the Workplace **455**
    Gary L. Crump, M.D. and Paul D. Schneider, M.D.

33. Hand Therapy for Occupational Upper Extremity Disorders **469**
    Connie Lane, P.T.

34. Return-to-Work Programs After Hand Injuries **479**
    Nancy P. McElwain, M.B.A., R.N.

35. Unable to Return to Work—Now What? **483**
    *Terri L. Wolfe, O.T.R./L., Mark S. DiPlacido, M.A., and
    John D. Lubahn, M.D.*

36. Cumulative Trauma Intervention in Industry: A Model Program for the
    Upper Extremity **489**
    Connie M. Rystrom, B.S. and William W. Eversmann, Jr., M.D.

37. Legal Considerations in Occupational Medicine **507**
    Susan J. Hauck, J.D.

38. Workers' Compensation—Legal Issues **515**
    Freeda M. Steinberg, J.D.

39. Ergonomic Design of Handheld Tools to Prevent Trauma to the Hand and
    Upper Extremity **527**
    Susan L. Johnson, O.T.R., C.V.E.

40. Ergonomic Considerations and Job Design **539**
    Bradley S. Joseph, Ph.D. and Donald S. Bloswick, P.E., Ph.D.

Index **569**

CONTRIBUTORS

JANNICE O. AARON, M.D.

Saint Anthony Medical Center Imaging Center, Louisville, Kentucky

PETER C. AMADIO, M.D.

Associate Professor of Orthopedics, Mayo Medical School; Consultant, Department of Orthopedics, Mayo Clinic and Mayo Foundation, Rochester, Minnesota

ELIN BARTH, M.D., Ph.D.

Lunceford-Moore Chair of Orthopaedic Research, Department of Orthopaedics, University of South Carolina School of Medicine, Columbia, South Carolina

MELISSA L. BARTON, M.D.

Attending Staff Surgeon, Metropolitan Hand Surgery Associates, St. Paul, Minnesota

ELLEN BEATTY, M.D.

Clinical Assistant Professor of Plastic Surgery and Orthopedic Surgery, University of South Florida; Staff, Florida Orthopedic Institute, Tampa, Florida

ROBERT J. BELSOLE, M.D.

Professor of Orthopaedic Surgery, University of South Florida Medical College; Staff, Florida Orthopedic Institute, Tampa, Florida

EDWARD W. BERG, M.D.

Professor of Orthopaedic Surgery, University of South Carolina School of Medicine; Chief of Orthopaedics, Dorns VA Hospital, Columbia, South Carolina

ANTHONY C. BERGER, M.B.B.S., FRACS

Former Fellow of the Christine M. Kleinert Institute for Hand and Micro Surgery, Louisville, Kentucky

SIDNEY J. BLAIR, M.D., FACS

Dr. William M. Scholl Professor and Chairman, Department of Orthopaedics and Rehabilitation, Stritch School of Medicine, Loyola University, Maywood, Illinois

DONALD S. BLOSWICK, P.E., Ph.D.

Assistant Professor, Department of Mechanical Engineering; Director, Ergonomics and Safety Program, Rocky Mountain Center for Occupational and Environmental Health; University of Utah, Salt Lake City, Utah

PAUL W. BROWN, M.D.

Clinical Professor of Orthopaedic Surgery and Clinical Professor of Plastic and Reconstructive Surgery, Yale University School of Medicine; Chief, Division of Hand Surgery, St. Vincent's Medical Center, Bridgeport, Connecticut

RONALD C. BURGESS, M.D.

Assistant Professor of Orthopaedic Surgery, University of Kentucky, Lexington, Kentucky

DANIEL G. CAMACHO, M.D., FACS

Associate Clinical Professor of Surgery, Wright State University School of Medicine, Dayton, Ohio

EDWARD R. CHAPLIN, M.D.

Attending Physician, Scripps Memorial Hospitals, La Jolla, California

LELAND R. CHICK, M.D.

Assistant Professor, Plastic and Reconstructive Surgery, University of Utah Medical Center, Salt Lake City, Utah

JANET R. CHIPMAN, M.D.

Resident (General Surgery), University of Louisville School of Medicine, Louisville, Kentucky

GARY L. CRUMP, M.D.

Arthritis and Orthopedic Center of Excellence, Humana Hospital—Surburban; Rheumatology Associates, Louisville, Kentucky

CHESTER L. DAVIDSON, M.D.

Associate Clinical Professor of Medicine (Dermatology), University of Louisville, Louisville, Kentucky

MARK S. DiPLACIDO, M.A.

Director of Work Hardening/Rehabilitation Coordinator, Hand & Arthritis Rehabilitation, Erie, Pennsylvania

DONALD M. DITMARS, JR., M.D.

Clinical Assistant Professor (Surgery), University of Michigan Medical School; Division Head, Plastic Reconstructive and Hand Surgery, Henry Ford Hospital, Detroit, Michigan

PAUL J. DONAHUE, M.D.

Attending Staff Surgeon, Metropolitan Hand Surgery; Staff, United Hospital and Children's Hospital, St. Paul, Minnesota

WILLIAM W. EVERSMANN, JR., M.D.

Hand Surgeon, Iowa Medical Clinic, Cedar Rapids, Iowa

DAVID P. FALCONER, M.D.

Attending Staff Surgeon, Metropolitan Hand Surgery Associates; Associate Clinical Instructor, Department of Orthopedics, University of Minnesota Medical School; St. Paul, Minnesota

JOEL B. GRAD, M.D.

Assistant Professor of Orthopaedic Surgery, New York University; Director of Hand Service, St. Vincent's Medical Center, New York, New York

FRED M. HANKIN, M.D.

Staff, Huron Valley Hand Surgery, Ypsilanti, Michigan

SUSAN J. HAUCK, J.D.

Attorney, Lynch, Cox, Gilman & Mahan, Louisville, Kentucky

JERI P. IRWIN, M.D.

Staff, Diagnostic Medical Imaging Associates; Staff, St. Anthony Medical Center, Louisville, Kentucky

RICHARD K. JOHNSON, PH.D.

Licensed Clinical Psychologist, Louisville, Kentucky

SUSAN L. JOHNSON, O.T.R., C.V.E., ASHT

Owner and Director, Institute for Hand Rehabilitation, Colorado Springs, Colorado

BRADLEY S. JOSEPH, PH.D.

Corporate Ergonomist, Industrial Hygiene Section, Ford Motor Company, Dearborn, Michigan

WILLIAM W. JOULE, M.D.

Staff, Diagnostic Medical Imaging Associates; Saint Anthony Medical Center, Louisville, Kentucky

ROBERTA M. KALAFUT, D.O.

Medical Director, Medical Rehabilitation Center of Maryland, Baltimore, Maryland

ANN S. KASDAN, R.N.

Surgical Nurse, Louisville, Kentucky

MORTON L. KASDAN, M.D., FACS

Associate Clinical Professor of Surgery (Plastic and Reconstructive Surgery), University of Louisville School of Medicine, Louisville, Kentucky; Associate Clinical Professor, Occupational Medicine, University of Kentucky Medical Center, Lexington, Kentucky

HAROLD E. KLEINERT, M.D.

Clinical Professor of Surgery, University of Louisville School of Medicine, Louisville, Kentucky and Indiana University School of Medicine, Indianapolis, Indiana

JAMES M. KLEINERT, M.D.

Assistant Clinical Professor of Orthopaedic Surgery, University of Louisville School of Medicine, Louisville, Kentucky

CONNIE LANE, P.T.

Physical Therapist, Hand Rehabilitation Service, Louisville, Kentucky

L. SCOTT LEVIN, M.D.

Chief Resident, Division of Plastic and Reconstructive Surgery, Duke University Medical Center, Durham, North Carolina

PAULA D. LEVINSON, B.S., P.T.

Director, Hand Clinic of The Physical Therapy Center, Fairfax, Virginia

CURT E. LIEBMAN, M.D.

Staff Physician, Department of Radiology, Saint Anthony Medical Center, Louisville, Kentucky

GRAHAM D. LISTER, M.B., CH.B.

Professor of Surgery, University of Utah School of Medicine, Salt Lake City, Utah

JOHN D. LUBAHN, M.D.

Chairman, Department of Orthopaedics, Hamot Medical Center; Hand, Microsurgery and Reconstructive Orthopaedics, Erie, Pennsylvania

CHARLES J. MacDONALD, M.D.

Associate Clinical Professor, Department of Family Practice, University of Minnesota Medical School, Minneapolis, Minnesota

MICHAEL MADISON, PH.D.

Staff, Orthopaedic, Research Laboratory, University of California, Davis, Davis, California

NANCY P. McELWAIN, M.B.A., R.N.

Director, Occupational Medicine, Humana, Inc., Louisville, Kentucky

SUE A. MOKRIS, O.T.R.

Coordinator for The Hand Rehabilitation Program, Alexandria Hospital, Alexandria, Virginia

LINDA H. MOSELY, M.D., FACS

Plastic-Reconstructive and Hand Surgeon, Alexandria, Virginia

DAVID T. NETSCHER, M.D.

Assistant Professor, Baylor College of Medicine, Houston, Texas

RAYMOND C. NOELLERT, M.D.

Associate, Huron Valley Hand Surgery, Ypsilanti, Michigan

GARY H. PETERSON, M.D.

Saint Anthony Medical Center Imaging Center, Louisville, Kentucky

ROBERT L. REID, M.D., FACS

Clinical Professor of Surgery, Uniformed Services University of the Health Sciences, F. Edward Herbert School of Medicine, Bethesda, Maryland; Staff Surgeon, Mercy Hospital, Owensboro, Kentucky

JOHN F. ROSE, M.D.

Assistant Clinical Professor, University of Louisville School of Medicine; Staff, Humana Hospital—Surburban, Louisville, Kentucky

RAMON O. RYAN, M.D., M.S.

Medical Director, Saint Vincent Occupational Health Center; Assistant Medical Director, Sports Medicine; St. Vincent Hospital and Health Care Center, Indianapolis, Indiana

CONNIE M. RYSTROM, B.S.

Director, Hand Therapy, Iowa Medical Clinic, Cedar Rapids, Iowa

LUIS R. SCHEKER, M.D.

Clinical Instructor of Surgery (Plastic and Reconstructive), Department of Surgery, University of Louisville School of Medicine, Louisville, Kentucky

PAUL D. SCHNEIDER, M.D.

Arthritis and Orthopedic Center of Excellence, Humana Hospital—Surburban; Rheumatology Associates, Louisville, Kentucky

STEVEN R. SONKOWSKY, O.P.A.-C., R.P.A.

Physician Assistant, Metropolitan Hand Surgery Associates, St. Paul, Minnesota

FREEDA M. STEINBERG, J.D.

Attorney, Steinberg & Steinberg, Louisville, Kentucky

MICHAEL R. SWENSON, M.D.

Associate Professor, Clinical Neurosciences, University of California, San Diego; Staff, Clinical Center, Adult Neurology, University of California, San Diego, Medical Center, San Diego, California

ROBERT M. SZABO, M.D.

Associate Professor, Department of Orthopedics; Chief, Hand and Upper Extremity Service, University of California, Davis, Davis, California

LOIS E. THOMPSON, R.N.

Staff Nurse, Division of Plastic Surgery, University of Utah School of Medicine, Salt Lake City, Utah

R. FREDERICK TORSTRICK, M.D.

Staff, Department of Orthopaedics, The Jackson Clinic, Jackson, Tennessee

FRANK P. VANNIER, M.D.

Assistant Clinical Professor of Family Practice, University of Louisville School of Medicine; President, Kentucky Occupational Medical Association, Louisville, Kentucky

DAVID R. VILLASANA, M.D.

Clinical Assistant Professor, University of California, San Diego, San Diego, California

MARK R. WILSON, M.D.

Staff, Huron Valley Hand Surgery, Ypsilanti, Michigan

TERRI L. WOLFE, O.T.R./L.

Staff, Hand and Arthritis Rehabilitation Center, Erie, Pennsylvania

KEVIN P. YAKUBOFF, M.D.

Assistant Professor, Plastic and Reconstructive Surgery, University of Cincinnati College of Medicine, Cincinnati, Ohio

PREFACE

For several years, I have felt there was a need for a general reference that would cover the problems of occupational hand injuries and diseases. The plant physician, nurse, industrial relations representative, workmens' compensation (insurance) adjuster, safety director, and anyone having to deal with occupational hand trauma will find useful information in the contents of this text.

We have tried to address the common problems that may be attributed to the work environment. We have covered the conservative and surgical management of most upper extremity injuries and diseases.

A number of chapters have been devoted to the very important peripheral problems of the patient with an injured hand. The reader is encouraged to take special note of the chapters on motivation, pain, psychology, legal aspects, back-to-work considerations, and ergonomics. I believe some of the chapters in this book will be considered classic references for many years.

Great respect must be given the injured upper extremity. It is important to recognize that what may appear to be a minor hand injury can produce devastating long-term effects. To restore function and gainful employment must be the ultimate goal of treatment. No matter how exacting and excellent the performance of an operative procedure, it can be considered successful only when the patient is returned to a productive life. To accomplish this goal, it takes not only a good medical team, but a well-motivated, cooperative patient. The best rehabilitation is a return to work.

I would like to thank my wife, Ann Kasdan R.N., for her encouragement to proceed with this book. I would also like to give a special thanks to my devoted secretary, Mrs. Bonnie Wood, who has given an incredible number of hours in the preparation of this work.

Morton L. Kasdan, M.D., FACS
Louisville, Kentucky

FOREWORD I

Even more than in the early decades of this century, when assembly lines revolutionized industry, workers of today are called to perform the same movements of the hand and upper extremity for hours on end. With the proliferation of computers and highly mechanized assembly lines, hands are trapped into performing a few specific movements, thousands of times a day, without the variety of motion afforded workers in the past. This problem has spread throughout the work force and across professions and occupations, increasing our sensitivity to the complex medical aspects of work-related injuries.

We have begun to realize that we must change our approach to health in the workplace to balance the goal of short-term productivity with the requirements of long-term health, safety, and productivity of the worker. Eventually, research and experience will lead us to better work patterns and improved equipment that will reduce the strain of repetitive motion and the incidence of traumatic injury.

Books such as this play a critical role in this process. This is one of the few books on occupational medicine edited by a hand surgeon, especially one who has devoted a great deal of his career to the treatment of occupational injuries of the hand and upper extremity. Morton Kasdan is exceedingly well qualified to edit this work. For 25 years he has devoted his time and energy to hand injuries and their treatment, including his career in Louisville, where he has subspecialized in occupational and workers' compensation injuries to the upper extremity.

The authors of the individual chapters have been carefully selected by Dr. Kasdan based on his personal knowledge of their work. These chapters represent many years of combined experience with occupational hand injury and disease. Covering all aspects of occupational hand and upper extremity disorders and their management, this book also contains chapters directed toward motivation of the patient, medicolegal issues, and ergonomics.

Because of its comprehensive nature and the experience of its many authors, I expect this book to serve a valuable function in expanding our knowledge and improving our ability to treat work-related medical problems of the upper extremity.

Harold E. Kleinert, M.D.
Louisville, Kentucky

FOREWORD II

The hand of man is in essence life itself. Of all the animals, man is the only one with a hand and the intellect to use it. It is never still except in sleep. The hand caresses in love, pats encouragement, greets in friendship, and clenches in anger. It can lift and support, restrain to protect, and sign to talk. It can demonstrate disgust or indicate approval. It feeds us, holds the glass to quench our thirst, and allows us to ply our trade.

The hand at work goes in harm's way. Daily we expose these fine-drawn yet tough members to injury or loss. For those of us unfortunate enough to damage severely digits, a hand, or a wrist, there is help.

Over the past 30 years, Morton Kasdan has dedicated his life to the preservation of function of the hand. His interest started in 1959 as a freshman medical student. He has learned, he has worked, and he has taught his skills to others through the years.

This book is the culmination of his efforts to communicate not only his technical but his psychosocial skills. The aim is the ultimate return of not only the hand but the entire person to maximum function.

Knowing Morton Kasdan is like watching an arrow fly true—one direction, slowing only when it hits the mark. In this text, he has hit the mark. He has assembled authors who are second to none in their fields. It goes far beyond instruction in the repair and care of the injured extremity. It delves into cause and effect of injury and the eventual return to function, not just physically, but spiritually and emotionally. Disability is explored as well as the approaches to legal ramifications of injury, recovery, and rehabilitation.

As you "thumb" through this volume, keep in mind what a marvelous gift we humans have been given.

Eugene H. Kremer, III, M.D.
Louisville, Kentucky
President,
American College of Occupational Medicine

Chapter 1

THE ROLE OF MOTIVATION IN THE RECOVERY OF THE HAND

Paul W. Brown, M.D.

There are two things that make man unique among living creatures—his psyche and his hands. This chapter deals with motivation, one aspect of the psyche, as it applies to the recovery of function in impaired hands. Though much of the chapter could apply to patients with low back pain, paraplegia, or other physical infirmity, hands have a special significance in that their function is so complex and because they are related to earning a living. It is also significant that the hands and the face are the only parts of the human anatomy bared to public scrutiny.

It is easier to describe motivation than to define it. This effort is akin to that description of pornography by a distinguished jurist, who said, "I can't tell you exactly what it is, but I know it when I see it." In attempting to define motivation, it helps to understand how and why people make decisions, and then to examine some examples of how the quality of motivation may affect people in health and in infirmity. The chapter then deals with those various factors that may affect a patient's fund of motivation—for better or worse. How to apply our knowledge of motivation to the recovery (i.e., rehabilitation) of the patient with a hand problem is finally addressed.

THE SELECTION OF ALTERNATIVES

Man's behavior is determined in part by influences beyond his control. His actions are inexorably programmed by his genetic heritage. He can not escape from this control system. It is implanted permanently, and although behavior may be modified, it is ever there calling out basic signals. Man's ancestors are always looking over his shoulder, influencing and sometimes dictating his actions.

Man is not a robot, however. Though his genes may direct him, they still allow him much leeway for decision-making and for maneuvering. His genes govern fundamental physiologic and psychologic responses, but they also allow some freedom for individual deviation from the basic hereditary program. It is this latitude that allows man to self-determine what type of person he becomes, what he does with his life, whether he produces or merely consumes, whether he rises or falls. The latitude allotted to him by his genes is manifested by his ability to moderate the program by conscious as well as subliminal thought.

We believe that man differs from all other forms of life by virtue of his imagination and his capability for abstract thought. His cerebral capacity enables him to consciously select a specific course of action from among many possible courses. The individual progresses through life making thousands of choices—decisions—each day. Most of the choices are mundane: which necktie to select, which route to take to the office, whether to walk quickly or slowly or to cross the street here—or there. Many of the choices are smudged by the overlay of habit and set patterns and require little thought, but some choices are much more complicated and affect not daily living patterns, but more important and complex issues such as character, life style, and achievement.

Deciding to take a course of action—or refusing to take an action—is basically a selection of one possibility from several alternatives. The very word "alternative" implies choice, and the word "choice" signifies a license to select. The selection may be decided by only one or two factors, or influenced by many—some obvious, some obscure, and some totally unrecognized.

Some decisions are simple and some extremely complex. Consider first an example of a relatively simple decision—not easy, but simple in that there are so few alternatives. Picture a frightened individual crouched on the ledge of a burning building. He is on the twentieth floor; the fire has entered his room and forced him outside onto the ledge. The heat behind him is becoming unbearable and threatens to overwhelm him. His choices are to jump and probably perish, or to remain on the ledge and most certainly perish. The influencing factors are a fear of jumping and the intolerable heat. Most would elect to jump, but a few will be incapable of making a choice, or will not be able to choose quickly enough—paralyzed by fear, as it were—and will perish in the flames. The jumpers have weighed the alternatives and have made a choice.

At the other end of the scale are complex decisions such as deciding on a career, picking a mate, or writing a book. In the last-mentioned example, the writer's brain functions as a computer examining hundreds of thousands of possibilities for selection of the right word, combining words into sentences, sentences into a plot or theme, and then all the combinations required to end up with a finished product—a book, a set of books, an encyclopedia.

How incredibly complex was the decision-making and the selection of alternatives in the creation of *War and Peace*! Why did Tolstoy select the words and ideas he did, and elect to string them together in a style that lesser authors have failed to achieve? What influenced The Bard to produce *The Merchant of Venice*? How did he decide on that theme and how many decisions on words and style did he make? How many brush strokes did El Greco elect to use on one of his works? How many colors, and in what combinations? How did he make his selections? And finally, how and why was he motivated to work that hard? The permutations and the possibilities in this sort of creative decision-making seem infinite.

Most of us are not involved in creating masterpieces of prose or art, but all of us are busy picking our way through life making thousands of decisions that influence our careers, our life styles, our relations with others, and our environment in general. These choices, these decisions, determine how happy we will be—or how unhappy; how successful we will be, or how we will fail. There are many factors that influence our decisions, some obvious and some outside our recognition. Our genetic makeup is beyond our control and so, to a large degree, are the influences of our family background and our formative years. We can't change our past experiences and how they have influenced us, but we can modify our interpretation of them, depending on our intelligence, our introspection, and our desire to do so. This quality of objective self-analysis varies greatly among individuals, but it determines how well we make decisions. This, in turn, depends on our *motivation* to do it; depends on our ability to recognize that there are always alternatives. Our challenge is to weigh those alternatives and select that which serves our *purpose* best.

WHAT IS MOTIVATION?

Purpose and motivation are so intertwined as to be inseparable; they can even be considered synonymous. Man's main purpose—aim, goal, objective—in life is to gratify himself. This is more complicated than just the seeking of pleasure and considerably more subtle than simple hedonism. It has to do with emotional satisfaction and is only peripherally concerned with physical pleasure.

Motivation is an abstract quality that we all know something about, but for which we have no clear definition—at least not a concise definition that most would agree on. Most members of the healing arts believe that a patient's desire to get well influences the getting well process, but we've given more lip service than study to the concept. Scientists prefer things they can measure and most physicians—particularly surgeons—are uncomfortable with abstractions. Abstractions can't be measured or graphed or catalogued or classified, and thus most physicians shy away from an in-depth examination of what motivation is and a realization of how useful it can be to them. The psychiatrists and psychologists dig into it and use it as a tool but have not made much progress in influencing other physicians to do the same. Various types of "therapists" use it to varying degrees; credentialed therapists, such as physical, occupational, hand, and speech therapists, are often more adept in using motivation as a therapeutic tool than the physicians who direct them. Other, less recognized, and sometimes less respectable, dealers in healing—faith healers, and quacks in general—are experts in exploiting the patient by manipulating his desire for something—usually his desire to get well.

Man does what he does because it gratifies him; he unerringly makes the choice he believes (rightly or wrongly) will please him the most—or that will spare him the most discomfort. The alternatives he may have to select from are not always pleasant. It is just as gratifying to avoid unpleasantness or to select the lesser of unpleasant alternatives as it is to select from pleasant ones. There is really no such thing as altruism; the only martyrs that exist are those defined in a political or religious sense. The martyr selects the course—albeit from horrible alternatives—that gratifies him or her the most, or harms him or her the least. For some, religious ecstasy is a perfectly logical choice even though it may mean awful suffering, mutilation, and death. The hero, who in combat deliberately sacrifices himself to save his buddies, does it because that course of action seems preferable to seeing them die, or seeing himself appear as a coward. His selection of action is based on which alternative gratifies him the most.

The mother who daringly risks her life to save her threatened child has decided that not to take that risk is an insupportable alternative. She doesn't like to risk her life, but of the possibilities she has to select from, the risk-taking course is the most acceptable. This most acceptable alternative—the one that pleases most, or threatens least—is the choice individuals always make. Their judgment may be faulty, and what seemed to offer the most gratification turned out to offer the least, but that doesn't change the premise.

In his quest for gratification, man may be seeking pleasant sensations or avoiding unpleasant ones. He may be responding to a conscience bequeathed to him by his background, religion, or upbringing. He may be reacting to a sense of benevolence towards his loved ones and does so because it gratifies him. Not to do so would be painful and perverse. Thus, benevolence belongs in the same category as altruism. How then does one account for a parent spanking a naughty child? Simply that the parent is more gratified by the thought that he is contributing positively to the child's upbringing and this overshadows any remorse he may feel at inflicting pain on his child. Or perhaps it is just basically satisfying to swat a bad kid—or because it assuages one's anger.

Motivation is the force that determines how a choice of alternatives will be made. It is an emotional component of one's character and exists to some degree in everyone. It may be a stimulus for achievement, though with some it may be a negative force. The achievers are easy to recognize; they have the same type of driving force that great artists, scientists, explorers, musicians, and authors have demonstrated. There are others who are highly motivated toward destructive ends, the tyrants and terrorists. Adolf Hitler had tremendous drive—another term for motivation—to accomplish what he did, no matter how horrible those accomplishments were. His choices of action—repugnant to most of the world—definitely gratified him.

THE SPECTRUM OF MOTIVATION

Where does a Hitler—or in a positive sense an Einstein—get his motivation? Surely, intelligence is only one factor. For every Milton there are hundreds of poets just as intelligent who don't, won't or can't drive themselves to the heights of expression he attained. Genetic makeup and family background offer some contribution to motivation but not always to siblings equally, and not always in a positive way. How can one account for the disparity between two brothers brought up in the same manner, by the same parents, and in the same environment, where one becomes a success and a pillar of the community and the other a black sheep, a failure, or a criminal? What made one go one way, and the other the opposite?

Though it is relatively easy to recognize highly motivated individuals—the achievers—we do not truly understand what it is in their makeup that causes them to be motivated. Motivation is a desire to do something, to get something.

In some it is a strong force easily recognized, as in the achievers, the doers, and the attainers. In others it may be weak and obscure, unrecognized by either the individual or by those around him.

If every individual must make a never-ending series of choices in life, and if those choices are predicated on a desire for something, and if that desire is tantamount to motivation, then it follows that every individual has some degree of motivation in his makeup. The allotment of motivation among individuals follows the usual bell-shaped curve. At one end are a few superachievers and at the other a few who seem to have little or no motivation for much of anything. In between these two extremes is the majority—people who to varying degrees have some motivation. As healers and rehabilitators, we must direct our efforts to where they will do the most good—the principle of triage. We will seldom have to expend much of our therapeutic skills on those highly motivated people at the extreme right hand side of the curve. All they need is our technical skills, and the chances are good that they will then supply all the impetus needed for their rehabilitation. On the other extreme, for those whose drive for achievement is so weak as to be unrecognizable, we are probably wasting our limited assets. Although it is true that these extreme cases of nonachievement may have some potential for rehabilitation, the effort and expense required to assist the individuals in mobilizing it would be so great as to detract from those who would have a much better chance of benefiting from our efforts. It has become apparent that our resources are not unlimited and that some type of rationing (i.e., optimal utilization) is necessary.

Outstanding examples of motivation for achievement can serve as sources of inspiration and may help us to better understand what this quality is and where it comes from. Ludvig von Beethoven is one such. Early in his career, while composing his Moonlight Sonata, he began to lose his hearing. Deafness was intolerable to him and almost led to a psychotic breakdown. He adjusted to his growing handicap and went on to compose his Second Symphony, followed by all the rest of his magnificent works, dying totally deaf some 26 years later. Such an affliction would totally disable most musicians, but he persevered. In 1802 he wrote, "I have been forced to accept a permanent infirmity in my sense of hearing—a sense which should be more perfectly developed in me than in others. This has brought me close to despair and I came near to ending my own life. Only my art held me back as it seemed impossible to leave the world until I have produced everything I feel has been granted to me to achieve."

People who are self-employed are usually well motivated to improve their hand problems. They wish to return as soon as possible to their preinjury state. There are many reasons for this. The fact that they own or run their own businesses or professions indicates that they are at least fairly high on the achievement scale. Their livelihoods depend on their return to a productive role. Often they have little or no disability insurance; also the longer they are out of work, the more at risk is their shop, business, office, or profession. Because they are achievers and because they have very specific reasons for returning to work, they are loathe to be idle. They find the concept of disability distasteful and its prospect frightening. They are basically quite uncomfortable in a nonproductive role.

This desire to return to productivity—this motivation to improve, to get well—is the key to their success in rehabilitation and the basic reason why the self-employed almost always go back to work sooner than the worker who is salaried or who is paid by the hour or piece work and is backed up by generous disability benefits. The self-employed and the professionals only need technical skills from the rehabilitation team. While it is true that communication and understanding are important in their therapy, seldom will much effort be needed to get their cooperation. Indeed, a more common problem is preventing them from moving too quickly and too aggressively in their recovery.

Of 185 surgeons who had lost parts of their hands (ranging from loss of a finger to multiple amputations in both hands, amputation of a hand, and several who had lost thumbs), only three failed to return to the active practice of surgery. Half of them had lost their digits after becoming surgeons, and most said they returned to the office a week or two after their injury—and to the operating room within a month. Most agreed that their rehabilitation consisted of getting back to work. None of the 182 felt they had any significant disability in their professions as surgeons or in their daily living activities, which included many types of sports and musical instruments. An eye surgeon who had lost a hand as a teenager, and who has become a very successful surgeon and now regularly performs eye surgery, when asked how he had achieved this, replied, "I taught myself to operate using a prosthesis to hold my instruments." He added, "Incentive is the key." And perhaps that says it all.

This desire to return to productivity—this motivation to get well—this desire to succeed—this distaste for disability—is what separates the doers from the nondoers. It is this quality that the rehabilitation team must seek out, strive to recognize, and learn to potentiate and to exploit in their patients. Without it the results will end up being evaluated by compensation commissions and measured by disability "awards."

At the other end of the spectrum is the slothful person who assigns himself the role of disability, sometimes without the presence of significant physical infirmity. He is unable or unwilling to think beyond a few bodily comforts. He will respond to physical pleasure or to discomfort, but can not, or will not, progress beyond satisfaction of these priorities.

Difficult to categorize are those who are perversely motivated to pursue socially unacceptable ways: deviants, criminals, and sociopaths—many of them high achievers, it is true, but in ways not morally acceptable by most of us. Occasionally, patients in this category demonstrate considerable motivation for recovery of function and prove to be cooperative. This is particularly true if their income depends on manual function, as with forgers, safe-crackers, and pickpockets.

Our efforts must be directed to the majority, those in the middle of the curve and its shoulders. If we can understand something of their motivational levels and learn how to stimulate and utilize them, then we should be able to use that knowledge and that skill as a tool for rehabilitation. Thus, except for the extremes— the very high achievers and the obvious losers—we can assume that all of our patients have some level of motivation that we should find a way to use. In some it will be obvious, and in others obscure. In those whose motivation is not immediately apparent, but who are not obvious losers (not so easy to be sure!), we must start with the assumption that they have a *latent motivation*, and it is our therapeutic challenge to uncover it and to show them how they can help themselves.

MOTIVATION AS A TOOL FOR RECOVERY

Many of us, medical and lay, alike, have noted that the *desire* to get well often influences the *ability* to get well. Motivation for recovery may not have a direct effect on disease, but it does have a direct effect on how the patient reacts to his disorder. It may affect his attitude and thus his life style—and life style is what rehabilitation is all about. We have all wondered how one patient with what seems to be a crushing illness or physical "handicap" can surmount it, and, if not able to cure himself, can at least modify the course of his disease or adapt and cope with it, whereas another, with the same or lesser problem will become "disabled."

Some patients are motivated to develop compensatory skills that help overcome unsolvable physical problems. Some of this is instinctive and some motivational. Witness the compensatory super touch and hearing that most blind patients develop. While it is true that most would develop some of this automatically, the degree of acuteness can be markedly augmented through training and persistence by training, the persistence depending on the degree of motivation. Helen Keller's level of motivation must have been phenomenal.

Most patients are motivated to get well. Most of them wish to be rehabilitated, once they understand what rehabilitation means. And most patients want to get back to work. Unfortunately, *most* doesn't mean *all*. There are many who don't want to or who are deterred by factors that impede our rehabilitative efforts. If we can find ways to challenge the patient to enlist his own resources, if we can uncover the latent motivation that we should assume most people have, we will be able to help them to cope successfully with their hands at work— and in life.

There are many tools for this at our disposal, and the best way to start is with good communication: a clear explanation of the physical problem, the limits it imposes on ability to perform, and a realistic projection of future performance. Only if our patient understands what is wrong, what he can do to correct or improve it, and what he can expect in the future, only then will he become a cooperating part of the rehabilitation effort. If he is not motivated to do this, we are wasting our time— and his—and society's.

Once communication has laid the foundation for cooperation, many paths for stimulating or exploiting the patient's motivation for recovery are available. Appeals to pride are fruitful for some. Praise, approval, and constant encouragement are useful, and so may be disapproval. Patients who have demonstrated obvious success in their recovery and patients who can infuse enthusiasm for the program in others can be useful in setting the example and leading the way. One must be careful, however, not to use the superachiever too much, as he may inhibit the patient who is fearful or unsure of himself. The program must be tailored to the individual patient and will depend not only on the specific physical problem inherent in his upper extremity, but also on his personality, his desire to get well, and also the nature of the job and life style to which he will be returning.

Very useful is an agreement with the employer to take the patient back on a limited work basis designed to fit in with his rehabilitation. This is dependent on good communication with the employer, the foreman, and sometimes with fellow workers. It also depends on the patient's desire to return to that particular employ. Some companies have come to realize that cooperation with these efforts pay off in tangible ways, i.e., less cost in the long run, and in less obvious, but nevertheless valuable, ways, such as employee morale, a more harmonious workplace, and the like. Sad to say, the degree of enlightenment in this regard in the manufacturing the business world is rather low. Some third party payers—mainly in the insurance industry, but not many in the government—are becoming involved in return-to-work programs. Further encouragement and education of the business world by the rehabilitators will help further such programs.

The rehabilitation team is basically tripartite: the patient, the physician, and the hand therapist. Family, friends, and other patients can be peripheral to the team and may be brought in to play important roles as required. The patient must understand that though his recovery will be greatly aided by such a team endeavor, it is his own desire for success—his motivation—that will determine the outcome. If the patient plays a passive role, if he expects that recovery will be granted to him, if he is disinterested or uninformed, then surely all attempts to rehabilitate him will fail. When this happens we often fault our methods, but that may be incorrect. It may well be that we have not understood what the patient really wanted—

what he was truly motivated for. In such an instance our error was in failure to recognize the patient's *goals*.

WHAT DO PATIENTS WANT?

It is natural, perhaps, to assume that the patient and the therapeutic team share the same goals. Usually this is true, but there are enough exceptions to this assumption to warrant some examination of the many reasons why patients may not want to get well, or to go back to work. These reasons may be potent deterrents to recovery.

Goals, objectives, aims, desires—all are related to gratification, and this, in turn, governs motivation. Some patients have a wish *not* to recover hand function and may deliberately, or unconsciously, frustrate the team in its attempts to help them get well, to improve their hand function, and to help them get back to work. It is not enough that the team understand the anatomy and function of the hand, or that it be skilled in surgery. The team must know something of its patient's personality, his life style, his family, and his work place. Knowledge of these things depends on good communication with him. If the team is unfamiliar with this background, the assumption by the team that they and the patient have the same goals may be quite wrong.

As a part of the therapeutic challenge it must be asked, "What do patients want?" Are the patient's goals the same as the team's: to get well, to go back to work, to go back to what he had before his injury or disease brought him to the team? Some would prefer sympathy to recovery. A deformed hand, obvious to all, may be much more gratifying to its owner than return to work. Most patients enjoy some sympathy and some attention; most don't want it at the expense of pride or independence, but some do. Recognition of his infirmity—and that is the way the patient may see it—may be more important to him than pride or respect or earning a living. He may do this quite unconsciously, without deliberate misrepresentation. He will pursue his unrecognized goal stubbornly and will not do well with his rehabilitation no matter how persistent or insistent the team.

There are other reasons for not wanting to get better. If the injured hand is the result of the abuse of another, it may be preferable to retain the residual of the injury as a constant reminder of the assault than to recover from it. The injured person may then use the injury as a weapon for vengeance, and this may be more rewarding than rehabilitation. I remember a seemingly stable patient of mine whose hand had been malaligned in a family brawl. She preferred to retain an obvious deformity rather than have it corrected, using it, to her immense gratification, to remind her abusive husband of his guilt for many years to come. Her disability became an instrument of power and influence, gratifying her more than would a functional and more attractive hand.

Some patients are more concerned with their disability rating than with a return to useful function. For them the rewards of compensation payment outweigh the benefits of return to work, or at least the return to work will be put off as long as possible pending a monetary award. The person poorly motivated for working for a living will derive a sort of perverse satisfaction for sustained disability if emphasizing his hand problem promises a greater cash reward. Workers' compensation laws were intended to protect the honest worker who wishes to return to work but who is truly unable to, or whose return is delayed until "maximum medical benefits" have been attained. Unfortunately these protective laws are subject to much abuse. The physician, supposedly the patient's advocate, is often forced to be the compensation arbiter and must decide who is entitled to benefits and who is not. The problem becomes even more complex in those instances where society is willing to pay the patient more for staying out of work than he could earn if he returned, as is sometimes the case with Scandinavian socialism. This perversion of protective labor laws discourages motivation for recovery by penalizing the ambitious, those motivated to achieve, and society in general—and rewarding the nonachiever. Contrast that with a society where survival is difficult or even marginal, where one must produce or starve. Such a harsh extreme is not compatible with civilized society but it is clear that where this is the case, then motivation for function is strong indeed!

The prospect of money often clouds the patient's perspective, and the greater the sum the darker the clouds. Litigation can be a potent deterrent to recovery; the more protracted the legal process the more obscured are normal motivational factors. A prompt return to function weakens the case for a reward for damages and thus is contrary to the objectives of the patient's attorney, whose motivation is often quite different from those of his client's physician. A patient with average motivation for improvement of his injured hand may find himself beset by several opposing forces; his own pride in productivity, his physician who wishes the best possible hand, and his attorney who realizes that the worse the hand is, the better his case. If the potential reward is very high, the best intentioned patient may be seduced from the path of effective rehabilitation. It's an old saw, but one with some meaning, that for some patients a greenback poultice is the most effective cure.

True malingering is rare. It implies a deliberate falsification of physical ills for some type of gain. Few patients are deliberate in their attempts to avoid or delay return to work, but many patients do not honestly define their goals and are unconsciously seduced by the temptations of a protracted holiday or a continued "disability" payment. If it is true that "everyone has a bit of larceny in his heart," then it is easy to understand why the patient with an unpleasant, dangerous, or low prestige job will unconsciously seek ways to avoid a return to it—particularly if there is a large monetary award involved.

HOW TO USE MOTIVATION IN REHABILITATION

1. Start Early

The sooner, the better. Immediately after the injury if possible. Influencing the patient to use the injured part for *something*, even if it is only as simple an act as lifting a piece of paper, or scratching his nose, will prevent him from adopting an "It's no good for anything" attitude. Help the patient understand that the sooner one starts, the more likely one is to succeed. Even the smallest start is something to build on.

2. Communication

a. Patient education: Cooperation by the patient depends on his understanding of what is wrong, what can be done to improve matters, what kind of results are *probable*, and what kind are *possible*. Explanation of the anatomy involved, the function of injured parts, a description of the surgical procedures, and most important, a clear-cut explanation of the rehabilitation program and his part in it—all these are necessary if he is to be motivated to succeed. All members of the rehabilitation team must contribute to this educational process, but it should be emphasized to the patient that his recovery is his own responsibility. He must realize that the result he ends up with will depend, in the main, on his own efforts.

b. Team Education: Rehabilitative goals should be clearly defined and all members of the team must understand them and agree with them. This requires clear and frequent communication among team members. It also requires direction and leadership. A leader should be designated at the start, usually the surgeon charged with prime responsibility for the patient's care. When the main surgical and medical problems have been taken care of, the role of leader can be passed to whoever then has the major involvement with the patient. If primary responsibility is not clearly designated, the patient will be in the sad position of having no one directing his care or, even worse, find that his care is by a committee whose members are not communicating with one another.

c. Definition of Goals: Everyone on the team must be aiming at the same target, and the only way rehabilitative goals can be clearly defined and supported is by good communication within the team. Cryptic, unintelligible, or vague prescriptions by the primary physician will confuse everybody. The physician must make his directions and intentions clear. If these goals are not defined to the therapist, she must insist on clarification. Confusion and contradiction by members of the team will dampen the enthusiasm of even the most highly motivated patient.

d. Group Communication: Regular meetings of all members of the rehabilitation team with the patient are essential for clarifying issues, methods, and goals. In these roundtable meetings, the patient's central role is repeatedly emphasized, questions are answered, and suggestions for improvement or change are considered. Such suggestions should be welcomed from all members of the team, especially those from the patient. There is no room for arrogance or surgical prima donnas in such a group setting. A patient is very favorably impressed that the team meets to consider and discuss his particular needs, especially if all members invite him to be a contributing member. This enhances whatever motivation the patient already has and serves to uncover latent motivation in the passive patient.

3. Recruiting Outside Help

Personnel peripheral to the immediate rehabilitation team may be very helpful in stimulating motivation. Family members, friends and clergy, or anyone whose approval is important to the patient may stimulate the patient to excel. Conversely, those whose disapproval he fears may be goads to further achievement.

Other patients with the same type of problem may serve as role models to be emulated. As coaches, their suggestions may be as valuable as any made by regular members of the team. One must be cautious, however, in using the super-achievers as examples or as helpers. They often tend to set goals too difficult for a patient with average motivation and thus may discourage or intimidate him.

4. Cultivating Latent Motivation

a. Build On Small Gains: Any gain, real or perceived, enhances enthusiasm for continued effort. Define realistic targets. Better a series of small gains with only an occasional letdown than aiming too high and sustaining a crushing failure.

b. Recognize and Reward Effort; Criticize Lack of Effort: This is the "carrot or the stick" approach. Caution is required in reproaching patients with tender egos or who are poorly motivated. Conversely, overpraise may invite complacency.

c. Positive Thinking: Optimism must be based on realistic expectations, but motivation for continued cooperation can only be sustained if patient remains in a positive frame of mind. It will help him to know that his attitude will definitely influence his result.

Dealing with failure and discouragement is difficult for all members of the team, but when it occurs it must be faced. Frank discussion and analysis by the rehabilitation team is required. Group discussion of failures gives an opportunity for a restatement of goals and a chance for all team members, especially the patient, to ask questions and clear up misunderstandings, i.e., to improve communications. Periods of adversity can thus be used to further stimulate motivation.

d. Dealing with Dependency: The patient who is passive about his treatment or who manifests overdependence on his physician or therapist must be dealt with firmly from the beginning. It is best to discuss such behavior frankly with the patient and make it clear that if he cannot or will not acquire a more positive attitude, little or no improvement is likely. If negative thinking, dependency, or passivity cannot be converted, serious consideration should be given to dropping the patient from the program. Where facilities are limited, others will profit from them more.

e. Program Discipline: Treatment schedules, meetings, and conference times should be clearly defined and adherence to them by all team members insisted on. Consistent program discipline not only makes for efficient use of time but helps deter the passive patient from falling by the wayside. Specific goals should be defined and a timetable for achieving them should be understood by everyone involved with the patient.

f. Pain Problems and Drug Dependence: Pain cannot be changed by attitude, but the interpretation of painful stimuli and the reaction to pain can be influenced by positive thinking. Severe pain problems such as causalgia must be faced realistically, but even they can be influenced to some degree. In fact, a high degree of motivation and dogged perseverance with rehabilitative efforts may be the only hope for improvement in patients with a reflex sympathetic dystrophy. Analgesics must be controlled by the physician and should be appropriate in type and dosage for the individual's pain and his reaction to that pain. Patients who are opiate-dependent will probably do poorly with any hand rehabilitation program. When severe drug dependence is recognized, and it is often difficult to do so, the patient must be faced with it frankly, and at the first sign of noncompliance dropped from the program. Such patients are not motivated for recovery, and it is unlikely that they can be.

5. Working With Employers

The longer the patient is away from work, the less likely that he will return to it. A patient's motivation to return to his job is greatly enhanced if he can return to some type of work early in the rehabilitation program. This requires an understanding by the company, its personnel department, and—especially—the foremen and supervisors at the patient's work place. Communication with the patient's co-workers, explaining the aims, purposes and methods of the "early return to work program," will not only ease his way but will increase general understanding and support for such a program by future candidates for it. Management must be convinced that this is not only

fiscally sound but pays dividends in improved worker morale and loyalty. Indications by the employer that an injured employee is still a valued one is a great potentiator of motivation to return to work. If the employer and supervisors—and often co-workers—understand the patient's hand problem and his capabilities and limitations, it may be possible to assign him duties compatible with his abilities. It may even be possible to tailor the job to be a part of his occupational therapy program. This understanding depends on clear communication between the rehabilitation team and the employer. Where there is a company nurse, she is often useful as a liaison person and can also help in reporting the patient's progress on the job. She will often have helpful suggestions for modification of the patient's job activities.

6. Settle Litigation As Early As Possible

Litigation is lengthy, expensive, and almost always in conflict with the get-well process. The lure of a cash reward or vengeance obscures the rewards of returning to work, particularly if that work is unpleasant, dangerous, or poorly remunerative. Usually there is a professional conflict between the physician and attorney, in that the former wants as good a result as possible, whereas the patient's lawyer knows that the more "disabled" his client, the better his chances are for a large settlement, and the more protracted the legal process, the greater his compensation.

It is important that members of the rehabilitation team refrain from giving their patient anything that smacks of legal advice, but it is almost always good medical advice to urge that legal matters be settled as promptly as possible. Attorneys who have their patient's best interests at heart support this concept, but where there is potential conflict it is advisable—with the patient's consent—to discuss the problem with the attorney.

In those instances where litigation concerning compensation, work-related injury, and the degree of disability is pending, the rehabilitation team should determine what the patient's goals are. If he is really motivated to return to work, it should become apparent in his approach to the treatment program. If he is not making progress, the reasons must be investigated. If it is decided that his primary goal is a cash settlement, or avoiding a return to work, it will be better for him and for other patients in the program if his rehabilitation program be ended. Motivation cannot be forced on someone. It is reasonable to try to cultivate it, but if results are not forthcoming it is realistic to quit. The difficulty lies in knowing when to persist and when to stop.

7. Dealing With Third Parties

Many individuals and agencies may be involved with the patient and his hand problem, with his rehabilitation, and his return to work. All may influence his motivation to succeed, for better or worse. Family, friends, co-workers, bosses, insurance companies, attorneys, compensation commissions, and other governmental agencies—all may influence the patient's recovery and his motivation to achieve it. Most of them will claim they are acting in the patient's best interest. Sometimes that's true, sometimes not.

Whether any of these third parties will aid the patient in his recovery and return to a productive role will depend in large part on how well they understand what is wrong with him, what is being done to help him, and what they can do to help him to help himself. That understanding will depend in turn on how well the rehabilitation team communicates with the third party. Again, explanation of the patient's problem and his rehabilitation program, as well as a realistic definition of goals, is essential.

8. Amputations and Prostheses

The patient who has lost an arm, a hand, or part of a hand has problems not generally shared by other hand patients. Most obvious is the difficulty in learning to use a functional prosthesis. More obscure, but as important, is the problem of altered body image. How well the amputee patient accepts the loss and deals with his emotional, esthetic, and functional problems depends on how well motivated he is to make the best of it and return to his former style of life. There is much the rehabilitation team can do to stimulate that motivation.

Open discussion of the concept of body image and the significance of appearance and altered function with all members of the team, as well as with other patients with a similar problem, helps the patient accept the loss. Loss acceptance is the most important step; it is not the same as resignation, but rather a facing up to reality. If he never really accepts the fact that the part is gone, he will not accommodate to its absence nor utilize a functional prosthesis well.

Priority must be assigned to either appearance or function. The pragmatist will choose to concentrate on function, but for others cosmesis may be a more suitable goal. Compromise prostheses that attempt to serve both are rarely successful, though some finger prostheses that look very lifelike have some functional use. If the choice is a functional prosthesis, the sooner it is attached to the patient and the sooner it is put to use, the greater the probability that it will be accepted and utilized. When a hand has been lost, an early fit of a simple functional hook prosthesis will abort the amputee's natural attempt to concentrate on increased use of the remaining hand. The goal is to stop him from becoming exclusively one-handed. Complicated prostheses depending on electronics or elaborate motor function are seldom the best choice for beginners. If the amputee can perform some function with this prosthesis, no matter how simple, he will be encouraged to continue. Small early successes enhance motivation to persist with prosthetic training.

CONCLUSION

The desire to get well is an important part of the healing process and is essential for successful rehabilitation of the impaired hand. An understanding of motivation and how it can be recognized, stimulated, and utilized is an important achievement for those involved in the treatment of patients with injury, disease, or deformity of the hand.

SUGGESTED READING

1. Brown PW: The role of motivation in patient recovery. Connecticut Medicine 42:555–557, 1978.
2. Brown PW: Less than ten—Surgeons with amputated fingers. J Hand Surg 71:31–37, 1982.
3. Bunnell S (ed): Hand Surgery in World War II. Washington, D.C., U.S. Government Printing Office, 1955.
4. Burkhalter WE, et al: The upper extremity amputee. Early and immediate postsurgical prosthetic fitting. J Bone Joint Surg 58A:46–51, 1976.
5. Grunert BK, et al: Early psychological aspects of severe hand injury. J Hand Surg 13B:177–180, 1988.
6. Haese JB: Psychological aspects of hand injuries— their treatment and rehabilitation. J Hand Surg 10B:283–287, 1985.
7. Johnson RK: The role of psychological evaluations in occupational hand injuries. In Kasdan ML (ed): Occupational Hand Injuries. Occup Med State Art Rev 4:405–418, 1989.

8. Kasdan AS, McElwain NP: Return-to-work programs following occupational hand injuries. In Kasdan ML (ed): Occupational Hand Injuries. Occup Med State Art Rev 4:539–545, 1989.

9. Kilgore ES, Graham WP III; Psychosocial aspects of hand disabilities. In The Hand: Surgical and No-Surgical Management. Philadelphia, Lea & Febiger, 1977, pp 468–473.

10. Wynn Parry CB: Rehabilitation of the Hand, 3rd ed. London, Butterworth, 1973.

Chapter 2

CHRONIC PAIN AND THE INJURED WORKER: A SOCIOBIOLOGICAL PROBLEM

Edward R. Chaplin, M.D.

Tomorrow, and tomorrow, and tomorrow,
Creeps in this petty pace from day to day,
To the last syllable of recorded time;
And all our yesterdays have lighted fools
The way to dusty death. Out, out, brief candle!
Life's but a walking shadow, a poor player
That struts and frets his hour upon the stage
And then is heard no more: it is a tale
Told by an idiot, full of sound and fury,
Signifying nothing.

—*Macbeth*

Pain is the most common complaint for which people consult physicians. The Nuprin Pain Report in 1985 found that 13.9% of people surveyed had backaches 30 or more days per year.[32] Likewise, 13.13% had headaches, 13.8% joint pain, and 9% muscle pain for 30 or more days per year. In the same study, 55% of respondents described themselves as experiencing back pain that significantly interfered with functioning for 1 or more days per year. However, fewer than 20% of the people who reported back pain sought professional help, suggesting that occasional pain is accepted as part of living.

Pain is a major problem in the workplace. Sixty billion dollars are spent annually in the U.S. on chronic pain syndromes, and 550 million sick days are lost annually because of chronic pain syndromes among the working popula-

tion.[10] Back complaints are second only to upper respiratory infections in accounting for absenteeism.[56] Seventy-four percent of workers who experience an acute injury resulting in low back pain are back to work within 30 days. An additional 19% or a total of 93% are back to work within 6 months. The residual 7% are absent from work for more than 6 months, and many never return to work. These latter patients account for 70% of work days lost owing to back injury and for 73% of the medical care given and 76% of the compensation payments made to people with low back injuries.[66]

Everyone experiences severe pain at one time or another. For most of us, the pain ends as the disorder producing it heals. There is, however, a small but significant population in whom pain persists for months or years. Why one injury completely resolves without residual pain or functional impairment and another produces chronic pain or long-term disability is not at all clear.

WHAT IS PAIN?

People have asked what pain is for centuries.[8,17] Aristotle considered pain an emotion—the opposite of pleasantness—and a quality of the soul.[8,17] With René Descartes, the human being was conceptually divided into mind and matter. To Descartes, a healthy person was like a well-made clock in perfect mechanical condition, and a sick person like a clock whose parts malfunction. Born in this tradition, modern Western medicine has looked upon the body in mechanical terms and has held pain to be a problem of sensory input. As a result, we now have numerous pharmacological agents that act on sensory pathways, anesthetics and alcohol to inject into nerves, and surgical procedures to disrupt sensory pathways at every possible site, from peripheral nerves to the cerebral cortex. No mechanistic attack on the sensory afferent system, however, has satisfactorily dealt with the chronic pain patient. Medicine is again focusing upon the awareness, behavior, and emotional state in people with chronic pain.

The International Association of Pain Study defines pain and pain-related syndromes as follows:

> Pain is an unpleasant sensory and emotional experience associated with actual or potential tissue damage, or described in terms of tissue damage. NOTE: Pain is always subjective. Each individual learns the application of the word through experience related to injury.[47]

This definition emphasizes that pain is an experience and therefore subjective. It also separates pain from tissue injury. Pain in general, and chronic pain in particular, is a multidimensional experience. Melzack and Casey[45] have proposed the following three distinct dimensions to the pain experience:

1. **Sensory-Discriminative Dimension**—Electrochemical reception of noxious stimulation, afferent transmission, and initial central processing. This dimension is composed of experiencing the location, quality, and intensity of the painful sensations; it can be mapped in time (e.g., constant versus intermittent, acute versus chronic) and space. This dimension includes the when, how long, and where (i.e., body location, central versus peripheral) of pain.

2. **Cognitive-Evaluative Dimension**—A dimension of ongoing perception and appraisal of the meaning of what is happening, or what might take place in relation to the sensation. This dimension is mapped in time (past, present, and future) and occurs at the level of the whole person within a social network.

3. **Affective-Motivational Dimension**—A dimension of moods and a sense of meaning and relationship to the desire to avoid harm or an expectation of harm; this dimension is also mapped in time and occurs at the level of the whole person within the social network.

Traditional medicine has focused on the sensory-discriminative dimension of pain. The anatomy, physiology, and chemistry of pain have been intensively studied and widely taught. These aspects of pain are not reviewed here. Suffice it to say that traditional medical training encourages a focus on the sensory-discriminative components of pain.

In the acute pain state, the sensory-discriminative dimension dominates the pain experience (Fig. 1A). The traditional, mechanistic approach to pain, addresses the major component

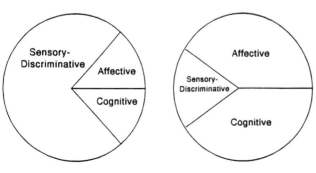

(A) Acute Pain   **(B) Chronic Pain**

FIGURE 1. Acute versus chronic pain. During the acute phase of chronic pain, the sensory-discriminative dimension dominates the pain experience. In chronic pain, however, the sensory-discriminative dimension is less important, and the motivational-affective and cognitive-evaluative dimensions dominate the experience.

of acute pain and, in almost all cases, proves to be an effective strategy. For most people, acute pain subsides and resolves over several weeks to a few months. In a small but significant percentage, however, pain persists. With the passage of time, the localized sensory-discriminative dimension of pain becomes vaguer and "makes less sense." At the same time the cognitive and affective dimensions become more prominent (Fig. 1B). With time, a type of behavior we now call the chronic pain syndrome is recognized.

Another way of visualizing the transformation from acute to chronic pain is presented in Fig. 2A. Assume that two workers sustain hyperextension injuries to the wrist resulting from falls; each worker has skin abrasions and stretch injuries to joint and ligamentous structures and to the median nerve. The "acute pain" experience includes (1) pain arising from the skin, (2) pain arising in joint and ligamentous structures, (3) pain secondary to peripheral nerve injury, and (4) pain associated with psychological, social, and environmental factors (Table 1). In acute pain, the "peripheral" aspects of the pain experience predominate. Now assume also that one worker completely recovers and returns to work within 3 weeks, whereas the other develops chronic pain syndrome and has not returned to work after 1 year. In the latter scenario, it is likely that the skin would have healed, the wrist sprain improved, and the median nerve stretch injury resolved. These structures would make a minor, if any, contribution to the chronic pain problem. Instead, central factors, including changes in pain perception and learned pain behavior, are likely to predominate (Fig. 2B). It is in people like the second worker that our traditional, everyday, commonsense approaches to pain (which focus on treating the sensory-discriminative aspects) break down.

TABLE 1. Categories of Pain Based on Location of the Stimulus[52]

1. External events, including those affecting skin
   Skin is always involved.
   The pain is usually short in duration, except when tissue injury results.
   The subject can usually localize and identify the pain source.
   The nervous system is intact.
   If not interfered with, conduction is intact and modulating factors are fully operational.
2. Pain due to internal events
   The skin is usually not involved except where directly injured, or in referred pain.
   Pain is longer in duration; the patient often cannot localize and identify its source.
   The nervous system is intact.
   Conduction is intact, and modulating factors are operational.
   Examples include events in the viscera, joints, and muscle.
3. Pain associated with lesions in the nervous system
   The skin is often involved; identification of external events is difficult, if not impossible.
   Localization of the source may be faulty.
   The pain is prolonged and may last years, even a lifetime.
   The nervous system is not intact.
   Conduction is faulty, and modulating mechanisms are disrupted.
   In contrast to categories 1 and 2 above, here the lesion is proximal to the afferent receptors.
   Peripheral nerves of the spinal cord or higher levels may be involved.
   The injury may be localized or systemic.
   Examples include post-herpetic neuralgia, causalgia, phantom limb pain, plexus avulsion, thalamic syndrome, and peripheral neuropathy.
4. None of the above
   Pain is associated with social or environmental factors.
   The nervous system is intact.
   Conduction is intact.
   Modulating systems are not structurally altered in a pathological sense.

Pain can be described and categorized by its point(s) of origin or *location* and by its temporality or *duration* (i.e., space and time). For example, pain can be classified as arising from:

FIGURE 2. Site of origin of pain and suffering in acute versus chronic pain. In the acute pain process, injuries to peripheral tissues, such as skin, joints, ligaments, and peripheral nerves, tend to dominate the experience. In contrast, in chronic pain, these latter components tend to be much less prominent and central processes dominate.

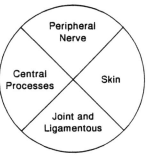

(A) Acute Pain

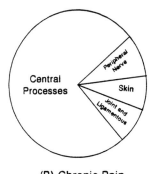

(B) Chronic Pain

1. External events, including those affecting skin

2. Internal events, such as those affecting viscera, joints, or muscle

3. Lesions of the nervous system

4. None of these factors—i.e., pain associated with psychological, social, or environmental factors (Table 1).

We, as health care professionals, are trained to use characteristics of the pain experience such as onset, location, quality, and duration to localize and identify its point of origin and find the underlying pathology. Our initial treatments are directed at alleviating "cause" and "curing" the symptoms of pain. Our acute interventions are predicated on our common-sense, conventional understanding of underlying disease processes and sensory mechanisms.

Pain can also be categorized by its temporality:

1. Acute pain

2. Acute recurrent pain (for example, arthritis, trigeminal neuralgia, and cancer pain);

3. Chronic pain

Chronic pain can be further subdivided as follows:

1. Pain associated with residual structural deformity after injury or disease

2. Pain that is part of a persistent disease process (for example, rheumatoid arthritis)

3. Pain with no residual structural deformity or evidence of disease[53]

Most physicians are accustomed to treating acute injuries that rapidly improve. And most don't know what to do with the chronic pain patient who has no evidence of residual structural deformity or disease. Patients with no measurable anatomical, physiological, or biochemical evidence of functional impairment who continue to feel pain despite rational treatment regimens are a major cause of frustration, burnout, and cynicism in today's health care professionals. This is particularly true for the health care professional who continues to look for a rational, mechanistic solution to the problem. To most of us, our inability to resolve the problem is merely a function of the lack of appropriate knowledge. Traditional medical thinking assumes that when our knowledge is more complete, we will be able to pinpoint the molecular problem, take effective action, and correct it. Part of the dilemma we face in "understanding" chronic pain and suffering, however, is understanding "ourselves."

> If the human brain were so simple we could understand it, we would be so simple that we could not.
>
> —Emmerson Pugh

If we look to the "hard" physical sciences, such as physics, we see that in the molecular realm, the mechanistic cause and effect explanations of Newton have been supplanted by a more uncertain and probabilistic quantum theory. Chronic pain may be the problem that forces medicine to abandon its 18th century Newtonian mechanistic cause-effect perspective for a more relativistic or quantum approach, as physics has done.[18] Einstein was quoted to have said, "The world we have made as a result of the level of thinking we have done thus far creates problems we cannot solve at the same level at which we created them."

If we are going to take on the issues of chronic pain, we, like Don Quixote, may have to take on the windmills of our own imagination and be prepared to look into the mirror of reality and behold ourselves and our contributions to the chronic pain state. More and more is being written about the iatrogenic component (resulting from the activity of physicians) of the chronic pain syndrome. Consider the simple and often routinely prescribed admonishment about acute pain, "If it hurts, don't do it." This rule literally interpreted by the chronic pain patient produces an ever-decreasing level of activity and increasing level of disability. The failure to establish an early diagnosis of a chronic pain disorder, the continued emphasis on repetitive diagnostic studies, the excessive and inappropriate use of medication, the prolonged use of passive physical therapy modalities, the prolonged immobilization and inactivation, and poorly conceived surgical intervention—all inevitably lead to perpetuation and augmentation of the chronic pain syndrome.

Likewise, there is an increased awareness of the "pistigenic" (resulting from the activity of insurance companies) and "normogenic" (resulting from the activity of attorneys) components of the chronic pain disorder. Chronic pain behavior and the chronic pain syndrome are part of the socioeconomic environment and culture of Western industrial society. As the definition of pain by the International Association of Pain Study[30] emphasizes, "Each individual learns the application of the word" [*pain*]. Learning appears to be very important in the chronic pain disorder. Our society has evolved an intricate feedback process that lives in our background culture, where suffering and pain behavior can result in both tangible and intangible rewards. On the one hand, we expect people to return to work; on the other hand, we pay them to be sick. In some settings, we are like the animal trainer who "tells" the sea lion to stop a certain behavior and then rewards the animal with a fish for the same behavior.

In a chapter in a recent textbook on pain, Berna and Chapman[4] have divided the development of chronic pain into three stages:

1. **Stage of Acute Injury.** At this stage, the sensory-discriminative dimensions predominate (Fig. 1A). The degree of physical impairment and social disability relate to or are at least correlated with identifiable physical and pathological impairments or with what has come to be expected with a given injury. (For definitions of impairment, disability, and handicap, see Table 2.)

2. **The Transition Period.** This is a critical period in the recovery process. In most pa-

tients, the injury heals, the person goes on to a "good recovery" and resumes a role in society, or the residual disabilities closely correlate with the residual impairments.

3. **The Learned Phase.** Through conditioning (learning), further impairments and disabilities result from drug misuse, inactivity, and deconditioning and from prolonged and repetitive functioning in a "sick" or unhealthy role. Here, the cognitive-evaluative and affective-motivational aspects of pain predominate.

The challenge we face as physicians treating acute pain disorders is identifying the "at risk" patients and the "transition" from acute pain behavior to chronic pain behavior and modifying management strategies accordingly. At first, the transition may be subtle and difficult to recognize. Where does acute pain end and chronic pain begin? In the past, chronic pain operationally was defined as pain existing beyond 6 months. It is becoming clear, however, that many chronic pain patients exhibit chronic pain behavior as early as 2–6 weeks after an injury.

THE PAIN GAME

After a few years in practice, most physicians readily recognize the well-established, "professional" chronic pain patient. Such patients tend to report pain and disability far out of proportion to their physical impairments and to have a long list of studies done and failed therapies. After several unpleasant experiences with persons for whom chronic pain is a lifestyle, many physicians become aware of what Richard Sternbach referred to as "the pain game"[67]: a conversation or dance that goes as follows:

PATIENT: I hurt. Please fix me. [At some level, the patient, however, knows you cannot.]
M.D.: I'll fix you.

After a period of time, numerous tests, and a number of tried therapies, with perhaps initially some improvement, but subsequently failure, the patient returns stating he or she is not better.

PATIENT: [in righteous indignation] Another incompetent quack.
M.D.: [defensively] Another crock.

In this interaction, the lack of trust between the participants is evident. It is my opinion, as

TABLE 2. Impairment, Disability, and Handicap[20]

Impairment
  The loss, loss of use, or derangement of any body part, system, or function
  An assessment of alteration of health, as determined by a medical expert
  Anatomical, psychological, chemical, and psychiatric dimensions
  Endogenous to the living system
  Does not necessarily equal disability
Disability
  The limiting, loss, or absence of the capacity to meet personal, social, or occupational demands, or statutory or regulatory requirements
  Exogenous; includes both the individual and the environment
  Essentially a social, not a medical, distinction
  A determination of the gap between what the person can do and what he or she needs to do to function in society
Handicap
  An impairment that substantially limits one or more activities of daily living
  A barrier, an obstacle to accomplishing
  Does not necessarily entail disability if, for example, barriers to accomplishing are overcome

a physician and a student of chronic pain, that the lack of trust is, in part, related to our commonsense misconceptions about chronic pain in particular and sensory experiences in general. These misconceptions are addressed, in part, in the following three sections of this chapter.

THE NATURE OF PERCEPTION

This section digresses from the subject of chronic pain as a specific entity and addresses the processes of perception in general. Take a few moments to read, study, and think about Figure 3. Unless you do that now, the rest of this section may not make sense.

Consider Figure 3 in the context of the patient-physician interaction and the different reactions each might have to the figure.

M.D.:   All your diagnostic tests are normal, so you do not have a serious physical problem producing your pain. [Pain is subjective.]

PATIENT: He is trying to tell me the pain is all in my head (not real). I feel it. It is real.

M.D. and   The background of the figure is blue.
PATIENT: Everyone can see it and would agree it is blue; therefore it really is blue. [Color is objective.]

The patient and the physician readily agree that the background of the figure is blue, and their common sense tells them that color is something objective, real. But here the communication often breaks down. Typically, the physician's scientific construction of reality is that pain is subjective, whereas color is objective. The patient, however, understands "subjective" as "mental, in my mind, all in my head, not real, I'm making it up." The conversation, therefore, collapses around the issue, "What is real?"

Webster defines *real* as

Not artificial, fraudulent, illusory, or apparent

Occurring in fact; having objective independent existence.

and *objective* as

Of, relating to, or being an object, phenomenon, or condition in the realm of sensible experience

independent of individual thought and perceptible by all observers; having reality independent of the mind.

Expressing or dealing with facts or conditions as perceived without distortion by personal feelings, prejudices, or interpretations.

Underlying these definitions is the presupposition that we have the ability to assess "objects" or "things" independently of ourselves—that is, not relative to ourselves. Let us explore this assumption. Look at the experiment of colored shadows. The experimental design is that of two lights focused on a white background (Fig. 4). In Figure 4A, the beam of light on the right is red and the one on the left is white. The two lights focused onto a white background result in a mixture of the two colors, or pink. If an object such as a hand is placed over the white light (Fig. 4B), the object casts a shadow that is a dark red. This is "logical"; it makes sense. The white light is obstructed, and the shadow is going to be darker and red. Now, if we place a hand in front of the red light, what color will the shadow be?

Note in the adjacent figure what color we perceive (Fig. 5). How can this be? This is called the simultaneous contrast phenomenon.[40,42,44] When asked how the shadow in this case can be green, most people fall into a discourse about primary and secondary colors, color subtraction, wavelength, and so forth. However, if we try to measure light composition in this experiment, "there is no predominance of the wavelength called green or blue in the shadow we see as blue-green, but only the distribution proper to white light."[44] Physicists such as Schrodinger have long understood that there is absolutely nothing in yellow light (i.e., light consisting of electromagnetic waves of wavelength 590 mμ) that has anything to do with the yellow that we see.[62] This may be hard to "understand." Let us consider Beham's wheel (Fig. 6A). Half of Beham's wheel is black, and the other half contains a series of black arcs on a light background. When the wheel spins, we see color.

How can this be? Where is the color? Our everyday common sense says there is an object out there that has color, and we see the color as it is (i.e., the color is objective, independent—not relative—to us). Pointing to experiences such as the one with colored shadows, Manturana, Varela and others[40,42,44,62] suggest that our experience of colored objects is not dependent on the wavelength, the composi-

FIGURE 3. Objective versus subjective perception. The background of the figure in the original text is blue and the lettering white.

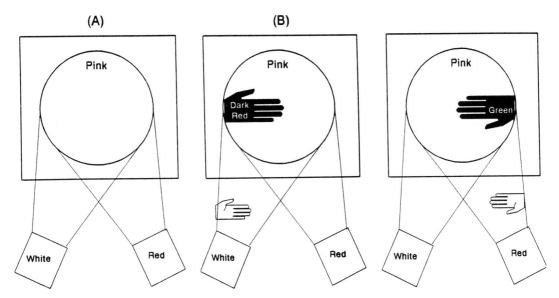

FIGURE 4. Colored shadows experiment. The design of the experiment is two light sources focused on the white background. The light source on the left is white, and that on the right is red. When they both project onto a white background, we perceive the background as lighter than the red light source, i.e., as pink (A). When an opaque object, such as a hand, is placed in front of the white light source, the shadow cast is darker and close to the original intensity of the red light source (B). What is the color of the shadow when the hand is placed in front of the red light source?

FIGURE 5. Colored shadow experiment. When an opaque object, such as a hand, is placed in front of the red light source, the shadow we perceive on the background is green. How can this be?

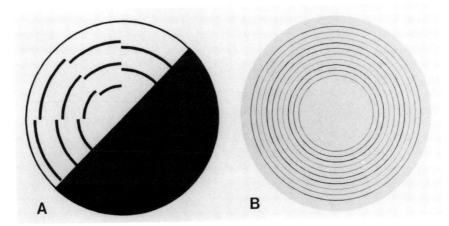

FIGURE 6. Beham's wheel (A) consists of a disk one-half of which is black, the other half white. The white half contains a series of arcs. When Beham's wheel spins (B), we perceive a series of colored circles. The colors include blue, green, yellow, and a red-brown. The resting wheel, or top, does not contain colors. That is, color is not inherent to the wheel. Where is it that we perceive the color?

tion, of the light coming from "the world out there" but, rather, our experience of color corresponds to specific patterns of activity in the nervous system, which the structure of the nervous system defines. That is, we correlate the naming of colors we perceive with states of electrical activity in the brain. When Beham's wheel spins, it stimulates rods and cones, generating a pattern of activity in the brain that we recognize as, see, and call color. Although the experiments discussed here concentrate on visual sensations and experiences, the principles of perception they reveal apply to other experiences of "the world" as well.

We assume that we see the world as "it really is" and that we *need* to see it as it is in order to live and survive in it. Is this really the case? Let us consider the living process. What is the living organization? What is the organization of living?[55] Again, using examples of Manturana and Varela,[43,44] let us consider a simple organism, the single-cell amoeba, and look at the qualities of its living organization. First, it has a structure within a boundary (cell membrane) that separates it from the environment. Second, it has an internal organization that maintains a relatively constant relationship between the components within the cell membrane (i.e., homeostasis—the tendency of the living system to maintain stability, owing to the coordinated response of its parts to any disruptive situation or stimulus). Maintaining these relations is critical for the continuing organization—that is, for survival.

We, as observers, can see the amoeba as a separate, individual unit interacting with its environment. We say that the amoeba is "stimulated" and "responds" (Fig. 7). For example, if we introduce a "nutrient particle," we, as observers, say the amoeba engulfs the stimulus of food for nutrition. If we introduce a "noxious chemical," we, as observers, say the amoeba flees noxious stimulation for survival. This domain of description, which explains or attributes purpose, is a perspective, however, that we, as observers, bring to the interaction. From inside the amoeba, there are only changes in organizational relationships followed by a series of reactions that, when effective, eventually bring the organism back to the set relationship points (homeostasis). From inside the cell, there are no stimuli, there is no purpose, only constant process, constant maintenance of homeostatic relationships within the living organization. From the amoeba's perspective, the actions executed correlate not with the purpose or explanation deduced by the observer outside the cell but only with changes in relationships within the cell.

Consider the pilot in an airplane that is descending through thick clouds over a city and an observer on the ground. When the plane descends into the clouds, the pilot no longer has any idea of what is going on outside; his vision is obscured. He must rely on the instruments within the airplane. From the pilot's perspective (from within the unit), he works to maintain certain relationships (homeostasis) with respect to the instruments monitored on his panel. These are relationships he has learned from past experience. The person on the ground, however, may describe the pilot as banking, turning, ascending, and so forth in order to go between hills or around hills and buildings. That is, the observer on the ground attaches a purpose to the plane's actions. In the pilot's perspective, however, all that he is doing is maintaining the dials constant.[44]

Within the amoeba and other individual cells, biochemical gradients and enzymatic processes

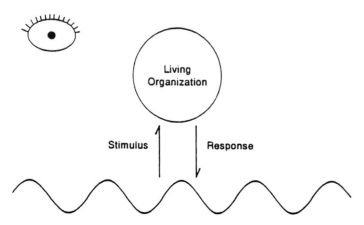

FIGURE 7. The living process, the environment, and the observer. The closed circle represents living organization, and the wavy line below, the environment. The observer, symbolized by the eye, can describe the living organization's interaction with the environment in terms of stimulus and response relationships.[43]

coordinate the living organization. With the evolution of multicellular organisms and increasing complexity of the living organization, the nervous system evolved to correlate internal relationships between cells (i.e., homeostasis of the multicellular organism) as well as to coordinate sensory and effector (motor) responses.[44] The nervous system is a network of cells that correlates stimuli (perturbations that change the organism and its resting relations) with effector responses (coordinated actions that reestablish resting relations, which are critical to survival—i.e., homeostasis). Maintaining relationships within the nervous system of the multicellular organism is to the multicellular organism what maintaining biochemical gradients and enzymatic processes in the nuclear/cytoplasmic soup is to the single cell.

As the nervous system becomes more complex, both "external" and "internal" stimuli perturb it. For example, consider chemoreceptors. Changes in blood CO_2 stimulate chemoreceptors (stimuli) that, via their connections, produce changes in patterns of activity within the central nervous system, triggering motor (behavioral) responses within the respiratory system. These motor responses, in turn, alter pCO_2, and as the pCO_2 approaches a set point, the activity in the sensory unit—the chemoreceptors that initiated the response—is itself changed by the behavior it initiated. In other words, there is a recursive loop. The nervous system is a recursive system. Sensory stimuli produce responses that are, in turn, stimuli to which the organism responds, and so on and so on. It's like the person standing between two opposing mirrors in which he sees reflections of himself and reflections of himself and so on ad infinitum (Fig. 8).

Our highly complex nervous system has evolved a capacity to perceive and represent the environment within it. Our ordinary everyday common sense tells us that these representations are exact representations of the way the environment is. However, the experiences with color vision suggest that how we see the world corresponds to specific patterns of states of activity, which the structure of the nervous system defines, and that we correlate naming of colors and other perceptions with specific states of activity of the brain. The nervous system is actually a closed, self-referential system; neither we nor the instruments we use can objectively perceive the world as it is. Begin-

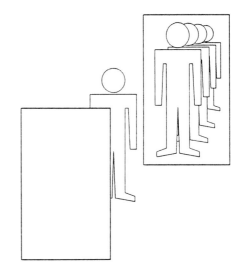

FIGURE 8. Standing between two mirrors. The person standing between two mirrors and looking into one sees the self and its reflection in the other mirror, the reflection of the reflection of the self in the other mirror, and so on and so on, recursively . . . ad infinitum.

ning with Einstein and his theory of relativity, physicists have understood this. The science of physics recognizes that we do not experience an objective reality independent of ourselves. We live in a world of relativity; our perceptions are relative to ourselves and our nervous systems. As Heisenberger stated, "We have to remember that what we have observed is not nature in itself, but nature exposed to our method of questioning"—in the above examples, our methods of examination and perception. We do not experience an objective reality independent of ourselves. "We do not see the 'colors' of the world; we live in our chromatic space,"[44] which we create and generate. "We do not see the 'space' of the world; we live in our field of vision."[44] Like the amoeba, our actions correlate as a function of how the world alters our living organization.[44]

DO WE DANCE WITH THE MAP OR THE TERRITORY?

Figure 9A shows a land formation, a territory. There are plains, hills, valleys, and a river. In time, people come along, build a road, divide the territory up into counties, districts, and states (Fig. 9B). In State Y (say it's Nevada), you may be able to smoke, drink, and gamble legally, and there may be open prostitution. A few feet away, in State Z (say it's California), you may be able to drink and smoke,

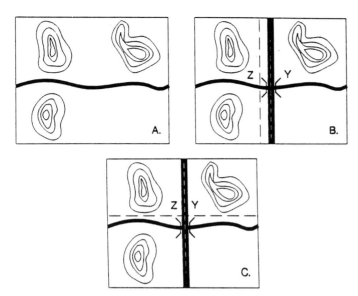

FIGURE 9. Map versus the territory. A,
The territory has inherent topographical
features, including hills, a plain, and a river.
B, As people appear on the scene, they
may develop territory with roads and also
separate it into states and counties. The
distinctions can affect inhabitants' actions.
In State Y, for example, an inhabitant may
be able to smoke, drink, and gamble legally, and there may be open prostitution.
A few feet away, in State Z, people may
be able to drink and smoke but not legally
gamble, and there may be no legal prostitution. The difference between Y and Z
is not something that is inherent in the
territory. Rather, the difference is the distinction that we as human beings create
and map onto the territory. C, The territory
could just as easily have been divided up
along the river as along the road. In this
reframed map of the territory, Y and Z would
be governed by a single set of rules and
regulations.

but you may not legally gamble and there is
no legal prostitution. The difference between
Y and Z is not something that is inherent in
the territory they occupy, as a river or valley
would be. Rather, the difference is in the distinctions human beings create and map onto
the territory. Within the limits the territory
allows, we can construct a variety of maps with
different distinctions and different representations. For example, the territory could have
just as easily been divided along the river instead of down the middle (Fig. 9C). Now, in
the left half of the figure, a person at point Z
may be able to gamble, whereas before he may
not have been. To the degree to which the
territory allows, our behavior and actions correlate with our representations (our maps), our
constructs of "the territory" or "the world."
Our representations result in certain patterns
of neuronal activity in the nervous system, and
our actions are correlated with the patterns of
neuronal activity (X is legal in Y but not in Z).
"I cannot do X because my pain will get worse."

IMPLICATIONS IN THE CONTEXT OF CHRONIC PAIN

Go back and reread Figure 3 and the reactions to the figure in the text. Which of the
two statements do you now think is invalid?

The presupposition that an objectivity really
exists independent of us—that is, an objectivity without subjectivity—collapses and becomes unimportant, as does a discussion whether
chronic pain is objective or subjective. In our
ordinary everyday way of living and thinking,

the tree out there exists and we see it as it is.
An alternative hypothesis, however, is that light
reflects from something we call a tree, hits the
retina, and stimulates the retina-brain complex; what we see is the result of the activity
of the retina-brain complex projected back into
the environment (Fig. 10). How we see it is a
function not only of the stimulus that interacts
with us, but also of the structure or organization of the nervous system.

If you have followed what has been presented in the preceding sections, you ought to
have at least some uncertainty about whether
the background of Figure 3 is really blue. If
our experience of color correlates with certain
patterns of neuronal activity, is it not possible
that, in the absence of malingering (lying), the
chronic pain and suffering that chronic pain
patients experience also correlate with certain
states of neuronal activity that are "physical"
and that may be as "real" and as "objective" as
the blue background in Figure 3? Furthermore, is it not possible that these states of neuronal activity and the patients' resulting actions
are related to how the world appears to their
nervous system—that is, according to their maps
of the territory?

In our interactions with chronic pain patients
and with chronic pain behavior, we need to
keep "in mind" that we see the problem only
as observers; we are like the ground observer
of the airplane descending through fog. We see
these people acting with respect to our maps
of the territory, through our virtues and our
values. There is, however, another perspective
that is unseen by us, the inner perspective at

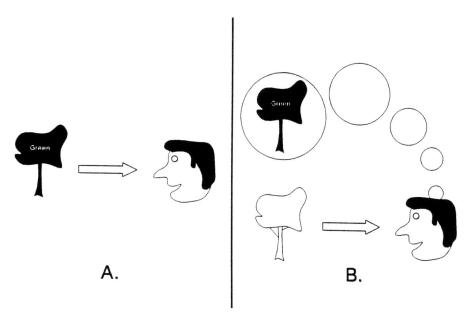

A.   **B.**

FIGURE 10. Our commonsense, everyday way of thinking is that a tree is inherently green and we see its inherent greenness (*A*). The data from the colored shadow experiment and Beham's wheel, however, suggest that the green we perceive may be inherent in the structure of the central nervous system and we perceive it as projected back into the environment (*B*).

the level of patterns of electrical activity that generate the chronic pain patients' representations (maps) within their central nervous systems. This is the perspective of the pilot who works to keep the dials and levers steady, i.e., "homeostatic." From our perspective as observers, the actions and behaviors of chronic pain patients may not make sense; however, from the inner perspective of the patients (the

pilot), the actions are in accord with their maps and presuppositions about the territory. All they may be doing is maintaining a "learned" stability within the living organization that they are. Their actions are based on the structure and function of their nervous system. They act according to their maps of the territory. We, as observers, can describe the behavior of chronic pain patients and attribute what is typ-

FIGURE 11. Impossible? We believe that the room is rectangular and see the figures as different sizes. This is what happens inside the Ames distorted room. We are so used to rooms being rectangular that we bet on the room's being normal and the person's being an odd shape.[31] The geometry of the Ames distorted room is shown in Figure 12. (Reprinted with permission from Eastern Daily Press, Norwich, England.)

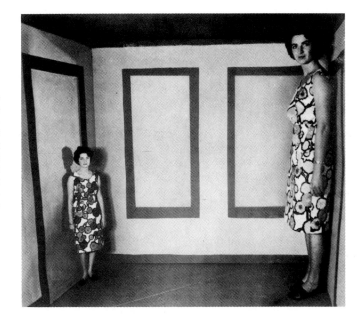

ically called secondary gain to their maladaptive behaviors. I am convinced, however, that some chronic pain patients truly do not see what we label as secondary gain. They see only one way of behaving and sense that any other way involves risk. They are acting according to their maps of the territory.

PERCEPTION AND THE HISTORICITY WE ARE

Look at Figure 11. What do you notice? One woman looks very large and the other very small, yet the configuration of the room looks rectangular. One woman is not a giant, nor is the other a midget. In this figure, we are simultaneously presented with two conflicting and contradictory perceptions that result in an optical illusion or paradox. Where do the illusion and deception take place?

The illusion is a product of our learned expectation that rooms are rectangular, which causes us to see the figures at different sizes. In fact, the room is not rectangular (Fig. 12). Evidently we are so accustomed to rectangular rooms that we see the figures—that is, the two people—as odd sizes rather than the room as an odd shape.[31]

What is remarkable about illusions involving perspective is that if the illusion is shown to people in societies without rectangular buildings and rooms, such as the Zulu, they do not see the paradox. It has also been reported that wives do not see their husbands as distorted by the Ames room. Rather, they see their hus-

bands as normal and the room in its true shape.[31] What is important about illusions involving perspective is that they demonstrate visually that during our development, on the basis of our sensory experiences, we unconsciously learn

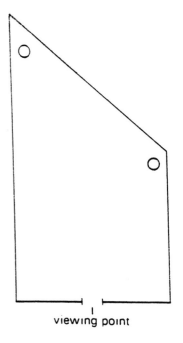

FIGURE 12. The geometry of the Ames distorted room. The farther wall, in fact, recedes from the observer (and the camera) to the left. The figure on the left is farther away, but the walls and windows are arranged to give the same retinal image as those of a normal rectangular room, and the figures appear to have different sizes. (Reprinted with permission from Gregory RL: Eye and Brain: The Psychology of Seeing. New York, McGraw-Hill, 1966.)

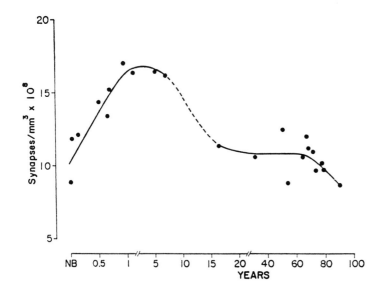

FIGURE 13. Synaptic connections. The counts of synapse in layer three of the middle frontal gyrus are shown as a function of age. The number increases from birth to 1–5 years and then decreases to the number and density found in the adult.[36] (Reprinted with permission from Huttenlocher PR: Synaptic density in human frontal cortex: Developmental changes and effects of aging. Brain Res 163: 195, 1979.)

to make a priori assumptions about how things—in this case, a room—should look. These a priori assumptions, which are probably hard-wired into our central nervous system, affect how we see things in the present—hence, the paradox.

The ultimate structure and functional relationships of the adult human brain are the product of genetic possibilities and environmental experiences. Both in the uterus and after birth, interaction with the environment helps to determine what genetic possibilities are manifested and stabilized. In this manner, the environment imposes an order on the structure of the nervous system. The structure of the nervous system is coupled to the environment through our interaction with the environment.[11,44]

Studies in intact animals and in tissue cultures indicate that during the development of the nervous system, there is a tremendous overproliferation of collateral axons and dendritic branches (connections between nerve cells). As the organism matures, "excess" connections decrease. Changeux and Danchin[11] and others[51] have put forth a selective stabilization hypothesis to describe this process and to explain how the environment imposes a higher order on the structure and function of the nervous system through experience. They postulate that early in development, connections between neurons are labile and that the early activity within the nervous system (spontaneous and evoked activity) results in preferential stabilization of certain circuits. In other words, the genetic environment of the organism generates spontaneously a multiplicity of internal variations of interactions within the nervous system. Subsequent activity within the nervous system selectively stabilizes some of these. In this manner, the environment indirectly, by a selective (Darwinian) mechanism, imposes a higher order upon the nervous system.[11] A number of biological systems that have been described support this hypothesis.[11]

This process probably also occurs in the nervous system of man. Studies in man indicate that synaptic density (an index of the number of neuronal connections) gradually increases during infancy, reaching a maximum by the age of 1–2 years that is 50% higher than in the adult (Fig. 13).[36] Between the ages of 5 and 16 years, synaptic activity steadily declines. The connections that persist are undoubtedly related to the connections that are activated and stimulated by our interactions with ourselves

and our environment—that is, by our experiences. Our interactions with the environment thus affect the structure of the nervous system. In primates, the occipital cortex (visual section of the brain) normally has what are referred to as ocular dominance columns (Fig. 14). When the eye of an adult monkey is surgically closed, there is no alteration in the pattern of ocular dominance (Fig. 14A). In the

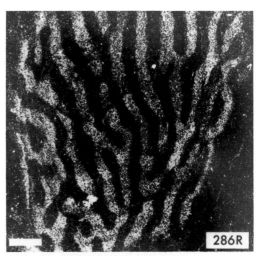

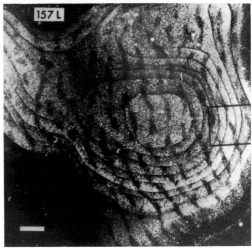

FIGURE 14. The effect of binocular vision on the structure of cortex from the monkey. Evidence of the importance of sensory inputs for cortical development can be seen clearly when the two photos are compared. Shown are the ocular dominance columns, columns of neurons that alternatively receive input from the right eye and the left eye. Top, relatively normal pattern (from a monkey whose right eye was closed in maturity); below, the pattern in a monkey whose right eye was closed at 2 weeks of age and kept closed for 1½ months; the columns for the functioning left eye obviously dominate. (Reprinted with permission from Hubel DH, LeVay S, Wiesel TN: The development of ocular dominance columns in normal and visually deprived monkeys. J Comp Neurol 191:1, 1980.)

developing monkey, however, surgically closing an eye dramatically alters the pattern of ocular dominance (Fig. 14B).[35]

In another study, kittens were trained to raise a forepaw repetitively to avoid an electric shock ("pain"). These kittens developed a much greater number of and more complex dendritic branches in the cerebral hemisphere contralateral to the paw that was shocked than in the other hemisphere. (Fig. 15).[58,65] Again, these studies indicate that sensory experiences early in development have profound effects on the ultimate structure and function of the brain. These studies as well as the illusions of perspective, such as Ames's distorted room (Fig. 11), indicate that past experiences determine how we see things in the present. It should, therefore, not be surprising that previous painful experiences, cultural background, family life, and personality traits all affect the pain experience. A review of 100 consecutive case histories at an inpatient chronic pain center indicated that 83 of the patients had a history of major psychological stress during growth and development. Many were sexually abused, battered, or grew up in family settings with destructive alcoholic behavior.[49] Such histories appear to be the rule rather than the exception among chronic pain patients and suggest that many of them may be "prewired" and, hence, predisposed to such problems.[7,21]

Pain plays a very important role in our development and learning. We learn that pain can alert us to damage to parts of the body and tissues. Pain and suffering are also intimately involved in our relationships to other human beings. Infants learn to cry when they are uncomfortable; crying elicits a response from the mother or some other close person. The injured child is often comforted by a parent. Although the pain in such examples may not be pleasant, we may come to learn to expect pain to be followed by relief from the interaction with another human being. During infancy and childhood, pain and crying (pain behavior?) get attention. In early childhood, pain and punishment may also become linked. Pain may be inflicted by a parent or another when the infant or child is "bad." After being punished, the child is often consoled by the parent. Therefore, pain may also become an important medium for the expiation of guilt.[7]

The structural coupling of the nervous system to the environment (including the internal environment of the body) does not cease when the animal reaches the adult state. Contrary to what was believed in the past, it is now apparent that the adult system is not rigid and permanently hard-wired but, rather, that synaptic density and internal neuronal connections change with experience well into adult life. Repetitive activities associated with learning are accompanied by biochemical and structural changes at the synaptic level.[41] It is quite probable that some of the disorders of behavior we see in adults, including chronic pain problems, are learned phenomena. Through conditioning, impairments and disabilities can be reinforced and new ones can develop. Observations in patients who undergo amputations and develop a painful, ischemic diabetic extremity indicate a higher percentage of phantom pain (pain that persists after the extremity is removed) in patients with relatively late am-

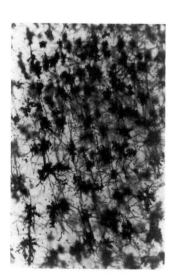 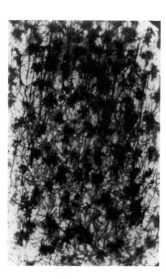

FIGURE 15. The effects of stimulation in learning on neuronal density in interconnections. The effects of learning on the cortex can be seen when these two photomicrographs are compared. They are from the somatosensory cortex of a kitten trained to raise a paw in response to a pattern of horizontal lines, a stimulus that signaled "danger" (application of a mild electrical shock—"pain".) A pattern of vertical lines signaled safety from the shock. The "trained" area of the somatosensory cortex (on the right) shows a much greater number of and more complex dendritic branches than the control on the left. (Reprinted with permission from Spinelli DH, Jensen EF, Dipresco: Early experience effect on dendritic branching in normally reared kittens. Neurology 62:1, 1980.)

putations compared to those who receive early amputations. This suggests that sensory input is important in the development of chronic phantom pain in these patients.[22]

Phantom pain raises an interesting question: Where do we perceive pain? Have you ever wondered how myocardial infarction produces pain in the inner aspect of the left arm? Or how pain occurs in an extremity that is not there, as in phantom pain? When you begin to look at pain and pain perception, the evidence suggests that what we call "pain" occurs in the brain, not in the area of the body where it is felt. That is, pain is projected not back into the tissues but, rather, on the brain's representation of the body (Fig. 16). How else can referred and phantom pain be explained? Again, it should not be surprising that past experience and body image affect the pain experience.

The preceding sections have explored some aspects of the living organization and perception, how the structure and function of the nervous system is influenced by experience and how our experiences impose a higher order on the living organization and the nervous system.

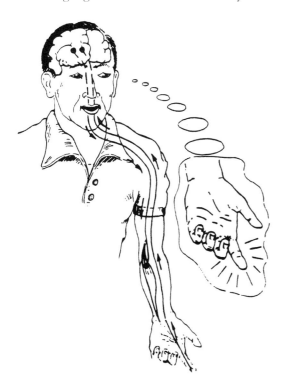

FIGURE 16. Noxious stimulation may be detected in the hand and transmitted to the brain, but the brain's awareness occurs on the brain's representation of the hand.[6] (Reproduced with permission from Chaplin ER, Kasdan ML: Hand Clin 2:514, 1986.)

The discussion has been primarily from the perspective of the individual. Although chronic pain behavior is a problem that becomes manifest in an individual, the "maladaptive" behavior of the chronic pain syndrome is not solely a disorder of the individual. It is a disorder that develops within society and becomes manifest as a breakdown between what is expected from the individual by society and how the individual actually behaves. The chronic pain problem cannot be explored without looking at society and its contributions. We are social animals, and we live in complex social networks.

SOCIETY, LANGUAGE, AND CHRONIC PAIN

In the single cell, ionic gradients and enzymatic reactions are the medium for *intra*cellular communication and coordination of actions. In the multicellular organism, the nervous and endocrine systems are mechanisms for *inter*cellular communication and coordination of actions. In human society, language is the medium for *inter*personal communication and for coordination of actions. The development of language has allowed us to coordinate our actions and make today's human social networks possible.

In our common, everyday way of thinking, we assume that language is a system for representing (labeling) the world. Language not only labels; it also commits us to specific actions in the present and future. Repeat the following expressions aloud:

Rhinoceros.

I promise I will complete this chapter in 1 hour.

What is the difference between the expressions? When you say "rhinoceros," you may have an image or thought, but no action takes place in the world outside you. You have not committed yourself to any action. When you say, "I promise to complete this chapter in 1 hour," you make a commitment to do something by a certain time. Your speaking, your words, change how the world may unfold before you. You are committing yourself to a specific action. Promises to perform a particular action and an intention to keep promises are implicit in the background that society is built on. We coordinate our social interactions on the basis of promises.

The philosopher Jay L. Austin developed a theory of categories of speaking based on the manner in which various acts of speaking coordinate our actions.[1] Austin's student Searle[61,62] and Searle's student Flores[32,74] have formalized these categories. As a result of my reading of these authors, I have come to listen for and anticipate the following types of speech acts in my conversations with patients:

An **intention** is a stated purpose that is declared to oneself or to others as a desirable goal. However, it does not commit the speaker to specific actions directed at achieving the goal.

A **promise** is a commitment from the speaker to the hearer (who may be the speaker or another) to do something by a certain time. That is, it is a commitment to do X by time Y. Promises are one way of committing intentions into actions.

A **request** (a directive) is an attempt by the speaker to get the hearer to do something, to commit to an action. For example, I request that you do X by time Y. To a request, a hearer can decline, accept, not respond, agree to respond later, or make a counterproposal. The pain patient often arrives in the physician's office or facility with a blanket request. Whether addressed or not, it usually is implicit.

A **fact** implies a promise by the speaker to produce evidence for the statement. For example, I state that the car would not start. My statement commits me to be able to demonstrate that the car will not start and that the car's not starting is something that can be observed.

Opinions, judgments, and assessments are statements about preferences, biases, and interpretations. They carry no commitment to provide evidence other than the implied commitment that people expressing them really feel or believe what they say they feel or believe—that is, that they are telling the truth.

When you learn and begin to listen for these distinctions in conversations, your effectiveness as a listener and as a speaker improves. You begin to listen to what chronic pain patients request of you and what they *want* or *intend* to do or not to do, as opposed to what they are actually making *commitments* to do or not do. You also begin to think and speak more clearly and directly about what you commit yourself to do or not to do in these relationships.

The discourse of language also allows us to be observers of ourselves and others.[43] As human beings, we have the capacity to observe ourselves and our actions within our environment. This capability to observe and describe ourselves within our environment, however, has arisen in a nervous system that is part of a living organization whose purpose is to maintain constant its internal relationships. In our ordinary everyday way of living, we do not stop to consider the effects that language—words or thoughts—has on and within our body. For example, recall a time when you heard something that embarrassed you. Did a change in skin color occur? Did you feel flushed? What about a time when you heard tragic news? Did you feel a tug or pain in your chest or abdomen? Language occurs within the structure and function of the nervous system, a system where one state of activity (a response) is, in turn, a stimulus that produces another response. Our thoughts are projected and appear to us in the domain of the ground observer; however, they arise in the domain of the central nervous system (the pilot in the clouds).

A stimulus or an event (external or internal) may result in a thought (a response). Thoughts are, in turn, stimuli to which the nervous system responds, and so on and so on . . . (Fig. 17). Again, it is like a person standing between two mirrors looking at a reflection of himself and a reflection of the reflection looking at himself and so on and so on (Fig. 8)—what Eastern philosophy has referred to as the vicious circle. The capacity for man to observe and communicate arose within the capacity for language. "In the beginning was the Word." Words also affect us: "And the Word became flesh."

Language is a powerful tool. Its development has profoundly altered the course of life on this planet. The ability to oppose thumb and forefinger is another great tool. It allows a manual dexterity that has also altered the course of the world. However, neither we nor primates, who also have thumb and forefinger opposition, go through life continually preoccupied, marveling at, and, in particular, stimulating ourselves with our thumbs and forefingers. We do, however, tend to continually stimulate ourselves with our internal conversations, our wants, desires, disappointments, and laments. This evaluation and judgmental self-stimulation is a major source of pain and suffering in our society. We become trapped by our moods, which are affected by our individual wants, desires, expectations, and continual self-evaluations.

As individuals with consciousness, we see ourselves as separate. Our perception of our-

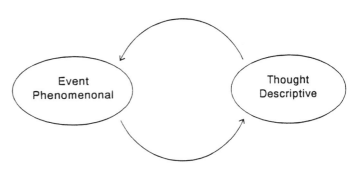

FIGURE 17. "In the beginning was the word . . . and the Word became flesh." The capacity for language, description, and thinking arises within the living organization. Events that occur in what we perceive in the phenomenal world are reflexively associated with phenomena in our cognitive (thought) descriptive capacities. These thoughts, descriptions, conversations, however, all occur within the living organization that perceives the initial phenomena and, in turn, are events, phenomena, to which we respond, and so on and so on, in a recursive manner.

selves as separate entities also creates problems for society as a whole. Einstein is reported to have said that "a human being is part of the whole that we call the universe, a part limited in time and space. We experience ourselves, our thoughts, and our feelings in a kind of optical delusion of our consciousness, as something separate from the rest. This delusion is a prison that restricts us to our personal desires and to affection for a few persons nearest us. Our task must be to free ourselves from this prison by widening our circle of compassion to embrace all living creatures and the whole of nature in all its beauty." Instead, for many of us and, in particular, for the chronic pain patient, life becomes

> . . . but a walking shadow, a poor player
> That struts and frets his hour upon the stage
> And then is heard no more: it is a tale
> Told by an idiot, full of sound and fury,
> Signifying nothing.

Why this emphasis on language? I request that you raise your hand. Do that now. How did you do it?

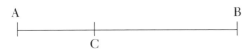

If we represent the entire amount of activity within the central nervous system that must take place for this act to occur as the line from A to B and the amount of activity that is actually involved in physically moving the arm up as the line from C to B, what is the activity in the central nervous system that is left? (i.e., What is the line from A to C?) The intention, the command, the thought, the words, the language that generates the action? "And the word became flesh." If a thought or language can do this, why does it seem so foreign to many physicians and laypersons that thoughts, language,

intentions, wants, desires, and so forth, may play a profound role in causing, exacerbating, reducing, or even healing "abnormal" body states? Perhaps it will be from this realm, these "soft and flaky domains," that our "new therapies" to compliment and assist the tremendous technological advances of the 20th century will emerge and advance the health and wisdom of the human being.

THE INJURED PARTY GAME

When people are seriously injured in automobile accidents or on the job, society has evolved mechanism such as disability insurance and workers' compensation insurance that excuse them from their expected roles and yet enable them to continue to meet financial obligations. Society also expects that, as the physical impairments heal, the associated disability will decrease. With the passage of time, these people are expected to resume their roles within society. The expectation is that when an injury is sustained, the injury will resolve, damages and medical expenses will be paid, and the injured person will reassume the role formerly played in society. However, more and more this is not the case. Newspaper reports suggest that as many as one in seven injured workers in the State of California enters into litigation against an employer or insurer. Some attorneys in the San Diego area have been reported to send runners down to meet incoming tuna boats to sign up injured workers as potential clients. Increasingly, the perception in southern California is that an injury is like a lottery ticket; if you play the game and get lucky, you can win big bucks.

Pooling risks and investments (i.e., accident or disability insurance) can offer common benefits only with the support of a *shared* social obligation. When physical impairment appears to have resolved but a major claim of disability persists, or when claims for damages seem disproportionate to an injury, the system breaks down and the injured party game may begin. The injured party game includes injured parties, their families, employers, physicians, insurance companies and their personnel, attorneys, and others. Initially, each player has a supportive commitment to the injured member of society, to himself or herself, and to society as a whole. With conflict, the commitment to society becomes less apparent and commitments to the self increase. This observation seems to be particularly valid when the injured party has chronic pain. For example, consider the injured worker who develops a chronic pain syndrome. Participants in the game may include:

Physician. The physician's initial commitments are to return the injured worker to health and to be compensated for services rendered. As chronic pain behavior becomes dominant, his skills often fail. The time required to work with these patients often exceeds what physicians can be reimbursed for unless they perform poorly conceived surgeries for which they are directly compensated, prescribe prolonged therapies for which they are indirectly compensated, or render forensic medical opinions.

Workers' Compensation Insurance Carrier. The carrier insures the employer against loss secondary to injury and compensates workers for temporary or permanent disability. The carrier also has a commitment to stockholders or a governing body and to other employers to remain economically viable and to show a profit. In cases where expenditures begin to seem excessive, it is in the insurer's self-interest to terminate the case and cut losses as soon as possible.

Workers' Compensation Case Workers. The initial commitments of case workers are to provide services to the injured worker and to their own employer. They expect to be paid for these services. Their job may involve quotas that keep case activity low and costs down. For them, "The only good case is a closed case."

Employer. The employer is committed to producing goods and services and returning a profit. It may not be in the employer's short-term interest to take an injured worker back. The employer looks not only at the worker's capability of returning and performing a task, but also at the risk of further loss of liability as a result of taking the worker back, particularly if the insured worker was a "problem worker" before the injury.

Plaintiff's Attorney. Plaintiff's attorneys are committed to their clients, the injured parties, and makes sure they receive all they are entitled to. They also expect to be compensated for their services. Frequently, the longer the case, the larger the attorney's compensation.

Attorney for the Insurance Carrier. The company attorney's initial commitments are to provide services to the insuring company and to be paid for his services. There is an implicit understanding that a continuing relationship depends on efficiency in keeping expenditures down.

Injured Worker. In the center of these conflicting commitments is the injured worker, who has the most to gain and, at the same time, the most to lose from the game. The anticipation of a big settlement can modify the injured worker's behavior. Physicians say there is nothing they can do to help, that the problem is one of attitude, that it is all in the worker's head, or they administer many tests and attempt many therapies and surgical procedures that fail. The attorney may tell the worker not to do anything that may indicate ability beyond what the worker acknowledges. "The insurance company may have hired someone who is watching you." This all takes place in the context of ongoing commitments to support family, pay bills, and so forth.

Like many chronic pain patients, the injured worker with chronic pain may have a predisposition to and a history of illness and illness behavior. The injury may be just another crisis that allows withdrawal from society's expected roles. Other workers, however, have functioned adequately in life. They do not have a history of multiple illness or illness behaviors; however, they become injured and may well fall into the injured party game. They may assume that they are expected to behave in a certain way, learn to behave in that way, and become stuck in the injured party game. Still others are attracted by the expectation of a large economic gain or a ticket our of a job they have learned to dislike, and they learn to behave accordingly.

The issue of malingering is one that almost always surfaces in the injured party game. Malingering is willful, deliberate, and fraudulent feigning or exaggeration of symptoms or illness or injury for the purpose of a consciously desired end. The distinction between *malingering* and *learned symptom exaggeration* can be difficult to make. Proof of malingering is difficult to come by short of proving the person is lying or committing perjury. The situation is further complicated by confusion concerning what we mean by "willful." As Schopenhauer stated, "A man can do as he will, but not will as he will."

MYTHS AND THE DANCE OF LIFE

In *The Hero with a Thousand Faces*, Joseph Campbell explores the myths of man's many cultures and reduces them to what he calls the "monomyth."[9] The hero of this monomyth is going along through life when he is interrupted by a stimulus, an event Campbell names "the call of adventure." The hero sets out on this grand adventure but soon descends into the abyss, where he is confronted by demons and monsters. Out of nowhere, a supernatural being appears and assists the hero. Together they conquer the adversity of the abyss, and the triumphant hero returns to the world to live happily every after.

Primitive culture acted myths out in ceremonies. During the ceremony, "the mind was radically cut away from the early attitudes and attachments"[9] and introduced to new responsibilities and goals. Such myths are apparent in modern culture as well. Jesus came to Earth as humankind's savior; he was tortured, crucified, buried, arose, and ascended back into Heaven. Similar themes can be found in Eastern religions, Judaism, and Islam.

We are all adventurers along the path of life (Fig. 18). We struggle for our individual identity. In the United States, we live the myth of the American Dream: "With enough guts and gumption, anyone can make it."[54] With hard work, we can defeat the enemy, have a perfect relationship and family, be rich and famous, and ride off into the sunset to live happily ever after.

Unlike daydreams and Hollywood movies, life usually does not offer us a reality that matches our ideals, and more often than not, some form of breakdown seems to happen. This breakdown may be an injury or painful illness. We are faced with pain and suffering and sadness that come with what we have lost or expect we may not now ever have. We become trapped in an abyss (Fig. 18). The central nervous system habituates to the pain and suffering—that is, we adapt to our new situation—we move on or remain stuck in the abyss. When stuck, we are in division. We no longer perceive ourselves as living up to our ideals of success and independence or as supporters of our family and relationships. In the present, we find ourselves stuck in the gap between our ideals and beliefs of the way it should be and the mess we perceive ourselves to be in. If we look back toward the past, we say, "If only . . . I should have . . . they should have . . . " If we look toward the future, we say, "What if . . . ?" In the present, these automatic and recurrent conversations may be associated with anger and guilt about what has happened in the past, or with anxiety and fear about the future. Here we confront the demons and monsters of our own psyche. We cry out for help. We are afraid to give up what we have had because we might not have it again and because we might not get what we perceive we are entitled to. In the setting of chronic pain, both the patient and the health care provider can be trapped in this abyss. The patient is in the abyss of loss and suffering, and the health care provider in the abyss of explanation, hypothesis, and a traditional medical model that does not provide a

FIGURE 18. The dance of life, the monomyth. The "hero" of the monomyth (A) is traveling through the path of life when an event occurs, what Joseph Campbell calls the call to adventure (in our context, injury, illness, disease). The individual then sets out on an "adventure" (C) and soon finds himself separated from the old and confronted by loss, fear, failure; i.e., he is in the "abyss." In the myth, the adventurer is helped by a supernatural hero (in modern Western society, the victim looks for "the answer"), and together they conquer the adversity. The adventurer attains a new identity and status in life, returns to society as "the triumphant hero," and lives happily ever after (B).[9]

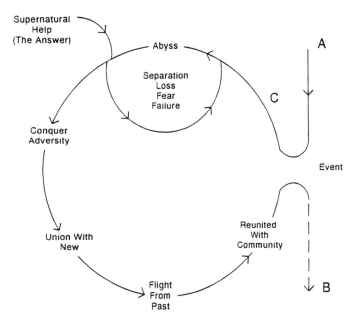

basis for effective action. For the health care provider, this, in turn, brings into question his own identity and effectiveness, widening the gap between himself and his ideals.

American culture is dominated by ideals.[54] Our ideals, our myths, live within the culture, and we, as individuals, inherit and incorporate them as our own. They become "hard-wired" into the nervous system during our development. They serve as reference points from which to interpret what we see and to judge the world in ourselves. We go through life trying to measure up to these ideals. We are also overtly or subliminally confronted with them in our everyday thinking and speaking, advertisements, news stories, novels, TV shows, movies, etc. We live in the gap between where we see ourselves in fact (in action) and where we see ourselves as ideals. It is in this gap that chronic suffering appears.

PROBLEMS AND OPPORTUNITIES FOR CHANGE

Life is a process that involves a dynamic equilibrium between forces for stability that preserve the living organization and forces of change that allow it to adapt and survive.[37]

$$\text{Stability} \longleftrightarrow \text{Change}$$

Since this is an equilibrium, if one side is changed, the other immediately offers resistance. For example, if you tell a chronic pain patient that he or she must change, you immediately get the reasons why change is impossible (forces of stability—in psychology, often referred to as resistance). If you say, "Okay, then stay the way you are," you immediately encounter the reasons why change is imperative (forces of change). The conversation often goes nowhere. It could be a scene from *No Exit*, the play by Sartre—a conversation about hell.

Each person seems to have a "safe or comfort zone." The process of learning is accompanied by the extinguishing of anxiety. Familarity is comfortable; uncertainty is not comfortable to most people. Situations or life-styles that may seem extremely irrational to the health care provider may be the most familiar and the most secure for the chronic pain patient. Despite the obvious benefits of change from the perspective of the health care provider or even the patient at the level of ground observer, change may be resisted because of the anxiety and risk associated with it at the level of pilot. For permanent change to occur, a new familiar or comfort zone must be learned. Such change must occur within the central nervous system at the level of the pilot, at the level of the synapse. However, as we, as health care providers, attempt to introduce change, we have to deal with the ground observer of the chronic pain patient.

The brain of mammals is divided into two halves or hemispheres. Each half receives sensory input from and effects motor control of the

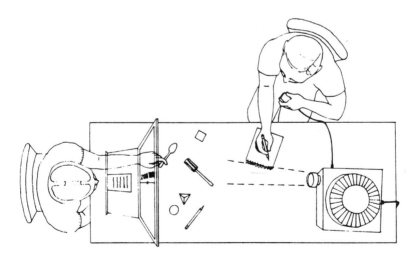

FIGURE 19. The tachistoscope presentation of different stimuli to the right and left hemispheres. The tachistoscope is a device used to present different images very briefly and simultaneously to the right and left sides of a screen while the subject concentrates on the dot in the center. (Reprinted with permission from Gazzaniga MS: The Integrated Mind. New York, Plenum, 1978.)

opposite side of the body. The hemispheres are connected by the corpus callosum. Experimental studies on patients in whom the corpus callosum has been sectioned as part of the treatment of epilepsy have led to some interesting insights into human behavior and logic. For example, consider studies using the tachistoscope (Fig. 19), a device by which different images are very briefly and simultaneously presented to the right and left sides of a screen while the subject concentrates on the dot in the center of the screen. The right half of the brain sees the image on the left side of the screen, whereas the left side of the brain sees the image on the right side. Without the corpus callosum, there is no communication between the hemispheres. Since the right hemisphere is nonverbal in right-hand-dominant people, these studies require the patient to point with the left hand to a picture or an object that matches what the right hemisphere has seen (i.e., the left hand controlled by the right brain matches what the right brain saw in the left visual field). Then the right-hand-dominant person is asked (language would be a left hemispheric function) to give an explanation of what the left hand chose (i.e., the left brain is asked why the right brain did what it did) even though the left hemisphere had no idea what, if anything, the right hemisphere had seen.[27,28,44] In one famous case, the left visual field contained a snowman and trees with snow on them, whereas the right visual field contained a chicken's foot (Fig. 20). The right brain saw the picture of the snow, and the left hand (right brain) picked a shovel. When the right-handed person was asked (i.e., the left hemisphere was asked) why he picked up a shovel, the person responded, "I saw a claw and I picked the chicken, and you have to clean out the chicken shed with the shovel."[28,29] Psychologists have come to refer to this area in the left hemisphere as "the interpreter."[27,29] This area seems to develop logical and rational interpretations for our every behavior. In addition to justifying or interpreting when our shortcomings are brought to light in the presence of others, we often become aggressive or withdrawn. These tendencies, along with the tendency for explanation and justification, are dramatically exhibited in chronic pain patients.

When we are stuck in the abyss, often with no one to point the way out, our society does not have an ancient medicine man or shaman to guide our souls through its trials and tribulations. For many in Western society, the

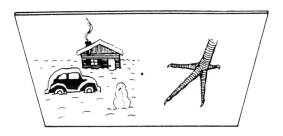

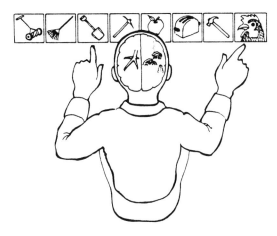

FIGURE 20. "The interpreter." In one famous case, the tachistoscope presented in the left visual field a snowman and trees with snow on them and in the right visual field, a chicken's foot. The right brain saw the picture of snow and the left hand (right brain) picked up a shovel. When the right-handed person was asked (i.e., the left hemisphere asked) why he picked up a shovel, the person responded, "I saw a claw and I picked the chicken and you have to clean out the chicken shed with the shovel." (Reprinted with permission from Gazzaniga MS: The Integrated Mind. New York, Plenum, 1978.)

clergy also can no longer fill this role. "In our society, the doctor is the modern master of the mythological realm, the knower of all the secret ways and words of potency. His role is precisely that of the wise man of the myths and fairy tales whose words assist the hero through the trials and terrors of weird adventure. He is the one who appears and points to the magic shining sword that will kill the dragon—the terror—tells the waiting bride in the castle of the many treasures, applies healing balm to the almost fatal wounds, finally dismisses the conqueror back to the world of normal life, following the great adventure into the enchanted night."[9] The problem is that modern medicine has evolved in such a way that the nonpsychiatrist, indeed even the psychiatrist, does not have time, opportunity, or training to assist such people in their passage. Hence, we again end up in the cynical, hopeless conversation and the dance outlined by Sternbach in what he called the pain game.

The physician, the chronic pain patient, insurers, attorneys, and society as a whole are looking for logical, mechanistic solutions to a problem that our common sense logic does not adequately explain. It is no wonder that many physicians, when faced with chronic pain, feel like Dante on his journey with Virgil as they come to the gates of hell: "Through me, you pass into the city of woe; through me, you pass into eternal pain." If the physician passes with the chronic pain patient into the abyss armed only with surgery and drugs, he has a low probability of transcending the abyss. Many well-intentioned health care providers retreat into their own city of woe, suffering, and burnout.

The theory of reciprocal determinism suggests that thoughts (cognitions), emotions, and behaviors are reciprocally interdetermined.[1]

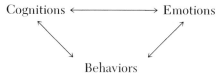

A shift in one is accompanied by changes in the other two. A simple example is the ability of an embarrassing word or statement (cognition) to change body posture, skin color, and body sensations (behavioral and affective responses). The cerebral cortices (cognitive system) is phylogenetically newer than the limbic (affective) system, but they are richly interconnected just as are thoughts and emotions.

Schacter and Singer's cognitive theory of emotional reaction contends that physiological arousal patterns are not in themselves specifically positive or negative phenomena.[58] Rather, they are context dependent. That is, feelings of exhilaration, palpitations, and mild tremulousness while skiing down an advanced ski slope would be cognitively labeled "excitement," whereas the same sensations felt while sitting in a chair doing nothing or walking down a darkened street would be labeled "anxiety" or "apprehension." A minor "discomfort" for a person fully engaged in life and society might be labeled a nuisance but would not result in major impairment. A similar "discomfort" for someone who is withdrawn, depressed, angry, or feeling "wronged" may become the major focus of life and produce what is perceived to be profound limitation. To paraphrase Shakespeare, "Things in life are not inherently upsetting. It is thinking that makes them so."

The human brain continually receives and perceives a myriad of stimuli from both outside and inside the body. These stimuli are processed, filtered, integrated, modified, and interpreted before reaching what we call human awareness or consciousness. What we, as humans, are conscious of is extremely limited compared to the amount of raw stimuli presented to and interpreted by the central nervous system. Only a small portion of these processed stimuli can achieve awareness at any one time. In the chronic pain patient, perceived impairment, pain, automatic conversations about "what if?" and "if only," and the resulting handicaps often totally dominate conscious life.

A major goal of the health care provider is to engage the chronic pain patient in a way that shifts them from their selective attention, generalizations, preoccupations, and errors of logic, all of which perpetuate their suppositions and prejudices. Many have elaborate, convoluted explanations of why they are the way they are and cannot change (the interpreter). All of our "psychotherapeutic" interventions can be viewed in the context of the reciprocal interrelationships between mood, behavior, and thought. We alter moods pharmacologically with antidepressants, neuroleptics, and antianxiety agents. We alter behavior by engaging patients in action within controlled or conditioning environments (behavioral therapy and operant conditioning therapy), and we shift thoughts or beliefs by conversation and relationship (cognitive therapy and psychoanalysis).

The chronic pain patient, from society's view, has an unhealthy equilibrium that is seen as self-perpetuating and self-restrictive. Their past determines how they interpret the present, and the present reinforces the past, in a self-fulfilling cycle. Outcome, as they see it, reinforces their presuppositions, beliefs, and expectations. Chronic pain patients are stuck. The charge to the health care professional who takes on such patients is to alter the equilibrium and get these patients moving again.

The stability side of the change-stability equilibrium shown above is composed of a series of subcomponents that, in turn, are interdependent and in equilibrium.

$$[\text{Change}] \leftrightarrow [(S_1) \leftrightarrow (S_2) \leftrightarrow (S_3) \leftrightarrow (S_N)]$$

In an equilibrium system, a change in one component has the potential to change the entire relationship.[37]

In medicine, we have limited categories of possible action that may potentially introduce a change into the structure and function of the organism[13]:

1. We can introduce change structurally; we call this surgery.

2. We can introduce change chemically; we call this pharmacology or drug therapy.

3. We can introduce change biophysically or biomechanically; we call this physical or occupational therapy, behavior modification, and operant conditioning.

4. We can introduce change linguistically; we call this cognitive therapy or psychiatry.

5. We can do nothing.

By definition, most chronic pain patients have failed surgery, or surgery is not available for them. Most are no longer being helped by analgesics, or they may be dependent upon them, and the dependency may aggravate the pain. Thus, we are usually left with trying to introduce change through experience, either by repetition under controlled conditions (retraining, behavioral modification, operant conditioning) or by generating moments of profound insight or angst (cognitive or insight therapy). Our goal is to introduce change where it will make a difference—at the synaptic level.

As we have seen earlier, the living organization is structurally coupled to the environment. With age, the magnitude of change that can be introduced appears to diminish, but it does not disappear. Lasting change needs to be introduced at the synaptic level, at the level of the pilot. Operant conditioning behavioral modification programs and cognitive behavioral modification programs have evolved as environments to accomplish this.

Behavioral or operant conditioning therapy assumes that physiological disorders represent some combination of biological determinants and learned factors. To the degree that dysfunctional behavior is the product of faulty or inadequate learning, it may be alleviated by applying techniques and principles of learning. For example, patients may be enrolled in graduated exercise programs under controlled settings in order to increase their activity and endurance. Repetition and conditioning are important. Improvements in functional behavior are reinforced while illness behavior is ignored or confronted. Through repetition, synapses undoubtedly change, the map of the territory changes, new behaviors (abilities) appear, and old maladaptive behaviors are extinguished.

Cognitive therapy assumes that symptoms and undesired behaviors are associated with specific underlying assumptions called schemata. Schemata are assumptions, prejudices, presuppositions, or beliefs derived from and based on previous interactions. They are unnoticed or silent rules for interpreting present events with respect to past interactions. A visual example of this is the Ames distorted room (Fig. 11). Our presupposition that rooms are rectangular causes us to experience the size of the people, not the shape of the room, as odd. Cognitive therapy holds that by careful observation, the therapist (facilitator, leader, or other) can become aware of what underlying schemata and assumptions are presenting problems for the patient.

Chronic pain patients appear to struggle with a variety, but a finite number, of issues. With time and experience, the therapist or other health care provider can become familiar with the maps and territories in which these patients struggle. As a culture of human beings, we bring forth our maps from which we coordinate our actions through our speaking and our behavior. Our judgments, biases, opinions, and assessments are reflections of our constructs (our maps) of the territory on the map. The nervous system is a differential system; that is, it is a difference detector. We perceive changes in what we are aware of as opposed to something else. For example, hot and cold are opposite points in the domain (territory) of temperature. Similarly, light versus dark is a map in the dimension of luminescence. By speaking and expressing our opinions, we declare our maps. Consider how chronic pain patients give their history. One patient may say, "They did this test, they did that operation, and they told me I had to . . ." Another person may say, "I told them I wanted this test, but I should not have let them do that operation. . . . I should have . . ." Each is revealing his or her map of a portion of the territory we call control. The first patient points to a map with an external locus of control (i.e., control is something outside the patient), whereas the second is likely constructing a map with an internal locus of control. Similarly, as we speak of our wants, desires, triumphants, disappointments, we do so with reference to (and we reveal) our ideals (myths) of how "it should be."

Cognitive therapy holds that therapists can develop an awareness in patients (overtly or covertly), through the process of reflection, of the impairments their maps produce for them.

The therapist can also engage the patient in dialogues or actions where the constructs of their maps fail to work, break down, and allow new constructs to be formed. For example, the technique of paradoxical strategy exemplified by the Zen Koan assumes that if the "rational" mind becomes trapped, confused, and inoperative, the "unconscious" mind will bring forth alternative constructs that may be more effective and healthy.[37] Positron emission tomographic scanning (PET scanning allows identification of areas of the brain that are more active as opposed to areas that are less active) indicates that when subjects perform a rote task, such as writing their names, the areas that are most active are posterior to the frontal lobes of the brain, in the motor and sensory cortex. When the subjects are asked to write creatively, more activity is seen forward in the frontal region. Subjects who are learning to perform new skills also show this initial frontal activity; but, with repetition, the activity shifts to a more posterior position as they become more   adept. Periods that we, as observers, regard as confused—that is, periods when our constructs of the world fail and break down—may be times of vigorous frontal activity and reformatting of our maps of territory. Cognitive theory also holds that such reinterpretation of the underlying beliefs and presuppositions about pain and ability can be associated with shifts in cognitive awareness, emotion, and behavior. Cognitive programs also typically contain positive coping skills designed to increase patients' self-observations, their actions, and their contributions to the problem and their environment.

Cognitively based programs lend themselves to treating large groups of patients and are relatively inexpensive to operate. Behavioral conditioning programs require a higher provider-to-patient ratio and tend to be more expensive. Controlled and uncontrolled studies using cognitive and behavioral therapy techniques in chronic pain report decreases in pain and depression and reduced analgesic use.[15,19,34,35,38,39,48,50,55,57] Operant conditioning behavioral programs have been successful in reducing pain behavior, increasing physical activity, returning patients to employment, and decreasing use of the health care system.[26,55,70,72] Other behavioral techniques, such as progressive relaxation, biofeedback and guided imagery are more successful as part of an overall cognitive or behavioral program than alone.[70,11] Nerve blocks, TENS (transcutaneous electrical neurostimulator) units, and acupuncture therapy all tend to be ineffective in the long term in hardened chronic pain patients unless they are used as part of an overall, multidimensional program.

After completing chronic pain programs, participants report decreases in pain intensity on self-rated pain scales and an overall increase in function.[14] The data shown in Figure 21 as well as those from other studies[50,71] demonstrate a statistically significant decrease in overall self-rated pain intensity. The magnitude of the reduction in pain, however, is relatively small—in the order of a 10–20% reduction. After completing such programs, this population is still reporting pain of an intensity that is slightly more than halfway between no pain at all and either the worst pain they have ever experienced or pain as bad as it could be. The magnitude of improvement on self-reported

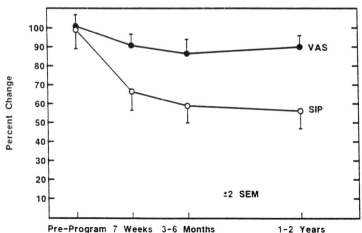

PAIN INTENSITY (VAS) AND DISABILITY (SIP)

FIGURE 21. Initial outcome measures for pain as measured by a visual analog scale (VAS) and illness behavior as measured by the sickness impact profile (SIP). Three separate groups of patients completed each scale before entering an 8-week, cognitive-behavioral, chronic pain management program. The scales were administered during the seventh week of the 8-week program and again at 3–6 months and 1–2 years. Significant changes ($p < 0.05$) were found on both measures. SEM, standard error of the mean.

disability scales is, in contrast, much larger than the reduction in pain. Chronic pain programs, therefore, do not "cure" pain and likewise do not change premorbid personalities. The change is that graduates become more functional. By our training, we are programmed to concentrate on and identify the characteristics of pain. This strategy can be very effective in the diagnosis and treatment of new and acute pain. However, it may be a trap in dealing with chronic pain. These follow-up studies suggest that dramatic improvement in function and behavior can occur without profound changes in chronic pain. Therefore, after the initial diagnostic evaluation of the chronic pain patient, we should shift our focus and conversations away from pain symptoms and concentrate on strategies that increase functional activity and wellness despite the persistence of pain.

This distinction is not well understood by many health care providers. To expect that after a chronic pain program, pain will no longer be a major issue is unrealistic. In populations where litigation is not an issue, such programs seem to pay for themselves.[12] To date, however, controlled data are lacking as to whether such programs are effective in reducing disability and enhancing function in settings where litigation or compensation settlements are pending. My bias is that these programs will be found to be much less effective in settings where disability payments are at issue or when unresolved monetary claims remain.

Patients are often initially reluctant to accept recommendations that they enroll in chronic pain programs. They take this as a sign that the physician is saying, "It is all in your head." It is often easier to get them involved in programs that have biofeedback and relaxation techniques. Patients look at these as being "physical treatment modalities." The conversation as to whether the pain is real is always present, either overtly or covertly, in one form or another in the patient-physician interaction. Chronic pain patients are, at some level, usually fearful that the pain is "all in their head"—that is, imagined and not real. Such cognitions are predicated on the Cartesian duality of mind and body. The pain is always very real for the chronic pain patient who is not an overt malingerer. A conversation between the physician and the patient with chronic hand pain concerning the mind-body duality—the "Is it real or imagined?" dilemma, or whether it hurts in the hand or the head—is like a conversation about the Ames distorted room (Fig. 11). The

physician may try to explain to the patient, "Can't you see that the room cannot be rectangular? One woman is not a giant, and the other is not a midget. It is really the room that is oddly shaped" (i.e., the physician is using a left-brain, logical rationale to suggest that things may not be the way they appear). The patient keeps stating, "The room is rectangular, I can see it is rectangular [spatial organization, right-brain function]; therefore, my pain is really in my hand and not in my head." This is another conversation from *No Exit*.

IDENTIFYING THE CHRONIC PAIN PATIENT

The *first step* in the treatment of chronic pain is to recognize it. Acute pain and acute pain behavior must be distinguished from chronic pain and chronic pain behavior. We in health care have all had experience with patients who come back over and over, demanding relief for the same problems, or those who travel from one health care provider to another over periods of years in search of "the right cure." These patients are fairly easy to recognize. The transition from behavior caused by acute pain to chronic pain behavior, however, may be difficult to recognize initially.

Pain by its nature is a perception and is not observable. It is also not easily quantified. Some investigators dissatisfied with unintelligible nosology of sensory experiences "were sufficiently fascinated by the problem to submit to having their own nerves crushed or cut and resutured in order to observe and describe the sensory experiences during the subsequent stages of reinnovation. Starting in 1905, these experiments were repeated by many in subsequent years. None of these investigators ever agreed with each other, thereby demonstrating it is impossible to convey the contents of a distorted message to the outside observer."[52] Pain behavior, on the other hand, is observable to the health care provider, the employer, and the chronic pain patient's family and peers.

Chronic pain behavior includes behaviors and coping styles that we have all probably employed at some time or other in our lives. Many behaviors in and of themselves are not necessarily abnormal in a qualitative sense. It is more the quantity of the behavior and the persistence in employing it despite its apparent ineffectiveness that is abnormal.

The medical profession as a whole has been slow to identify chronic pain as a specific medical disorder. Only recently have attempts been made to define and categorize essential characteristics of the chronic pain syndrome. In acute pain, particularly that arising from peripheral lesions of skin or viscera, there is relatively good agreement as to the kind of pain that is associated with a specific pathological process. On the other hand, as pain becomes more central, particularly in learned pain, the descriptions become more vague and are reported with more elaborate imagery and dramatization. Although chronic pain patients by no means constitute a homogeneous group and in some instances are difficult to define, we are coming to recognize many common features.

Blumer and Heilbronn[7] strongly argue that pain is a variant of a depressive state. They define what they refer to as a pain-prone disorder. Their comments are based on observations and evaluations of 900 patients with chronic pain of obscure origin. Many had a history of illness behavior. They also had a history of doing well under "physical stress." During such periods, they were likely to function at their best and to be pain free, but they relapsed later as demands on them decreased. Some of these patients described terrible pain in elaborate descriptive terms but presented little or no evidence of concurrent suffering. Indeed, this dramatic quality and the relish with which stories of difficult problems, trials, and tribulations are recounted should alert the physician that the person may be one for whom pain and suffering is a safe and secure way of life. Patients also often recount a history of "multiple physician contacts and many nonproductive diagnostic procedures; excessive preoccupation with the pain problem; and altered behavioral patterns with some of the features of depression, anxiety and neuroticism and, in particular, no realistic plans for the future."[5] Many of these patients seem prone to choose a spouse who turns out to be particularly brutal, alcoholic, promiscuous, or otherwise brings on prolonged suffering. About half of these patients have a history of a next of kin who is crippled or deformed by some injury or disease. An increased incidence of alcoholism and clinical depression in the patients themselves as well as in their relatives has also been noted.[7]

In citing the close relationship between chronic pain and depression, Blumer and others noted sleep disturbances, appetite changes, decreased libido, irritability, withdrawal of interest, weakening of relationships, somatic preoccupations, and other signs of depression.[7,68] Blumer and Heilbronn[7] have argued that the pain-prone disorder is something distinct from other chronic painful states, such as rheumatoid arthritis. They compared what they termed a well-defined somatic disease (rheumatoid arthritis) with chronic pain and cited distinct clinical, psychological, biographic and genetic differences between the patients.

Typically, chronic pain patients present as "solid citizens." They strongly resist any suggestion of and deny any difficulties in their interpersonal relationships. Rather, they often describe their family relationships in idealized, even mythical, terms. They tend to view themselves as independent and not needing help. The ideals they cling to include the need to be independent, the need to be active, and the need to care for others, whereas, in practice, their behaviors show them as dependent, passive, and needing to be cared for. They are, in other words, in the abyss or gap between their cultural ideals on the one hand and their actual behaviors on the other.

Blumer et al. built on contributions of Engle and proposed clinical features for the chronic pain disorder (Table 3). The clinical features of the pain-prone disorder include reports that pain is continuous and a lifestyle of preoccupation with bodily pain. The pain is often viewed as the only problem in life; if only the pain were resolved, things would be great. They

TABLE 3. Clinical Features of the Pain-Prone Disorder as Described by Blumer and Heilbronn[7]

Somatic Complaint
   Continuous pain of obscure origin
   Hypochondriacal preoccupation
   Desire for surgery
Self-image of "solid citizen"
   Denial of conflicts
   Idealization of self and family relations
Ergomania (prepain)
   "Workaholism"
   Relentless activity
Depression anergia (postpain)
   Lack of initiative
   Inactivity
   Fatigue
   Alexithymia: inability to appreciate and verbalize feelings
   Anhedonia: inability to enjoy social life, leisure, and sex
   Insomnia
   Depressive mood and despair
History
   Family (and personal) history of depression and alcohol and drug abuse
   Past abuse by spouse
   Crippled relative
   Relative with chronic pain

have a need to idealize their spouse (often after having suffered abuse in a previous marriage). Before the onset of pain, they often exhibit relentless work habits (ergomania and workaholism). Following the onset of chronic pain, they exhibit signs of a depressive state with a past history and family history of overt depressive episodes.

An appendix to the third edition of *Guides to the Evaluation of Permanent Impairments*[20] suggests that a chronic pain disorder should be considered when two or more of the following characteristics (the six Ds) are seen:

1. **Duration.**   Pain persists and progresses long after tissue damage should be expected to have healed; disability persists long after the impairments should have resolved. In the past, chronic pain syndrome was reserved for pain greater than 6 months in duration; however, now it is recognized that chronic pain syndrome can be diagnosed as early as 2–4 weeks after onset, particularly in the patient with the premorbid history.

2. **Dramatization.**   These patients use emotionally charged words to describe pain and suffering. They exhibit exaggerated histrionic behavior, including theatrical display of pain with moaning and groaning.

3. **Drugs.**   Substance abuse in the form of prescription drugs or alcohol is a flagrant stigma of chronic pain.

4. **Despair.**   Chronic pain results in a major emotional upheaval. The four manifestations include depression, apprehension, irritability, and hostility. These patients become embittered, defensive, and rigid.

5. **Disuse.**   Pain of musculoskeletal origin frequently results in prolonged and excessive immobilization. Such immobilization can be associated with secondary reaction to pain or with acquired pain occurring with attempts to resume normal activities. Such attempts further aggravate and perpetuate the chronic pain cycle.

6. **Dysfunction.**   Chronic pain patients tend to withdraw from the fabric of society. They disengage from work activities and recreation, and they tend to alienate friends and family.

The *second step* in the treatment of the chronic pain patient is to distinguish which type of chronic pain patient is at hand. A framework is needed that is descriptive and operative in nature and allows strategies and actions to be constructed from it, rather than one that is steeped in hypothesis and explanatory principles.

I have found the framework described by Gildenberg and DeVaul in their monograph on chronic pain patients to be helpful.[30] They divide patients who take on a sick role as a lifestyle into four categories:

The Overwhelmed Patient.   These patients develop a chronic pain response to overwhelming problems. They have a past history of responding to major stresses by escape or withdrawal. Injury and illness allow them to escape their adult responsibilities. Their explicit behaviors are rewarded usually by time off or disability payments. These rewards reinforce the illness behavior. Gildenberg and DeVaul estimate that 70% of the patients they see in their chronic pain clinic fall into this category.

The Need-to-Suffer Patient.   These patients often have a long history of unsuccessful and disappointing experiences. They relate long histories of suffering in anguishing terms and dwell in the past. Gildenberg and DeVaul estimate that these patients make up 20% of their clinic population.

The Assigned Patient.   These patients, about 5% of Gildenberg and DeVaul's population, become chronic pain patients because they believe that is what is expected of them. From their perspective, they are following what the physician or other health care provider has prescribed for them. (As physicians, we must come to realize that we not only prescribe medications, but we can also prescribe "diseases" and "disabilities.")

The Psychogenic Patient.   In these patients, approximately 5% of Gildenberg and DeVaul's population, pain is a symptom of an underlying psychiatric disorder. They are further divided into the following categories:

1. Pain as a symptom of depression
2. Pain as a symptom of anxiety
3. Pain as a symptom of hysterical or conversion reaction
4. Pain as a symptom of unresolved grief
5. Pain as a delusional symptom of psychosis

EVALUATION AND TREATMENT OF CHRONIC PAIN

Initial Evaluation.   The first step in the treatment of a chronic pain disorder is an adequate initial evaluation to ensure that previous diagnoses are appropriate and that conventional treatment interventions that have a *high probability* (not an outside possibility) of success have been adequately explored. In chronic pain centers in tertiary medical facilities, it is estimated that fewer than 5% of chronic pain patients seen have a disorder that is readily treated surgically. During the initial evaluation, particularly in occupation-related disorders, it is important to distinguish among impairment, disability, handicap, employability, and disability from work. Impairment, disability, and handicap are defined in Table 2. Employability is a function of job demands, conditions of industry, and the employer. The employer looks not only at the worker's capability of performing a task, but also at the risk of further loss or liability as a result of taking back an injured worker. Employability includes medical status, capacity to perform, capacity to travel to and from work, and capacity to be at work.

If an injured worker can travel to and from therapy, he is probably capable of traveling to and from work. Most injured workers have the capacity to do some kind of work, although they may not be able to do the work they previously did. The issues of employability and disability from work, then, often come down to: (1) what the person is capable of (performance capacity); (2) cost to the employer; and (3) risk to the employer. Performance capability is really the ability to complete defined tasks. The employer has to decide whether to pay the person for performing some task at work that he can do—that is, whether to modify the job or to pay the worker not to work. Employability, therefore, is decided more by the employer or by industry in general than by the physician.

A Shift in Perspective. When the initial evaluation is complete and it is clear that the patient has a chronic pain syndrome, the next, and often most difficult, step is to give up the role of healer. Mr. Fix-It, who continues to search for logical, mechanistic solutions for the hard-core, chronic pain patient remains stuck in the pain game, in a conversation around the mind-body duality, in the abyss. The physician needs to stop playing healer, who focuses on a section or part of the body, and begin playing rehabilitator, who takes into account the whole person and the social environment. Questions such as, "Why does this person have pain?" "What causes the pain?" and, "What can I do to relieve the pain?" need to be replaced by questions on the order of, "What are the patient's impairments?" and, "What can be done to reduce the disability and impairment?"

Acute versus Chronic Pain. It is important to draw contrasts for these patients between acute and chronic pain. Chronic pain does not necessarily involve continued tissue injury. Analgesics that may work in acute pain do not work in chronic pain. Chronic pain patients need to come to learn that in chronic pain, unlike acute pain, "Hurt does not equal harm." Treatment options available for chronic pain and the evidence for what works and what does not work should be presented. I discuss the gate theory of pain control with the patient and suggest that a number of factors that may seem totally unrelated to pain may open or close the gate—that is, increase or decrease pain. The current popular approach, borrowed from such tribal ritual as walking barefoot across hot cinders, demonstrates that the brain can alter pain perception and local responses to pain.

Drugs. Most pain centers report that one of the most effective actions that can be taken is to withdraw sedatives, hypnotics, and narcotics from chronic pain patients. Such agents work in acute pain for a short time, but they do not work in chronic pain. What happens is that when the patient hurts, he or she takes the drug. The concentration of the drug rises temporarily and then begins to fall. As the concentration falls, receptors are "unblocked," the pain accentuates, and more medication is needed. Some patients go through recurrent "mini-withdrawals." The risk-benefit ratio for narcotics in chronic pain is such that, with very few exceptions, these agents should not be used in its management. For example, narcotics should never be prescribed for chronic, recurrent, or continuous headaches.

Narcotic analgesics are initially prescribed in acute pain to suppress or block the input of the sensory afferent system. Although initially they may be effective, tolerance develops with time. Potential benefits of narcotics for chronic pain patients include dulling awareness, blunting the automatic conversations about chronic pain, and altering mood—that is, using the analgesics to affect cognitive-evaluative and motivational-affective components of pain. Blumer and Heilbronn[7] suggest a role for antidepressants in the treatment of chronic pain states. If medication is to be used, anti-inflammatory agents and antidepressants should be used in place of analgesic tranquilizers or other narcotic analgesics. Acutely sedating antidepressants given at night may help these patients sleep. In 3–6 weeks, some also experience anti-depressive effects as a change in mood. My experience, however, is that these benefits are short term unless the drug therapy is accompanied by other modalities that affect the patient's map of the territory and style of coping with life problems.

Listen for the Hidden Agenda. Attempt to elicit the patient's hidden agenda and expectations. Many elderly patients with chronic pain fear that an underlying cancer has not been detected. What is the occupational pain patient's problem at work? Job satisfaction correlates with the rate of return of the injured worker to work.[63] Motivation is an important factor. Professional athletes frequently play with injuries that would be serious handicaps to the average worker. Workers whose disability payments approach their full-time pay are more reluctant to return to work than workers who are paid for productivity, as in piecework, in which disability payments or light-duty earnings do not approach the usual salary. The issues of compensation and litigation are ever present in the injured chronic pain patient, particularly the worker.

Is This Person Ready to Change? To my eye, the population of chronic pain patients includes some who are ready to give up their illness role. These patients need a socially accepted vehicle for "getting well." Some are not sure if they are ready to change or not. They may sustain benefits from a chronic pain program. Some chronic pain patients are definitely not ready to change. This is not to say that any chronic pain patient does not have the capacity to change. Every human being has the biological capacity to change behavior. However, not every human being is sufficiently motivated to change, sufficiently willing to commit to the actions necessary for change, or willing to take the risk that change may entail.

When, from the chronic pain patient's perspective, things get "bad enough," a willingness to change may develop. By "bad" I refer, not to the patient's description of the pain, but to what is happening in the social support network. When the social support system begins to collapse and no longer supports the illness behavior, the benefits and secondary gains begin to disappear, the patient becomes uncomfortable and may be open to the possibility of change. Listening to these patients express themselves often reveals the map they have painted of the territory, where they see themselves within the map, and what possibilities for change exist within the territory. When the entire conversation is one opinion after another, without any intention or expression of commitment, and the patient refuses direct requests to commit to some action, it is unlikely that the patient is ready for change. The person who continually expresses likes and dislikes, wants, desires, and so forth is not committing to any action. On the other hand, the person who states, "Yes, I will begin walking 10 minutes a day beginning tomorrow and by the end of the month I will be walking 30 minutes a day," is committing to a specific action by a specific time to reach a specific goal (a promise). In speaking, the person is shaping how the future will unfold.

Early on in relationships with chronic pain patients, I develop a simple agreement that requires them to take some form of action. My goal is to give them an opportunity to break out of their chronic patterns by committing themselves to some action for change. Those who declare themselves ready for possible change through such actions are those I am willing to make a commitment to work with.

Rehabilitation Contract. The time and energy required in dealing with these patients is such that the busy medical or surgical physician cannot manage them alone. Some form of rehabilitation program needs to be designed, whether it involves a hand therapist, an occupational therapist, or a comprehensive multidimensional pain program. It is important to spell out to the patient what the goals and expectations are and what the treating professional's role is. Rehabilitation programs should focus on active therapies, not passive modalities.

Why a Contract? A contract is a promise one party makes to another to perform specific actions to accomplish defined goals by a set time. The specific conditions that need to be met to satisfy the contract are spelled out. When chronic pain patients present themselves for medical care, they arrive in a historical perspective that includes the expectation that the physician or health care provider will take care of their entire problem and meet all their needs. Such expectations are open-ended and unlimited. Commonly, chronic pain patients expect the provider to "fix" them. In our technology-oriented society, people have come to believe that almost anything can be done surgically or pharmacologically. A patient may ask, "If you can put a new heart in someone, why can't you stop my pain?" However, by definition, patients with chronic pain are people for whom there are no further surgical procedures or conventional treatment interventions. A contract that spells out their responsibility often helps them to confront the reality of their situation and to resign themselves to the lack of a magical fix. As noted earlier, the breakdown that occurs around chronic pain is usually a breakdown between society's expectation and the individual's performance. A contract is one way to make explicit what is implicit in society—that society functions through coordinated actions and mutual promises and requests.

The contract commits the patient to specific actions. The essence of the contract is a commitment to actions that have a probability of narrowing the gap between what the patient is doing or not doing and what the patient needs to do or not do to achieve agreed-upon goals. The contract also defines the health care provider's role. If no progress is made, the health care provider can look back at the contract and assess whether patient and provider have fulfilled their commitments. The contract thus provides an alternative to the open-ended, unlimited expectations of the patients as a means of judging the effectiveness of therapy. Such a process is important to the health care professional's sanity and well-being. Everyone's dance with life is filled with expectations, ideals, and fantasies, and the health care provider also has an "interpreter" complete with presuppositions, explanations, and biases.

Commit to Actions, Accept the Results. Learn to distinguish between actions and the results they produce. Focus on specific actions and accept the results. This has been a difficult distinction for me to make during my initial endeavors in chronic pain. Health care providers who persist in demanding results that conform to their own expectations, biases, value systems, and ideals are setting themselves up for frustration and burnout. You can promise a specific action that is highly probable to produce a result in the direction of the desired goal. But what actually happens next as a result of the action is a function of the chronic pain patient's structure and functional organization. For example, consider the simple action of flicking the switch of a television set. What determines what happens next? Is it the structure and function of your finger? Is it how you turn the switch on? Or is it the structure and function of the television set?

Content of Contract. The contract should spell out specific goals, specific actions required to achieve them, a specific time table, and the conditions that need to be achieved for satisfying the contract. Not uncommonly, with chronic pain patients, the contract needs to be renegotiated from time to time in order to keep it relevant to where the patient is. Contracts should specifically address the issues of drugs, exercises, nutrition, and commitment to participate in either individual therapy programs or a comprehensive multidimensional pain program.

CONCLUSION

A traditional Western technological approach designed to intervene at the level of the individual as a separate and independent entity does not work in the case of chronic pain. Our "optical delusion" of objective and subjective realities and our illusion that we are separate as individuals from the world and society are handicaps to our effectiveness in interacting with chronic pain. Our current strategies are designed to attack the problem at the level of the individual, to induce change by altering intracellular and intercellular homeostatic mechanisms. Chronic pain, however, is a disorder not just of an individual organism, but a disorder that appears in the coordination of human interactions and individual responsibilities within our social networks.

Chronic pain does not exist solely within the body of the affected individual. The disorder appears within the social network and fabric of our society. It is not solely a disorder of anatomy and physiology but rather is a discourse of our culture. Chronic pain and suffering are endemic in our society. Social programs and cultural environments often reinforce them. The best treatment of the chronic pain patient is likely to prove to be anticipation and prevention of the pain through social interactions. A recent study suggests that being clear and direct about the nature of the injury, prescribing a duration for recovery, defining expectations up front, and prescribing medications for a finite number of days results in better long-term outcome and less disability than most of the traditional haphazard treatments.[25] Training more specialists will not reduce the incidence of chronic pain. This primary health care provider needs a new understanding and effective means of action. This physician is often the initial treating physician for chronic pain patients and is, in any case, the physician who treats their other acute and chronic medical problems. Whether they complete a chronic pain program or not, these patients often need constant attention and reassurance. I specifically recall a patient who had not worked in several years and who, during the chronic pain program, quit a two-pack-a-day cigarette habit and began exercising on a regular basis. This patient wanted to return to some form of employment, but his physical impairments precluded a return to his former trade. On a visit to his regular physician, the patient expressed his desire for employment. The physician appropriately, I thought, recommended job retraining through various local and state agencies. The patient pursued retraining, only to return frustrated by the bureaucracy and reporting that his pain was increased and he was getting nowhere. At this point, the primary care physician again prescribed a synthetic narcotic, and the two returned to the abyss.

Wall, in his introduction to a major textbook on pain, pointed out, "Our concepts of pain are changing."[73] The old concept that pain is the result of a single, isolated sensory system of afferent and central cells is dead. We now recognize that the afferent signal passes through gated controls, which are influenced by peripheral events as well as by the sensory posture of the central nervous system at the time. We also appreciate that the central connections are not rigid but change with time. "Pain is now coming to be considered one of the many modes of behavior exhibited by a single sensory-emotional-behavioral system of the living organism we call the human being."[73] Although we are unable to measure the afferent sensory component of the pain process, we are able to observe its behavioral consequences. Chronic pain is beginning to be associated with an abnormal output rather than just with an abnormal sensory input. As Wall has suggested, pain may be better classed with bodily sensations such as hunger and thirst, which are need states associated as much with imperative for action as with the need to modify the stimulus.[73] Instead of trying to fix the problem by cutting, adding a gadget, or giving a drug, we are beginning to ask what is missing to fulfill the need? What specific action or actions are required to get this patient moving in the desired direction?

The chronic pain problem is an interesting and fascinating one that is unlikely to disappear in the near term. Wilbert Fordyce, who has written and published extensively on chronic pain and suffering, recently ended a review of the subject with the following statements: "Pain behaviors are interesting social communications (the meaning of which remains to be discovered in the individual case)" and, "People who have something better to do don't suffer much."[24] The patients are their own Rosetta stones.

Parts of this chapter are metaphorical, and parts are descriptive. For example, the colored shadows illustration (Figs. 4 and 5) and Beham's wheel (Fig. 6) are included to provoke the reader to question some everyday, commonsense ways of "seeing" (perceiving) the world and ourselves. The issue is not whether the tree is really green or how it is that we see green. Both of these questions miss the direction to which our paradoxical experiences and metaphorical perceptions point. Understanding that "our experience is moored in our structure in a binding way"[44] and that our structure is, by its nature, recursive and self-referential, makes such questions as, "What color is it really?" illogical.

Within the limits of the environment and the capacities of our structure and organization, we continually invent a world complete with joys and pains. However, the points of reference we use to define a human order out of a "natural" chaos of the universe are not our own. We have inherited them from our culture. The basic tenets of our presuppositions, our biases, our values, and our ideals existed before we appeared. We inherit and incorporate them during our "formative years." They are embodied in the structure of and they affect the functional organization of the nervous system.

With the incorporation and use of language, self-awareness and self-consciousness appear.[43] With self-awareness appear narratives. Our self-narratives, the narratives of the interpreter, the ground observer, explain what we did or did not do (and why) in the past, what we can or cannot do in the present, and what we will or will not do in the future. These stories and explanations, however, are already based on our presuppositions and biases. Not only that. These linguistic events occur within and affect the structure and function of the nervous system in which they arise. They affect how we view the past and the present and how we anticipate the future. They affect our moods and our emotions. Current speculation is that they also can affect the structure and function of our immune system, and thus our very health and well-being. In our ordinary, everyday cultural way of being, we do not see this.

As health care providers we have learned that we have a blind spot in our field of vision. "How come we don't go around with a hole that size all the time in our field of vision? Our visual experience is of continuous space. The fascinating thing about the blind spot is that we do not see that we do not see [in it]."[44]

The profoundness of many of these self-referential relationships is often very hard to hear. It contains a death knell for the ego, which, with its constructs of the world, is revealed as a house of cards. Furthermore, exploring this circularity gives us a dizzy sensation; "we are using the instrument of analysis to analyze the instrument of analysis."[44]

A major goal of this chapter has been to prompt the reader to question underlying presuppositions upon which understandings of chronic pain are based. The chapter does not, however, succinctly put into language a new paradigm with reference points to replace the old. We as a culture and medical tradition are only beginning to address this need; it is a task for the future.

Earlier in this chapter, the metaphor of the pilot and the ground observer was used to point out different aspects of knowing and awareness. It is important to understand that they are not separate beings. Rather, they point to different aspects of the same process. In the final analysis, there is no pilot, no ground observer, no doer of the deed; there is only the process.

Acknowledgments

I thank the many friends, teachers, colleagues, and patients who have contributed to my experience in the realm of chronic pain and suffering, and in medicine in general. I especially thank Dr. Ephraim Roseman, who generously funded the study that provided the data in Figure 21. As I think of him now, my thoughts (these words) are associated with sadness (an emotion with bodily feelings). He recently died after a long illness. Not only did "Rosey" literally see the world different from most of us because he was blind to color, he articulated and demonstrated very clearly many aspects of chronic pain and chronic pain behavior that only years later I hear and see.

REFERENCES

1. Austin JL: How To Do Things with Words. Cambridge, Harvard University Press, 1984.
2. Bandura A: The self-system in reciprocal determinism. Am Psychol 33:344, 1978.
3. Bergner M, Bobbitt RA, Pollard WE, et al: The sickness impact profile: Validation of a health status measure. Med Care 14:57–67, 1976.
4. Berna SF, Chapman SL: Pain and litigation. In Wall PD, Melzack R (eds): Textbook of Pain. New York, Churchill Livingstone, 1984, p. 832.
5. Black RG: The chronic pain syndrome. Surg Clin North Am 55:999, 1975.
6. Bloom FE, Lazerson A: Brain, Mind and Behavior. New York, W. H. Freeman, 1988.
7. Blumer D, Heilbronn M: Chronic pain as a variant of depressive disease. J Nerv Ment Dis 170:381, 1972.
8. Bonica JJ: The Management of Pain. Philadelphia, Lea & Febiger, 1953, p 1533.
9. Campbell, J: The Hero with a Thousand Faces. Princeton, NJ, Princeton Univerity Press, 1968.
10. Casey KL, Melzack R: Neural mechanisms of pain: A conceptual model. In Way E, Leon G (eds): New Conceptions of Pain and Its Clinical Management. Philadelphia, F. A. Davis, 1967, pp 13–31.
11. Changeux JP, Danchin A: Selective stabilization of developing synapses as a mechanism for the specification of neural networks. Nature 264:705, 1976.
12. Chaplin E, McCarberg W, Adams J: Southern California Permanente Medical Group, San Diego. Data Collection supported by The Ephraim Roseman Foundation.
13. Chaplin, ER: Chronic pain: A difficult problem. Occup Med 4:483, 1989.
14. Chaplin ER, Kasdan ML: Occupational neurology and the hand. Hand Clin 2:513–529, 1986.
15. Chappell MN, Stevinson TI: Group psychological training in some organic conditions. Mental Hygiene 20:588, 1963.
16. Crick F: Do dendritic spines twitch? Trends Neurosci 44–46, Feb 1982.
17. Dallenbach KM: History and present status. Am J Psychol 52:331, 1931.
18. Dorsey L: Space, Time and Medicine. Boston, Shimbhala, New Science Library, 1985.
19. Draspa LJ: Psychological factors in muscular pain. Br J Med Psychol 32:106, 1959.
20. Engelberg AL (ed): Guides to the Evaluation of Permanent Impairment, 3rd ed. Chicago, IL, American Medical Association, 1988.
21. Engle GL: "Psychogenic" pain and the pain-prone patient. Am J Med 26:899, 1951.
22. Finch DR, MacDougal M, Tibbs DJ, Morris PJ: Amputation for vascular disease: The experience of a peripheral vascular unit. Br J Surg 67:233, 1980.
23. Flores CF: Management and Communications in the Office of the Future. San Francisco, Hermenaz, 1982.
24. Fordyce WE: Pain and suffering: A reappraisal. Am Psychol 43:276, 1988.
25. Fordyce WE, Brockway JA, Bergman JA, Spencer D: Acute back pain: A control-group comparison of behavioral versus traditional management methods. J Behav Med 9:127, 1986.
26. Fordyce WE, Shelton JL, Dundore DE: The modification of avoidance-learning pain behaviors. J Behav Med 5:405, 1982.

27. Gazzaniga M: Fires of the Mind: The Infinite Voyage. Kent, OH, PTV Publications, 1988.
28. Gazzaniga MS: The Integrated Mind. New York, Plenum, 1978.
29. Gazzaniga MS: The Bisected Brain. New York, Appleton-Century Crofts, 1980.
30. Gildenberg PL, DeVaul RA: The Chronic Pain Patient. In Gildenberg PL, DeVaul RA (eds): Pain and Headache, Vol 7. New York, Karger, 1985.
31. Gregory RL: Eye and Brain: The Psychology of Seeing. New York, McGraw-Hill, 1966.
32. Harris L, et al: The Nuprin Pain Report. New York, 1985.
33. Holuryd KA, Androsik F: Coping and self-control of chronic tension headache. J Consult Clin Psychol 46:1036, 1928.
34. Holuryd KA, Androsik F, Westbrook T: Cognitive control of tension headache. Cogn Ther Res 1:21, 1977.
35. Hubel DH, LeVay S, Wiesel TN: The development of ocular dominance columns in normal and visually deprived monkeys. J Comp Neurol 191:1, 1980.
36. Huttenlocher PR: Synaptic density in human frontal cortex: Developmental changes and effects of aging. Brain Res 163:195, 1979.
37. Keeney BP: Aesthetics of Change. New York, Gilford, 1983.
38. Khatami M, Rush AJ: A pilot study of the treatment of outpatients with chronic pain: Symptom control, stimulus control and social system intervention. Pain 5:163, 1978.
39. Khatami M, Rush AJ: A one-year followup of the multimodal treatment for chronic pain. Pain 14:45, 1982.
40. Land E: The retinex theory of color vision. Sci Am 237:108, 1977.
41. Lee KS, Schottler F, Oliver M, Lynch G: Brief bursts of high-frequency stimulation produce two types of structural change in rat hippocampus. J Neurophysiol 44:247, 1980.
42. Livingston M, Hubel D: Segregation of form, color, movement and depth. Anat Physiol Percept Sci 240:740, 1988.
43. Manturana HR, Varela FJ: Autopoiesis and Cognition. Boston Studies in Philosophy of Science, Vol 42. Boston, Reidel, 1972.
44. Manturana HR, Varela FJ: The Tree of Knowledge. Boston, Shambhala, New Science Library, 1988.
45. Melzack R, Casey KL: Sensory, motivational and central control determinants of pain: A new conceptual model. In Densholo D (ed): The Skin Senses. Springfield, IL, C. C Thomas, 1968, p 427.
46. Melzack R, Wall PD: Pain mechanism: A new theory. Science 150:971, 1965.
47. Merskey H: Classification of chronic pain. Pain 3(suppl):215, 1986.
48. Mitchel KR, White DG: Behavioral self-management: An application to the problem of migraine headaches. Behav Ther 8:213, 1977.
49. Morgan C, Director, Pain Program, Scripps Memorial Hospital, La Jolla, CA: Personal communication.
50. Moore JE, Cheney EF: Outpatient group treatment of chronic pain: Effects of spouse involvement. J Consult Clin Psychol 53:326, 1985.
51. Nass MN, Copper: A theory for the development of feature detecting cells in visual cortex. Biol Cybern 1:275, 1975.
52. Noordenbos: In Wall PD, Melzack P (eds): Textbook of Pain. New York, Churchill Livingstone, 1984.
53. Ostarweis M, Kleinman A, Mechanic D (eds): Pain and Disability Institute of Medicine Committee on Pain, Disability and Chronic Illness Behavior. Washington, National Academy Press, 1987.
54. Reich R: Tales of a New America. New York, Random House, 1987.
55. Roberts A, Reinhardt L: The behavioral management of chronic pain: Long-term followup with comparison groups. Pain 8:151, 1980.
56. Rowe ML: Low back pain industry: A position paper. J Occup Med 11:116, 1969.
57. Sachs LB, Feverstein M, Vitale JH: Hypnotic self-regulation of chronic pain. Am J Clin Hypn 20:106, 1977.
58. Schacter S, Singer J: Cognitive, social and psychological determinants of emotional state. Psychol Rev 60:379, 1962.
59. Scheffer CB, Donlon PT, Bittle RM: Chronic pain and depression. Am J Psychiatry 137:118, 1980.
60. Schrodinger E: The Mystery of the Sensual Qualities in What Is Life, Mind and Matter. Cambridge, UK, Cambridge University Press, 1967.
61. Searle JR: Speech Acts. Cambridge, UK, Cambridge University Press, 1969.
62. Searle JR: A taxonomy of illocutionary acts in language, mind and knowledge. In Dunderson K (ed): Minneapolis, University of Minnesota, 1975.
63. Sevensson HO, Anderson GB: Low back pain in forty-to forty-seven-year-old men: Work history and work experience factors. Spine 8:272, 1983.
64. Spinelli DH, Jensen EF: Plasticity: The mirror of experience. Science 203:75, 1979.
65. Spinelli DH, Jensen EF, Dipresco: Early experience effect on dendritic branching in normally reared kittens. Neurology 62:1, 1980.
66. Spitzer WO, et al: Rapport du Groupe de Travail Quebecois sur les aspects cliniques des affections vertebrales chez les travaillieurs. L'Institut de Recherche en Santé et en Securité du Travel du Quebec, February 1986.
67. Sternbach RA: Pain Patients: Traits and Treatments. New York, Academic Press, 1974.
68. Sternbach RA: The psychology of pain. New York, Raven, 1978.
69. Turk D: Cognitive behavioral techniques in the management of pain. In Foret J (ed): Cognitive Behavior Therapy: Research and Application. New York, Plenum, 1978.
70. Turk D, Flor H: Etiological theories and treatments for chronic back pain. II. Psychological models and interventions. Pain 19:208, 1984.
71. Turner JA: Comparison of group progressive-relaxation training and cognitive behavioral group therapy for chronic low back pain. J Consult Clin Psychol 50:757, 1982.
72. Turner JA, Chapman CR: Psychological interventions for chronic pain: A critical review. II. Operant conditioning hypnosis and cognitive behavioral therapy. Pain 12:23, 1982.
73. Wall PD: Introduction. In Wall PD, Melzack P (eds): Textbook of Pain. New York, Churchill Livingstone, 1984.
74. Winegrad T, Flores CF: Understanding Computers and Cognition. New Jersey, Ablex, 1986.
75. Woolsey TA, Wann JR: Area changes in mouse cortical barrels following vibrissal damage at different postnatal ages. J Comp Neurol 170:53, 1976.

Chapter 3

PREVENTION OF OCCUPATIONAL HAND INJURIES

Sidney J. Blair, M.D., F.A.C.S.

This chapter discusses the incidence and the prevention of occupational injuries of the upper extremity. Some statistics on disabling work injuries in the United States are presented in Tables 1 and 2. Both tables are from *Accident Facts* published by the National Safety Council.[2] Table 1 shows that about a third of disabling work injuries are related to the upper extremity but that injuries to this bodily area have decreased over the last 8 years. Statistics gathered from the presidents of hand societies throughout the world confirm this finding.[5]

With this brief statement about incidence, I should mention the present regulating mechanism in the U.S. that deals with safety in the workplace. In 1970, Congress passed the Occupational Safety and Health Act with the purpose "to assure so far as possible every working man and woman in the nation safe and healthful working conditions, and to preserve our human resources." The Occupational Safety and Health Administration (OSHA) was established within the Department of Labor to encourage employers and employees to attempt to reduce hazards in the workplace, to initiate and implement safety and health programs, and to develop and enforce job safety health standards. OSHA also establishes reporting and record-keeping procedures to monitor job-related injuries and illnesses and inspects workplaces for violation of health and safety standards. Its duties range from enforcement to implementation to the development of standards.

The National Institute for Occupational Safety and Health (NIOSH) was also established under the OSHA Act. It is part of the Department of Health and Human Services and the Centers for Disease Control of the United States Public Health Service. This agency investigates health and safety standards in various workplaces upon request. It identifies and evaluates hazards and recommends procedures for prevention and control. NIOSH develops criteria and prepares reports. These are sent to the Department of Labor and OSHA then sets standards.

In 1983 NIOSH published the following list of 10 leading work-related diseases and injuries:

1. occupational lung disease
2. musculoskeletal trauma
3. occupational cancers
4. severe occupational traumatic injuries
5. occupational cardiovascular diseases
6. diseases of reproduction
7. neurotoxic disorders
8. noise-induced hearing loss
9. dermatological conditions
10. psychological disorders

Hand injuries, which mainly fall in items 2 and 4 above, account for a larger number of days lost from work than any other kind of occupational injury. Days lost mean money lost: wages, medical expenses, insurance administration, and fire loss. Table 2 shows an increase in the annual cost of hand injuries from $32.5 billion in 1981 to $42.4 billion in 1987. The total cost of arm, hand, and finger injuries constitutes about 20% of all the compensation costs of all injuries.

47

TABLE 1.   Disabling Work Injuries

Year	Total Injuries	Arms	Hands	Fingers	Total Upper Extremity
1979	2,300,000	210,000	160,000	340,000	710,000
1982	1,900,000	170,000	130,000	280,000	580,000
1985	2,000,000	180,000	100,000	280,000	560,000
1986	1,800,000	160,000	90,000	250,000	500,000
1987	1,800,000	180,000	90,000	230,000	500,000

Reprinted with permission from Accident Facts. Chicago, National Safety Council, 1989.

The occupational physician needs to be aware of the classification system for work accidents that was recommended and has been adopted by workers' compensation boards in many states. The system depends on the events that caused the injury. This classification of injuries includes:

1. struck by object
2. overexertion
3. fall from elevation
4. fall from the same level
5. caught in, under, or between
6. motor vehicle accidents
7. other causes

One of the more important injuries is that classified as "caught in, under, or between." Such injuries cause crushing, squeezing, or pinching of the body part between two moving objects. This type of injury is associated with power press and metal-stamping machines and is one of the more distressful injuries seen in hospital emergency rooms.

Thomas Anton in his book, *Occupational Safety and Health Management*, describes three essentials for accident prevention programs[3]:

1. leadership by the employer
2. safe and healthful working conditions
3. safe work practices by employees

If these three essentials are missing, he says, accidents on the job are likely to occur. The results are increased damage to property, loss of production, increased expenditure of insurance and compensation, and other costs.

A company with one of the best safety records in the U.S. is the E.I. duPont de Nemours and Company. The duPont safety philosophy is the keystone of its company-wide safety programs. This philosophy includes these beliefs:

1. All injuries and occupational illness can be prevented.
2. All deficiencies must be corrected properly.
3. Management is directly responsible and accountable for preventing injuries and illnesses.
4. It is essential to investigate all unsafe practices and incidents with injury potential, as well as all injuries.
5. Working safely is a condition of employment.
6. Safety off the job is as important as safety on the job.
7. Training is an essential element for safe workplaces.
8. It is good business to prevent illnesses and injuries.
9. Safety audits must be conducted.
10. People are the most critical element in the success of a safety and health program.

Hazard recognition and identification lead to:

1. control of a worker's performance
2. control of tools and machines
3. control of the working environment

The cause of accidents is either environmental or behavioral and, frequently, a combination of both factors. The key to accident prevention is determining the cause and preventing recurrences. Some of the more commonly found unsafe acts observed in the workplace include:

1. using broken or defective hand tools
2. not following safety procedures or obeying safety rules

TABLE 2.   Cost of Work-Related Accidents Involving the Upper Extremity*

1981	$32.5 billion
1982	31.5 billion
1984	33.0 billion
1985	37.3 billion
1986	34.8 billion
1987	42.2 billion

Reprinted with permission from Accident Facts. Chicago, National Safety Council, 1989.

*Costs include wages lost, medical expenses, insurance administration, and fire loss.

3. not wearing the prescribed personal protective safety equipment

4. poor housekeeping practices

Anton[3] has listed four distinct parts of the anatomy of an accident: (1) contributing causes, (2) immediate causes, (3) the accident, and (4) the result of the accident.

POWER PRESS AND STAMPING MACHINE INJURIES

The function of power press and stamping machines is to shape materials such as a piece of plastic or sheet metal between two dies. The material is placed on the lower die, and the upper die closes down on it with tremendous force to form the desired shape. Severe crushing may occur when any part of the body is between the dies.

In the early 1970s, Congress passed a law to prevent any worker from placing his extremities in a die press. Manufacturers, however, felt that compliance was too difficult, and the law was amended to require only careful guarding of die presses.

Criteria for guarding standards that are used today were set up by a committee of the American National Standards Institute (ANSI). This organization is responsible for recommending designs for the safety of various types of machinery in the U.S. Safety guards recommended by ANSI include pull-back devices, various screens, push button devices, and electronic sensory devices.

Etherton[7] reported a study indicating that two-hand devices are an increasingly important factor in injuries. Further study of causality, in particular, information about the distance between palm buttons and press dies, is needed in order to evaluate the effectiveness of protection with two-hand devices.

The NIOSH group issued a bulletin, entitled "Injuries and Amputations Resulting from Work with Mechanical Power Presses,"[8] stating that in 1986 the estimated 151,000 operators of mechanical power presses in the United States were still at risk of injury.

In addition, data from the Bureau of Labor Statistics indicated that 20,000 amputations occur every year and that between 1600 and 2000 or 10% of these amputations occurred among power press operators.

Research reported by NIOSH in 1987[8] indicated that young male workers appeared to be at a greater risk than other operators. Inadvertent activation of the power press while the operator's extremities were in the operating zone of the press is one of the risks. Inadvertent press activation may increase as the cycling rate increases.

Injuries occur as a result of "after reach" among operators who start up power presses while using dual controls. Attention should be given to individual operators' hand speed. Injuries may also occur as a result of activation or overriding safeguards. Guarding devices are used to prevent extremities from being placed in hazardous areas (Fig. 1). Various electronic devices are used as sensors that can prevent the operation of a machine while hands are in the danger zone.

Maintenance activities such as cleaning and repairing the machines are frequently the cause of injuries. These operators are particularly at risk because of the necessity of removing guards in order to reach sections that require maintenance. This activity should only be performed when the machine is in a nonpowered state. This is done by a special lockout switch that would prevent the machine from being started during the servicing procedures.

Recently OSHA put out strict regulations about lockout devices that must be in place in plants with presses and stamping machines. On October 31, 1989, OSHA announced a new rule regarding lockout devices that would require employers to install locks to prevent accidental activation of equipment during repairs or to place warning tags on the power source

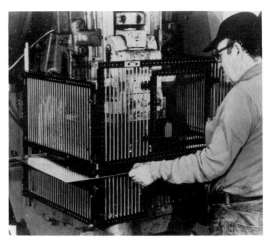

FIGURE 1. Operator using a Gap series 300 Guard. (From Rockford Systems, Inc., Rockford, IL, Safeguarding Power Presses (SPP) catalog, p. 44, with permission.)

to alert workers that the machinery is being worked on and must not be activated. It was estimated that about three million workers who service the equipment would be affected. The standard applies to most machinery used in manufacturing and in services such as industrial laundries.

OSHA data showed that packaging and wrapping equipment, printing presses, and conveyors account for the highest proportion of accidents due to failure to cut off power during major maintenance and repairs. The new regulation will prevent an estimated 60,000 in-injuries a year, about 28,000 of which are serious injuries such as loss of limbs or crushed bones.

Another helpful practice is to post safety rules on bulletin boards, especially near drinking fountains and locker rooms, where employees can see them (see Appendix I).

WOODWORKING INJURIES

Injuries are commonly sustained by workers using woodworking machinery and hand tools.[10] The table saw is probably the most dangerous of these machines. Significant factors involved in injuries include failure to use properly installed guards, fatigue, and postprandial somnolence.

RING INJURIES

In many occupational accidents a worker catches a ring on an object and then falls from a height. All the soft tissues of the digit in-

volved may be avulsed. The digit most commonly affected is the ring finger. A ring can strip back the soft tissues of the finger and disrupt the skin flap. This may result in an amputation of various parts of the digit.

Dr. William Frankelton, formerly of the Columbia Hospital, Department of Surgery in Milwaukee, Wisconsin, developed modifications to make a ring safer for its wearer (Fig. 2).[5] His simple, inexpensive method slots the ring into three quadrants so that, caught on a projection, the ring spreads open and the finger is spared. Workers in plant areas where they can catch their fingers on devices should be encouraged to use this modification of rings.

Meagher[11] has recommended that full- or part-time occupational physicians can apply their professional talents in preventing occupational trauma (see Appendix II). Physicians can make rounds in the workplace and carefully inspect machines, work stations, and job performance movements. They can also examine all incoming machinery to help mechanical and safety engineers look for hazardous areas. Stop controls must be in the operator's reach, and available mechanical guards or other safety systems must be in place.

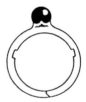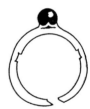

FIGURE 2. Safety ring slotted in three quadrants, designed by Dr. William H. Frankelton. Ring stretches if caught. (From Blair SJ, Allard KM: Prevention of trauma: A cooperative effort. J Hand Surg 8:649–654, 1983, with permission.)

APPENDIX I

Twelve Safety Rules for Conveyors[16]

These 12 universal safety rules for anti load-handling conveyor systems should be prominently posted on bulletin boards, near drinking fountains, and in locker rooms where employees can see them when they are momentarily at leisure.

1. Keep clothing, fingers, hair, and other parts of the body away from the conveyor.
2. Know the location and function of all stop/start controls.
3. Keep all stopping/starting control devices free from obstructions to permit ready access.
4. Operate conveyor with *trained personnel only*.
5. Make sure all personnel are clear of obstructions.
6. Keep area around conveyors clear of obstructions.
7. Service conveyor with authorized maintenance personnel only.
8. *Report all unsafe practices* to your supervisor.
9. Don't perform service on conveyor until motor disconnect is locked out.
10. Don't load conveyor beyond its design limits.
11. Don't climb, step, sit, or ride on the conveyor at any time.
12. Don't remove or alter conveyor guards or safety devices.

APPENDIX II*

Improper Control Design Elements to be Noted during a Machine Inspection

Safety switch guards
Unguarded activation controls
Unilateral stop switch
Open pedals
Safety pedal on movable cable
Lack of color identification
Lack of control function labels
Lack of individual stop controls on multi-station machines
Use of dual buttons without an additional machine guarding system

Start and stop by the same switch
Safety control not within reach
Small-size stop switch
Unguarded console
Low resistance activation control
Failure to guard activation controls by location
Absence of lock-out control for servicing of the machine

REFERENCES

1. Absoud EM, Harrop SN: Hand injuries at work. J Hand Surg 9B:211–215, 1984.
2. Accident Facts. Chicago, National Safety Council, 1989 and prior years.
3. Anton TJ: Occupational Safety and Health Management, 2nd ed. New York, McGraw-Hill, 1989.
4. Blair SJ, Allard KM: Prevention of trauma: A cooperative effort. J Hand Surg 8:649–654, 1983.
5. Blair SJ, McCormick E: Prevention of trauma: Cooperation toward a better working environment. J Hand Surg 10A (6, Pt 2):953–958, 1985.
6. Concepts and Techniques of Machine Safeguarding. U.S. Department of Labor (OSHA) publication no. 3067, 1980 (reprinted 1981).
7. Etherton J: Factors Reported in Amputation and Other Injury Cases at Mechanical Power Presses between 1976 and 1984. Trends in Ergonomics/Human Factors V. New York, Elsevier North-Holland, 1988, pp 629–638.
8. Injuries and Amputations Resulting from Work with Mechanical Power Presses. Current Intelligence Bulletin 49, NIOSH, May 1987.
9. Investigation and analysis of fifty reports of injury to operators of mechanical power presses. U.S. Department of Labor (OSHA), Office of Standard Development, final report, November 1975.
10. Justis EJ, Moore SV, LaVelle DG: Woodworking injuries: An epidemiologic survey of injuries sustained

---

* Reprinted with permission from Meagher S: Human factors engineering: A primer for the surgeon's participation in industrial injury prevention. Contemp Orthop 8(3):76, 1984.

using woodworking machinery and hand tools. J Hand Surg 12A (5, Pt 2):890–895, 1987.

11. Meagher SW: Appliance design hazards. J Prod Liabil 2:267–270, 1978.

12. Meagher SW: Human factors engineering. A primer for the surgeon's participation in industrial injury prevention. Contemp. Orthop 8(3):76, 1984.

13. OSHA: Recordkeeping Requirements under the Occupational Safety and Health Act of 1970. U.S. Department of Labor (OSHA) publication no. 200, 1978.

14. Power Presses Safety Manual, 3rd ed. Chicago, National Safety Council, 1979.

15. Schulzinger: The Accident Syndrome. Springfield, IL, C. C Thomas, 1956.

16. Tuinstra BJ: Effective conveyor safety programs must be tailored to specific design. Occup Health Saf 104–106, 1989.

Chapter 4

ETIOLOGIES AND PREVALENCE OF OCCUPATIONAL INJURIES TO THE UPPER EXTREMITY

Frank P. Vannier, M.D., and John F. Rose, M.D.

Epidemiology has classically been defined as the field of medicine concerned with distribution and determinants of disease in circumscribed populations.[11] It has traditionally provided the methodology for studying disease epidemics. Currently, epidemiology has a broader scope—namely, the study of health and illness in human populations. The purpose of epidemiological research can include the quantification of disease occurrences and the definition of disease etiology.[26]

The identification of upper extremity disorders related to work activity is becoming a major focus of occupational medicine. Since the hand is used in many occupations, upper extremity injuries in the workplace are a common finding. For example, traumatic injuries to the upper extremities are a well-known consequence of foundry work, assembly line manufacturing, and meatpacking. In recent years, the number of patients with upper extremity injuries due to overuse, repetitive motion, and vibratory tool-related motions of the extremity has markedly increased. The Bureau of Labor Statistics' 1988 Annual Survey of Occupational Injuries and Illnesses reported more than 240,900 new cases of all types of occupational illness among workers in private industry. The number is a 25% increase over 1987. Disorders associated with repeated trauma (due to repeated motion, pressure, or vibration, such as carpal tunnel syndrome) accounted for more than 80% of this increase.[48]

Occupational upper extremity injuries represent a major economic burden. In 1976, approximately one-third of work-related injuries involved the upper extremity; 66% involved the hand. Nearly 80% of the hand injuries involved lacerations, puncture wounds, or fractures. The index finger and thumb were the most frequently affected digits.

Insurance and administrative costs associated with occupational upper extremity injuries approximated $630 million in 1980. Other costs associated with a workplace injury to the upper extremity include the monetary value of time and effort involved in investigating accidents, preparing reports, and training replacement workers, as well as time lost because production schedules are disrupted. These indirect costs totaled approximately $3.75 billion in 1980.[22]

The risk of upper extremity injuries in the workplace is increased by alcohol and drug abuse among employees. Employees with substance abuse problems are two to four times more likely than others to be involved in an industrial accident. The result of accidents is increased absenteeism as well as loss of productivity. The documented increase in the costs associated with workers' compensation injuries in recent years is attributable to substance abuse.

In 1980, the economic burden of alcohol and drug abuse was estimated at $140 billion, 55% of which was due to decreased productivity. Because one-third of industrial injuries involve the upper extremity, the economic impact of substance abuse on that extremity is significant.[19,39]

A review of epidemiological data can be helpful in pinpointing occupations at risk for certain types of upper extremity injuries. These data can be applied in a practical manner to specify the etiological factors. Ergonomic evaluations that study the integration of people into the work environment can then be applied to change a specific work activity, thus preventing the injury. For example, studying a worker as he operates a machine can reveal motions at risk of causing an injury and can lead to the development of specific alternate motions that may prevent an occupational injury.[27] The following discussion of occupational injuries of the upper extremities is an overview of their etiologies and prevalence in certain high-risk occupations.

CUMULATIVE TRAUMA INJURIES

Chronic upper extremity pain is epidemic in occupations involving repetitive work. Chronic incapacitating arm pain has been well recognized in Australian factory and office workers, where the terms "overuse syndrome" and "repetitive strain syndrome" have been

---

SURVEILLANCE CASE DEFINITION FOR WORK-RELATED CARPAL TUNNEL SYNDROME (CTS)

A. One or more of the following symptoms suggestive of CTS is present*: paresthesias, hypoesthesia, pain, or numbness affecting at least part of the median nerve distribution[†] of the hand(s).

B. Objective findings consistent with CTS are present in the affected hand(s) and wrist(s):
EITHER
1. Physical examination findings—Tinel's sign[§] present or positive Phalen's test[¶] or diminished or absent sensation to pin prick in the median nerve distribution of the hand.
OR
2. Electrodiagnostic findings indicative of median nerve dysfunction across the carpal tunnel.**

C. Evidence of work-relatedness—a history of a job involving *one or more* of the following activities before the development of symptoms[††]:
1. Frequent, repetitive use of the same or similar movements of the hand or wrist on the affected side(s).
2. Regular tasks requiring the generation of high force by the hand on the affected side(s).
3. Regular or sustained tasks requiring awkward hand positions on the affected side(s).[§§]
4. Regular use of vibrating hand-held tools.
5. Frequent or prolonged pressure over the wrist or base of the palm on the affected side(s).

---

*Symptoms should have lasted at least 1 week or, if intermittent, have occurred on multiple occasions. Other causes of hand numbness or paresthesias, such as cervical radiculopathy, thoracic outlet syndrome, and pronator teres syndrome, should be excluded by appropriate clinical evaluation (1).
[†]Generally includes palmar side of thumb, index finger, middle finger, and radial half of ring finger; dorsal (back) side of same digits distal to PIP joint; and radial half of palm. Pain and paresthesias may radiate proximally into the arm.
[§]Paresthesias are elicited or accentuated by gentle percussion over the carpal tunnel.
[¶]Paresthesias are elicited or accentuated by maximal passive flexion of the wrist for one minute.
**Criteria for abnormal electrodiagnostic findings are generally determined by the individual laboratories
[††]A temporal relationship of symptoms to work or an association with cases of CTS in co-workers performing similar tasks is also evidence of work-relatedness.
[§§]Awkward hand positions predisposing to CTS include the use of a pinch grip (as when holding a pencil), extreme flexion, extension, or ulnar deviation of the wrist, and use of the fingers with the wrist flexed.

FIGURE 1. Surveillance case definition for work-related carpal tunnel syndrome; developed by the Sentinel Event Notification System for Occupational Risks (SENSOR).

used.[13,28] In the United States, this clinical syndrome has classically been called tenosynovitis or tendinitis. A cumulative trauma disorder can include tendinitis, but it can also refer to various neuropathies and degenerative joint diseases involving the upper extremities. In 1989, Gerald F. Scannell, Assistant Secretary of Labor, Occupational Safety and Health Administration, stated that virtually every workplace in the United States has the potential to cause cumulative trauma disorders.[6]

PERIPHERAL COMPRESSION NEUROPATHIES

When the body is stressed beyond its physiological work capacity, neurological syndromes related to overuse and entrapment of peripheral nerves tend to manifest themselves.[25] Cumulative trauma disorders as they relate to overuse syndromes present as tendinitis, joint inflammation, degenerative joint disease, bursitis, ligamentous (muscle) strain, and neuritis. These symptoms are due to the stresses of the repetitive motions required to perform many work activities. Nerve entrapment syndromes can manifest themselves when a peripheral nerve is compressed in a confined area.[25]

Carpal tunnel syndrome is a nerve entrapment syndrome in that it develops in the carpal tunnel at the wrist. The median nerve is compressed or irritated as it passes between the carpal bones and the transverse carpal ligament. Systemic diseases such as diabetes and rheumatoid arthritis can predispose a worker to carpal tunnel syndrome. Multiple precipitating factors are associated with work activity. These include grasping or pinching of tools or objects, awkward positions of the hand and wrist, direct pressure over the carpal tunnel, and use of vibrating, hand-held tools. Patients with nonoccupational risk factors for carpal tunnel syndrome, as in pregnancy, diabetes mellitus, or rheumatoid arthritis, are also at risk of developing work-related carpal tunnel syndrome.[7]

The Sentinel Event Notification System for Occupational Risks (SENSOR), a collaborative effort involving the National Institute for Occupational Safety and Health (NIOSH), the Centers for Disease Control (CDC), and 10 state health departments, stipulates the surveillance case definition for work-related carpal tunnel syndrome shown in Figure 1. This definition assists in the surveillance and reporting of carpal tunnel syndrome as an occupational disease at the state and local levels.[7]

Workers known to be at risk for carpal tunnel syndrome include textile workers, butchers, grocery checkers, electronics assembly workers, typists, musicians, packers, and carpenters.[7] Numerous other occupations have also been associated with carpal tunnel syndrome. Working with the wrist in flexion and ulnar or radial deviation is associated with an increased incidence of carpal tunnel syndrome.[44]

The entrapment of the ulnar nerve at the elbow is called cubital tunnel syndrome and has been found to occur in workers who lean on their elbows: brass polishers, locksmiths, jewelers, and many workers who use fine hand movements.[25]

There is also an entrapment syndrome that involves the ulnar nerve at the wrist. It generally occurs in Guyon's canal and can selectively involve the deep branch of the ulnar nerve within the hand. This finding is associated with gardeners, machine tool fitters, typists, bicycle deliverers, and mechanics.

Radial tunnel syndrome occurs with radial nerve entrapment distal to the elbow joint and involves the posterior interosseous nerve. This type of nerve entrapment is related to repetitive forceful twisting (supination or pronation) of the forearm in association with poor positioning of the elbow when it is used for leverage.[18] It is seen in musicians, assembly line workers, and mechanics.

Thoracic outlet syndrome is compression of the brachial plexus and is commonly associated with work activity requiring repetitive shoulder movements. Examples include operation of video display terminals, assembly line work, and playing the violin or double bass. A previous hand injury can have a direct role in the etiology of thoracic outlet syndrome in that it can cause the worker to change his shoulder posture and thus the anatomy and can lead to brachial plexus compression. Poor posture while watching a video display terminal can result in spasm of the scalene musculature, which can also occur with cervical strain (i.e., whiplash).[25]

UPPER EXTREMITY INJURIES IN MUSICIANS, GARMENT WORKERS AND DATA PROCESSORS

The development of cumulative trauma syndrome and related upper extremity discomfort is a common occupational problem of musicians. A survey of musicians in eight orchestras revealed that the incidence of cumulative trauma syndrome is greater than 50%. This problem is described in the literature as an overuse syndrome.[14]

The specific anatomical area involved tends to vary according to the instrument played. Symptoms manifested include pain, tenderness, and decreased function of the involved muscles and ligaments.[14] Keyboard players tend to develop symptoms in the lumbrical muscles of the hand and the extensor tendons of the wrist and fingers. Stringed instrument players have symptoms in the extensor and flexor musculature of the hand, wrist, forearm, and shoulder. Clarinet and English horn players tend to have overuse symptoms in the web spaces between the digits of the hands. Oboe musicians and orchestra conductors develop entrapment of the radial nerve with subsequent neuropathy.[46] Entrapment of the median nerve or carpal tunnel syndrome can be associated with violin playing. Pianists have also been reported at increased risk for carpal tunnel syndrome.[25]

If the musician continues to perform and to practice for long hours, the symptoms begin to spread to other areas of the upper extremities. The diagnosis is based on a history of playing a musical instrument and on the type of overuse syndrome associated with the particular instrument. Treatment is aimed at providing symptomatic medications, which can include nonsteroidal anti-inflammatory drugs, rest programs for the involved upper extremity, and efforts at modification of the musician's technique.[15]

Garment workers have been noted to experience upper extremity symptoms of pain and paresthesias. The prevalence of these symptoms has been said to be as high as 42%. Treatment involves ergonomic evaluation of the specific work activity and implementation of appropriate changes. A medical evaluation is necessary to rule out a systemic disease or a treatable nerve or tendon problem.[32]

The use of computers has resulted in an increase in the number of employees performing rapid data entry. The job activity of keying data at a video display terminal for long hours has resulted in a marked increase in musculoskeletal complaints. Typical symptoms are pain, stiffness, and paresthesias. Contributing factors are poor posture, poorly designed work stations, and psychological factors. The number of workers presenting with these findings is expected to increase in the 1990s as the demand for this type of work continues to increase.[47]

HYPOTHENAR SYNDROME

Another type of injury that can occur while working involves the palm of the hand; it is especially likely to occur when the palm is used to beat or pound an object. This type of activity has the potential to produce ischemic changes along the distribution of the ulnar artery referred to as hypothenar hammer syndrome. Ulnar artery thrombosis or aneurysm with possible embolization to the second through fifth digits can result, causing claudication of the hand, paresthesia, cold hypersensitivity, and pain. Diagnosis is confirmed with arteriography or Doppler mapping. Workers at risk include metal workers, lathe operators, and mechanics.[9,42,45] Prevention of hypothenar syndrome through worker education is critical. Ergonomic evaluation of the occupations carrying high risk can offer alternative means of performing these activities.

VIBRATION WHITE FINGER SYNDROME

Raynaud's phenomenon and Raynaud's disease are associated with a pathological vasospastic response. The diagnosis requires that at least two of three classic skin color changes—pallor, cyanosis, and erythema—occur.[21] The vasospasm can be referred to as Raynaud's disease if it is idiopathic and there is no history of underlying disease.[21] In Raynaud's disease both hands typically are affected symmetrically, and the feet may also be involved.[5] When the vasospasm is a manifestation of a pre-existent factor or disease state such as a connective tissue disorder (i.e., rheumatoid arthritis, systemic lupus erythematosus), a vascular disorder (i.e., peripheral vascular disease, thoracic outlet syndrome), hematological abnormality (i.e., cryoglobulinemia), medications (i.e., beta-adrenergic blockers), mechanical factors (i.e., vibratory tools), or toxins (i.e., vinyl chloride), it is referred to as Raynaud's phenomenon.[16,21]

If the causes of Raynaud's phenomenon can be excluded in workers who use vibrating tools, vibration white finger syndrome is the commonly accepted diagnosis. Research studies in the early 1900s in the United States revealed that up to 90% of various types of stone cutters experienced Raynaud's phenomenon, and it was concluded that the tools of the trade were responsible for the symptoms. However, the medical community failed to recognize the magnitude of the problem. As recently as 1960, one study concluded that Raynaud's phenomenon was not an occupational problem.[30] Subsequently, several well-designed research studies have clearly demonstrated the magnitude of this problem.[5]

Workers who use vibratory tools are at risk of developing the vasospastic symptoms of Raynaud's syndrome. Workers at highest risk include foundry workers and forestry employees. Any workers who use chipping and grinding tools, pneumatic hand tools, power drills, and chain saws are at risk. A Canadian forestry study demonstrated that 28% of these employees had symptoms of vibration white finger syndrome. Over the 15 years that these workers were followed, the prevalence of this syndrome was 50%.[33]

The gray iron foundries exhibited a prevalence of vibration white finger syndrome that was nearly 47%. A shipyard foundry demonstrated a 19% prevalence. Time span from first exposure to vibratory tools to development of vibration white finger syndrome at these foundries varied. The eventual difference in the percentage of workers in the two types of foundries who developed symptoms was thought to be related to incentives for good work practices the foundries offered.[4]

The diagnosis of vibration white finger syndrome is determined by a history of Raynaud's phenomenon and of exposure to vibratory tools. No condition known to be associated with Raynaud's syndrome can be present.

Ergonomic design of tools to attenuate vibration has been helpful. Education and instruction of employees in proper gripping and safe use of vibratory tools are also beneficial. A proper schedule of rest breaks and, in particular, job rotation that decreases worker exposure to vibratory tools can reduce the frequency and severity of the symptoms of vibration white finger syndrome.

OCCUPATIONAL INJURIES OF THE WRIST

Wrist injuries are commonly associated with various occupations. De Quervain's disease is most common in occupations requiring repetitive, twisting ulnar and radial deviation. The abductor pollicis longus and extensor pollicis brevis tendons are involved.[10,37]

Industries associated with this form of tenosynovitis include the electronics industry. A predominance of de Quervain's disease was reported among workers using needle-nose pliers that required repetitive gripping and deviation of the wrist joint. Modifying the handles of the pliers sometimes can eliminate the offending motion and reduce the incidence of de Quervain's disease.[28]

Similarly, a high incidence of de Quervain's syndrome was demonstrated in a poultry processing plant. Ergonomic investigation revealed a thigh-boning procedure that required workers to grip with force and to flex and ulnarly deviate the wrist repetitively. A modified knife design was recommended to decrease the incidence of this problem.[2] De Quervain's disease also occurs in certain assembly line manufacturing processes and various packing operations.

OCCUPATIONAL INJURIES OF THE ELBOW

Occupational injuries to the elbow can occur from isolated or cumulative trauma. Machine shop workers, construction workers, meatpacking plant workers, and persons involved in food preparation are among those affected.

One form of repetitive strain injury to the elbow is **lateral epicondylitis** (tennis elbow). The actual lesions are small ruptures and incomplete tendinous repairs of the extensor carpi radialis brevis tendon fibers distal to the origin of the lateral epicondyle of the humerus. Any activity or occupation that involves repetitive forearm motion and wrist extension with the palm rotating can predispose to lateral epicondylitis. Workers at significant risk include house painters, carpenters, and those who use screwdrivers and wrenches extensively.[34]

Medial epicondylitis is caused by stress on the flexor pronator musculature at its tendinous origin on the medial humeral epicondyle. Active flexion of the wrist or pronation of the forearm against resistance generally causes discomfort if medial epicondylitis is present. This form of cumulative trauma injury is found in professional athletes, animal skinners, and fish scalers.[40,41,43]

Treatment approach to occupation-related epicondylitis should be ergonomic evaluation of the workplace and appropriate changes in job design. This preventive approach helps reduce the cause of this overuse syndrome of the upper extremity.

Another type of elbow injury is **olecranon bursitis**, which can occur as a result of constant elbow pressure, repeated minor trauma, or bacterial infection. Olecranon bursitis can be traumatic or septic in origin. Predisposed workers include plumbers, carpenters, construction workers, and people who lean on their elbows. Hemorrhagic fluid and effusion associated with trauma are often found in the bursitis. The effusion from septic olecranon bursitis may be turbid or grossly purulent and is usually caused by the common microorganism *Staphylococcus aureus.*[41]

OCCUPATIONAL INJURIES OF THE SHOULDER

In physically demanding work, the shoulder is vulnerable to injury; the rotator cuff is the most common site of trauma leading to injury. Elevation of the arm can impinge on the rotator cuff and bursa. Workers at risk include warehouse workers, whose tasks include overhead lifting of materials, and painters who use repetitive overhead motions. Hairdressers, musicians, and clerical workers, who work with their arms abducted, can sometimes alleviate symptoms by lowering their arms to the side of the body from time to time.[29,34]

DERMATOLOGICAL DISEASES OF THE HAND

Dermatological conditions commonly occur in various occupations. Approximately 90% of occupational dermatitis involves the hands. This disease can occur in the form of an irritant or allergic contact dermatitis. Dermatitis of the hands is prevalent in workers with significant exposure to water and surfactants, which disrupt the barrier function of the skin. Dishwashers and bartenders frequently develop dermatitis.[8]

Allergic contact dermatitis is the cell-mediated immunological response of delayed hypersensitivity that occurs after sensitization. Allergic hand dermatitis can be seen in electroplaters, who may exhibit chrome sensitivity, and in dentists, who can develop allergic contact dermatitis to local anesthetics. Forestry-related occupations are at increased risk of phytodermatitis; numerous plants are a primary cause. Farmers are also subject to phytodermatitis and to contact dermatitis from exposure to insecticides and fungicides.

Butchers and those working in the meat-packing industry demonstrate an increased incidence of viral, bacterial, and fungal hand infections. In the plastics industry, a unique phenomenon occurs in workers in contact with vinyl chloride. Vasospastic changes (Raynaud's phenomenon), sclerodermoid-related skin changes, and bone resorption (osteolytic changes) occur in the hand.[1,8,17]

OCCUPATIONAL BURN INJURIES OF THE UPPER EXTREMITY

Many workers are at risk for burn injuries, which can be caused by thermal, chemical, electrical, or radiation contact.

Thermal origin represents the most common type of burn. The chemical industry is associated with the risk of explosion, which can produce blast, flame, and chemical burns. A hot press in the laundry industry can produce a combination of crush and thermal burn. Workers in a foundry or forge shop are at risk for very deep burns.[3,20]

Chemical burns may be classified as either alkali or acid in origin. An example of an acid that causes burns is phenol (carbolic acid), which is used in the health care industry and in the manufacture of plastics. The systemic toxic effects of phenol supersede its ability to cause a surface burn. Percutaneous absorption at the site of the phenol-related burn injury can cause toxic cardiovascular and central nervous system effects, including grand mal seizures.[35]

Sulfuric and nitric acid are used in manufacturing with nitrators and acid dippers and in steel production. Generally, acids are water soluble and penetrate the subcutaneous tissue. Some acids also tend to create a tough, indurated eschar.

Hydrochloric acid burns of the upper extremity occur in chemical and refinery work. Picric acid is used in the manufacture of explosives and by tannery workers and dye makers. Acetic acid, which may produce dermatitis and skin ulceration, is used in acetate rayon synthesis, in the hat industry, and in printing and dyeing.[23]

Hydrofluoric acid is a common cause of chemical burns of the upper extremity. It deserves special mention because it has potentially life-threatening effects. Hydrofluoric acid has many industrial applications, including the manufacture of silicon chips for computers, glassmaking, ceramics manufacturing, photography, and masonry. It is extensively used in the petroleum industry, in fertilizer production, in the plastics industry, and in the production of drugs and dyes. The fluoride ion has a great affinity for calcium and characteristically penetrates tissue, causing hypocalcemia, unless appropriate treatment is initiated.

Treatment of hydrofluoric acid exposure and related chemical burn injuries involves removing the worker's contaminated clothing and copious irrigation of the wound with water. Soaks with Zephiran (active ingredient, benzalkonium chloride) can be employed. Subsequent definitive treatment involves application of calcium gluconate gel or local injections of calcium gluconate. In localities with industrial plants where the potential for hydrofluoric acid burns exists, all local emergency rooms should be alerted.[12,36]

Alkaline caustics may be an overt entity or a component of a compound. For example, cement is comprised of lime (calcium oxide) and alkali oxides, which form caustic hydroxides when in contact with water. Ammonium hydroxide is used in fertilizer manufacture, refrigeration, and textile and paper industries. Sodium hydroxide is used by tannery workers, in the petroleum industry, and by soap and dye manufacturers. Potassium hydroxide is used in the electroplating industry, paper production, and soap manufacture.

Alkaline caustics tend to penetrate the burn injury significantly. In addition, they penetrate less painfully than do acid compounds. Thus the victim may be less aware of the evolving injury and less likely to seek immediate medical care. Prevention, through employee training and the use of protective equipment, is a critical factor in dealing with chemical burns of the upper extremities.[23]

Electrical burn injuries are particularly significant. Industrial and residential electricians are at risk for this type of injury. Public utility employees working in power plants where high voltage currents are generated are at risk for serious electrical injury.[17,20]

MICROWAVE INJURY OF THE UPPER EXTREMITIES

Microwave energy is a nonionizing form of radiation used in food preparation, drying of products, and sealing plastics. After a microwave injury, the skin may appear relatively unharmed, but underlying structures may be significantly damaged. Nerve damage may be quite severe as these structures are susceptible to microwave injury. Pain and paresthesias are consistent symptoms. Treatment is generally conservative. Surgical intervention involves decompression and debridement.[17]

FROSTBITE INJURY

Workers who come in contact with refrigeration equipment, such as in the food preparation industry, are predisposed to injury related to excessive or prolonged cold exposure. Letter carriers, utility workers, and baggage handlers need to be educated about the hazards of frostbite. Treatment is conservative and involves rapid rewarming of the affected area. Surgical procedures should be delayed as long as possible.[17]

INJECTION AND LACERATION INJURIES OF THE UPPER EXTREMITY

Significant hand trauma can occur in the workplace from high-compression injection injuries. These occur from high-pressure grease guns, paint and solvent guns, or any high-pressure line or container[24] (see Chapter 18).

Simple lacerations of the upper extremities as well as lacerations involving tendon, digital nerves, or joint capsules may occur in the workplace. The construction industry and other occupations involving moving machinery have a high incidence of these injuries.

CONCLUSION

The upper extremities are called upon to perform myriad tasks in the workplace. There is a significant incidence of injury to the upper extremities among a wide variety of workers. Such injuries are best combatted by ergonomic changes that decrease their incidence. Prevention of accidents is the best way to contain the medical costs of workplace injuries.

REFERENCES

1. Adams RM, Emmet EA, Pincus SH: What's new in occupational dermatitis? Patient Care 21:151–171, 1987.
2. Armstrong RJ, Foulke JA, Brady J, Goldstein S: Investigation of cumulative trauma disorders in a poultry processing plant. Am Ind Hyg Assoc J 43:103–116, 1982.
3. Baux S: Thermal and chemical burns in the hand. In Tubiana R (ed): The Hand. Philadelphia, W. B. Saunders, 1988, pp 756–774.
4. Behrens V, Taylor W, Wasserman D: Vibration syndrome in workers using pneumatic chipping and grinding tools. In Brammer, Taylor W: Vibration Effects on the Hand and Arm in Industry. New York, John Wiley, 1982, pp 147–155.
5. Behrens V, Taylor W, Wilcox T, et al: Vibration syndrome in chipping and grinding workers. J Occup Med 26:766–773, 1984.
6. Bruening JC: Scannell charts OSHA'S future course. Occup Hazards 51:27–30, 1989.
7. Cummings K, Maizlish N, Rudolph L, et al: Current trends: Occupational disease surveillance: Carpal tunnel syndrome. MMWR 38:485–488, 1989.
8. Davidson CL, Cost KM: Occupational dermatology of the hand. Hand Clin 2:457–466, 1986.
9. DiBenedetto MR, Nappi JF, Ruff ME, Lubbers LM: Doppler mapping in hypothenar syndrome: An alternative to angiography. J Hand Surg 14A:244–246, 1989.
10. Field J: De Quervain's disease. Am Fam Physician 20:103–104, 1979.
11. Fletcher RH, Fletcher SW, Wagner EH: Clinical Epidemiology: The Essentials, 2nd ed. Baltimore, William & Wilkins, 1988, p 4.
12. Flood S: Hydrofluoric acid burns. Am Fam Physician 37:175–182, 1988.
13. Fry HJH: Overuse syndrome, alias tenosynovitis/tendinitis: The terminological hoax. J Plast Reconstruct Surg 78:414–417, 1986.
14. Fry HJH: Overuse syndrome in musicians: Prevention & management. Lancet ii:728–731, 1986.
15. Fry HJH: The treatment of overuse syndrome in musicians. J Royal Soc Med 81:572–575, 1988.
16. Grisanti J: Raynaud's phenomenon. Am Fam Physician 41:134–142, 1990.
17. Hankin FM: Contact injuries to the hand. Occup Med State Art Rev 4:473–484, 1989.
18. Harter, BT Jr.: Indications for surgery in work-related compression neuropathies of the upper extremity. Occup Med State Art Rev 4:485–496, 1989.
19. Harwood H, Napolitano D, Kristiansen P, Collins J: Economic Cost to Society of Alcohol and Drug Abuse and Mental Illness: 1980. RTI:2734:00-01FR, 1984, pp 1–12.
20. Hentz V: Burns of the hand. Emerg Med Clin North Am 3:391–403, 1985.
21. Kahl L: Raynaud's phenomenon: It may signal systemic disease. Diagnosis 7:30–38, 1985.
22. Kelsey J, Pastides H, Krieger N, et al: Upper Extremity Disorders: A Survey of their Frequency and Cost in the United States. St Louis, C. V. Mosby, 1980, pp 17, 33–34.
23. Kunkel D: The toxic emergency. Emergency Medicine 3:165–172, 1984.
24. Lewis, RC Jr.: Hand injuries from injections and crushing force. Diagnosis 7:101–110, 1985.
25. Mandel S: Neurologic syndromes from repetitive trauma at work. Postgrad Med 82:87–92, 1987.
26. Maylack FH: Epidemiology of tennis, squash and racquetball injuries. Clin Sports Med 7:233–243, 1988.
27. McGrath S; World War II: Ergonomics begins. J Forms Mgmt 10:13–15, 1985.
28. Miller MH, Topliss DJ: Chronic upper limb pain syndrome (repetitive strain injury) in the Australian workforce: A systematic cross sectional rheumatological study of 229 patients. J Orthop Res 15:1705–1712, 1988.
29. Neviaser RJ: Treating patients with rotator cuff tears. J Musculoskel Med, 4:17–23, 1985.
30. Pecora LJ, Udel M, Christman RP: Survey of current status of Raynaud's phenomenon of occupational origin. Am Ind Hyg Assoc J 25:80–83, 1960.
31. Percy E: Tennis elbow: A common overuse syndrome. Drug Ther 12:139–154, 1982.
32. Punnet L, Robins JM, Wegman DH, Keyserling WM: Soft tissue disorders in the upper limbs of female garment workers. Scand J Work Environ Health 11:417–425, 1985.
33. Pyykko I, Korltonen OS, Frankkila MA, et al: A longitudinal study of the vibration syndrome in Finnish forestry workers. In Brammer AJ, Taylor W: Vibration Effects on the Hand and Arm in Industry. New York, John Wiley, 1982, pp 157–167.
34. Rowe C: Tendinitis, bursitis, impingement, snapping scapula and calcific tendinitis in the shoulder. In Rowe C: The Shoulder. New York, Churchill Livingstone, 1988, pp 105–129.
35. Stewart C: Chemical skin burns. Am Fam Physician 31:149–157, 1985.
36. Tepperman P: Mortality due to acute systetmic fluoride poisoning following a hydrofluoric acid skin burn. J Occup Med 22:691–692, 1980.
37. Thorson EP, Szabo RM: Tendinitis of the wrist and elbow. Occup Med State Art Rev 4:419–431, 1989.
38. Tichauer E: Some aspects of stress on forearm and hand in industry. J Occup Med 8:63–71, 1966.
39. Vickary J, Resnik H: Prevent Drug Abuse in the Workplace. Drug Abuse Monogr Ser, Public Health Service, 1982, pp 1–10.
40. Walker LG, Mealo RA: Tendinitis: A practical approach to diagnosis and management. J Musculoskel Med, 5:24–54, 1989.
41. Watrous BG, Ho G: Elbow pain. Prim Care 15:732–735, 1988.
42. Wernick R, Smith DL: Bilateral hypothenar hammer syndrome. Am J Emerg Med 7:302–306, 1989.
43. White P, Laukaitis J: Diagnosis and management of shoulder and elbow complaints. Occup Probl Med Pract 3:1–6, 1988.
44. Wieslander G, Norback D, Gothe CJ, Juhlin L: Carpal tunnel syndrome (CTS) and exposure to vibration, repetitive wrist movements, and heavy manual work: A case-referent study. Br J Ind Med 46:43–47, 1989.
45. Ischemic fingers that point to the workplace. Emergency Medicine 21:119–121, 1989.
46. The medical care of musicians. Emergency Medicine 21:125–130, 1989.
47. Council on Scientific Affairs: Health effects of video display terminals. JAMA 257:1508–1512, 1987.
48. United States Department of Labor News. Bureau of Labor Statistics. USDL publication no. 89-548, 1989, pp 2–3.

Chapter 5

ANATOMY OF THE UPPER EXTREMITY

Joel B. Grad, M.D.

A thorough knowledge of upper extremity anatomy is essential for those of us involved in the care of injuries and other problems affecting the hand and arm. Initial frustrations of study evolve into a rewarding experience as the serious student realizes the great importance of his efforts in acquiring such knowledge to every aspect of clinical work. Understanding problems of and developing diagnoses for the upper extremity, especially the hand, are essentially an exercise in applied anatomy.

SKELETON

The anatomy of the upper extremity is best understood by considering it as three parts: arm (brachium), forearm (antebrachium), and hand. It is appropriate to discuss the skeletal architecture first, because many of the soft tissue relationships are based upon this bony framework.

The arm's one bone is the cylindrically shaped humerus. The humerus divides the arm into anterior (flexor) and posterior (extensor) compartments. The body's most mobile joint, the shoulder, lies proximally; despite its extensive soft tissue supports, the shoulder is the most frequently dislocated great joint. The elbow lies distally and is essentially a hinge joint more prone to fractures than to dislocations. The forearm consists of the radius and ulna. Only the radius articulates with the elbow and wrist; the ulna articulates solely with the elbow via its olecranon. The triangular fibrocartilage complex separates the ulna from the wrist. An-

atomically, this complex is simply a meniscus-like structure that, along with the wrist ligaments, supports and stabilizes the ulnar wrist (carpus).

The radius and ulna, along with the interosseous membrane between them, separate the forearm into three compartments: anterior, posterior, and lateral. The parallel relationships of the radius and ulna, with rotation and flexion-extension joints proximally and distally, is unique. The forearm's anterior compartment contains the flexion-pronation muscles, and the posterior compartment contains the extensor-supinator group. Interestingly, the anterior musculature takes origin primarily from the ulna, and the posterior extensor musculature primarily from the radius. The lateral compartment contains three muscles: the brachioradialis and the extensors carpi radialis longus and brevis. These three muscles often are referred to as the "mobile wad."

The hand's basic architecture is composed of 27 bones, 8 of which are carpal bones usually referred to as the wrist complex; clinically, however, wrist considerations should include all the metacarpal bases as well as the distal radius and ulna.

After birth, it takes approximately 10 years for the 8 bones of the wrist to calcify sufficiently for radiographic appearance. The wrist is a frequent site of accessory bones, coalitions, and bipartitions. The possibility of anatomic variations must be considered to avoid incorrect diagnoses following injuries. Fortunately, a mirror-image variation is usually found on the contralateral wrist, which can be checked radiographically. The most common variation is

61

a congenital coalition between the lunate and triquetrum. The lunula is an accessory ossicle immediately distal to the ulnar head. Appreciating its presence is important because the ulnar styloid is a frequent site of fracture and nonunion.

The wrist has three axes of motion: flexion-extension, pronation-supination, and radial-ulnar deviation. These are motions in the sagittal, axial, and frontal (coronal) planes, respectively. The two primary functions of the wrist are strategic positioning of the hand and modulating the amplitude of the digital flexor and extensor tendons via tenodesis effect. The wrist has the distinction of being our most complex joint; it is described radiographically as having two horizontal (proximal and distal) carpal rows. The proximal row consists of the scaphoid, lunate, triquetrum, and pisiform. The scaphoid, formerly called the navicular, being a mechanical link between the two rows, is often injured and in fact, accounts for approximately 70% of all carpal bone fractures. The pisiform is a sesamoid bone within the substance of the flexor carpi ulnaris tendon and, strictly speaking, is not an active participant in wrist mechanics. The bones of the distal carpal row from lateral to medial are the trapezium, trapezoid, capitate, and hamate.

Conceptualizing the carpal bones as three columns is helpful when studying wrist mechanics. In a normal wrist, the columns move and alter their orientations to one another in a predictable pattern. The scaphoid is the radial or mobile column. It is the stabilizing strut between the proximal and distal carpal rows. Scaphoid fractures that do not unite or complete tears of the scaphoid ligaments may produce a disabling instability pattern with eventual diffuse degenerative arthritis. The central column is the most important for flexion-extension. It is formed by the lunate and the four bones of the distal row. The wrist's center of motion lies within the head of the capitate. The triquetrum alone is the medial column and is essential to stable rotatory motions of the wrist. The triquetrum is the second most commonly fractured carpal bone, accounting for approximately 20% of carpal fractures. Normally, with ulnar deviation of the wrist, the proximal row translocates radially. With this motion, the scaphoid and lunate tilt dorsally and the triquetrum assumes a low position on the hamate. The reverse occurs with radial deviation of the wrist. Disruption of the synchronous motion

causes painfully restricted mobility of the wrist complex.

The hand's bones form three arches—two transverse and one longitudinal. The former are the carpal and metacarpal arches. The thick transverse carpal ligament by attaching to the four bony pillars of the carpal arch (pisiform, hamate, scaphoid, and trapezium) forms the oval carpal tunnel. Though only 1 inch in diameter, the carpal tunnel is a busy area anatomically. It contains the median nerve—the most important structure in the upper extremity—and nine digital flexor tendons. The carpal tunnel is the most frequent site of entrapment neuropathy—the carpal tunnel syndrome. The ulnar wrist tunnel—Guyon's canal—lies adjacent to the carpal tunnel. Its bony walls are the pisiform and hamate; the volar carpal ligament forms the roof of Guyon's canal. This ulnar wrist tunnel contains only two structures, the ulnar artery and nerve.

Studies using computerized topography have shown that this fixed and unyielding structure, the carpal tunnel, is normally oval in configuration; it becomes circular after surgical division of the transverse carpal ligament in the treatment of carpal tunnel syndrome. Not only does the volume of the tunnel increase by approximately 20%, but postoperative division of the transverse carpal ligament changes the shape of Guyon's canal from triangular to oval. This may be the reason why patients with carpal tunnel syndrome and sensory symptoms on the palmar aspect of the little finger (ulnar nerve territory) often experience relief of symptoms after division of the transverse carpal ligament alone.

The mobility and stability of the wrist are dependent upon skeleton and soft tissue supports—that is, ligaments and capsule. The wrist ligaments are complex, and although their integration into the joint capsule makes them appear ill defined, each of them is functionally critical. After trauma, injury to the wrist ligaments must be considered as suggested by the mechanism of injury and physical findings in order to request documented diagnostic tests and to formulate treatment plans. To facilitate understanding, the ligaments may be considered as either intrinsic or extrinsic. Intrinsic ligaments are those whose origin and insertion are between the carpal bones. The scapholunate and the lunotriquetral ligaments are the most important; their integrity is essential to synchronous motion. Loss of these passive restraints alters the relationship of the proximal carpal row to the distal radius and ulna as well as to the distal carpal row.

The extrinsic ligaments originate outside the wrist proper—that is, at the distal radius and ulna. The volar deep extrinsic ligaments are the most important stabilizers of the wrist. They consist of the radioscaphocapitate, radiolunotriquetral, and ulnar carpal ligaments (Fig. 1). If any of these ligaments is disrupted, the bones may shift in a troublesome instability pattern.

On the ulnar side of the wrist is the triangular fibrocartilage complex (TFCC), which, much like the knee's meniscus, functions as a stabilizer and shock absorber for the ulna carpus. The major portion of the complex is the triangular cartilage, a segment of fibrocartilage originating at the radius and inserting at the ulnar styloid. This is a frequent site of traumatic tears that may cause chronic wrist pain. Degenerative tears in the TFCC are found with

increasing frequency after age 40 and are not necessarily associated with pain.

Distal to the carpal bones are the five metacarpals, each of which articulates with one or more of the bones of the distal carpal row. The thumb metacarpal is the shortest, and its adjacent index metacarpal the longest. The metacarpals decrease in size from the index to the small finger. The first carpometacarpal joint is extremely mobile, whereas the index and middle finger carpometacarpal joints are almost immobile.

The first metacarpal articulates proximally with the trapezium. This articulation, the basal joint of the thumb, is critical to strategic positioning and strength. The basal joint has a saddle-like configuration, and because it is the most mobile of the hand's joints, it is vulnerable to injury and painful arthritis. The second and third metacarpals have almost immobile articulations with the trapezoid and capitate to comprise the fixed functional unit of the hand. Normally, only a few degrees of motion in the anteroposterior plane are present at these articulations, whereas the articulations of the fourth and fifth metacarpals with the hamate are mobile enough to allow cupping of the palm. Approximately 30 degrees of anteroposterior motion are usually present at the carpometacarpal articulations of the ring and small fingers.

The interosseous muscles originate from the metacarpals and give the fingers abduction and adduction. Littler[4] has beautifully described how, with the fingers in full extension-abduction, the fingertips lie on the circumference of a circle whose center is the head of the third metacarpal.

The 14 phalanges are the bones distal to the metacarpals. The proximal phalanges of the index, middle, ring, and small fingers form ball-and-socket (condyloid) loose-fitting joints with their metacarpals. The thumb's metacarpophalangeal (MCP) joint is more like a hinge; in the radioulnar (coronal) plane it has little motion and a highly variable degree of flexion-extension. The MCP joints have soft tissue supports, which, along with their skeletal configurations, give them stability. The collateral ligaments are located on the radial and ulnar sides of the joint and are really lateral oblique ligaments because of their acentric origin and insertions. The volar plate is a specialized thickening of the joint's capsule anteriorly between the metacarpal head and flexor tendons. Unlike

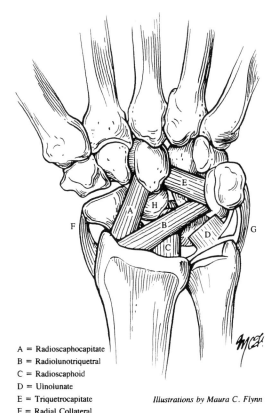

A = Radioscaphocapitate
B = Radiolunotriquetral
C = Radioscaphoid
D = Ulnolunate
E = Triquetrocapitate
F = Radial Collateral
G = Ulnar Collateral
H = Space of Poirier

Illustrations by Maura C. Flynn

FIGURE 1. Wrist ligaments. (Reprinted with permission from Grad JB: Hand anatomy and physical examination, Pt 1. Surg Rounds Orthop 3(6):26, 1989.)

the interphalangeal joints, the digital MCP joints can hyperextend because the volar plates are only loosely attached proximally to the metacarpal necks. The so-called collateral ligaments of the MCP joints arise dorsally at the metacarpal necks, and because the metacarpal heads widen in a dorsal-to-volar direction, flexion occurs with a cam effect at the MCP joints. The collateral ligaments are stretched over the condyles of the metacarpal heads with MCP flexion. In the protective (intrinsic plus) position, the collateral ligaments are maximally stretched over the condyles; their shortening is thus prevented and troublesome extension contractures avoided.

In the hand, the ligament most frequently injured is the ulnar collateral ligament of the thumb's MCP joint. This is the classic skier's thumb injury, and the tear may be partial or total. Interestingly, the ulnar collateral ligament of the thumb at this level usually ruptures or avulses from its insertion or distal attachment. In contrast, the much less frequent tears of the radiocollateral ligament at the thumb's MCP joint usually occur at its origin.

The digital interphalangeal (IP) joints are basically tight-fitting hinge (ginglymus) joints (Fig. 2). They also have collateral ligaments and volar plate supports, but these elements have a different arrangement from those of the MCP joints. Because the IP joints are concentric, the collateral ligaments do not undergo significant length changes between flexion and ex-

tension. In contrast to the MCP joints, the volar plates of the IP joints are attached firmly both proximally and distally and thus must fold when the joint flexes. The best position for immobilization of the IP joint is just to the extension side of neutral. Most people have little hyperextensibility of the IP joints because the volar plates, acting as check ligaments, prevent extension past neutral. The common "jammed finger" injury is an avulsion or tear of the IP volar plate from the base of the middle phalanx. With rare exception, the ligament tears distally; often a bony fleck is avulsed and can be radiographically demonstrated.

MUSCULOTENDINOUS SYSTEM

The muscles of the arm are separated into anterior (flexor) and posterior (extensor) compartments. The humerus as well as the medial and lateral intermuscular septi divide these two functional groups. Three muscles occupy the anterior compartment: the biceps, brachialis, and coracobrachialis; all are innervated by the musculocutaneous nerve. The biceps is the prime elbow flexor when the forearm lies supinated and is the only one of the three muscles to cross both the elbow and the shoulder. Forearm supination is also a biceps function when the elbow is flexed, because the biceps inserts on the radial tuberosity. The biceps tendon can be easily palpated in the antecubital fossa and

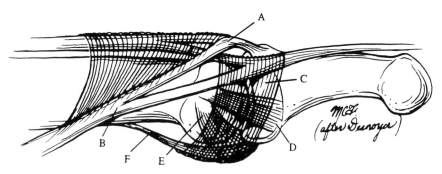

A = Central Slip
B = Lateral Band
C = Transverse Retinacular Ligament
D = Collateral Ligament, Proper
E = Accessory Collateral Ligament
F = Volar Plate

FIGURE 2. Digital interphalangeal joint. (Reprinted with permission from Grad JB: Hand anatomy and physical examination, Pt I. Surg Rounds Orthop 3(6):30, 1989.)

serves as an important anatomic landmark. The brachial artery is immediately medial to it, and the median nerve just medial to the artery. The lateral antebrachial cutaneous nerve is lateral to the biceps tendon. The deeply situated brachialis is the prime elbow flexor when the forearm is pronated, because it inserts on the coronoid process of the ulna. The coracobrachialis assists in flexion of the arm, but its prime function is adduction.

The triceps with its three heads (medial, lateral, and long) is the sole muscle occupant of the posterior compartment. It is the prime elbow extensor and is innervated by the radial nerve. Only the long head of the triceps crosses the shoulder joint.

The muscles providing power and control to the hand are divided into intrinsic and extrinsic groups. The extrinsic muscles (flexors and extensors) originate in the forearm, whereas the intrinsic musculature originates within the hand proper. There are 21 extrinsic muscles and 19 intrinsic muscles. The extrinsic group is comprised of 5 pronation-supination muscles, 6 muscles of wrist flexion-extension, and 10 muscles that provide finger flexion or extension. The intrinsic muscles are the 7 interossei, 4 lumbricals, the adductor pollicis, the 4 thenar and 3 hypothenar intrinsics, plus the highly variable, rudimentary, and functionless palmaris brevis.

Extrinsic Muscles

The extensor-supinator group is innervated by the radial nerve; these muscles originate at the distal humerus and its lateral epicondyle. This is a frequent site of elbow pain due to lateral epicondylitis (tennis elbow). The "mobile wad" consists of the three muscles that originate in the area of the lateral epicondyle: the brachioradialis and the extensors carpi radialis longus and brevis. Persistent pain in this area that is recalcitrant to conservative or even surgical treatment of "tennis elbow" may be due to a neuritis of the nearby radial nerve.

The extensor muscles in the posterior compartment of the forearm can be anatomically divided into a superficial and a deep layer. The superficial layer consists of the digital extensors as well as the extensors carpi radialis longus and brevis (Fig. 3). In the deep layer, which lies on the interosseous membrane, are the muscles of thumb abduction-extension as well

as the extensor indicis proprius. The posterior interosseous nerve lies in the deep compartment and courses through the forearm between the abductor pollicis longus and extensor pollicis longus. The extensor muscles narrow into tendons in the middle and distal forearm. These 12 units course beneath the extensor retinaculum at the wrist, where they are separated into 6 compartments. Roughly corresponding to the finger flexor fibero-osseous canals ("finger pulleys") anteriorly, the extensor retinaculum keeps the digital extensor tendons close to the axis of rotation of the wrist dorsally to prevent bowstringing or tendon prolapse. Gliding of both the extrinsic flexor and extensor tendons is facilitated and occurs with minimal friction, because a thin layer of paratenon covers the tendons in unrestricted areas. Interestingly, in restricted areas—beneath the extensor retinaculum or within the carpal tunnel and fibro-osseous canals of the fingers—the tendons are covered by synovium. Inflammation of this very vascular synovium is often masked early on by the restricting fibrous tissue surrounding the tendons.

The thumb extensors pass through the first and third dorsal compartments. The two tendons of the first compartment, abductor pollicis longus and extensor pollicis brevis, are prone to tendinitis or entrapment beneath the unyielding extensor retinaculum (de Quervain's tenosynovitis). The thumb's long extensor, the extensor pollicis longus (EPL), lies in the third dorsal compartment. As it passes around Lister's tubercle, the line of pull is changed. Hyperextension of the thumb's IP joint is not possible without a functioning EPL. The EPL is the sole resident of the third dorsal extensor compartment; as such, it has a great tendency toward early retraction when lacerated. The tendons of the first and third compartment are the volar and dorsal borders of the radial (anatomical) snuff box, which forms an important landmark for identification of the radial styloid, scaphoid, and thumb basal joint. The wrist extensors lie in the second (extensor carpi radialis longus and brevis) and sixth compartments (extensor carpi ulnaris). These tendons modulate, by wrist tenodesis effect, the amplitude of the extrinsic finger flexor system. Active contraction of the wrist extensors places the extrinsic finger flexors at a biomechanical advantage for manipulating small objects or gripping. Wrist extension essentially removes slack from the flexor system, allowing strong finger flexion.

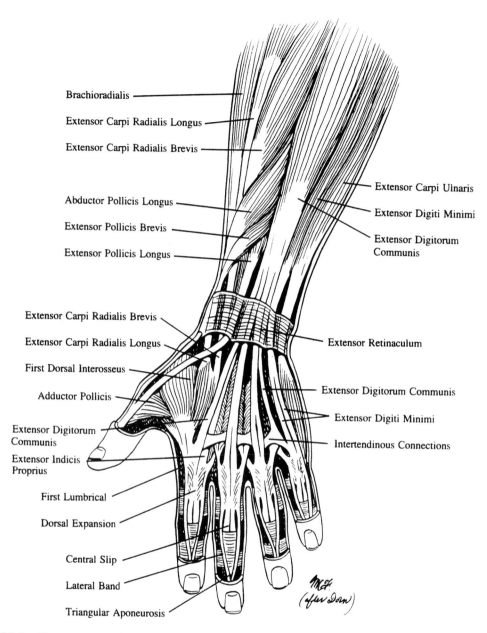

Brachioradialis

Extensor Carpi Radialis Longus

Extensor Carpi Radialis Brevis

Abductor Pollicis Longus

Extensor Pollicis Brevis

Extensor Pollicis Longus

Extensor Carpi Radialis Brevis

Extensor Carpi Radialis Longus

First Dorsal Interosseus

Adductor Pollicis

Extensor Digitorum Communis

Extensor Indicis Proprius

First Lumbrical

Dorsal Expansion

Central Slip

Lateral Band

Triangular Aponeurosis

Extensor Carpi Ulnaris

Extensor Digiti Minimi

Extensor Digitorum Communis

Extensor Retinaculum

Extensor Digitorum Communis

Extensor Digiti Minimi

Intertendinous Connections

FIGURE 3.   The extensor muscles of the forearm. (Reprinted with permission from Grad JB: Hand anatomy and physical examination, Pt II. Surg Rounds Orthop 3(7):27, 1989.)

Simultaneously, relaxation of extrinsic digital extensors, the antagonists, facilitates grasping large objects. The extensor carpi radialis brevis is the prime wrist extensor. Its insertion at the base of the third metacarpal is more central and the greatest distance from the axis of rotation of the wrist. The extensor carpi radialis longus and extensor carpi ulnaris are primarily deviators of the wrist; they insert at the bases of the second and fifth metacarpals, respec-

tively. The extensor carpi ulnaris contracts synergistically with the two radial wrist extensors when the forearm is supinated. When the forearm is in a position of pronation, the extensor carpi ulnaris acts synergistically with the flexor carpi ulnaris.

Palpating Lister's tubercle (the small prominence on the dorsal aspect of the radius immediately proximal to the wrist joint) facilitates individual identification of the extensor compartments. The second compartment lies on the radial side, and the third compartment, containing the EPL, on the ulnar side of the tubercle. Recognizing this is helpful when making diagnoses or planning surgical incisions for wrist procedures.

The extensors of the fingers lie in the fourth (extensor digitorum communis and extensor indicis proprius) and fifth (extensor digiti minimi) compartments. They are the extensors of the MCP joints and contribute to IP extension when the MCP joints are stabilized in flexion. The extrinsic extensors attach to the sagittal fibers, the extensor hood of the MCP joints, as well as the dorsal capsule. Their bony attachment is at their insertion into the extensor tubercle at the base of the middle phalanx via the central slip. Traumatic disruption of the central slip or its attenuation due to chronic synovitis at the proximal IP joint leads to a "boutonnière" deformity.

A similar disruption of the extensor system at the distal IP joint results in an extension lag or "mallet finger." This is often the initiating cause of a swan-neck deformity, which is characterized by an extension lag at the distal joint and a hyperextension or recurvatum at the proximal IP joint. It is essentially the reverse of the boutonnière deformity.

The flexor muscles occupy the anterior compartment of the forearm. They originate from the area of the medial epicondyle of the humerus and proximal ulna. Functionally these muscles are known as the flexor-pronator group. All are innervated by the median nerve except the flexor carpi ulnaris and flexor digitorum profundi of the ring and small fingers, which are controlled by the ulnar nerve. The flexor-pronator muscle group is arranged in the anterior compartment such that the pronator teres and wrist flexors (flexor carpi radialis, palmaris longus, and flexor carpi ulnaris) are most superficial and lie just deep to the antebrachial fascia. The digital superficial flexors form the next layer, and the profundi along with the EPL lie deep within the compartment on the interosseous membrane and forearm bones.

The muscles of the extrinsic digital flexors become tendons chiefly in the distal third of the forearm. These nine tendons (four sublimi, four profundi, and the single flexor pollicis longus) along with the median nerve comprise the contents of the carpal tunnel. As stated previously, the carpal tunnel is a small and rigid compartment that is the most frequent site of median nerve compressions. In the classic carpal tunnel syndrome, the compression is due to inflammation and swelling of the musculotendinous structures. Within the carpal tunnel, the median nerve lies palmar to the nine flexor tendons; it is vulnerable to repetitive stress because the finger flexor tendons press upon it. Its vulnerability is pronounced with activities involving simultaneous flexion of the wrist.

After passing through the carpal tunnel, the flexor tendons transverse the palm through loose tissues until they enter the digital fibro-osseous sheaths at the level of the distal palmar crease on the surface. The fibro-osseous canal has five strong, transversely oriented annular pulleys and three flexible cruciate components, which are obliquely oriented (Fig. 4). These structures are biomechanically essential to function because they prevent bowstringing and flexor tendon prolapse during active digital flexion.

From a biomechanical and clinical standpoint, the second and fourth annular portions of the digital flexor tendon sheaths are the most important. These critical "pulleys" are located at the proximal aspect of the proximal phalanx (A2) and the middle of the middle phalanx (A4). Great care always must be taken to preserve these structures because secondary reconstruction never completely restores normal finger mechanics. The superficialis tendons decussate at the base of each finger to form two broad and flat slips that cross deep to the profundus tendon and insert into the middle phalanx. The profundus tendon, which is the more superficial tendon in the finger proper, inserts into the proximal half of the distal phalanx distal to the volar plate attachment. Whereas isolated rupture of a sublimis tendon is a most rare occurrence, rupture of the profundus tendon is not uncommon; it happens often in contact sports such as football.

Strong grasp is dependent upon stabilization of the MCP joints and contraction of the extrinsic finger flexors, which are three times as powerful as the extensors. This is synergistically accompanied by wrist extension, except for objects of very large diameter. Although the extrinsic wrist flexors are very much stronger than the wrist extensors, the biomechanical effect of wrist tenodesis—that is, extension of the wrist with grasp—is the factor of greatest importance. Flexion of the fingers normally proceeds from the proximal interphalangeal (PIP) joints to the MCP joints and finally to

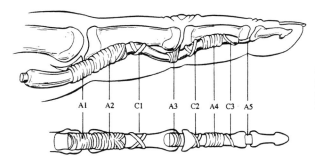

FIGURE 4. The fibro-osseous pulley system. (Reprinted with permission from Grad JB: Hand anatomy and physical examination, Pt II. Surg Rounds Orthop 3(7):29, 1989.)

the distal IP joints. These closely synchronous movements of the normal hand are dramatically changed in the presence of intrinsic palsies resulting from median and ulnar nerve lesions. With palsy, flexion begins at the distal IP joint and proceeds to the PIP and finally the MCP joint. The finger is "rolled up" because the IP joints are fully flexed before MCP joint flexion begins, and space for effective gripping is essentially lost. Clawing or hyperextension of the MCP joints causes even greater loss of the important digital flexion arc. This is so despite the seemingly small contribution— only 5%—to the flexion arc that occurs at the distal joint; 20% at the PIP level, and 75% at the MCP joint level.

Intrinsic Muscles

The intrinsic muscles of the hand proper may be divided into functional and anatomic groups— that is, thenar, hypothenar, and interosseous-lumbrical. The thenar intrinsics, controlling thumb position and power, are both median and ulnar innervated. The median-innervated group, lying radial to the flexor pollicis longus tendon, are the opponens pollicis, abductor pollicis brevis, and flexor pollicis brevis (superficial head). They are primarily positioners of the thumb's basal joint. The adductor pollicis, flexor pollicis brevis (deep head), and first dorsal interosseous, all ulnar innervated, give the thumb its characteristically powerful key pinch. The flexor pollicis brevis has a superficial median-innervated and deep ulnar-innervated portion. The deep portion of the flexor brevis lies ulnar to the flexor pollicis longus along with the adductor pollicis and first dorsal interosseous muscles. The thumb's unique ability for power pinch is primarily a function of the flexor pollicis longus and adductor pol-

licis muscles. It is important to realize that a 1-kg force of pinch at the thumb's tip generates a joint compression force of 12 kg on the carpometacarpal articulation at the thumb's base. This explains why the thumb's basal joint is the most frequent site for symptomatic arthritis to develop.

The hypothenar intrinsic muscles are ulnar innervated. They control opposition of the small finger as well as MCP flexion and IP extension. The hypothenar intrinsics are the opponens digit minimi, flexor digiti minimi, and abductor digiti minimi.

The interosseous-lumbrical group controls finger abduction-adduction as well as MCP flexion and IP joint extension. The seven interosseous muscles lie between the metacarpals, and their tendons, the lateral bands, run volar to the axis of rotation of the MCP joints. Like the lumbricals, the interossei are MCP flexors and IP joint extensors. The four dorsal interossei are bipenate abductors, whereas the three volar interossei are unipenate adductors. These movements are named in relation to the middle finger position. Although the interossei contribute to IP joint extension, the lumbricals are the prime intrinsic extensors. The four lumbricals originate from the profundus tendons in the palm just distal to the carpal tunnel. Those of the index and middle finger are median innervated, whereas those of the ring and small fingers are ulnar supplied.

The contributions of intrinsic and extrinsic extensors vary with MCP joint positioning, but the intrinsic system is the IP extensor. Lacerations of the median and ulnar nerves result in a complete intrinsic palsy and anesthesia to the hand's working surface. Impairment is so severe as to be almost a physiological amputation of the hand. It is impossible either to grasp large objects effectively or to conduct precision manipulations.

NEUROLOGICAL SYSTEM

The upper extremity receives its nerve supply through five peripheral nerves that are extensions of the brachial plexus. The roots of the nerves are cervical 5 through thoracic 1. The roots form three cores—medial, lateral, and posterior—named for their relationship to the axillary artery. Medial and lateral cords represent the anterior divisions of the nerve trunks, and the posterior cord represents the posterior divisions.

The medial cord gives rise to the ulnar nerve and part of the median, and the lateral cord gives rise to the rest of the median and the musculocutaneous nerve. The radial and axillary nerves are extensions of the posterior cord. Although variations exist, the usual root contribution to each nerve is the following: C5–6, axillary nerve; C7–8, radial nerve; C5–6, musculocutaneous nerve; C8–T1, ulnar nerve. Because the median nerve is formed by both the medial and lateral cords, it usually receives fibers from the entire plexus, cervical 5 through thoracic 1.

The axillary nerve innervates the deltoid muscle for shoulder abduction. The musculocutaneous nerve supplies the three muscles of the arm's anterior compartment. The coracobrachialis has adduction of the arm as its primary function, and the biceps and brachialis are elbow flexors. The radial nerve innervates the triceps, which extends the elbow via its insertion into the olecranon process of the ulnar.

Sensibility of the upper extremity is essentially supplied by four cervical routes. The midline of the sagittal plane of the arm and forearm is the root supply division. For the arm, C5 and T2 are the primary roots for skin sensibility of the lateral and medial aspects, respectively. The distribution terminates at approximately elbow level. Forearm sensibility is innervated by routes C6 and T1 for the lateral and medial aspects, respectively. These are the areas supplied by the medial and lateral antebrachial cutaneous nerves from the elbow to the wrist.

The hand receives innervation from three major nerves: the radial, median, and ulnar. Functional names describe simply the complex and important contributions of each. Myriad variations of these nerves are possible; knowing the terminal muscle supply and the autonomous zone of sensibility for each is essential for clear interpretation of physical findings. The radial nerve is appropriately termed the "preparatory nerve." It strategically positions the hand in preparation for a task. It courses distally in the arm beneath the triceps and pierces the intermuscular septum at the distal third of the humerus. The nerve enters the anterior compartment of the arm, where it lies between the brachialis and brachioradialis muscles. The radial nerve innervates the 12 muscles of wrist and extrinsic finger extensions. Whether loss of these functions is partial or complete depends on the exact site of injury—that is, on whether the radial palsy is "high" or "low." The muscles of the mobile wad (the brachioradialis and the extensors carpi radialis longus and brevis) are innervated by the branches of the radial nerve arising from it proximal to the elbow. A "high" radial palsy results in a complete loss of wrist and thumb extension as well as finger MCP extension. Sensibility is also lost on the dorsoradial aspect of the hand. A "low" radial palsy is exclusively a motor loss causing inability to extend the fingers at the MCP level and the thumb at the IP joint. "Low" radial palsy is due to injury or compression of the posterior interosseous nerve, a branch of the radial nerve that takes origin usually about 3 cm distal to the elbow. The superficial radial nerve is solely sensory and is not affected with a "low" (posterior interosseous nerve) radial palsy. Sensibility on the dorsal surface of the hand remains normal.

The posterior interosseous nerve lies beneath the supinator muscle in the proximal forearm and, somewhat like the cauda equina, branches at the muscle's distal aspect. It then innervates 10 of the 12 extensor muscles of the forearm, whose tendons course distally beneath the extensor retinaculum. Only the radial wrist extensors of compartment II (the extensors carpi radialis longus and brevis) are not innervated by the posterior interosseous nerve. With a complete low radial palsy, wrist extension is preserved, yet it occurs with noticeable radial deviation of the hand because of loss of the counterbalancing force with extensor carpi ulnaris paralysis.

The median nerve is the most important structure in the upper extremity and is functionally named the "precision manipulator." In the arm it lies anterior to the brachial artery and courses medial to the coracobrachialis and biceps muscles. The median nerve with the brachial artery enters the forearm through a sphincter formed by the lacertus fibrosus (anteriomedially), biceps (laterally), and pronator teres. The nerve courses in the forearm in the intermuscular plane between the superficialis and profundus muscles. At the wrist it is very superficial, directly under the palmaris longus tendon and the antebrachial fascia. Its entrance to the carpal tunnel is immediately radial to the tendon of the superficial flexor of the middle finger.

The median nerve provides sensibility to the working surfaces of the thumb, index finger, middle finger, and usually the radial half of the ring finger. The median nerve controls the radial group of thenar muscles involved with thumb opposition or positioning and all of the functionally independent sublimi, the flexor pollicis longus, and the profundi of the index and middle fingers.

A high median palsy causes loss of sensibility to the radial three fingers along with intrinsic muscle and extrinsic flexor palsies. A low median palsy results in a similar pattern of anesthesia, but IP (proximal and distal) thumb-finger flexion is not affected. The low median palsy such as is seen with injuries at the level of the carpal tunnel causes loss of median innervated thenar intrinsic function and paralysis of the radial two lumbricals. Compression of the median nerve can occur at various levels of the forearm or at the carpal tunnel. The palmar cutaneous branch of the median nerve separates from the main trunk at approximately 6 cm proximal to the distal wrist crease. It gives skin sensibility to the base of the thenar eminence immediately radial to the major thenar crease. Because this area is not affected by median nerve compression at the carpal tunnel alone, disturbance of skin sensibility in this area indicates that at least some component of the neuropathy is proximal to the wrist. The pronator teres syndrome is essentially a "high" carpal tunnel syndrome. It involves disturbance of sensibility in the radial three-and-one-half fingers as well as in the area supplied by the palmar cutaneous branch of the median nerve. The pronator teres syndrome can be caused by median nerve compression in the proximal forearm at various sites—for example, the lacertus fibrosus, pronator teres, or the fibrous arch of origin of the sublimis muscles. Nerve disorder of an established carpal tunnel syndrome is typically an axonotmesis, whereas proximal compression more often resembles neurapraxia.

The anterior interosseous nerve is a branch of the median nerve that arises from its posterior side in the proximal forearm, usually at about 5–8 cm distal to the elbow. The anterior interosseous branch innervates four muscles: the flexor pollicis longus, the profundi to the index and middle fingers, and the pronator quadratus. Disturbances of this nerve cause loss or weakness of terminal flexion of the thumb or index finger. Remember that selective injuries or neuropathies of the anterior interosseous nerve do not cause disturbance of skin sensibility, because this nerve is exclusively a motor nerve.

Functionally, the ulnar nerve is the power coordinator. It courses through the arm in a common neurovascular bundle, along with the brachial artery, median, and medial antebrachial cutaneous nerves, between the coracobrachialis and triceps. The ulnar nerve is medial to the brachial artery and posterior to the brachial vein. In the distal forearm, the nerve passes through the intermuscular septum before entering the cubital tunnel of the elbow. Immediately distal to the elbow, the ulnar nerve enters the forearm between the two heads of the flexor carpi ulnaris and descends toward the wrist between flexor carpi ulnaris and profundus muscles. In the midforearm, the ulnar artery joins with the ulnar nerve and is anteromedial to it as they enter Guyon's canal of the wrist.

The ulnar nerve innervates the profundi and lumbrical muscles of the ring and small finger. In addition, the ulnar nerve controls the hypothenar intrinsics, the adductor pollicis, the first dorsal interosseous, and the two ulnar lumbricals. The seven interosseous muscles are also ulnar-innervated. The ulnar nerve provides sensibility to the small finger and the ulnar half of the ring finger on both their palmar and dorsal aspects.

It is important to note that the ulnar nerve also has a palmar cutaneous branch, which, however, is much more variable in size than the corresponding branch of the median nerve. This sensory nerve branches from the main ulnar nerve in the distal forearm and follows a course superficial to the ulnar artery. It distributes to part of the hypothenar eminence and with injury can form symptomatic neuromas.

It is usually possible to differentiate clinically a "high" (elbow level) from a "low" (wrist level) ulnar palsy. A low ulnar lesion disturbs sensibility to the volar surface of the small finger and weakens or destroys ulnar-innervated intrinsics. Ulnar intrinsic strength is best assessed by measuring key pinch between thumb and side of index finger. If compression is solely at the wrist level, sensibility is normal over the dorsum of the fifth metacarpal as the dorsal branch of the nerve leaves the main trunk proximal to the wrist. A high ulnar palsy is present when sensibility is disturbed on the dorsal ulnar surface of the hand as well as the working surfaces of the small finger and the small finger profundus is weak.

In summary, the autonomous zones of sensibility for the three nerves are as follows: radial nerve, dorsoradial aspect of the first web; median nerve, tip of the index finger; ulnar nerve, tip of the small finger. The terminal muscle supplied by the radial nerve is the extensor indicis proprius. The terminal muscles supplied by the median and ulnar nerves are the abductor pollicis brevis and first dorsal interosseous muscles, respectively.

NEUROVASCULAR SYSTEM

The brachial artery is the primary vessel of the upper extremity. It is the direct continuation of the axillary artery and is so named when it exits from the axilla at the lower border of the teres major. The brachial artery bifurcates in the proximal forearm into the radial and ulnar arteries. Although the radial artery is usually more readily palpable at the wrist, the ulnar artery is the dominant vessel to the hand.

The radial artery's first-named branch at the wrist is the palmar carpal artery, which supplies the distal radius and the proximal carpal row. The next main branch is the superficial palmar artery. This artery is often palpable at the base of the thenar eminence and is particularly vulnerable during falls upon the heel of the hand. The main branch of the superficial palmar artery is the princeps pollicis artery. The radial artery courses through the snuff box between the scaphoid and trapezium, where it may be vulnerable to injury during surgical procedures on the radial aspect of the carpus. After passing between the two heads of the first dorsal interosseous muscle, the radial artery turns toward the palm and is then termed the princeps pollicis (Fig. 5). This gives rise to the proper digital arteries of the thumb, which usually are two in number but the radial side may be absent. The princeps pollicis terminates with a contribution to the superficial palmar arterial arch.

The radial artery and nerve lie near each other at the elbow but are separated at the wrist. This is the reverse of the relationship between the ulnar artery and nerve. In the distal forearm the ulnar artery is superficial and just radial to the ulnar nerve. The ulnar nerve lies beneath the flexor carpi ulnaris tendon, which is a helpful landmark for ulnar nerve anesthetic blocks at the wrist. Within Guyon's canal the artery remains anterior to the nerve and then courses laterally around the hook of the hamate to give rise to the superficial palmar arch. The arch lies beneath the palmar aponeurosis and traverses the palm, approximately 1 cm proximal to the proximal palmar crease. The superficial palmar arch gives rise to the common and proper digital arteries, which in the palm are superficial to the corresponding nerves.

Each finger has a dominant artery, usually on the ulnar side of the radial two fingers and on the radial side of the ulnar two fingers. As noted, arteries to the fingers are anterior to the nerves in the palm, but at the level of the natatory ligaments, which are immediately distal to the distal palmar crease, the nerves become superficial. Throughout the finger the digital nerves are anterior to the arteries. The neurovascular bundles in the fingers lie within a compartment formed by skin ligaments. Anteriorly these ligaments are named Grayson's ligaments, and they have an oblique orientation; dorsally they are Cleland's ligaments, which are oriented transversely. Recognition of these ligaments during surgery facilitates rapid identification and safe dissection along the neurovascular bundles.

Venous drainage of the upper extremity occurs in a retrograde fashion via deep and superficial systems. The latter is of greater importance and is readily apparent on the dorsoradial aspect of the hand. The veins have check valves that permit flow only proximally toward the heart's right atrium. Although hand elevation is helpful to reduce edema, venous return is effective only when elevation is accompanied by active muscle contractions. The lymphatic drainage of the hand has a random

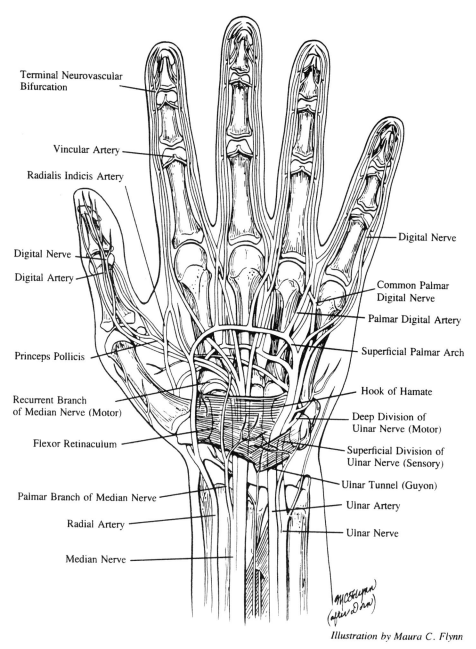

Terminal Neurovascular
Bifurcation

Vincular Artery

Radialis Indicis Artery

Digital Nerve

Digital Artery

Princeps Pollicis

Recurrent Branch
of Median Nerve (Motor)

Flexor Retinaculum

Palmar Branch of Median Nerve

Radial Artery

Median Nerve

Digital Nerve

Common Palmar
Digital Nerve

Palmar Digital Artery

Superficial Palmar Arch

Hook of Hamate

Deep Division of
Ulnar Nerve (Motor)

Superficial Division of
Ulnar Nerve (Sensory)

Ulnar Tunnel (Guyon)

Ulnar Artery

Ulnar Nerve

Illustration by Maura C. Flynn

FIGURE 5. The neurovascular system of the hand. (Reprinted with permission from Grad JB: Hand anatomy and physical examination. Surg Rounds Orthop 3(8):37, 1989.)

arrangement. It travels basically with the venous system proximally in a rather predictable course toward the nodal collections at the elbow and axilla. The lymphatics of the radial three fingers drain primarily to the axillary nodes, whereas the ulnar two fingers drain into the epitrocheal elbow region. This drainage pattern is apparent in the patient with an infection accompanied by an ascending lymphangitis.

SKIN AND FINGERNAILS

The palmar and dorsal skin of the hand are quite different. Fibrous septae from periosteum firmly attach to the palmar skin, making it less mobile than dorsal skin and enhancing the hand's abilities during forceful grasp. The palmar skin is thick and inelastic compared with skin on the dorsal side, and its blood supply is oriented vertically. Dorsally the vascular orientation is basically horizontal branching, which makes elevation safe and rotation of flaps easier.

The palmar skin has a dense concentration of sensory end organs, which can be readily apparent when the patient's static two-point discrimination is assessed. A distance of 5 mm or less is normal for fingertips compared with approximately twice that distance at the corresponding areas of the dorsum of the hand.

The fingernail, a specialized skin appendage, is an important structure. The nailbed, which forms the nail plate, has two major components. The primary area of metabolic activity, cell growth, and plate production is the germinal matrix. Most of the germinal matrix is proximal to the cuticle, and its most distal extension is the opaque lunula. The pink portion beneath the nail plate, distal to the lunula, is the sterile matrix, which makes only a small contribution to nail growth but provides secure plate fixation. Fortunately, it is the sterile rather than germinal matrix that is most often injured.

CONCLUSION

As experienced is gained, the serious student of the hand becomes increasingly impressed with the beauty and complexity of hand function. A carefully elicited history followed by a physical examination based on thorough knowledge of anatomy are the most important steps toward consistently correct diagnosis and optimal treatment of hand disorders.

REFERENCES

1. Beasley RW: Hand Injuries. Philadelphia, W. B. Saunders, 1981.
2. Grad JB: Hand anatomy and physical examination, parts I–III. Surg Rounds Orthop 3(6):25, 3(7):27, 3(8):37, 1989.
3. Hollinshead WH: Textbook of Anatomy, 4th ed. New York, Harper & Row, 1985.
4. Littler JW: Reconstructive Plastic Surgery, Vol. VI. Philadelphia, W. B. Saunders, 1977.
5. Tubiana R: The Hand, Vol. I–III. Philadelphia, W. B. Saunders, 1981–1988.

Chapter 6

PSYCHOLOGICAL EVALUATION OF HAND PAIN

Richard K. Johnson, Ph.D.

Pain behaviors are interesting social communications, the meanings of which remain to be discovered in the individual case.

Fordyce, "Pain and Suffering"

There are few problems more worthy of human endeavor than the relief of pain and suffering.

Melzack, The Puzzle of Pain

Recovery from injury or disease is a multifaceted process involving physical, psychological, social, economic, and legal factors. Psychological evaluations of the psychosocial factors that can either complicate recovery or aid in rehabilitation add valuable diagnostic and therapeutic information about a patient.[22,23] Boyes encourages hand surgeons to appreciate the variety of psychological problems experienced by patients with hand disabilities and injuries and voices his hope that the surgery of the hand not become "an exercise in mechanics."[5]

Oliver Sack, a neurologist, wrote his "neurological novel," *A Leg to Stand On*, to recount his experiences after a hiking accident in which he sustained severe injuries to the muscles and nerves of one leg.[38] He describes the "business of being a patient," illuminating many psychological processes and problems he faced in his rehabilitation. "One had to go back, one had to regress, for one might indeed be as helpless as a child, whether one liked it, or willed it, or not" (p. 165).

Mendelson et al. describe the psychological impact of traumatic amputations, highlighting issues of identity and competence.[32] They show that the patient's perception of loss, acceptance of deformity, and ability to adapt determine the degree of disability. They quote Grant: "We pursue our vocation—and perhaps our avocation—as bimanual creatures. We caress our loved ones with the hand, we greet a friend or acknowledge an individual with the right hand. Loss of these capabilities diminishes the inner individual (p. 578)."

Recovery from a physical injury or disease requires more than physical healing. Issues of body image and identity, employability and physical activity, and possible changes in ability to fulfill familial and social roles need to be evaluated and dealt with. Anxiety, depression, pain, discouragement, faulty thinking, distrust, and noncompliance are some of the factors that many exacerbate or prolong physical illness or injury.[8]

75

As Millon points out, "Depending on prior experience, health status, and personality disposition, one individual may interpret a series of potentially troublesome circumstances as a positive challenge rather than as a disruption that portends danger. In essence, objective 'stress' means nothing unless the person apprehends it as such."[33] An evaluation of how that individual perceives his or her physical damage as affecting functioning is critical.

Psychological assessments need to be made in a timely and sensitive fashion. Timely psychosocial evaluations have been seen as critical ingredients in the successful and cost-effective care of back pain.[40] Deyo argues that an early identification of psychosocial factors contributing to an injured worker's rehabilitation enhances outcome and reduces long-term incapacitation and disability.[12] The rationale for a psychological evaluation needs to be communicated. It should be explained that the medical personnel want to understand how the disease or injury has affected the patient in order to develop the most effective treatment intervention in view of the patient's unique needs and coping resources. The referral for assessment can communicate to patients that they are being taken seriously and personally and not as just more injured hands or arms. The role of stress in health should be outlined to the patients to let them know that there are common reactions to stressful injuries and illnesses and that discussing and understanding them can be beneficial.

A referral to a psychologist sometimes triggers the thought: "They think I'm crazy and the pain is all in my head." People who have experienced a physical injury already have a lowered sense of personal effectiveness. They feel especially apprehensive about participating in a psychological evaluation at a time when their own self-worth has been damaged. Usually when it is explained that no two people react to the same injury in exactly the same way and that the medical treatment team want to discover the best way of treating this patient by obtaining thorough information, the patient's anxiety declines. Such an assessment allows patients to explore and to see how a variety of psychosocial factors affect their condition and improvement.

For patients known as somatizers, any referral to a mental health professional is seen as an insult or challenge to the authenticity of their somatic symptoms. Wickramasekera points out that somatizers prefer a medical diagnosis to a psychiatric or psychological one.[47] He argues that the perception of psychosocial conflicts as physical symptoms in these patients is reinforced by potent personal, social, vocational, and financial consequences. The somatic packaging of psychosocial conflicts increases their reimbursability and social acceptance as true patients.

Wickramasekera, in describing somatizing patients as ones who experience mental conflicts as physical symptoms and who seek medical diagnoses, therapy, and cure, suggests that referrals for psychological services are unacceptable to these patients because they may be unaware (1) that psychosocial factors operate in their situation, (2) that mental and emotional changes can trigger physiological responses, and (3) that they may be in a "fight-or-flight" stress mode.

I have previously discussed my experience indicating that patients receive relief through participating in psychological evaluations after injuries because the process is the first time they thoroughly tell their story.[22] They describe not only their injury and pain, but also the complications and disruptions the injury caused in their lives. One injured worker, after an extensive medical diagnostic workup, used the psychological evaluation to relate his feeling that the medical team, insurance adjustors, and his company's officials were only interested in isolated aspects of his situation. He thought that medical and work personnel were not interested in hearing how traumatic and stressful the hand injury was, not only to his physical functioning, but also to his mental and social health.

DIAGNOSTIC ISSUES

Three articles in the occupational medicine/hand surgery and therapy literature serve as an introduction to diagnostic issues involved in assessing patients with physical injuries who display psychological symptoms.

Simmons and Vasile describe the "clenched fist syndrome," which they view as a conversion phenomenon.[39] The patient presents for an evaluation of swelling due to trauma, which often is of a rather benign nature. The fingers are noted to be tightly held within the palm, and the wrist is also held in a flexed position. Attempts to extend the fingers result in pain, although the finger flexors can be felt to contract when passive extension is attempted. Laboratory tests are normal, as are an electromyogram (EMG) and nerve conduction studies. Under anesthesia, the hand easily falls into extension. In reflex sympathetic dystrophy (RSD), however, the hand has limited flexion and extension even under anesthesia. Simmons and Vasile conclude that the clenched fist is a symbolic expression of repressed anger. "The hand bound into a fist symbolically expresses anger, yet keeps it in check by 'paralyzing' the dominant hand" (p. 426).

Hardy and Merritt, in a study examining psychological and pain factors in patients with reflex sympathetic dystrophy (RSD), conclude that emotional factors are important in this medical condition.[18] RSD is a symptom complex characterized by chronic unexplained pain and associated evidence of autonomic nervous system dysfunction that is out of proportion to the extent of injury. The pain in RSD is variable (it can occur at rest or with motion, is aggravated by single or multiple stimuli, and radiates proximally or distally or both) and may be an indication of malingering or compensation neurosis. RSD resembles hysteria in that symptoms spread beyond known anatomical limits. The withdrawn position of the arm has been given the name "hysterical hand" by psychiatrists. Hardy and Merritt find RSD patients anxious and depressed, they complain more frequently of somatic distress, and they relate poorly interpersonally, as compared with hand-injured patients without signs of RSD.

Stokes reports an objective method of documenting real, as opposed to fictitious, loss of grip.[43] He describes malingerers as those with psychological rather than organic disability; they can voluntarily record lower grip measurements in the so-called injured hand than in the normal hand. He reports that the patient who voluntarily demonstrates weakness of grip applies the same minimal pressure at each of the adjustable handle positions of the sealed hydraulic dynamometer.

Conversion reaction, hysteria, and malingering have been mentioned in the three previous studies. Definitions and diagnostic distinctions need to be made among those terms, as well as among factitious disorders, somatoform disorders (the somatizers previously mentioned), compensation neurosis, Munchausen syndrome, hypochondriasis, and psychogenic pain disorder.

Post-traumatic stress disorder can develop in people who have been seriously traumatized by an injury. Psychological symptoms of anxiety and depression can develop as a response to traumatic injury. Workers who have sustained extensive burns or lost extremities genuinely experience phobic reactions to situations like those in which the injuries occurred. I have evaluated utility linemen who have been electrocuted on the job and whose fear of returning to work on the lines prevents them from continuing as linemen. Doubts about their safety as well as the safety of their co-workers permeate their thinking. Intrusive thoughts and recollections of the accident can interfere with daily functioning. Recurrent dreams of the trauma, as well as feeling that the traumatic event is recurring, are symptoms of increased arousal, manifested as sleep difficulties, exaggerated startle responses, and increased irritability. Psychological intervention is warranted to assist the person to cope with the symptoms and to overcome a developing avoidance behavior pattern.

The **factitious disorders** are characterized by a pattern of complaints of psychological or physical symptoms that is totally intentionally produced or feigned. People who enjoy and seek out illness and find the role of a patient emotionally rewarding may or may not be motivated by financial gain. The **Munchausen syndrome**, the classic factitious disorder, usually focuses on physical rather than psychological symptoms. The motivation is idiosyncratic, usually unconscious, and typically involves a need to gratify dependency needs through being cared for in a medical setting. Munchausen patients inject themselves with substances to cause infection, take drugs to produce body rashes, and feign bodily pains to imitate medical conditions such as heart attacks or kidney stones. The total fabrication, self-infliction of damage, or exacerbation of an existing injury implies serious psychopathology, usually a personality disorder. (The syndrome gets its name from Baron Karl Friedrich von Munchausen, an 18th-century German cavalry officer who lied extravagantly.)

Malingering patients also produce symptoms intentionally, but their goal is more easily recognized; they usually want to avoid standing trial or going into the military. Sometimes the secondary gain is not avoidance but the receipt of some form of financial remuneration. The motivation is largely conscious to the patient.

Compensation neurosis is a need to be rewarded for being sick or injured. Walsh and Dumitru suggest that financial compensation may discourage a return to work.[46] During litigation, the patient's pain behavior may be reinforced, maximized, and groomed with the intent of increasing the final settlement. As a result of this reinforcement, the pain behavior develops into a learned response and becomes the disability for which the patient seeks compensation. Walsh and Dumitru argue that compensation factors may delay recovery, prolong symptoms, and reinforce sick-role behavior. If patients believe they need to continue to demonstrate injury, pain, and suffering, their lack of recovery and continued reporting of pain experiences have probably become associated with an effort to show their loss.

Conversion reactions, hypochondriasis, somatization disorders, and psychogenic pain disorders are classified as **somatoform disorders** in the Diagnostic and Statistical Manual of Mental Disorders, 3rd edition, revised (DSM-III-R).[2] The symptoms are not intentionally produced, as in malingering and factitious disorders. They are not under voluntary control. The somatic symptoms suggest a physical disorder for which there are no organic findings or identifiable physiological bases. The process involves converting emotional stresses and pressures into physiological responses. In many cases, the referral for psychological assessment is not so much to help with the diagnosis, which is more or less apparent, as to help identify the sources of the stress and offer interventions to patients that will help them learn better ways of handling the stress.

Conversion disorders, sometimes referred to as hysterical neuroses, conversion type, involve the alteration or actual loss of physical functioning. Patients are not consciously aware of their responsibility for the change in physical functioning. The symptoms are related to a significant conflict. Patients can use somatic symptoms to express deeper emotional tensions or to compensate for some intense emotion. Histrionic (hysterical) or dependent personality traits may be present.

Patients exhibiting conversion disorders deny psychological difficulties in spite of conflicts that are apparent to others. The conflicts are often expressed in a body language that symbolizes the actual problem. Impairments such as blindness, deafness, or paralysis are associated with things that are not to be seen, heard, or enacted. The clenched first syndrome is a good example of this process in an injured hand.[39]

Hypochondriacal patients are preoccupied with the fear of getting, or the belief that they already have, a serious disease, despite repeated medical reassurance to the contrary. Patients are so absorbed in the experience of illness that little else enters into their thinking or emotional life. Being ill compensates for a number of unfulfilled dependency needs and tends to occur in people with a personal or family history of illness. Strained doctor-patient relationships and doctor shopping are frequent. Interviews with such patients turn into monologues as the patients present "organ recitals" of their symptoms. Sternbach points out that most pain patients whose pain has a physical origin become somewhat hypochondriacal over a period of time.[42] Pain makes the patients so conscious of their bodies that they begin to notice and worry about other physical symptoms. When the pain persists, they start suspecting that they may have some serious disease that no one has found.

A somatization disorder is diagnosed when a patient presents recurrent and multiple somatic complaints of several years' duration and does so in dramatic and exaggerated ways. The DSM-III-R requires the presence of at least 13 symptoms from a list of 35, involving multiple body systems.[2] Some of the prototypic symptoms in this disorder include vomiting, shortness of breath when not exerting, difficulty swallowing, burning sensation in sexual organs other than during intercourse, and painful menstruation.

In somatoform (or psychogenic) pain disorders patients become preoccupied with pain in the absence of adequate physical findings to account for either the presence or the intensity of the pain. The patient refuses to consider the contribution of psychological factors, such as dependency, feelings of inadequacy, or family conflicts. Frequent visits to physicians to obtain relief despite medical reassurance, excessive use of analgesics without relief of pain, requests for surgical relief of pain, and the assumption of an invalid role can all be indications of a somatoform pain disorder.

When there is some related organic pathological condition, the complaint of pain is grossly in excess of what would be expected from the physical findings. According to the DSM-III-R, there is some evidence that among people with somatoform pain disorder, a greater proportion than would be expected began working at an unusually early age, held jobs that were physically strenuous or overly routinized, were workaholics, and rarely took vacations.[2]

PAIN AND SUFFERING

To avoid pain is to detour the essence of life itself—the choice for all of us is not if we will accept pain, but how.

Hansel, You Gotta Keep Dancin'

There's no coming to life without pain.

Jung

In clinical settings, the concepts of pain, suffering, and disability can become confounded. Fordyce distinguishes suffering as belonging to the person; disability, in contrast, is a legal judgment based on medical information regarding the extent of pain-related work dysfunction.[15] Drawing upon Loesser's formulation of pain,[28] Fordyce discusses four dimensions of the concept of pain.

Nociception is the mechanical, thermal, or chemical energy impinging on specialized nerve endings that in turn activate Aδ and C fibers to initiate a signal to the central nervous system that aversive events are occurring.

Pain is thought of as the sensation arising from the stimulation of perceived nociception. There is not a direct, one-to-one connection between nociception and the experiencing of pain. It is possible for pain to be perceived in the absence of nociception, as in phantom limb pain, and nociception may occur without being perceived, as when a soldier wounded in combat is unaware of the event for several hours.

Suffering is the affective response in the central nervous system triggered by nociception or other aversive event such as the loss of a loved one. Suffering is observed only indirectly from behavior that might imply it.

Pain behavior consists of the things people do when they suffer from pain. The actions may arise because of nociception or for other reasons.

Nociception and pain may be thought of as the input system, whereas suffering and pain behaviors may be seen as the response or output system. One can have severe pain with minimal functional limitation or disability; one can also have minimal pain with severe limitation.

Flor and Turk have shown that the empirical evidence supporting postulated pain mechanisms (e.g., inflammatory, structural, traumatic, muscular) is neither necessary nor sufficient for there to be complaints of chronic low-back pain.[14] Deyo, Diehl, and Rosenthal demonstrate that 2 days of rest for back injury leads to a better outcome than do 7 days of rest.[13] The prevention of chronicity studies by Fordyce have shown that specifying time points for an end to prescribed rest and the resumption of activity leads to a better outcome.[15] Fordyce argues that hurt (pain) and harm are not the same. That one hurts on moving does not necessarily mean that healing has not occurred or that residual injury is present. How much better a chronic pain patient gets depends mainly on how much the patient does. To remain convinced that pain and suffering are a symptom only keeps the patient coming back to the health care system for assistance. Fordyce, based on years of research and practice with pain patients, believes that "people who have something better to do don't suffer much."[15]

Sturgis points out that our society, which prizes success, comfort, speed, and efficiency, is not geared to settle for repair, pain, gradual recovery, or partial restoration of functioning.[44] How people deal with the loss involved in injury or disease of the arm or hand is a function of what meaning they attach to the loss and to the future. Suffering is not the inevitable consequence of painful stimulation. Some chronic pain patients appear to be totally defeated by their suffering, while others actually appear to live more meaningful lives as a result of their experience. Some make a career of suffering.

Brown's survey of surgeons who lost parts of their hands is relevant here.[6] Only 3 of 183 surgeons surveyed gave up surgery because of the amputation. Brown concluded that the motivation of the patient is more important to hand function than the actual number of digits retained. One surgeon said, "The important thing is what I have left and what I can do—not what I have lost and what I cannot do." This is similar to the quote attributed to Hubert Humphrey: "Some people look on any setback as the end. They are always looking for the benediction rather than the invocation. But you can't quit."

Pain researchers have demonstrated that the use of analgesics and complaints of pain are significantly less in combat situations, where a wound usually means leaving the scene of danger. In the safer context of a hospital, however, where a wound only means continued noxious stimulation and the presence of fear and anxiety, more complaints of pain are heard and more analgesics used. Soldiers wounded during the battle at Anzio in World War II needed far less morphine than did civilians with similar wounds.

As pain researchers have theorized, pain is a complex psychophysiological phenomenon involving sensory, neurochemical, cognitive, affective, and motivational components.[15,31,45] Pain is certainly influenced by antecedent and consequent variables. Mediating variables include anxiety, depression, and hypochondriacal thoughts that can intensify pain; sexual and cultural role expectations; the context and meaning of the pain; and reinforcement in the form of additional attention and avoidance of noxious situations. An injured worker's pain threshold can be affected by feelings of being wronged. Workers who blame the company for the injury and believe the employer was negligent in some way and has not accepted responsibility for that negligence find it harder to let go of their pain. Perceived injustice can lead to harbored resentment and anger, which increase pain and suffering.

An assessment of the consequences of pain behaviors can help in understanding what maintains the experience of pain and reports of suffering. The common directly reinforcing consequences of pain behaviors include prescription of pain medication on a pain-contingent basis (PRN) and special attention from others for the reporting of pain. Pain behaviors may lead to sanctioned constraints in activities that give the person "time out" from responsibilities, demands, or situations seen as noxious or threatening. The concept of secondary gain refers to the payoff a patient receives from an injury, including personal attention and sympathy, monetary gain, disability benefits, and release from or avoidance of certain responsibilities.

Pain, suffering, and pain behaviors tend to increase when issues of disability payments and litigation are present. If patients believe that they need to continue to demonstrate suffering to authenticate their pain in order to win or keep disability funding, the direct linkage be-

tween the original physical trauma and their demonstrations of pain will eventually disappear.

Aronoff et al.[3] summarized the conditions predicting that an injured worker will return to work in spite of pain:

1. early intervention and rehabilitation
2. positive hospital course: high motivation, effective mastery of pain, and success in stress-reduction strategies
3. positive work history, in which employment offers purpose and satisfaction and worker has high incentive to return to work
4. no major psychopathology
5. no narcotic/analgesic dependency
5. primary/secondary/tertiary gain factors not operative in perpetuating pain
7. no litigation
8. expeditious return to work after hospital discharge.

These researchrs believe workers' attitude and motivation, coupled with their support systems, determine whether they will allow pain to be totally disabling.

STRESS AND "HARDINESS"

Dana,[8] Wickramasekera,[47] and Kobasa[25] are examples of researchers in the stress literature who have proposed models that examine the various factors at work in order to determine how a person will respond to stress and whether or not the stress will defeat the person or will be mastered.

Dana argues for a model of health assessment in four domains: personal responsibility, life stresses, personality dispositions, and psychiatric symptoms.[8] Because many physical situations require shared responsibility for management and effective treatment, it is important to assess the patient's beliefs in personal power and responsibility. The patient's ability to assume responsibility for problems and their solutions addresses issues of compliance. Some patients expect the total treatment to come from the medical experts; as patients they see themselves as ill and believe it is inappropriate to expect them to be responsible for their recovery.

The domain of life stresses needs to be assessed to see whether the patient views stresses as catastrophic and overwhelming or as a challenge and an opportunity for growth. An examination of personality dispositions provides an assessment of whether coping techniques used allow the person to exacerbate an illness or injury or to adapt to it. An assessment of the presence of psychiatric symptoms is necessary to see what role they might play in the treatment.

Wickramasekera's high-risk model assesses predisposers, triggers, and buffers.[47] Predisposing conditions include negative affectivity or neuroticism; catastrophizing cognitive habits (e.g., "I can't stand this," "This is horrible"), which can allow amplification of the aversive properties of even minimally noxious sensory stimuli; and hypersensitive physiology. Triggers are both major life changes or the accumulation of minor hassles (microstressors). Buffers are positive elements that counteract predisposers and triggers. A person can be buffered against stress by a significant social support system and a high degree of satisfaction with it and also by coping skills and competencies acquired throughout life.

Kobasa's research indicates that the concept of psychological hardiness is a mediating factor that aids in preserving general health and in buffering the debilitating effects of stressful life events.[24,25] Some of the elements in this concept include: a person's estimate of self-esteem and self-worth; individual coping skills in dealing with past stressful events; the network of social supports of family, friends, and organizations; and the extent of investment in activities that are not work-related, such as hobbies or leisure activities that provide a sense of purpose and enjoyment.

Kobasa's concept of hardiness combines these mediating variables into three:

1. commitment to self, work, family, and religious faith
2. a sense of personal control over one's life, rather than feeling like a victim
3. the ability to see changes in one's life as challenges rather than as threats

The challenge for persons with an injury or an illness of the arm or hand is to take control of their attitude and outlook. People can choose whether to remain focused on their pain and emit much suffering and pain behavior response, or to redirect their energies, accept their pain, and develop goals for their lives that will take their limitations into account but not be stopped by them. Hansel's pronouncement,

"Pain is inevitable, but misery is optional," is accurate.[17]

METHODS OF ASSESSMENT

In addition to the clinical interview, which explores the patient's history and psychosocial factors, a psychological evaluation employs a variety of instruments. These range from structured formats that measure the contributions of psychosocial variables, measures of clinical symptoms of anxiety and depression, comprehensive symptom checklists, inventories of life stresses, and inventories of personality and psychopathology.

Measures of intelligence and reading skills are sometimes used when there are questions of a patient's level of understanding and comprehension of questions presented both orally and in written form. Reading skills below a sixth grade level indicate patients who will have difficulty completing written inventories on their own and will need to have them presented orally. A measure of intelligence can reveal whether the patient understands the medical information presented regarding diagnosis, treatment planned, and personal role in rehabilitation.

Heaton et al.[20] have published a standardized interview format for assessing psychosocial factors related to pain. Their Psychosocial Pain Inventory (PSPI) investigates forms of secondary gain, avoidance of performance demands, and other stresses.[19] A pilot study suggests that high scores on the PSPI predict poor response to medical treatment for pain.[20] The inventory rates whether pain behavior is sufficiently dramatic to have a major influence on interpersonal relationships and rates the existence of stressful life events that may contribute to subjective distress or promote avoidance learning. Items are included that rate past learning history that could familiarize a patient with the chronic invalid role. The inventory has a standardized scoring system.

Checklists

Two commonly used self-report mood inventories are the Beck Depression Inventory (BDI) and the State-Trait Anxiety Inventory (STAI). The BDI consists of 21 multiple-choice items reflecting specific behavioral signs of depression.[4] It can be administered orally as part of the clinical interview or can be part of the battery of tests patients complete on their own. The STAI measures two dimensions of anxiety: state or situational anxiety, which indicates how a person feels "right now," and trait or generalized anxiety, which measures how a person usually feels.[41] The discrimination may help in determining whether a patient is only tense in the evaluative session or whether there are signs of chronic apprehension.

The SCL-90-R is a multidimensional self-report system inventory that is widely used in medical settings. A prototype version of the scale was developed in 1973, and the completed instrument was published in 1975.[10] It is a 90-item inventory that provides a brief summary of psychiatric distress. The global severity index provides an overall measure of symptomatology. An administration and scoring manual was published in 1977.[11]

The Schedule of Recent Experience is derived from Holmes and Rahe's research on stress-producing life events.[21] It asks a person whether a variety of life events, including death, divorce, and job dismissal, have been experienced in the recent past. The events on the schedule were chosen because they require some adaptation by the individual and because they have been found to occur in patients preceeding the onset of illness.

Personality Inventories

The four most commonly used personality inventories are the Clinical Analysis Questionnaire (CAQ), part I of which is the Sixteen Personality Factor Questionnaire (16PF); the Millon Clinical Multiaxial Inventory; the Millon Behavioral Health Inventory; and the Minnesota Multiphasic Personality Inventory.

The CAQ was developed to measure both normal and pathological traits of an individual's personality structure.[26] It has 28 scales. Sixteen of the scales measure normal personality traits, and the remaining 12 measure various dimensions of psychopathology.

Millon has developed two instruments to assist health care workers in assessing and treating people with emotional, interpersonal, and health difficulties.

The original Millon Clinical Multiaxial Inventory (MCMI) and its revision (MCMI-II) were developed to coordinate with the psychiatric diagnostic system in the DSM-III and the DSM-III-R.[1,2,34,35] Separate scales have been constructed in line with the DSM-III model to distinguish the more enduring personality characteristics of patients (axis II diagnoses) from the acute clinical disorders they display (axis I). Profiles based on the 13 scales of clinical personality disorders and the 9 scales of clinical symptoms display the interaction between longstanding characterological patterns and the distinctive symptomatology shown under stress.

The Millon Behavioral Health Inventory (MBHI) was specifically designed for physically ill patients and medical-behavioral decision-making issues.[36] It is referenced against general medical populations rather than normal or psychiatrically normative groups. It consists of eight basic coping styles, six psychogenic attitudes, three psychosomatic correlates, and three prognostic indices.

Green reports that the MBHI has been useful in predicting behavior such as isolation, hostility toward health personnel, and excessive complaining and emotionality.[16] For example, sensitive coping-style patients typically react negatively to reassurance and often report that efforts to minister to them produce more, rather than less, trouble. The psychogenic attitude scales reveal patients' feelings and perceptions that might increase psychosomatic susceptibility or aggravate the course of a current illness or injury. The prognostic indices week to identify future treatment problems. The MBHI literature spells out specific treatment methods for dealing with patients' different coping styles.

The MMPI has become the most widely used and researched instrument for personality assessment.[7] It was developed in the late 1930s by Hathaway and McKinley and was published in 1943. The Minnesota Multiphasic Personality Inventory-2 (MMPI-2) was published in 1989.[37] It contains items concerning attitudes, behavior, and experiences with a variety of somatic and psychological factors. The basic profile consists of three validity scales that identify test-taking attitudes such as the desire to exaggerate or minimize symptoms and ten clinical scales. In addition, the MMPI literature contains hundreds of special scales, such as ones focusing on addictions and low back pain.

The MMPI, in addition to assessing the presence or absence of psychopathology, also assesses personality characteristics that can be useful in predicting responses to medical and surgical interventions. Long[29] examined the relationship between surgical outcome and MMPI profiles in chronic pain patients. The greatest percentage of surgery failures—that is, patients who continued to report pain postoperatively and did not return to their usual activities—was in people with MMPI profiles indicating hypochondriasis and hysteria.

Another study using the MMPI highlights its utility in understanding levels of low back pain chronicity in patients receiving workers' compensation. Levenson et al.[27] found elevations on the hypochondriasis, depression, and hysteria scales in this group, characterizing them as patients manifesting diffuse somatic complaints and depression and using the defense mechanisms of denial and repression.[27] The researchers concluded that workers' compensation patients who are disabled for two or more years evidence significantly more depression and psychopathology than those who are disabled for less than one year. Workers who have been disabled longer tend to have more diffuse somatic symptoms. The researchers argued that the results underscore that continued disability serves to heighten depression and feelings of helplessness and the need for early psychological assessment before the pattern becomes chronic.

Clinical Case Examples

Psychological evaluations can be helpful in selecting good-risk candidates for surgery and excluding those who would be poor surgical risks. Included in the poor-risk group are people who are psychotic or too anxious or depressed to be able to comply with medical care follow-up and those who have somatoform disorders such as conversion reactions. Deaton and Langman[9] point out that presurgical screening does not produce a dichotomous decision of surgery or no surgery.[9] Other options include: (1) delay surgery until the patient is in a better emotional state and can handle stress more effectively as a result of psychological or psychiatric treatment, (2) suggest psychological counseling regarding expectations and possible outcomes to prepare the patient for surgery, and (3) make surgery contingent upon counseling before and after to provide support and stress management skills. Surgeons are interested in knowing if they have a patient who might have technically excellent surgery but would continue to report pain and lack of full

functioning and would not return to preinjury work owing to psychosocial variables.

Patient A.   In a previous article[23] (p. 415, patient 2) I described a psychological evaluation conducted as a preoperative measure to determine if the patient was a good candidate for surgery.[23] The patient was a 47-year-old man who had three fingers amputated at work while repairing an engine. He was facing the prospect of surgery to straighten out tendons and further amputate the remaining part of his little finger. The patient desired more flexibility in the use of his fingers in order to eventually use hand tools; he was positive that surgery could allow him to return to work as a mechanic. The evaluation included the Beck Depression Inventory and the MMPI, both of which fell within normal limits, and concluded that the patient would recover from surgery successfully and that emotional factors would not compromise his recovery or participation in rehabilitation. A follow-up check with his surgeon several years later confirmed that the surgery had been successful and the patient had a good recovery.

Here I will describe some case studies from previous articles to illustrate diagnostic issues and the role of psychosocial variables in understanding patients referred with hand injuries and pain.[22,23]

Patient B.   The patient was a 32-year-old man referred for psychological assessment before surgery for carpal tunnel syndrome. His MMPI profile, which fell within normal limits, described him as extroverted, sociable, uninhibited, and energetic. He fit a sterotyped view of a "macho he-man." His profile indicated that he did not use physical symptoms to control and manipulate others and that he did not exaggerate physical complaints to seek sympathy from others. The interpretation of the MMPI profile was that his energy level was an indication that he would find access to physical activity after surgery to be highly reinforcing. It was concluded that he would not report continued and persistent pain and that he would not find a passive, inactive life-style attractive.

He was seen as a cooperative and motivated patient who would recover from surgery successfully and return to work. Follow-up information revealed that he did return to work after his surgery and that he resumed his usual jobs in a foundry except that he did not use vibrating tools. A one-year follow-up revealed that although he had reported the return of some mild symptoms of the carpal tunnel syndrome, he was still employed in his job and was not restricting his activities or reporting pain.

Patient C. The patient, a 38-year-old man, was injured on his job as a construction worker. The psychological assessment was part of the comprehensive evaluation of his current physical and psychological condition requested by the insurance company responsible for his employer's workers' compensation program. He sustained a fractured hand and, when the cast was removed, maintained his hand in a clenched-fist position.

The neurological evaluation conducted as part of the comprehensive workup revealed no objective abnormalities or neuronal injury. The neurological report stated that needle examination of the muscles resisting extension of the digits showed increased motor activity with a normal firing rate; this report suggested that the patient was resisting extension of the digits.

The psychological assessment required more than the usual amount of time. After many medical evaluations and uncertainty about the probabilities of regaining the use of his hand, the patient had accumulated a wealth of intense feelings regarding his situation, including discouragement, anger, and anxiety. He used the assessment session to voice his bitterness and resentment against his former company and what he perceived to be harmful medical practices that he had undergone.

His MMPI profile indicated a man who expressed feelings of anger and hostility in indirect ways. The Beck Depression Inventory revealed a moderate level of clinical depression. His sense of discouragement and demoralization was apparent. His personal satisfaction, pleasure, and livelihood for almost 20 years had been derived from using his hands, one of which he now viewed as useless. To lose the use of his hand, which had been tied up so intrinsically with his self-identity and self-worth, was extremely depressing and anger arousing because he viewed it as a result of a needless work accident.

The psychological assessment recommended a psychotherapy program to reduce depression and demoralization. With the help of therapy, he might feel a sense of support, encouragement, and motivation to follow through with a difficult course of physical therapy, the outcome of which was unpredictable. Several of the surgeons who had examined him said that

if he did not begin physical therapy, there would be little likelihood of his ever regaining the use of his hand and being employed again in a skilled trade.

The patient agreed to participate in psychotherapy but failed to keep his first appointment. A second appointment was also not kept, and no notification was given. Several months after the psychological assessment, the patient was reported as having not kept any of his appointments for either psychotherapy or physical therapy rehabilitation. This patient fits the "clenched-fist" syndrome reported by Simmons and Vasile.[39] There was an absence of neurologic and organic factors to explain his fist, and there was evidence from a psychological perspective of intense anger and psychological conflict. Simmons and Vasile report that patients respond with ambivalence to starting treatment; often when they do begin, they refuse to adopt treatment recommendations. One wonders what would have happened to Patient C if psychological assessment and intervention had occurred early in his course of injuries and encounters with medical personnel, rather than as the last evaluation in a series conducted over a period of almost one year. The likelihood of defusing his anger would have been greater earlier in the process rather than later, when it had become entrenched and well defended.

Patient D. The patient, a woman in her midtwenties, was injured at work when a shelf fell on her left arm and hand. Before psychological evaluation, several surgeons, radiologists, and physical therapists had seen her. The psychological evaluation was included as part of a comprehensive workup by a hand surgeon who was providing an opinion for her workers' compensation insurance company. Surgery was contemplated for thoracic outlet and carpal tunnel syndromes. The patient reported sensations of arm numbness and burning in the shoulder area. Her normal morning routine of showering, washing hair, applying makeup, brushing teeth, and curling hair all produced considerable pain. For a year after her work injury, she came to work only when she was not hurting in the mornings. She reported that when her arm hurt considerably she took a pain pill, lay down, and rested for a couple of hours or all day. The patient reported that before her injury she shared household responsibilities and duties with her roommates. As a result of her pain, she ceased performing any of those duties.

On the MMPI four of the ten clinical scales were elevated above normal limits. There were highly significant elevations on the first four scales describing chronic personality disorder. The patient sought nurturance and support from others and was prone to admit pain readily. Her validity scales on the MMPI indicated an attempt to maintain a facade of adequacy and control and to admit no psychological or social difficulties. This deliberate defensive orientation stood in contrast to her elevations on the clinical scales. Measures of current distress were not elevated. Both her psychasthenia score on the MMPI and her responses to the State-Trait Anxiety Inventory revealed an absence of general tension or apprehension. The patient indicated that she almost always felt satisfied with herself and was happy, secure, and content. She almost never worried too much or had disturbing thoughts.

The patient's elevations on the hysteria and hypochondriasis scales indicated a person who seriously lacked insight, denied psychological problems, and looked for simplistic solutions to life's problems. She was similar to people who are excessively concerned with somatic complaints and use physical symptoms to manipulate and control others. Her MMPI profile indicated a conversion reaction. Even when there is an initial physical injury, the person's response and reaction are more determined by emotional functioning and psychological makeup than by the objective physical findings.

The other significant feature of the young woman's MMPI profile was her indirect discharging of hostile and angry feelings. Although she tried to appear outwardly conforming, there were indications of serious passive-aggressiveness. Individuals with such profiles are seen as very demanding and have an inordinate need for attention and affection. The passive-aggressive qualities with significant elevations of hysteria described a woman who, while superficially sociable and vehemently denying hostile feelings, was adept at enraging others without any real understanding on her part.

Her MMPI profile was classified as similar to those of people who are surgery failures. All five of Long's diagnostic signs[29] were met.

This patient's DSM-III-R diagnoses were axis I, conversion disorder with axis II, mixed personality disorder with dependent and passive-aggressive features. She was seen as a woman who was not conscious of intentionally producing the symptoms of numbness and pain and thus was not seen as a malingerer. Issues of primary and secondary gain were more at issue in her diagnoses. The patient was seen as actively repressing long-standing emotional and psychological conflicts. She vigorously disagreed that her difficulties were psychological in nature, and she tenaciously clung to the concept that her work injury was the sole determinant of her continued pain and physical symptoms. The psychological evaluation revealed the patient as receiving secondary gain from her injury in that she was excused from household responsibilities and from reporting for work. She received attention in a sanctioned way for her disability. It is also possible that taking pain medication on an as-needed basis allowed a direct reinforcement of the pain complaints. It was predicted that the patient would escalate the intensity and frequency of pain complaints if she believed her symptoms were seen as having an unrealistic basis.

The evaluation recommended psychological treatment to assist the patient in recognizing the sources of her emotional conflicts and to aid in her recovery to preinjury functioning, both vocationally and socially. Treatment would be needed to help assist her to develop strategies to manage her pain better and to find vocational activities that would permit a more normal working life. In this patient's case it was unfortunate that psychological evaluation occurred more than a year after injury.[12,40]

Patient E. One of the diagnostic questions in this case was whether the patient's complaints were factitious. The patient was a 37-year-old woman who reported sharp pain in her left arm whenever she pulled a cart at work with considerable weight on it. The psychological evaluation was part of a comprehensive assessment of her work-related injury. Medical records indicated that she had been seen by several surgeons. There was a notation that her nerve conduction studies were normal and that testing for carpal tunnel syndrome was negative. Another surgeon was unable to find anything surgically correctable and raised the possibility that her complaints were factitious. One surgeon commented that the patient might have sustained some strain of the carpus in an initial injury several months before his examination, but he found no significant pathologic change. He further noted that findings on rapid exchange grip-strength testing showed incomplete cooperation with the examination.

The patient had finished only the tenth grade of school and had not earned a GED. Her reading performance was below third-grade level. The Beck Depression Inventory, State-Trait Anxiety Inventory, and MBHI were administered orally. Although the patient spoke openly about her arm injury and her life stresses, she did not communicate a sense of being distressed by them.

The picture that emerged from the psychological instruments was that of a woman without obvious signs of clinical distress or psychopathology. Her responses to the Beck Depression Inventory fell in the normal mood level. Her trait anxiety score, compared to other medical and surgical patients, fell only at the 19th percentile. Her profile on the MBHI described a person who felt minimal pressure and responsibilities and had a low probability of developing tension-related illness. Although in the interview she described her past year as a stressful one, on the questionnaire she presented herself as a person who was quite calm, confident, and sociable. The MBHI indicated that the patient was likely to be friendly and cooperative with health personnel but, at times, would reverse roles and sound like a know-it-all who was able to self-diagnose and recommend treatment for her problems. Issues of noncompliance were mentioned as a result of her tendency not to give up control to others.

The evaluation revealed an absence of serious current emotional distress. The patient had not been in a position to avoid usual household responsibilities. Her recent stresses involved caring for her daughter, who had been hospitalized for a kidney infection, and caring for her father, who had sustained a heart attack. It appeared to the psychologist that the patient had been the one caring for others and that she might have been overwhelmed by that responsibility and have used her slight work injury to reverse the roles in order to receive attention and sympathy. She was seen as having a factitious disorder with a good likelihood of a histrionic personality disorder and a deep psychological need to assume the sick role, without any obvious external incentives for that behavior. The total fabrication of symptoms or self-infliction of pain was seen as a viable explanation of her continued complaints. Psychiatric treatment was recommended.

Patient F. The psychological evaluation of this patient revealed the significance of a work injury on a worker's self-esteem. The patient was a 62-year-old man who injured his right wrist at work when climbing down from a truck. He underwent surgery, including a bone graft, several months after his injury. The patient reported that his surgeon said recent x-rays showed no significant increased bone growth and did not recommend future surgery. Surgery for carpal tunnel syndrome was being contemplated with the expectation that it might decrease the numbness the patient experienced. The patient reported very limited motion with his right wrist and hand and said he had little grip or strength left. He reported difficulty sleeping through the night as a consequence of hand numbness. As a result of his injury, his activities had undergone a number of significant changes. He reported not being able to do yard work or engine and car maintenance. His surgeon informed him that he probably would not be able to return to his truck-driving job. That was a crushing pronouncement. The patient prided himself on being an excellent driver and valued maintaining his ICC driver's permit over the years. He reported a sense of loss from not being able to work for two years after his injury, "after all those years of working."

On the two self-report mood inventories, the patient indicated mild depressive features and average levels of tension and apprehension. His profile on the MMPI was a valid one. All of his validity, clinical, and supplemental scales fell within normal limits, with the exception of a slight elevation on the hypochondriasis clinical scale, which indicated excessive concern with physical and somatic symptoms. It was likely that the patient tended to exaggerate his ills and used symptoms to command attention and some sympathy from others. His score on the depression scale indicated dissatisfaction and discouragement about his life situation; it was in a range typically obtained by patients who have learned to make an adjustment to a chronically unsatisfying situation. It appeared that the patient was focusing his grief over loss of his job in terms more of physical pain than emotional hurt. The evaluation concluded that a considerable amount of the patient's self-worth and self-esteem was wrapped up in his work and that he was in the process of adjusting to the loss of employability. His pain complaints were viewed as a disguised form of depression and as a substitute way of dealing with the loss of his hand functioning and his job.

The psychological evaluation of a patient who

has sustained a hand injury can be considered part of the complete care. Early intervention can help the employer and physician return the injured worker to his job with fewer emotional and social conflicts.

REFERENCES

1. American Psychiatric Association: Diagnostic and Statistical Manual of Mental Disorders, 3rd ed (DSM-III). Washington, D.C., American Psychiatric Association, 1980.
2. American Psychiatric Association: Diagnostic and Statistical Manual of Mental Disorders, 3rd ed, revised (DSM-III-R). Washington, D.C., American Psychiatric Association, 1987.
3. Aronoff G, McAlary P, Witkower A, Berdell M: Pain treatment programs: Do they return workers to the work place? Occup Med State Art Rev 3:123–136, 1988.
4. Beck A: Depression: Causes and treatment. Philadelphia, University of Pennsylvania Press, 1972.
5. Boyes J: We are first physicians, then surgeons: A view of the whole patient. J Hand Surg 5:103–104, 1980.
6. Brown P: Less than ten: Surgeons with amputated fingers. J Hand Surg 7:31–37, 1982.
7. Dahlstrom W, Welsh G, Dahlstrom I: An MMPI Handbook. Vol. 1. Clinical Interpretation. Vol II. Research Applications, Minneapolis, University of Minnesota Press, 1972, 1975.
8. Dana R: Assessment for health psychology. Clin Psychol Rev 4:459–476, 1984.
9. Deaton A, Langman MI: The contribution of psychologists to the treatment of plastic surgery patients. Prof Psychol 17:179–184, 1986.
10. Derogatis L, Lipman R, Covi L: SCL-90: An outpatient psychiatric rating scale. Preliminary report. Psychopharmacol Bull 9:13–27, 1973.
11. Derogatis L: SCL-90-R: Manual. Baltimore, Clinical Psychometrics Research, 1977.
12. Deyo R (ed): Back Pain in Workers. Occup Med State Art Rev 3: viii, 1988.
13. Deyo R, Diehl A, Rosenthal M: How many days of bed rest for acute low back pain? A randomized clinical trial. N Engl J Med 315:1064–1070, 1986.
14. Flor H, Turk D: Etiological theories and treatment for chronic back pain. I. Somatic models and interventions. Pain 19:105–121, 1984.
15. Fordyce W: Pain and suffering: A reappraisal. Am Psychol 43:276–283, 1988.
16. Green C: Psychological assessment in medical settings. In Millon T, Green C, Meagher R (eds): Handbook of Clinical Health Psychology. New York, Plenum Press, 1982, pp 339–375.
17. Hansel T: You gotta keep dancin'. Elgin, IL, David Cook, 1985.
18. Hardy M, Merritt W: Psychological evaluation and pain assessment in patients with reflex sympathetic dystrophy. J Hand Ther 1:155–164, 1988.
19. Heaton R, Lehman R, Getto C: Psychosocial Pain Inventory. Odessa, FL, Psychological Assessment Resources, 1980.
20. Heaton R, Getto C, Lehman R, et al: A standardized evaluation of psychosocial factors in chronic pain. Pain 12:165–174, 1982.
21. Holmes T, Rahe R: The social readjustment rating scale. J Psychosom Res 11:213–218, 1967.
22. Johnson R: Psychological evaluations of patients with industrial hand injuries. Hand Clin 2:567–575, 1986.
23. Johnson R: The role of psychological evaluations in occupational hand injuries. Occup Med State Art Rev 4:405–418, 1989.
24. Kobasa S: The hardy personality: Toward a social psychology of stress and health. In Sanders G, Suls J (eds): Social Psychology of Health and Illness. Hillsdale, NJ, Erlbaum, 1982.
25. Kobasa S, Hilker R Jr, Maddi S: Who stays healthy under stress? J Occup Med 21:595–598, 1979.
26. Krug S: Clinical Analysis Questionnaire Manual. Champaign, IL, Institute for Personality and Ability Testing, 1980.
27. Levenson H, Glenn N, Hirschfeld ML: Duration of chronic pain and the Minnesota Multiphasic Personality Inventory: Profiles of industrially injured workers. J Occup Med 30:809–812, 1988.
28. Loeser J: Perspectives on pain. In Proceedings of the First World Conference on Clinical Pharmacology and Therapeutics. London, Macmillan, 1980, pp 313–316.
29. Long C: The relationship between surgical outcome and MMPI profiles in chronic pain patients. J Clin Psychol 37:744–749, 1981.
30. Melzack R: The puzzle of pain. New York, Basic Books, 1973.
31. Melzack R, Wall P: The Challenge of Pain. New York, Basic Books, 1982.
32. Mendelson R, Burech J, Polack E, Kappel D: The psychological impact of traumatic amputations: A team approach: physician, therapist, and psychologist. Hand Clin 2:577–583, 1986.
33. Millon T: On the nature of clinical health psychology. In Millon T, Green C, Meagher R (eds): Handbook of Clinical Health Psychology. New York, Plenum Press, 1982, pp 1–27.
34. Millon T: Millon Clinical Multiaxial Inventory Manual. Minneapolis, National Scoring Systems, 1982.
35. Millon T: Millon Multiaxial Inventory, II. Manual. Minneapolis, National Computer Systems, 1987.
36. Millon T, Green C, Meagher R: Millon Behavioral Health Inventory Manual. Minneapolis, Interpretive Scoring Systems, 1982.
37. MMPI Restandardization Committee. Minnesota Multiphasic Personality Inventory, 2. Minneapolis, University of Minnesota Press, 1989.
38. Sack O: A Leg to Stand On. New York, Summit Books, 1984.
39. Simmons B, Vasile R: The clenched fist syndrome. J Hand Surg 5:420–427, 1980.
40. Snook S: Approaches to the control of back pain in industry: Job design, job placement, and education/training. State Art Rev Occup Med 3:45–59, 1988.
41. Spielberger C, Gorsuch R, Lushene R: The State-Trait Anxiety Inventory Manual. Palo Alto, Consulting Psychologists Press, 1970.
42. Sternbach R: Mastering Pain: A Twelve-step Program for Coping with Chronic Pain. New York, Ballantine Books, 1987.

43. Stokes H: The seriously uninjured hand: Weakness of grip. J Occup Med 25:683–684, 1983.

44. Sturgis E: The relationship between a personal theology and chronic pain. In Miller W, Martin J (eds): Behavior Therapy and Religion. Newbury Park, CA, SAGE Publications, 1988.

45. Turk D, Meichenbaum D, and Genest M: Pain and Behavioral Medicine: A Cognitive-Behavioral Perspective. New York, Guilford Press, 1983.

46. Walsh N, Dumitru D: The influence of compensation on recovery from low back pain. Occup Med State Art Rev 3:109–121, 1988.

47. Wickramasekera I: Enabling the somatizing patient to exit the somatic closet: A high risk model. Psychotherapy 26:530–544, 1989.

Chapter 7

HOW THE RADIOLOGIST CAN HELP TO EVALUATE INJURIES AND DISEASES OF THE UPPER EXTREMITY

Jeri P. Irwin, M.D., William W. Joule, M.D., Gary H. Peterson, M.D., Curt E. Liebman, M.D., and Jannice O. Aaron, M.D.

Occupational injuries of the upper extremity are a common clinical problem. After a careful physical examination, radiographic evaluation should proceed in an organized manner, with plain film imaging as the first step in the workup. Radiographic investigation is used to recognize fracture, characterize displacement, joint involvement, and foreign bodies, and detect old previously unreported or unrecognized injury. Previous trauma can lead to degenerative change. If an injury requires surgery, the initial radiographs are an important baseline and a medicolegal record.

The procedure to use after the initial plain film evaluation depends upon what abnormality, if any, is found. Subsequent evaluation may include nuclear medicine, fluoroscopy, tomography, computed tomography (CT), arthrography, ultrasound, angiography, or magnetic resonance imaging (MRI). This chapter discusses the radiological evaluation of work-related injuries and conditions of the upper extremity. An overview of technical principles is followed by separate discussions of the shoulder, the elbow, the forearm, the wrist, and the hand.

GENERAL TECHNICAL PRINCIPLES

Successful imaging of the upper extremity depends upon a combination of important elements, including film screen combinations, film processing and chemistry, filming technique, and personal interaction with the patient.

Probably the most important factor is the choice of film-screen imaging systems. Of the very broad choices available today, we advocate a system designed for extremity radiography—one that includes a high-detail screen and the use of single-emulsion film. While many good combinations are marketed, we have found the combination of Fuji MI-NH film and Kyokko Ultrasharp 100-speed screens to be a cost-effective, yet superb extremity system.

The second most important factor is filming technique. Collimation is critical to good radiographs. Detail is improved in a geometric progression as smaller filming windows are used. Certainly the smallest field size necessary to see the area of interest should be used. Coned-down views are obtained if additional information is needed. Kilovoltage ranges of between 50 and 60 kvp are essential, and the small focal spot should be used routinely.

Good, consistent positioning is the responsibility of the radiographer, especially for exacting elbow, wrist, and hand images. Even slight flexion or extension on lateral wrist views, for example, can change carpal alignment and make the exams difficult to interpret. Additional views tailored to the patient's symptoms may occasionally be the only way to demonstrate pathological changes.

Finally, faulty film processing and chemistry selection can damage or destroy an otherwise perfect exam. The modern automated processors do an excellent job; however, their development temperature must be carefully controlled, and the processors must be cleaned and maintained properly.

BONE SCAN (RADIONUCLIDE IMAGING)

Technetium-99m–labeled phosphorus complexes—polyphosphates, pyrophosphates, and diphosphonates—are excellent agents for bone scanning. With intravenous injection of the radionuclide, uptake of the isotope by bone is dependent on blood flow to the region and on the extraction of the isotope. This process is related to metabolic activity, capillary permeability, and extracellular fluid volume.

Ordinary bone scans are obtained 3 to 4 hours after injection of isotope to allow for clearance of the nuclide from blood and soft tissues. Three-phase bone scans include both images of the flow of isotope and blood-pool images in soft tissue. The area of interest is placed under the camera, and serial 3-second exposures are obtained postinjection (phase 1). The blood-pool images (phase 2) are obtained at 5–7 minutes after injection and reflect soft tissue uptake in the area. Because metabolic activity accounts for bone uptake, increased uptake normally is seen in the infused epiphysis, costochondral junctions, sacroiliac joints, and sternoclavicular joints.

About one-third of the injected radionuclide dose is excreted through the kidneys into the urine. Thus, the kidneys and bladder should be seen on the bone scan.

Indications

Indications for bone scanning include:
1. Evaluation of bone pain when plain films are normal
2. Evaluation of patients with a known malignancy to rule out bone metastasis
3. Evaluation of possible early osteoarthritis (this can be very important to the occupational physician because early osteoarthritis may only be demonstrated on bone scan)
4. Early diagnosis of stress fractures
5. Evaluation of joint disease
6. Evaluation of initial diagnosis of Paget's disease
7. Detection of avascular necrosis
8. Evaluation of painful joint prosthesis
9. Evaluation of bone graft

MAGNETIC RESONANCE IMAGING

Magnetic resonance imaging (MRI) is the newest tool in the diagnostic workup of many pathological entities. No ionizing radiation is used. Instead, the part to be examined is placed in a high-strength magnetic field. When a relatively stable magnetic reorientation of some of the hydrogen molecules in the area to be examined occurs, additional energy in the form of radiofrequency (RF) waves is added. As this energy is lost from the area, a returning RF echo can be sampled. Using complex computer calculations and changing the time when energy is added and echos sampled, different information can be obtained. Today we are only able to base our analysis on the concentration of hydrogen molecules in the area examined. In the future, we may be able to sample the total chemical composition of the area.

MRI offers better soft tissue resolution than CT. It also allows for imaging in virtually any plane or section. Its limitations include relatively long exam times during which the patient must remain motionless and a cost that is between two and three times greater than that of CT studies.

THE SHOULDER

William W. Joule, M.D.

ANATOMY

The glenohumeral joint—the proximal end of the humerus—consists of the head, the anatomic neck, the surgical neck, and the greater and lesser tuberosities. The tuberosities provide insertion for the muscles of the rotator cuff—the subscapularis, supraspinatus, intraspinatus, and teres minor. Between the tuberosities lies the bicepital groove, in which runs the tendon of the long head of the biceps.

The glenoid cavity faces anteriorly and is shallow. The fossa is deepened by a fibrocartilaginous labrum that attaches to the rim of the glenoid and is continuous with the joint capsule at the neck of the scapula.

The acromioclavicular (AC) joint is a true synovial joint surrounded by a capsule. The coracoclavicular ligament connects the distal clavicle to the coracoid process of the scapula and keeps the clavicle and acromion in contact. The AC ligament extends from the acromion process to the superolateral border of the cor-

acoid process and provides additional support for the humeral head. Motion at the AC joint includes forward and backward gliding and rotation about the long axis of the clavicle. The AC joint space is normally between 2 and 5 mm in width.[7,8,17]

SHOULDER INJURIES AND DISEASES

Figure 1 presents an algorithm for radiological diagnosis of shoulder injuries.

When evaluating **acromioclavicular joint separation,** the bony margins are usually smooth but may be straight or notched, concave, convex, or asymmetrical in appearance. Most injuries result from a fall onto the point of the involved shoulder; less common ones arise from a force transmitted from a fall on the elbow or outstretched hand.[8] The radiographic examination should include anterior–posterior (AP) views of both shoulders with the beam angled 15 degrees toward the feet (allowing better vis-

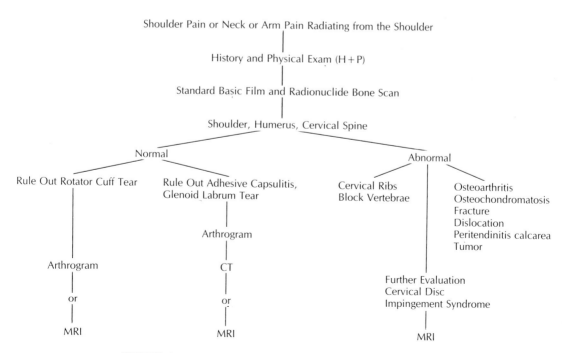

FIGURE 1. An algorithm for radiologic diagnosis of shoulder injuries.

ualization of the subacromial space), both with and without 5–15 pounds of weight suspended from each wrist.

In a **grade I sprain**, soft tissue swelling is present around the joint, but there is no separation. Follow-up may show subperiosteal new bone formation.

A **grade II sprain** is referred to as a **subluxation**. The clavicle is higher than the acromion, usually by less than the width of the clavicle. The coracoclavicular space is increased up to 4 mm above the normal (Fig. 2).

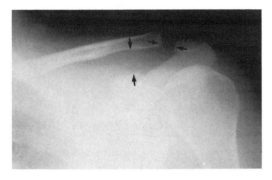

FIGURE 2. Acromioclavicular separation grade II.

A **grade III sprain** is referred to as a **dislocation**. The distal end of the clavicle is above the superior aspect of the acromion. The distance between the clavicle and the coracoid process is increased by more than 40–50% of normal. Associated fractures of the coracoid process may be seen.[28]

Fractures of the osseous structures of the shoulder girdle following trauma are common in all age groups. They can be as simple as a fractured clavicle or more complex and unusual, such as fracture of the scapula and ribs. AP views of the shoulder with the humerus in internal and external rotation plus axillary views are basic views to obtain following trauma. These can be supplemented by transthoracic lateral, transscapular, Grashey, sternal, and West Point views, as well as stress views of both shoulders in suspected AC separation. The Grashey view is obtained with the patient supine and 45 degrees oblique. It is a good view for showing the glenoid fossa in profile. In complex trauma to the chest and upper shoulder area, CT may be the quickest and most efficient way to detect fractures and evaluate position and alignment.[58]

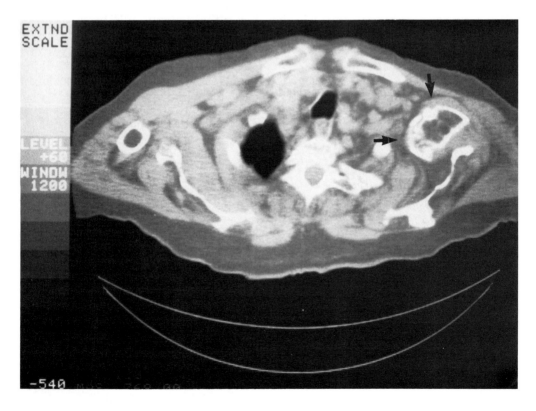

FIGURE 3. CT demonstration of anterior medial dislocation of humeral head with osteoarthritic changes involving the humeral head.

Anterior humeral dislocation occurs when the humeral head moves anteriorly, medially, and inferiorly (Fig. 3). The humeral head usually comes to rest below the coracoid process. This type of dislocation represents about 97% of all glenohumeral dislocations, most of which are due to trauma. They are usually easy to diagnose on routine shoulder trauma films; however, if associated with a fracture or lung injury, CT of the chest is a quick method of identifying the various damaged structures.[22,41]

Impacted fractures of the posterior humeral head are often seen with this type of dislocation and are called Hill-Sachs fractures (Fig. 4). Less commonly, fractures of the inferior glenoid rim, called Bankart fractures (Fig. 5), are seen, particularly with repeated dislocations.[46,56] A small number of anterior humeral dislocations also have fractures of the greater tuberosity. Because of the traumatic etiology of anterior humeral head dislocations, fractures of the ribs, scapula, clavicle, and humerus are often noted as well.

Posterior dislocations are seen in about 3% of glenohumeral dislocations. They are medically important but are often missed both clinically and radiographically. These dislocations are best seen with CT of the shoulder or with the axial view on the preliminary films. On the plain film with AP projection, posterior dislocation can be suggested if the humeral head has a rounded or cystic appearance and there

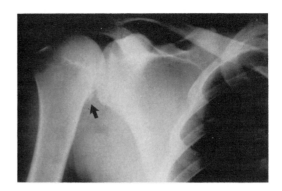

FIGURE 5. Bankart fracture of inferior glenoid rim.

is an increased distance between the medial portion of the humeral head and the deepest portion of the glenoid fossa. The crescent sign is thereby thinned down or absent. The crescent sign is formed by increased bone density as a result of overlapping of the humeral head and glenoid. With separation of the humeral head from the glenoid in posterior dislocation, this double-density crescent of bone becomes thinner on the AP projection. Occasionally, a vertical impacted fracture line is seen on the anterior head of the humerus.

Rotator cuff tears can produce shoulder pain with some inability to abduct the upper arm. These injuries are usually seen in adults over the age of 40. Trauma and degenerative changes in the rotator cuff are by far the most common etiologies.[58,63] Plain film examination of the shoulder gives some hint of possible rotator cuff tear. Indications include narrowing of the acromiohumeral space to less than 7 mm sclerotic and/or cystic changes in the area of the greater tuberosity, and sclerosis and concavity of the undersurface of the acromion. Contrast arthrograms of the glenohumeral joint dramatically demonstrate complete tear with filling of the subacromial bursa (Fig. 6). A noninvasive diagnosis of rotator cuff tear can be made with MRI.[23,48,63] These images are obtained in multiplanar sections in the frontal oblique position using both T1 and T2 modes. T1 and T2 modes produce different contrasts of various types of tissues registered on the film. With T1, water is black; with T2, water is white. Many factors affect the contrast, including strength of the magnetic field, type of pulse sequence, timing of pulses, thickness of slices obtained, signal-to-noise ratio, and others. Some of the findings indicating rotator cuff tear would include: increased signal in the distal 2 cm of the supraspinatus tendon, fluid in the subacromial bursa,

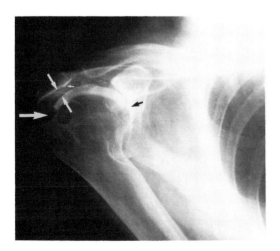

FIGURE 4. Hill-Sachs fracture of humeral head (large white arrow). Also, marked osteoarthritic changes of shoulder (black arrow) and impingement syndrome (bracketing white arrows). Note the marked narrowing of the acromial humeral joint space and the spur underneath the acromion process (smallest white arrow).

and retraction of the supraspinatus muscle medially. Ultrasound examination has been used to diagnose rotator cuff tears; however, it is operator-dependent and so far does not appear to be as accurate as an arthrogram or a good MRI examination of the shoulder.

Peritendinitis calcarea (Fig. 7) is one of the commonest pathological abnormalities seen on plain films of the shoulder. It is most commonly seen in the supraspinatus tendon near its attachment to the greater tuberosity.[28] It is seen most often in patients complaining of pain in the shoulder with some limitation of motion.

However, on occasion it is present in the soft tissues of the shoulder without acute symptoms. This radiographic density is commonly created by calcium phosphate or carbonate. However, other calcium complexes are often present. With the proper treatment, it can resolve within a matter of weeks.

Degenerative osteoarthritis of the shoulder (see Fig. 4) develops after a fracture or dislo-

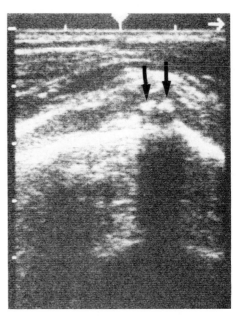

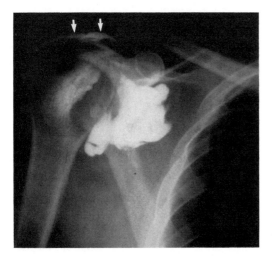

FIGURE 6. Arthrogram of shoulder. Contrast in the subacromial bursa indicates rotator cuff tear.

FIGURE 7. Peritendinitis calcarea demonstrated with ultrasound.

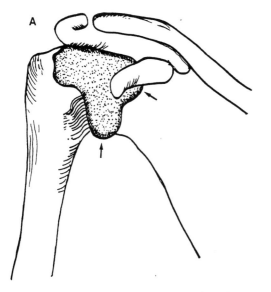

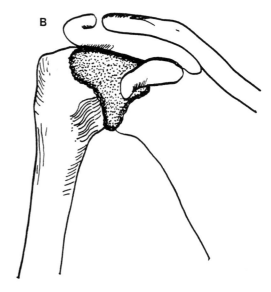

FIGURE 8. A, Drawing of normal shoulder arthrogram with good filling of axillary subscapular recess (arrows). B, Drawing of shoulder arthrogram in patient with adhesive capsulitis. There is diminished capsular volume, irregular capsule outline, and shallow axillary subscapular recess.

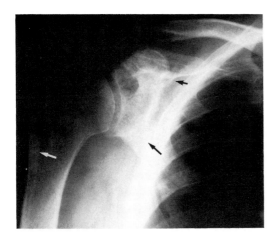

FIGURE 9. Metastatic disease of the shoulder from cancer of the colon.

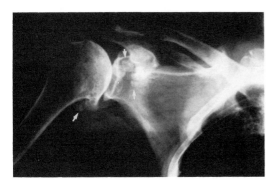

FIGURE 10. Osteochondromatosis involving the shoulder.

cation through the osseous structures of the shoulder girdle. It also can result from severe soft tissue trauma or inflammation. Chronic injury or tear of the rotator cuff sometimes produces osteoarthritis,[21,58] especially in older patients. Initially, the joint space narrows. Sclerosis of the opposing bony surfaces, marginal spurs, geode formation, and dystrophic calcification ensue. Resulting pain, tenderness, and limitation of motion can occasionally result in osteoporosis.

Adhesive capsulitis or frozen shoulder can result in pain and limitation in movement at the shoulder joint. Plain film findings of osteopenia and osteophyte formation are nonspecific, but adhesive capsulitis results in decreased volume of the glenohumeral capsule. A normal volume of 11–15 cc can be reduced to an abnormal volume of 4–8 cc. A single-contrast arthrogram offers the best evaluation.[8,17,58] An abnormal arthrogram shows a re-

duced capsular volume, irregular capsule outline, and decreased filling of the axillary subscapular recess and biceps tendon sheath (Fig. 8).

Shoulder impingement (see Fig. 4) is a common cause of chronic shoulder pain in patients past 50. It is also the commonest cause of rotator cuff tear. Plain films of the shoulder show narrowing of the acromiohumeral joint space to less than 7 mm, sclerosis and osteophytes involving the under surface of the acromion, and clavicle cystic and sclerotic changes in the

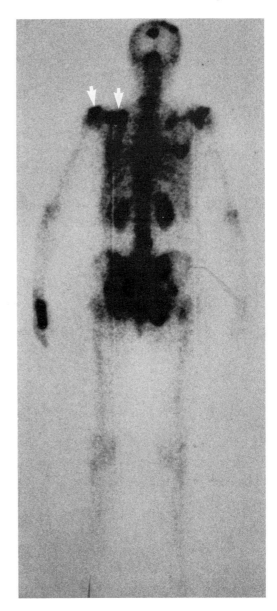

FIGURE 11. Breast cancer metastasis to the right shoulder shown on bone scan.

area of the greater tuberosity of the humerus. On occasion, dystrophic calcifications in the soft tissues of this area can be seen.[35,47]

In most patients presenting with **shoulder pain**, the basic disorder is bursitis, tendinitis, ligament strain or tear, fracture, or dislocation. However, primary or secondary tumor of the bone can, on occasion, cause initial symptoms in the shoulder girdle area (Fig. 9). This patient's main complaint was severe pain in the left upper arm and shoulder. The patient's previous history included colon resection for carcinoma. Radiographs reveal a sclerotic and lytic defect in the upper outer third of the left humerus and extension of the tumor mass into the soft tissues. Soft tissue calcification in the tumor is noted. In addition, sclerotic and lytic defects are noted in the scapular body, neck, and glenoid area. Often, metastatic disease to the shoulder occurs from the breast, prostate, lung, kidney, or thyroid.[17,28,56]

Synovial osteochondromatosis (Fig. 10) is an uncommon cause of shoulder pain, swelling, and limitation of motion. It is most common in middle-aged men and is usually monoarticular and almost always benign. It is usually found in the knee.

Repeated minor trauma to the joint may cause **synovial metaplasia**, which results in cartilaginous nodule formations that eventually enlarge and multiply. In about 40% of cases, these nodules calcify and eventually ossify. If ossification does not occur and osteochondromatosis is clinically suspected, then arthrogram, CT, or MRI can reveal the cartilaginous nodules.[28] Surgical removal of the nodules with most of the synovium often relieves symptoms.

Radionuclide bone scanning is a relatively quick way to assess the shoulder girdle and surrounding bone and soft tissue structure for areas of disease. A bone scan is positive long before radiographic evidence of a lytic or sclerotic defect can be seen. Figure 11 is from a patient with shoulder pain from widespread breast cancer metastasis; x-rays of the shoulder area were normal.

Unfortunately, bone scans can be falsely positive in the dominant shoulder, generally in the glenohumeral, AC, sternoclavicular, and rib cartilage joints and at the inferior scapular angle with few signs or symptoms of radiographic evidence localized to these areas.[56]

In addition, plasma cell disease of the bone often does not show up on bone scans, and extreme bone disease (e.g., metastatic areas) can be overlooked because of a moderate-to-marked overall increase in uptake that produces a superscan effect.

In general, it should be noted that a bone scan can be very sensitive but not particularly specific (indicating, for example, a severe bursitis, but not specifically locating it).

ELBOW AND FOREARM

Jeri P. Irwin, M.D.

ELBOW

Anatomy

The elbow, a hinge joint, has relatively limited range of motion, particularly by comparison to the shoulder. Approximately 6% of all fractures and dislocations involve the elbow. These injuries are usually the result of indirect trauma transmitted through the bones of the forearm as an angular force or as direct impact of the radius and ulna against the opposing articular margins of the humerus.[59]

The elbow articulation is composed of three distinct joints: the humeroulna, humeroradial, and radioulnar. All three are contained within a single cavity known as the capsule, which is lined with synovial membrane. The humeroulnar joint is considered the principle joint of the three.

The humerus flares at the distal end to form the medial and lateral condyles. The flexion and pronator muscles of the forearm arise from the more prominent medial condyle; the extension muscles of the forearm arise from the lateral. The distal articulating surface of the humerus consists of the trochlea medially and the capitellum laterally. The capitellum articulates with the radial head. The ulna proximally has a deep, concave articulating surface known as the trochlear notch. The anterior margin of the notch is a triangular projection called the coronoid process. This process serves as the insertion of the brachialis muscle. The posterior margin of the notch is the olecrannon process, which is the insertion of the triceps muscle. On the lateral and anterior aspect of the trochlear notch is the articulation with the head of the radius, known as the radial notch.

The brachial artery courses along the medial border of the biceps brachii muscle. It passes into the antecubital fossa at the level of the head of the radius. The brachial artery is susceptible to injury in association with a supracondylar fracture of the humerus, especially when the fracture is displaced. Injury to the brachial artery can lead to Volkmann's contracture of the muscles of the forearm and hand.

The median nerve lies just lateral to the brachial artery. It is infrequently injured. The ulnar nerve lies superficially on the posterior surface of the medial condyle in a groove between it and the olecrannon. This groove is known as the cubital tunnel (Fig. 12). It is palpable and susceptible to injury. Fractures of the medial condyle or medial epicondylar apophysis may result in injury to the ulnar nerve, which may also become trapped within the joint space after reduction of elbow dislocation.

Flexion of 150 degrees is possible from the neutral position. The radioulnar joint allows 180 degrees of pronation and supination of the forearm.

Plain Films

Plain film examination of the elbow should include AP, lateral, and both oblique views (Fig. 13). The injured elbow should be analyzed by evaluating the bony mineralization, development, and alignment. The examiner should search for displaced fat pads or other soft tissue abnormalities. The positioning of ossification centers should be evaluated, and osseous structures closely observed for fracture.

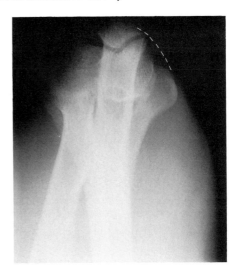

FIGURE 12.   Normal elbow–cubital tunnel view. The ulnar nerve lies in a tunnel bridged by the arcuate ligament (dashed line).

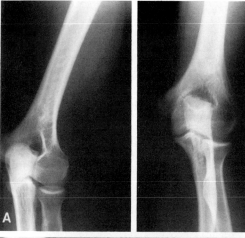

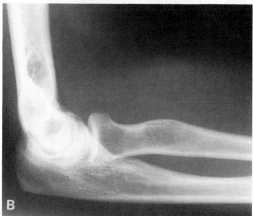

FIGURE 13. *A,* Normal elbow, AP and oblique views. *B,* Normal elbow, lateral view.

Fractures

An additional view of the elbow may be needed to visualize a fracture line. The radial head capitellum view may be valuable in evaluating trauma to the radial head. This view is obtained by positioning the patient for a lateral view and angling the beam 45 degrees to the forearm. The resultant image projects a slightly magnified radial head clear of the overlying ulna with an elongated capitellum. In one series, this view gave a 21% confirmation of radial head fractures.[13,14]

Dislocations

Dislocations of the elbow occur with some frequency. This joint is the third most common site of dislocation in adults (after the shoulder and the interphalangeal joints of the fingers)

and the most common site of dislocation in children. Elbow dislocations are classified according to the displacement of the radius and ulna in relationship to the humerus; 85–90% are posterior or posterolateral (Fig. 14). In practically all dislocations, both bones of the forearm are displaced simultaneously. Elbow dislocation is usually due to hyperextension upon a fall on the outstretched hand. Many dislocations are associated with fractures. The most common fracture of the elbow is of the medial epicondyle; fractures of the radial head and neck are somewhat less frequent. Elbow fractures associated with dislocation may be missed. Postreduction views should always be obtained.

Anterior dislocations are rare, but they raise the possibility of damage to the brachial artery or nerve. On the lateral view, the olecranon process impinges on the anterior aspect of the distal humerus.

Medial and lateral dislocations are most easily identified on A–P radiographs. The lateral view may not be strikingly abnormal. Alignment between the radius and capitellum and between the ulna and trochlea should be checked on every examination.

Rarely, the radius and ulna may dislocate in different directions. Of the two types of dislocation—AP and mediolateral—the AP is more common though it rarely occurs in an adult; it consists of posterior dislocation of the ulna and anterior dislocation of the radius. Recurrent dislocation is a rare complication and is usually of the posterior type.

Soft Tissue Abnormalities

Soft tissue abnormalities of the elbow most commonly are myositis ossificans, displace-

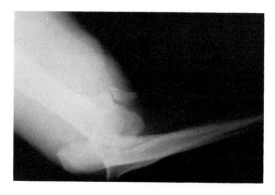

FIGURE 14. Posterior dislocation of elbow with avulsion fracture of medial epicondyle of distal humerus, lateral view. The patient was a 28-year-old man.

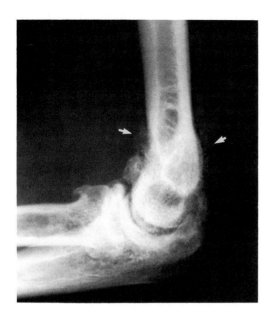

FIGURE 15. Myositis ossificans following trauma, lateral view. The patient was a 61-year-old man.

ment of the fat pads, and bursitis, and loose bodies.

Myositis Ossificans. Myositis ossificans occurs as a complication in 3% of all elbow injuries and 30% of radial head fractures. The cause of this heterotopic bone formation is presumed to be dystrophic in nature (Fig. 15). Small areas of myositis cause no problems, but more extensive areas may limit the range of motion. Myositis ossificans is increased if not treated; definitive treatment should be done in the first 24 hours to avoid this complication.

Displaced Fat Pads. Displaced fat pads were first described by Norell in 1954 as the posterior fat pad sign.[34] A lateral view of the normal elbow should not show the posterior fat pad, which is held against the posterior humerus by the triceps tendon. The anterior fat pads are normally visible. Displacement of the anterior fat pad was first described by Bledsoe in 1959.[33]

The anterior fat pad is a summation of the radial and coronoid fat pads. During extension, these pads are pressed into their fossa by the brachialis muscle. During flexion, their shape is determined by articular volume, surface tension, flexibility of capsule, and the limits of bone. Both fat pads are extrasynovial and intracapsular.

An abnormal anterior fat pad sign results from an intracapsular collection of fluid or issue, which increases the intra-articular space and dis-

places the fat pad superiorly and ventrally. The resulting configuration has been called a "ship's sail." A false negative anterior fat pad sign occurs with poor positioning, extracapsular fracture, and capsular rupture.

A false-positive posterior fat pad sign may occur with extension of the elbow. In extension, the posterior capsule is lax and the triceps relaxed, and the olecrannon process displaces the fat pad from the olecrannon fossa. Normal displacement of the posterior fat pad in extension should not be mistaken for a sign of joint disease.

Olecranon Bursitis. This is another soft tissue abnormality that can be demonstrated radiographically. Distention of the bursa is most often associated with trauma or rheumatoid arthritis. It produces a homogeneous soft tissue density on the x-ray and is best seen in the lateral view.

Cartilaginous or Osteocartilaginous Loose Bodies. These may be found in the elbow, usually as a consequence of osteoarthritis or osteochondritis dissecans (Fig. 16). Less frequent causes include fracture, synovial osteochondromatosis, and neuropathic joints. Loose bodies are most commonly found in the anterior portion of the joint but may lodge posteriorly in the olecranon fossa. The diagnosis is suggested if ossification or calcification overlies the inspected area of the joint capsule on standard x-rays. It is confirmed by arthrography. Loose bodies may lodge in the coronoid recess, the olecranon recess, or the periradial recess. They can grow because they are nourished by synovial fluid blocking full extension of flexion and can lead to further degenerative changes.[38]

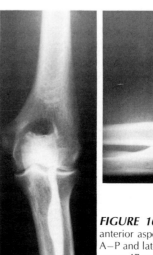
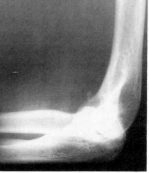

FIGURE 16. Loose bodies in the anterior aspect of the elbow joint, A–P and lateral views. The patient was a 47-year-old man.

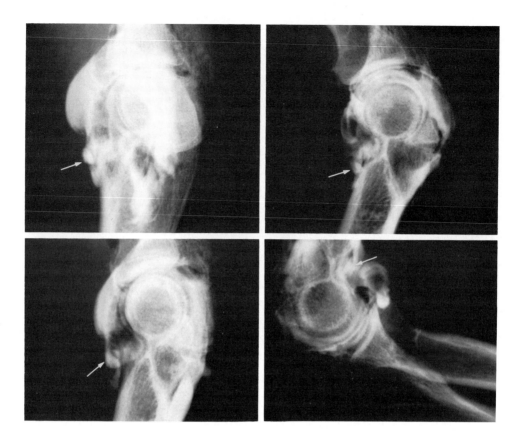

FIGURE 17.   Elbow arthrogram confirming loose bodies within elbow joint, four views. The patient was a 47-year-old man.

Arthrography is most useful to verify the presence of intra-articular loose bodies (Fig. 17). When periarticular calcific densities are seen in plain films, the arthrogram can help to determine which ones lie within the joint cavity and which are in the periarticular soft tissues.[18] The articular cartilage may be evaluated, especially in patients with osteochondral fractures, osteochondritis dissecans, or osteochondrosis. Arthrography may also demonstrate the increased joint capacity and irregularity of the synovial lining associated with rheumatoid arthritis, pigmented synovitis, and other proliferative synovial diseases.

An accurate elbow arthrogram may require considerable time to perform completely. Tomography is frequently a helpful follow-up.

Inflammatory Conditions

Inflammatory conditions of the elbow may occur with occupational stress. One of the most frequent of these is lateral epicondylitis, commonly known as tennis elbow. The condition

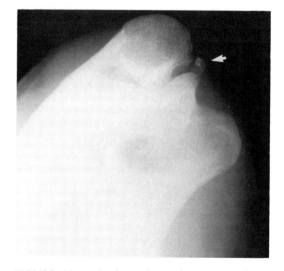

FIGURE 18.   Cubital tunnel view showing osteophytes impinging upon ulnar nerve.

can occur on the medial side of the elbow, but it is seven times more common on the lateral side. The commonly accepted disorder is a tear in the common extensor origin of the humerus

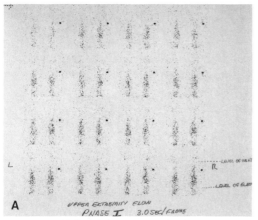

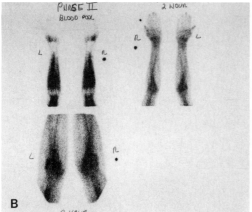

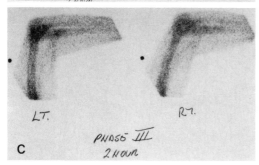

FIGURE 19. Normal three-phase bone scan of a 49-year-old woman with pain in the right elbow radiating to the hand and wrist. *A,* Phase 1 demonstrates regional blood flow to the upper extremities. *B,* A–P views of phases 2 and 3, upper extremities. *C,* Phase 3, lateral views of both elbows.

at the epicondyle level. Lateral epicondylitis is most commonly seen in the fourth decade.[53]

Vascular Conditions

Vascular conditions such as aneurysm or thrombosis of a small artery may give rise to pain due to local ischemia or to compression of a nerve in a confined space. These injuries are frequently related to repeated episodes of blunt trauma such as the use of a hammer. Vascular abnormalities may require angiography. Digital subtraction angiography gives excellent detail of vascular structures by subtracting out the underlying bony structures.

Other Conditions

Osteoarthritis changes of the bones of the elbow may be painful. An osteophyte projecting into the cubital tunnel may impinge upon the ulnar nerve (Fig. 18).

Olerud et al. described a prominent **radial tubercle** that limited pronation. It was diagnosed by CT and corrected surgically.[36] The proposed etiology was repeated forearm rotation caused by work demands. The motion was repeated several thousand times per day.

Pain of uncertain etiology that is not adequately explained by conventional radiographs or examination should be evaluated with radionuclide bone scanning. Three-phase studies

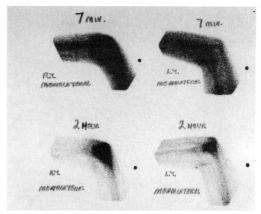

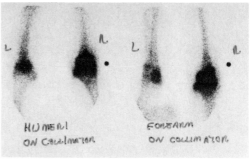

FIGURE 20. Capsulitis in a 17-year-old woman with pain and swelling of the right elbow. *A,* Lateral views of both elbows at 7 minutes (phase 2) and 2 hours (phase 3). *B,* A–P views of both elbows at 2 hours (phase 3).

yield the most information, because they include information about perfusion and soft tissues in addition to bone (Fig. 19). Inflammatory arthritis, noninflammatory arthritis, tendinitis, subtle fracture, or tumor may be revealed (Fig. 20).

Magnetic Resonance Imaging

MRI of the elbow has a variety of potential roles: evaluation of suspected traumatic inflammatory or degenerative joint disorders; investigation of bone marrow lesions; and study of abnormalities of the neurovascular structures traversing the joint (Fig. 21).

FOREARM

Injuries to the forearm are classified according to the bones involved. Fractures of both the radius and the ulna are usually associated with severe trauma and are obvious. AP and lateral views permit determination of comminution and deformity. Radiographs of the forearm must include both the wrist and the elbow, because fractures in one area are often associated with a dislocation at the other. The Galeazzi fracture is a fracture of the middle to distal radius with an associated dislocation or subluxation of the radioulnar joint. If the triangular fibrocartilage complex is not torn, an avulsion fracture of the ulnar styloid occurs. These fractures almost always require open reduction and fixation.

The Monteggia fracture-dislocation is a fracture of the proximal third of the ulna with an associated posterior dislocation of the radial head. The dislocation is often not recognized. A simple check is to draw a line through the

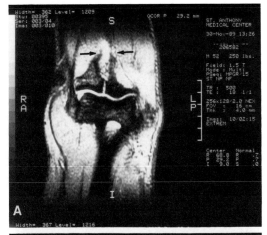

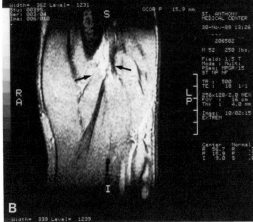

FIGURE 21. *A*, MRI of the elbow in a 52-year-old man with partial tear of the biceps tendon at its insertion. *B*, Same patient.

midshaft of the radius exiting perpendicularly through the radial head. Normally the line intersects the capitellum on both the AP and lateral views.

THE WRIST

Curt E. Liebman, M.D.

Acute or chronic wrist pain as a result of occupational injury is a common clinical problem. Determining the source of the pain can be a diagnostic challenge. Radiographic evaluation may be facilitated by the use of an algorithm developed by Pin et al. (Fig. 22).[39] Use of the algorithm is, of course, preceded by careful physical examination and involves plain film radiography (including fluoroscopy and tomography), radionuclide imaging, arthrography, CT, and MRI. Below brief review of wrist anatomy is followed by a discussion of radiographic evaluation of wrist pain.

ANATOMY

The anatomy of the wrist is quite complex, and definition of the joint varies. Most authors consider the wrist to include the distal radius and ulna, two rows of four carpal bones each, and the bases of the five metacarpals. The first row of carpals (from the radial side to the ulnar) includes the scaphoid, lunate, triquetrum, and pisiform, and the second row includes the trapezium, trapezoid, capitate, and hamate (Fig. 23). The radius and ulna have connecting lig-

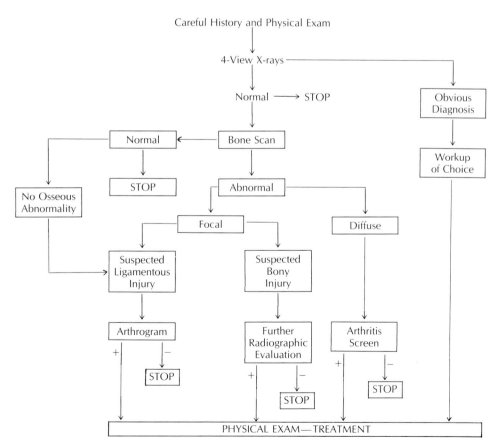

FIGURE 22. Wrist pain algorithm. Each step in the algorithm provides either a "normal" or an "abnormal" result. Abnormal results are either treated or pursued with further testing. Normal results are followed by either the cessation of tests or further testing as outlined, dependent on clinical judgment. The significance of abnormalities noted on radiographic studies must be determined by reviewing the mechanism of injury and examining the patient again. (From Pin, et al: Wrist Pain: A systematic approach to diagnosis. Plast Reconstr Surg 85(1): 1990, with permission.)

aments and cartilage, including the triangular fibrocartilage. The anatomy of the interosseous ligaments of the carpus is particularly complex and varies from patient to patient; diverse terminology for these ligaments is noted throughout the literature. The osseous-ligamentous complex of the wrist provides for its complex mobility and stability. Detailed anatomy of the wrist, including its vascular supply, is not included here because many excellent texts cover the topic.[19,24,51]

PLAIN FILMS

Plain film radiography begins with four routine views of the wrist. These are obtained in the initial workup of all patients with wrist pain. They include a standard PA view to delineate the scaphoid or navicular bones (Fig. 24), all of which are centered on the wrist rather than the hand. The PA view shows the radioulnar, radiocarpal, midcarpal, and scapholunate joints. The lateral views provide the proper positioning for evaluation of the relationship of the metacarpals, capitate, lunate, and radius and are particularly important in lunate and perilunate dislocations. The scaphoid or navicular view elongates this bone on the film and more readily demonstrates fractures or aseptic necrosis. These four views often demonstrate an obvious

diagnosis, such as fracture or dislocation, and treatment can be initiated. If, however, the routine views are normal, spot films of painful areas may be obtained.

Specific views of the carpal bones follow the standard four views and may include the carpal tunnel view or a semisupination view obtained off-laterally. The carpal tunnel view (Fig. 25) allows visualization of the hook of the hamate, the trapezium, the pisiform, and the ventral surface of the capitate or lunate. It also allows differentiation among the os styloideum, a bony prominence attached to the second or third metacarpal at its base, the opposing bony surface of the capitate or trapezoid, and degenerative spur formation. The semisupinated oblique view of the carpus (Fig. 26) has been developed by Papilion et al. to better diagnose rotatory subluxation of the scaphoid. It permits excellent visualization of the hook of the hamate.[37]

PLAIN FILM TOMOGRAPHY

Polycycloidal plain film tomography may follow if there is a questionable bone abnormality on routine or detailed spot views. Thin sections are obtained at 2- or 3-mm intervals, usually in two separate positions obtained at a 90-degree angle to each other. Fluoroscopic evaluation can aid in positioning for tomography to best define the proper bony profile. Computerized tomography has replaced plain film tomography in many institutions.[42]

RADIONUCLIDE IMAGING

Radionuclide imaging is performed after normal radiographs, usually when clinically suspicious injury persists. If the three-phase bone scan is normal (Fig. 27), a clinically significant abnormality is unlikely, though not impossible. Rolfe et al.[45] recently studied 95 patients with suspected scaphoid fractures and negative radiographs. On radionuclide bone scan, 47 had increased uptake in the wrist. In approximately half, activity was localized to the scaphoid. Of the 47 patients, 19 had subsequent radiographic evidence of a wrist fracture. When a traumatic lesion is suspected, focal superimposed changes can be particularly confusing. Positive findings on bone scan are highly sensitive, though not specific. A wide variety

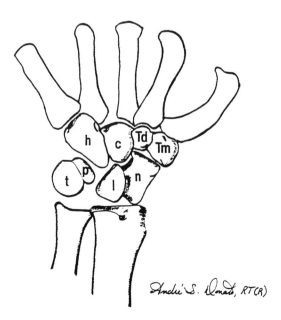

FIGURE 23. Anatomy of the wrist: *n*, navicular (scaphoid); *l*, lunate; *t*, triquetrum; *p*, pisiform; *Tm*, trapezium; *Td*, trapezoid; *c*, capitate; *h*, hamate.

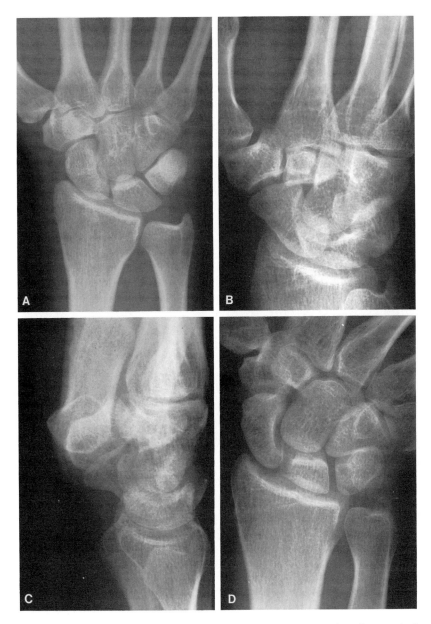

FIGURE 24.   Four routine views of the wrist. *A*, P–A; *B*, oblique; *C*, lateral; *D*, navicular.

of abnormalities show up as positive focal areas of activity.

ARTHROGRAPHY

The workup may then proceed directly to arthrography or to a ligamentous instability series. The routine instability series includes an AP clenched fist view as well as PA views obtained in neutral position and with radial and ulnar deviation. Instability series also include a semipronated oblique view obtained 30 degrees from P–A lateral views in neutral full extension and full flexion, and supinated off-lateral and oblique views obtained 30 degrees from lateral. Comparison views of the contralateral wrist may assist in assessing normal anatomic variation. The most common ligamentous injuries with instability include dorsal intercalated segment instability (DISI), volar intercalated segment instability (VISI), ulna translocation, and dorsal carpal subluxation. Effective treatment of carpal instability re-

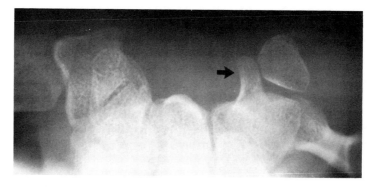

FIGURE 25.   Carpal tunnel view of wrist demonstrating hook of hamate (arrow).

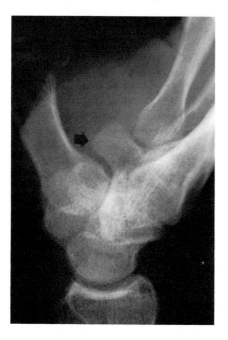

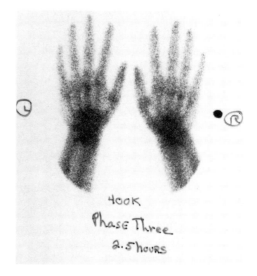

FIGURE 27.   Normal bone scan after injection of 19.8 m of technetium-99m–labeled copper, MDP IV, obtained at 2½ hours.

FIGURE 26.   Hamate view of wrist with hook (arrow).

quires early detection, and the instability series can be helpful.

Arthrography of the wrist may be performed before, after, or in conjunction with the instability series. It may be obtained earlier in the evaluation of the occupationally injured wrist if clinical judgment dictates. Wrist arthrography has undergone considerable progress in recent years and is indicated for evaluation of injury to the triangular fibrocartilage or the scapholunate and lunotriquetral ligaments and of tears of the capsule. It is also used to localize symptomatic calcifications. The wrist is divided into a series of three joints separated by a fibrous capsule; each joint is lined by synovium. These joint spaces include the distal radioulnar joint, the radiocarpal joint, and the midcarpal joint. A tear of the triangular fibrocartilage or the scapholunate, or other ligaments allows contrast material to flow into the adjacent compartment.

Routine wrist arthrography involves injection of 2–4 cc of contrast medium in a 25-gauge needle into the radiocarpal joint under fluoroscopic guidance. This is useful in determining the site of tears, specifically tears of the triangular fibrocartilage (Fig. 28). More recently, Tirman et al.[54] described an additional midcarpal injection for the detection of tears in the scapholunate and lunotriquetral ligament. Levinsohn et al.[26] present a three-compartment injection technique to include the radiocarpal injection and midcarpal and distal radioulnar joint injections. This examination can be quite time-consuming, but it is often the best way to determine the site of ligamentous

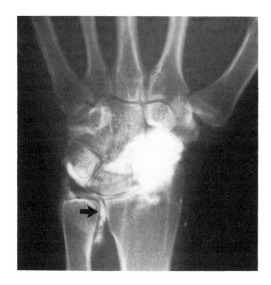

FIGURE 28. Athrogram demonstrating abnormal collection of contrast in the radioulnar joint (arrow) after injection of 3 cc of contrast into the radiocarpal joint.

injury, especially when contrast flows in one direction from one compartment to another.

COMPUTED TOMOGRAPHY

Routine computed tomography or three-dimensional CT, as well as postarthrography CT, may be useful in the radiographic evaluation of a patient with wrist pain who has had a previously normal workup. When transaxial images are obtained, the wrists are imaged together (Fig. 29).

Sagittal and coronal images may be obtained when the diagnostic problem requires them. The plane of imaging selected is at a 90-degree angle to the fracture of fusion plane. In a recent report by Quinn et al.,[43] a total of 173 wrist CTs were performed over 4 years at three institutions for follow-up of bone fusion procedures or in the evaluation of fracture healing and complication. A fracture of the waist of the scaphoid is best evaluated with coronal or sagittal imaging, and scapholunate fusions with transaxial or coronal images.

CT imaging of the wrist is also helpful in the evaluation of midcarpal dislocations,[5] radioulnar dislocations,[31] and cases of foreign bodies. CT is particularly helpful in evaluation of patients with overlying casts[43] when other modalities aren't completely satisfactory. Three-dimensional CT reconstructions are performed in some institutions and are particularly useful

in complex surgical cases, especially those involving prostheses.[2] With computer manipulation, individual bony structures can be eliminated from final images to facilitate detection of suspected abnormalities.[57]

MAGNETIC RESONANCE IMAGING

As MRI has proven its worth in the central nervous system, attention has increasingly turned to the musculoskeletal system. MRI has superior soft tissue resolution and has become increasingly useful in imaging of the wrist (Fig. 30). MRI has demonstrated effectiveness in the evaluation of tears of the intercarpal ligaments—specifically, the scapholunate ligament—disruptions of the extrinsic ligaments, articular cartilage defects, tears of the triangular fibrocartilage, subluxations of the distal radioulnar joint, and nonunion and avascular necrosis.[1,12,62]

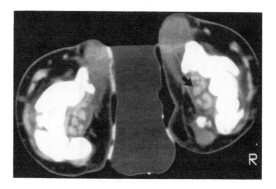

FIGURE 29. CT of wrists demonstrating carpal tunnel with median nerve (arrow).

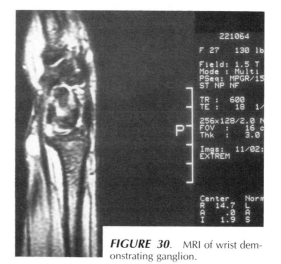

FIGURE 30. MRI of wrist demonstrating ganglion.

In carpal tunnel syndrome,[29,30] MRI findings include swelling and flattening of the median nerve, volar bowing of the flexor retinaculum, and increased signal intensity of the median nerve itself.[29] Zlatkin et al.[62] even suggest that MRI is the preferred choice (in lieu of arthrography), following the normal four views of the wrist, in a patient with chronic wrist pain who is thought to have a triangular fibrocartilage tear or ligamentous disruption. If MRI is negative or equivocal and intercarpal ligamentous injury is clinically suspected, they suggest follow-up with arthrography. They further suggest that if arthrography is necessary, a single midcarpal injection should be sufficient.

With the development of dynamic MRI techniques, it should be possible in the future, though not for several years, to replace the fluoroscopic instability series.

CONCLUSION

Evaluation of the wrist in occupational injuries provides a diagnostic challenge. The most important component is the careful physical examination. The radiographic evaluation may be made easier by the use of the algorithm described here and presented graphically in Figure 22. Any diagnostic algorithm, however, should be used only as a guide; additional imaging dictated by clinical information should be done. The importance of communication between the clinician and the radiologist cannot be overemphasized.

THE HAND

Gary H. Peterson, M.D.

Injuries to the hand represent a significant proportion of hospital emergencies and in many institutions comprise 15% of trauma cases.[10] Hand injuries also represent a significant proportion of occupational injuries. The hand is the most commonly injured area of the upper extremity. Prompt, accurate diagnosis and treatment of occupational injuries of the hand are vital in preventing serious, long-term disability, which can be functionally devastating to the patient and financially disastrous to the company employing the injured worker.

PLAIN FILMS

A minimum plain film study must include dorsopalmar (PA), oblique, and lateral views (Fig. 31).[40] In addition, spot views of individual fingers provide better detail and a truer lateral orientation (Fig. 32). Although the wrist and hand are thought of as a unit, they must be filmed separately. Positioning aids are readily available. The most useful are the precut sponge blocks used for separating the fingers in oblique and lateral projections.

The thumb requires special attention because an AP projection of it is not ordinarily obtained with the three routine views of the hand. The frontal view is obtained with the forearm midway between pronation and supination and the thumb extended away from the volar surface of the hand.

The Norgaard projection is an AP view made with the fingers held in mild natural flexion. Centering is at the metacarpophalangeal (MCP) joints, the primary area of interest. This view provides better visualization of the MCP joints. The Brewerton view is used for detecting small, often occult fractures of the metacarpal head or base.[20]

ANATOMY

Anatomic references to the hand should ideally refer to the thumb, index, long, ring, and small or little fingers in order to avoid the potential confusion of numbering the digits. More

practically, important aspects of hand anatomy relate to the nutrient arterial canals (medullary foramina), which are sometimes confused with incomplete fractures. They are located near the midpoints of the phalangeal and metacarpal shafts and enter the bones obliquely from the sides. Their margins are smooth and sclerotic and are parallel. The sesamoids are round, small bones embedded in certain flexor tendons. Their number is variable, but commonly five are found in the hand. They are characterized by dense, smooth cortical margins and a normal trabec-

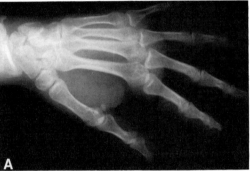
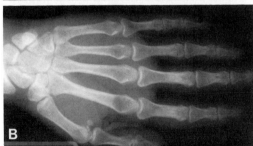
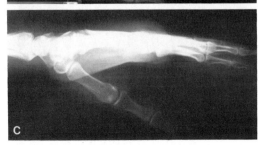

FIGURE 31. Oblique (*A*), PA (*B*), and lateral (*C*) views of the hand. Note that a fracture in the proximal shaft of the metacarpal of the long finger can only be seen on the lateral view.

ular pattern. Fractures of the sesamoids can occur (Fig. 33) and must be carefully evaluated along with signs of tendon injuries. Epiphyses or growth plates may be confused with fractures in the evaluation of hand films in a young person. Comparison films of the opposite extremity are of value and should be obtained in questionable situations.

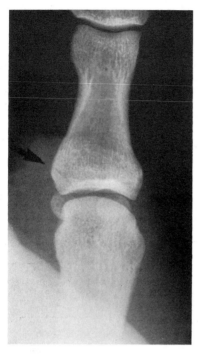

FIGURE 32. A very subtle fracture in the base of the proximal phalanx of the thumb (arrow) seen well on coned down views of the area of injury.

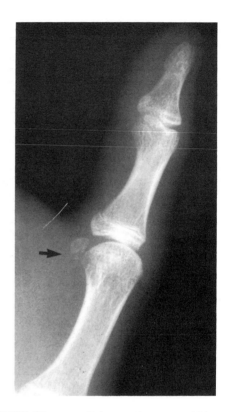

FIGURE 33. A small fracture in a sesamoid bone of the thumb.

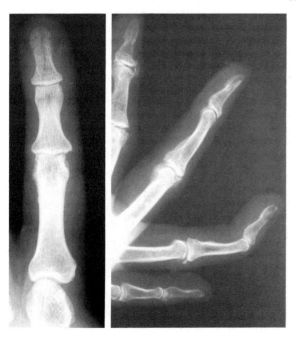

FIGURE 34. (left). Comminuted crush fracture of the distal phalanx of the index finger.

FIGURE 35. (right). Mallet deformity of the distal interphalangeal joint of the ring finger. Note the fracture at the dorsal base of the middle phalanx.

FOREIGN BODIES

The ease or difficulty of evaluating the hand for foreign bodies can be wide-ranging. Obviously, metallic densities are easily seen on standard or soft tissue studies.[49] Glass is generally fairly easy to visualize, especially if high-contrast images are available.[52] Vegetable matter or wood producing penetrating wounds can be difficult to identify. Xeroradiography, if available, can be invaluable in identifying this type of material.[6,55,61]

FRACTURES

The most common fracture of the hand involves the distal phalanges. Fractures of these bones result from crush injuries and are easily seen on standard plain films (Fig. 34). A careful assessment of articular alignment must be made.

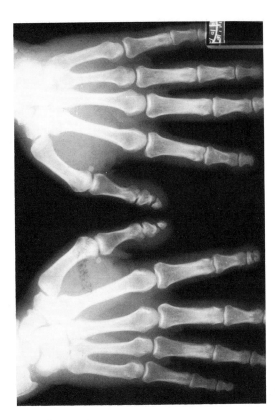

FIGURE 37. Acro-osteolysis in a vinyl chloride worker. Note the loss of the bone in the distal portions of multiple fingers.

The radiographic changes of mallet finger (Fig. 35) and boutonnière deformity (Fig. 36) are indications of significant underlying tendon injuries requiring immediate treatment.

Mallet finger is a flexion deformity at the distal interphalangeal joint caused by damage to the extensor tendon or by an avulsion fracture from the dorsal base of the distal phalanx. It generally is secondary to sudden forced flexion of the distal portion of the affected finger.[15]

Boutonnière deformity is seen most often as a result of rheumatoid arthritis. In trauma, it results from avulsion of the central extensor tendon from the dorsal aspect of the base of the middle phalanx.[4]

Fractures involving the **articular surface** of a joint are especially important. They must be diagnosed and treated promptly to avoid disability.

BONE LOSS

Acro-osteolysis of bone is now a rare, yet fairly well-known entity. It can be caused by

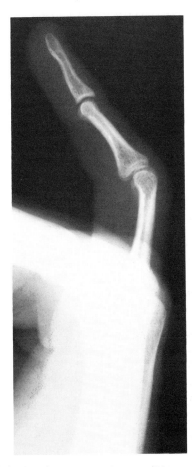

FIGURE 36. Boutonnière deformity of the ring finger; no fracture is present.

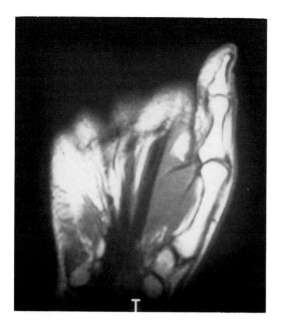

FIGURE 38. MRI of the hand. Note the exquisite soft tissue detail allowing visualization of flexor tendons of the fingers.

a variety of conditions; occupationally, it is seen in the hands of workers exposed to vinyl chloride and polyvinyl chloride materials.[60] It results in the loss of bone from the tufts of the distal phalanges (Fig. 37).

MRI AND CT

MRI has, up to now, had little use in evaluation of the hand. It can image in the multiplanar projections and can define the smallest anatomic details of the fingers (Fig. 38). The volar plates, the flexor, and the extensor tendons can be seen with great detail. In situations in which incomplete tears are suspected, MRI may be helpful. CT is of limited value in evaluating the hand unless a specific question cannot be answered in any other way.

REFERENCES

1. Binkovitz LA, Ehmna RL, Cahill DR, Berquist TH: Magnetic resonance imaging of the wrist: Normal cross-sectional imaging and selected abnormal cases. Radiographics 8:1171–1202, 1988.
2. Biondetti PR, Vannier MW, Guila LA, Knapp RH: Three-dimensional surface reconstruction of the carpal bones from CT scans: Transaxial versus coronal technique. Comput Med Imaging Graph 12:67–73, 1988.
3. Bunnell DH, Fisher DA, Bassett LW, et al: Elbow joint: Normal anatomy on MR imagings. Radiology 165:527–531, 1987.
4. Burke EN, Lanigan WN: Butterhole rupture of the extensor tendon: X-ray findings. Radiology 91:520, 1968.
5. Bush CH, Gillespy T III, Dell PD: High-resolution CT of the wrist: Initial experience with scaphoid disorders and surgical fusions. AJR 149:757–760, 1987.
6. Carneiro RS, Okunski WJ, Hefferman AH: Detection of a relatively radiolucent foreign body in the hand by xerography. Plast Reconstr Surg 59:862–863, 1977.
7. Clemente CD: Anatomy: A Regional Atlas of the Human Body. Philadelphia, Lea & Febiger, 1975.
8. Cofield RH, Berquist TH: The shoulder. In Berquist TH (ed): Imaging of Orthopedic Trauma and Surgery. Philadelphia, W.B. Saunders, 1986, pp 449–566.
9. Cone RO, Szabo R, Resnick D, et al: Computed tomography of the normal radioulnar joints. Invest Radiol 18:541–545, 1983.
10. Frazier WH, Miller M, Fox RS, et al: Hand injuries: Incidence and epidemilogy in an emergency service. J Am Coll Emerg Phys 7:265–268, 1978.
11. Gilula LA, Weeks PM: Post-traumatic ligamentous instabilities of the wrist. Radiology 129:641–651, 1978.
12. Golimbu CN, Firooznia H, Melone CP Jr, et al: Tears of the triangular fibrocartilage of the wrist: MR imaging. Radiology 173:731–733, 1989.
13. Greenspan A, Norman A: Radial head-capitellum view: An expanded imaging approach to elbow injury. Radiology 164:272–274, 1987.
14. Grundy A, Murphy G, Barker A, et al: The value of the radial head–capitellum vie in radial head trauma. Br J Radiol 58:965–967, 1985.
15. Hallberg D, Lindholm A: Subcutaneous rupture of the extensor tendon of the distal phalanx of the finger: "Mallet finger." Acta Chir Scand 119:260–267, 1960.
16. Hawkins RJ, Neer CS II, Pianta RM, Mendoza FX: Locked posterior dislocation of the shoulder. J Bone Joint Surg 69A:9–18, 1987.
17. Helms CA: Fundamentals of Skeletal Radiology. Philadelphia, W.B. Saunders, 1987.
18. Hudson TM: Elbow arthrography. Radiol Clin North Am 19:227–241, 1981.
19. Kaver JMG: Functional anatomy of the wrist. Clin Orthop Rel Res 149:9–20, 1980.
20. Kaye JJ, Lister GD: Another use for the Brewerton view. J Hand Surg 3:603, 1978.
21. Kieff GJ, Bloem JL, Rozing PM, Obermann WR: Rotator cuff impingement syndrome: MR imaging. Radiology 166:211–214, 1988.
22. Kieff GJ, Bloem JL, Rozing PM, Obermann WR: MR imaging for recurrent anterior dislocation of the shoulder: Comparison with CT arthrography. AJR 150:1083–1087, 1988.
23. Kneeland JB, Middleton WB, Carrera GF, et al: MR imaging of the shoulder: Diagnosis of rotator cuff tears. AJR 149:333–337, 1987.
24. Landsmeer JMF: Atlas of Anatomy of the Hand. Edinburgh, Churchill Livingstone, 1976.
25. Lane CS: Detecting occult fractures of the metacarpal head: The Brewerton view. J Hand Surg 2:131–133, 1977.
26. Levinsohn EM, Palmer AK, Coren AB, Zinberg E: Wrist arthrography: The value of the three-compartment injection technique. Skeletal Radiol 16:539–544, 1987.
27. Macrander SJ: The elbow: In Middleton WD, Lawson TL: Anatomy and MRI of the joints. A Multiplanar Atlas. New York, Raven Press, 1989, pp 56–81.
28. Meschan I: Roentgen Signs in Clinical Practice. Philadelphia, W.B. Saunders, 1966.

29. Mesgarzadeh M, Carson DS, Bonakdarpour A, et al: Carpal tunnel: MR imaging. Pt II. Carpal tunnel syndrome. Radiology 171:740–754, 1989.
30. Middleton WD, Kneeland JB, Kellman GM, et al: AJR 148:307–316, 1987.
31. Mino DE, Palmer AK, Levinsohn EM: The role of radiography and computerized tomography in the diagnosis of subluxation and dislocation of the distal radioulnar joint. J Hand Surg 8:23–31, 1983.
32. Munk PL, Holt RG, Helms CA, Genalt HK: Glenoid labrum: Preliminary work with the use of radial-sequence MR imaging. Radiology 173:751–753, 1989.
33. Murphy WA, Siegel MJ: Elbow fat pads with new signs and extended differential diagnosis. Radiology 124:659–665, 1977.
34. Nerell HG: Roentgenologic visualization of the extracapsular fat. Acta Radiol 42:205–210, 1954.
35. Newhouse KE, El-Khoury GY, Montgomery WJ: The shoulder impingement view: A fluoroscopic technique for the detection of subacromial spurs. AJR 151:539–541, 1988.
36. Olerud C, Sahlstedt B, Olerud S: Prominent radial tubercle causing limited pronation: Brief report. J Bone Joint Surg 70B:297–298, 1988.
37. Papilion JD, Dupu TE, et al: Radiographic evaluation of the hook of the hamate: A new technique. J Hand Surg 13A:437–439, 1988.
38. Pavlou H: Sports-related elbow injuries. Skeletal Radiol 5: Chapter 16, 1986.
39. Pin PG, Young VL, Gilula LA, Weeks PM: Wrist pain: A systematic approach to diagnosis. Plast Reconstr Surg 85 (1), 1990.
40. Poznanski AK: The Hand in Radiographic Diagnosis. Vol. 1. Philadelphia, W.B. Saunders Co., 1974.
41. Pring DJ, Constant O, Bayley JIL, Stoker DJ: Radiology of the humeral head in recurrent anterior shoulder dislocations: Brief report. J Bone Surg 71B:141–142, 1989.
42. Quinn SF, Murray W, Watkins T, Kloss J: CT for determining the results of treatment of fractures of the wrist. AJR 149: 1987.
43. Quinn SF, Belsole RJ, Green TL, Rayhack JM: Advanced imaging of the wrist. Radiographics, 9:229–246, 1989.
44. Rogers LF: The elbow and forearm. In Rogers LF: Radiology of Skeletal Trauma. New York, Churchill Livingstone, 1982, pp 435–497.
45. Rolfe EB, Garvie NW, Khan MA: Isotope bone imaging in suspected scaphoid trauma. Br J Radiol 54:762–767, 1981.
46. Rosenbaum HD, Hildner JH: Basic Clinical Diagnostic Radiology. Baltimore, University Park Press, 1984.
47. Seeger LL, Gold RH, Basset LW, Ellman H: Shoulder impingement syndrome: MR findings in 53 shoulders. AJR 150:343–374, 1988.
48. Seeger LL, Ruszkowski JT, Basset LW, et al: MR imaging of the normal shoulder: anatomic correction. AJR 148:83–91, 1987.
49. Smoot EC, Robson MC: Acute management of foreign body injuries of the hand. Ann Emerg Med 12:434–437, 1983.
50. Stark D, Bradley WG: Musculoskeletal system. In Stark D, Bradley WG: Magnetic Resonance Imaging. St. Louis, C.V. Mosby, 1988, p 1323.
51. Taleisnik J: The ligaments of the wrist. Hand Surg 1:110–118, 1976.
52. Tandberg D: Glass in the hand and foot: Will an x-ray film show it? JAMA 248:1872–1874, 1982.
53. Thorson EP, Szabo RM: Tendonitis of the wrist and elbow. Occup Med State Art Rev 4:419–432, 1989.
54. Tirman RM, Weber ER, Snyder LL, Koonce TW: Midcarpal wrist arthrography for detection of tears of the scapholunate and lunotriquetral ligaments. AJR 144:107, 1985.
55. Tountas CP, MacDonald CJ, Artman R: Detection of foreign bodies in the hand utilizing xeroradiography. Minn Med 63:296–297, 1978.
56. Vogler JB III, Helms CA, Callen PW: Normal Variants and Pitfalls in Imaging. Philadelphia, W.B. Saunders, 1986.
57. Weeks PM, Vannier MW, Stevens WG, et al: Three-dimensional imaging of the wrist. J Hand Surg 10A:32–39, 1985.
58. Weissman BNW, Sledge CB: The shoulder. Weissman BNW, Sledge CB: Orthopedic Radiology. Philadelphia, W.B. Saunders, 1986.
59. Weissman BNW, Sledge CB: The Elbow. Weissman BNW, Sledge CB: Orthopedic Radiology. Philadelphia, W. B. Saunders, 1986, pp 169–214.
60. Wilson RH, McCormick WE, Tatum CF, et al: Occupational acro-osteolysis. JAMD 201:577–581, 1967.
61. Woesner MF, Sonders I: Xeroradiography: A significant modality in the detection of nonmetallic foreign bodies in soft tissues. Radiology 115:636–640, 1972.
62. Zlatkin MD, Chao PC, Osterman AL, et al: Chronic wrist pain: Evaluation with high-resolution MR imaging. Musculoskel Radiol 173:723–229, 1989.
63. Zlatkin MD, Dalinka MK, Kressel HY: Magnetic resonance imaging of the shoulder. Magn Reson Q 5:3–22, 1989.

Chapter 8

NEUROLOGIC EVALUATION OF THE UPPER EXTREMITY

Michael R. Swenson, M.D. and David R. Villasana, M.D.

Clear clinical descriptions of upper extremity neurologic disorders began in the 1800s. S. Weir Mitchell, working with Civil War wounded, first used the term *causalgia* for a syndrome of limb pain, wasting, and trophic changes noted to follow gun-shot wound injuries of major nerves;[17,18] this is a syndrome now recognized as part of the reflex sympathetic dystrophy complex. Missile wound and laceration injuries were studied during the major wars of the next 100 years and resulted in accurate descriptions of peripheral nerve anatomy and the nerve supply to muscles. During the first 50 years of this century, civilian nerve entrapments and compressions were studied with the promise for surgical repair. Attempts to explain "thenar wasting" sparked speculation about the cervical rib syndrome,[12] scalenus anticus, scalenus medius, and other thoracic outlet syndromes, opening a confusing literature that is only now becoming rational.[7,8]

Clear understanding of common nerve entrapments and compressive neuropathies such as carpal tunnel syndrome and ulnar elbow neuropathy awaited the localizing capabilities of electromyography and nerve conduction techniques, which grew from the electronic technology of World War II and were made practical in the 1960s with transistors and noise-free biological amplifiers.

In the present day, upper extremity pain sits with headache and low back pain on the list of most common ambulatory complaints. A public awareness of occupationally related nerve entrapments and cumulative trauma syndromes has exploded; for example, front-page attention followed reports of affliction of newsroom workers at the *LA Times*.[14] Carpal tunnel syndrome related to prolonged keyboard use is described even in personal computer trade journals.[11]

Despite the prevalence of upper limb nerve injuries and entrapments, confusion still surrounds these common problems. (This is painfully evident in the medicolegal testimony of malpractice, personal injury, and industrial injury cases.) However, the hard facts of neuroanatomy form the underpinnings of neurologic localization. When skillfully employed, a neurologic history and examination along with clinical neurophysiologic testing should often yield a clear diagnosis and allow a reasonable management plan for the majority of patients.

The neuromuscular specialist, armed with a knowledge of nerve and muscle anatomy, and with training in electromyography and neurophysiologic techniques, has a uniquely powerful capability to localize nerve lesions. The referring nurse or physician should be aware, however, that expertise in neuromuscular disease is a recognized subspecialty often with postresidency training. Electromyography and clinical neurophysiology are board certifiable skills, with written and oral examinations usually following a year or two of fellowship study and active practice.[2]

NEUROLOGIC ANATOMY

The nervous system (Fig. 1) is composed of six parts: the brain, brainstem, cerebellum,

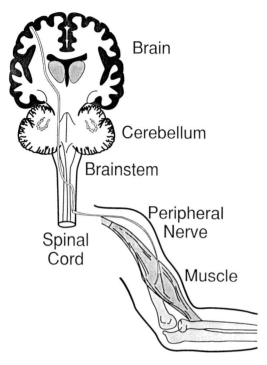

FIGURE 1.   The six major parts of the nervous system.

spinal cord, peripheral nerves, and muscles. The thoughtful clinician must bear in mind that a lesion in any of these structures may lead to upper extremity dysfunction.

Central nervous system (CNS) lesions may cause motor impairment, sensory symptoms or both. **Motor dysfunction** manifests as weakness or incoordination and implies a lesion in either the pyramidal or extrapyramidal motor systems. The *pyramidal system* has *upper motor neurons* with cell bodies in the frontal lobe of the brain. These extend filamentous axons downward, which cross in the brainstem and descend in the lateral column of the spinal cord to synapse on *lower motor neuron* cell bodies in the anterior horn of the spinal cord gray matter. These send axons anteriorly, which fuse to form nerve roots, then exit the spine and, in the neck and shoulder, combine to form the brachial plexus and nerves of the upper extremity. The motor axons within these nerves eventually synapse on muscle fibers of the limbs.

An intentional movement originates in the frontal lobe of the brain and a signal that traverses this pathway and activates lower motor neurons in the spinal cord. The lower motor neurons then propagate action potentials that reach and activate target muscle fibers via elec-trochemical processes at the neuromuscular junction.

Lesions at any point along this pathway can cause weakness. Examples include stroke, brain tumor, or spinal cord tumor affecting the upper motor neurons of the CNS. Brachial plexus stretch injury or nerve entrapment at the elbow or in the carpal tunnel can impair the lower motor neuron function in the *peripheral nervous system* (PNS).

The *extrapyramidal system* of the CNS includes the basal ganglia and cerebellum. Lesions here impair motor coordination without true weakness. Examples include *Parkinson's disease*, a basal ganglia disorder manifested by hand tremor, increased muscle tone, unsteadiness, and gait impairment. Symptoms often start with limb stiffness and a lack of arm swing when walking. Multiple sclerosis is a disease that often affects the cerebellum causing tremor and incoordination of the hands and arms, also without weakness. Signs of cranial nerve and spinal cord impairment are frequent accompaniments.

Sensory impairments are more difficult to localize, primarily due to the greater complexity of the sensory pathways. Sensory neuron cell bodies are grouped in *ganglia* of the dorsal roots that occupy the vertebral neural foramina. From these dorsal root ganglion cells, lengthy axons extend centrally into the dorsal spinal cord and peripherally to sensory receptors in the skin and other tissues of the limb. Small diameter axons subserve *temperature and superficial pain sensation*. They enter the spinal cord posteriorly and synapse in the dorsal grey columns. Second-order neurons then cross locally and ascend in the spinothalamic tracts of the opposite lateral white column of the spinal cord, destined for the thalamus with subsequent connections to the cerebral cortex of the parietal lobe. Large fibers carry sensation *joint movement, joint position, touch,* and *vibration.* They enter the spinal cord posteriorly and ascend ipsilaterally to synapse in the brainstem. The second-order neurons then cross in the brainstem and ascent to the thalamus.

These CNS pathways cannot be ignored when evaluating a patient with upper extremity sensory complaints. Illustrative clinical syndromes include *thalamic syndrome* causing numbness or pain in the limb opposite a stroke deep in the brain, and *syringomyelia*, a degeneration of the central core of the spinal cord affecting the sensory fibers crossing in the anterior commissure and causing a *cloak deficit* of pain and temperature sensation, sparing position and vibratory sense—a so-called *dissociated sensory loss* (Fig. 2A).

The CNS pathways are segregated: motor tracts remain anterior and sensory tracts posterior. The tracts cross at different levels, allowing lesion localization. *Brown-Séquard syndrome* (Fig. 2B) is a classic example: a hemilesion of the spinal cord causes spastic paralysis on the same side as the lesion and loss of pain and temperature on the contralateral trunk and limbs. This isolation of motor from sensory pathways continues into the nerve roots, but after joining to form the spinal nerves, the sensory and motor fibers intertwine.

Occupational, industrial, and medicolegal neurologic issues involving the upper extremity most often concern PNS injury of impairment. Peripheral nervous system neurology thus comprises most of this chapter.

The tissue elements of the PNS include the following:

1. Sensory receptors and sensory neurons and their connections with CNS structures.

2. Autonomic afferent (inbound) neurons and their central connections.

3. Autonomic efferent (outbound) neurons for control of nonvolitional activity (cardiac, gastrointestinal, sweat, salivation, and other glandular functions).

4. Lower motor neurons with cell bodies in the anterior horn; each sends an axon outward connecting the CNS to muscle.

5. Neuromuscular junctions connecting nerve to muscle.

6. Muscle cells.

7. PNS vasculature, connective tissue, and other supporting elements.

These ingredients are woven into the major parts of the PNS:

1. Cranial nerves.

2. Dorsal (sensory) nerve roots containing the dorsal root ganglia.

3. Ventral (motor) nerve roots.

4. The paravertebral sympathetic chain of ganglia.

5. Cervical, brachial, lumbar, and sacral plexuses.

6. Nerves of the extremities and intercostal and radicular nerves.

7. The muscles.

The unique features of the PNS make it susceptible to physical injury. Consider a sensory neuron. The axon, about 10 microns thick, extends about 2 meters from the brain stem to the toes, making it 200,000 times longer than wide. It depends on the nerve cell body in the dorsal root ganglion for replenishment of spent subcellular organelles and for supply of some nutrients. The axon is first vulnerable to phys-

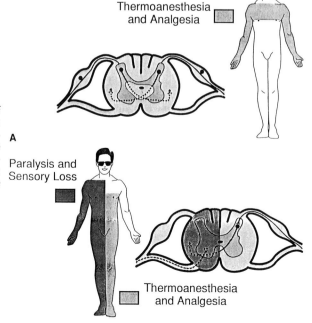

FIGURE 2. *A*, Syringomyelia is a degeneration of the central spinal cord causing a cloak pattern of pain and temperature sensory loss. *B*, Brown-Séquard syndrome results from an injury affecting one half of the spinal cord. Weakness occurs on the side of the lesion and sensory loss for pain and temperature on the opposite side, reflecting the local crossing of the latter pathway.

Thermoanesthesia and Analgesia

A

Paralysis and Sensory Loss

Thermoanesthesia and Analgesia

B

ical injury as it exits the spine by disc or bone-spur impingement. Further along, entrapment or stretch injury can occur as the brachial plexus traverses the thoracic apex. Compression, stretch, angulation, heat, cold, and blunt or sharp trauma may injure the nerves as they traverse joints. Also, the cellular components of nerve are metabolically active living tissue requiring a blood supply. The nerves tend to travel with the major vessels, receiving branches that terminate the *vasa nervorum*—small longitudinal vessels within the nerve sheath. Vascular injury ranges from transient numbness due to pressure occlusion of the capillaries and vasa nervorum to frank nerve infarct following major vessel thromboses or emboli.

A cross-section of nerve (Fig. 3) shows the internal organization. *Epineurium* ensheathes and protects the *fascicles* and arterioles and imparts tensile strength to the nerve. *Renaut bodies* are found at joints and points of compression, acting as shock absorbers or as a reaction to stress.[3] The fascicles interweave in ropelike array, are wrapped in a sleeve of flat *perineurial* cells joined in a tile-work by tight junctions, and form the *blood-nerve barrier*. The barrier isolates the endoneurial environment from the blood, but allows entry of necessary nutrients and outward diffusion of metabolic wastes.

Schwann cells wrap the larger diameter motor and sensory axons in layers of myelin (Fig. 4), a double sheet formed by fusion of the cell membranes, investing them with segments of insulation that raise membrane resistance. A *node of Ranvier* lies between each adjacent pair of Schwann cells. *Myelination* allows nerve action potentials to jump from one node of Ranvier to the next in a *saltatory conduction* at high velocity. Unmyelinated smaller diameter

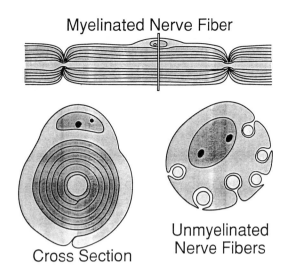

FIGURE 4.   Myelinated and unmyelinated nerve fibers.

fibers (subserving pain, temperature, and autonomic functions) conduct action potentials in a slower continuous fadhion. They lie grouped without myelin layers in Schwann cells that probably play a sustentacular role.

Segmental Anatomy

Nerve roots (8 cervical, 12 thoracic, 5 lumbar, and 5 sacral) exit from each vertebral interspace. At each exit, the dorsal sensory root joins the ventral motor root to form a spinal nerve (Fig. 5) that leaves the spine via the neural foramen. A *dural sleave* surrounds the roots and dorsal root ganglion and joins the *pia-arachnoid membranes* to become the epineu-

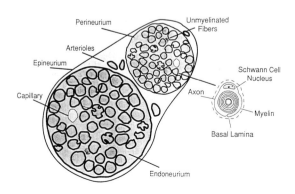

FIGURE 3.   The internal organization of peripheral nerve seen in cross section.

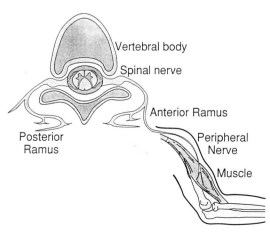

FIGURE 5.   Cross-section of the spinal cord showing exiting spinal nerve.

TABLE 1.   Nerve Root Innervation of Upper Extremity Musculature

	C5	C6	C7	C8	T1
Supraspinatus	◆	◆			
Infraspinatus	◆	◆			
Deltoid	◆	◆			
Biceps	◆	◆			
Ext. carpi radialis	◆	◆			
Brachioradialis	◆	◆			
Supinator		◆	◆		
Pronator teres		◆	◆		
Flex. carpi radialis		◆	◆		
Triceps			◆	◆	
Ext. digitorum comm.			◆	◆	
Flex. pollicis longus			◆	◆	
Pronator quadratus			◆	◆	
Abd. pollicis brevis				◆	◆
Dorsal interossei				◆	◆
Abd. digiti minimi				◆	◆

rium surrounding the nerve. Spinal nerves each divide into a small dorsal ramus, supplying the paraspinal region and paraspinal muscles, and a larger ventral ramus destined for the limb or anterolateral trunk. In the thoracic region, these form intercostal nerves. In the neck and lumbar region, the ventral rami weave into plexuses (Table 1).

The *brachial plexus* originates from cervical segments C5, C6, C7, C8, and T1 (recall that

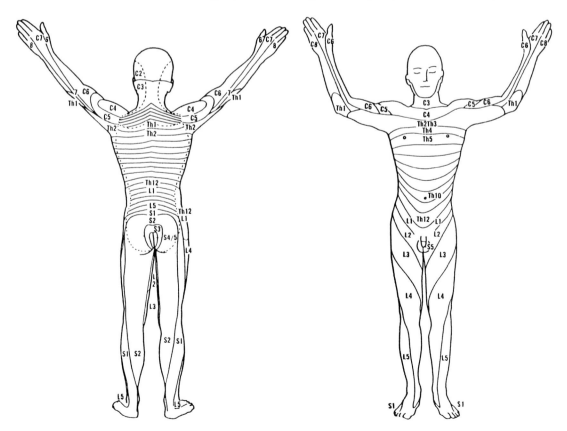

FIGURE 6.   Sensory dermatomes of the upper extremity.

one extra nerve root, C8, exits at the cervicothoracic junction). These intermingle elaborately and traverse the base of the neck, thoracic apex, and subclavicular region to divide near the axilla into the major nerves of the shoulder, arm, forearm, and hand.

Disc herniation, apophysial joint arthritis, vertebral body injury, or other cervical spine disorders may irritate or impinge upon nerve roots and manifest as pain, numbness, and reflex change in the limb. The location of symptoms and pattern of physical findings identifies the specific nerve root involved, often more accurately than x-rays, CT, or MRI scans. Table 1 lists the distribution of nerve root motor supply, and the sensory dermatomes are seen in Figure 6.

Figure 7 shows the brachial plexus. The spinal nerves join to form upper, middle, and lower trunks. These each divide into anterior and posterior divisions. The three posterior divisions fuse into the posterior cord, which, after giving off small nerves to the shoulder region, divides into the axillary nerve (to the deltoid and teres minor) and radial nerve (supplying all of the posterior extensor muscles of the arm and forearm). The anterior divisions of the upper and middle trunks join to form the lateral cord, and the anterior division of the lower trunk becomes the medial cord. The medial and lateral cords unite to form the median nerve, but, before joining, the musculocutaneous nerve branches form the lateral cord and the ulnar nerve from the medial cord.

The Individual Nerves

The **median nerve** is composed of motor fibers from the C6, C7, C8, and T1 roots, which traverse the brachial plexus and form the median nerve shown in Figure 8. The nerve trav-

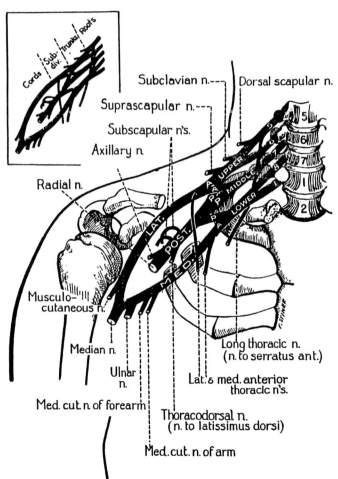

FIGURE 7. Diagram of the brachial plexus. The components of the plexus are depicted (out of scale) in the upper left. (From Haymaker W, Woodhall B: *Peripheral Nerve Injuries.* Philadelphia, WB Saunders, 1953, with permission.)

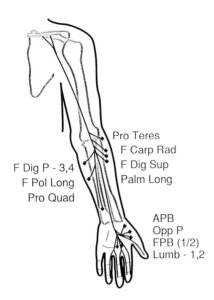

FIGURE 8. The median nerve.

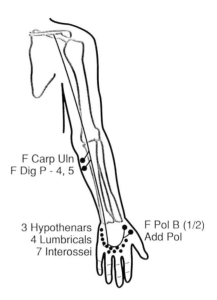

FIGURE 9. The ulnar nerve.

els medially down the arm, coursing anterior to the medial humeral epicondyle to the antecubital region with the radial artery. A *ligament of Struthers* occurs rarely just above the medial epicondyle and has been described as a rare cause of high median nerve entrapment. In the forearm, entrapments occur as the nerve passes through the *pronator teres* muscle or as the *anterior interosseus* branch passes below the sublimis arch. The nerve supplies seven muscles in the forearm, four from the main branch and three via the anterior interosseus nerve. The main branch enters the hand through the carpal tunnel beneath the *flexor retinaculum*, gives off a recurrent motor branch to the three thenar muscles, and then supplies the first two lumbricals. The final branch supplies sensation to the palmar surfaces of the first $3\frac{1}{2}$ digits. A palmar cutaneous branch comes off above the wrist and passes volar to the flexor retinaculum, explaining palmar sparing in the carpal tunnel syndrome.

The axons of the **ulnar nerve** (Fig. 9) derive from the C7, C8, and T1 nerve roots, traverse the inferomedial aspects of the brachial plexus, and travel medially in the arm to the medial epicondyle of the humerus, uniquely traversing the extensor aspect of the elbow in the medial epicondylar groove. Figure 10 shows detail of the true cubital funnel formed by the two heads of flexor carpi ulnaris, under which the ulnar nerve enters the deep forearm. Entrapments and chronic compressions may occur at the condylar groove, the cubital tunnel,

or both.[13] Only two muscles (flexor carpi ulnaris and flexor digitorum profundus to digits 4 and 5) are supplied in the forearm. The anatomic detail at the wrist is of importance: a tunnel is formed (the canal of Guyon) by the hamate and pisiform bones with a ligamentous roof. Three branches occur in this area: the hypothenar branch, the deep motor branch, and the cutaneous branch to the last $1\frac{1}{2}$ digits. Entrapments and compressions are common at this point, especially in association with sports ("handlebar palsy") and industrial tool use. The ulnar nerve supplies 15 of the intrinsic hand muscles: three in the hypothenar group, seven interossei, two lumbricals to digits 4 and 5, adductor pollicis, the deep belly of flexor pollicis brevis, and palmaris brevis. A cutaneous palmar branch and a dorsal cutaneous branch leave the ulnar nerve in the distal forearm and are spared from entrapment at the wrist, a point of value in electrodiagnostic localization.

The posterior cord of the brachial plexus branches into the **axillary nerve** and the larger **radial nerve** (Fig. 11). The axillary nerve travels posteriorly through the quadrangular space (a site of purported entrapment), supplies the deltoid and teres minor muscles of the shoulder, and is subject to injury with shoulder dislocation and high humeral fractures. The radial nerve leaves the axilla posteriorly, gives off branches to the triceps, and then twines around the humeral shaft in the spiral groove, a vascular watershed where the nerve can be injured with prolonged compression, the "Sat-

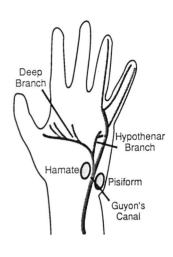

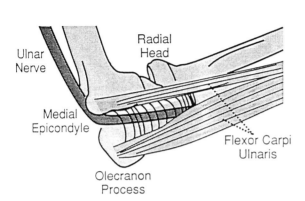

FIGURE 10.   Detail of the ulnar nerve at elbow and wrist.

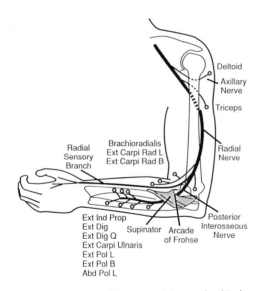

FIGURE 11.   The radial nerve and the arcade of Frohse.

urday night palsy." Branches to the mobile wad muscles (brachioradialis and extensors carpi radialis longus and brevis) and the main sensory branch leave as the nerve passes the elbow anterior to the lateral epicondyle and lateral to the biceps tendon. The posterior interosseus nerve dives below a fibrous entrance to the deep forearm, the *arcade of Frohse*, passes under the supinator muscle, and serves the digital extensor muscles and extensor carpi ulnaris. Compression beneath the arcade can cause digit extensor weakness, largely sparing wrist extension and sensation. The sensory branch to the dorsum of the hand can be injured with tight hand cuffs or bracelets (*cheiralgia paresthetica*).

Brachial Plexus

The brachial plexus traverses the most mobile joint in the body and is susceptible to stretch injury with extreme downward thrusts or hyperextension of the upper extremity as seen in motor vehicle accidents. Location of the plexus also makes it liable to missile wound, injury with shoulder dislocation or clavicle fracture, and surgical injury during orthopedic procedures. Upper plexopathy occurs as a birth injury with undue pressure applied to free a shoulder from beneath the pubic bone (Erb's palsy); shoulder weakness may be a permanent result. Localization of a lesion to the brachial plexus is usually done by exclusion; i.e. if the deficits found on physical examination are beyond a nerve or root distribution, then "think plexus."

Lymphoma or metastatic tumors may directly affect the plexus; axillary dissection and radiation add further risk of injury. Injury to the lower plexus during sternotomy for open heart surgery is a distressingly common occurrence, causing pain and hand/forearm weakness that usually resolves in 6 to 8 weeks.[15]

Parsonage and Turner first reported *brachial plexitis* (brachial neuritis, neuralgia amyotrophy), as observed in soldiers of World War II. They described a syndrome of sudden onset with marked upper limb pain occurring in the phase of convalescence from wounds or other illnesses. Pain wanes in a few weeks to reveal weakness and wasting of the limb in a distribution referable to the brachial plexus. Motor function recovers in 12 to 18 months.[6] This condition is uncommon, often following a cold or flu, and may affect both upper extremities in 40% of cases. Misdiagnosis seems to be the rule on first encounter, with the condition mistaken for a nerve, root, or shoulder joint affliction. Treatment is supportive.

Thoracic outlet syndrome (TOS) is best divided into vascular and neurogenic types.[22] The true or classical neurogenic TOS is rare, usually associated with a rudimentary cervical rib, a small projection from the transverse process of the seventh cervical vertebra that projects a fibrous band from its tip to the first rib. In affected individuals the brachial plexus is stretched or angulated over this band (Fig. 12) causing dysfunction of the lower elements,

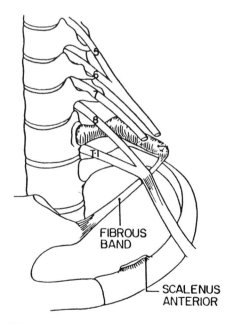

FIGURE 12. Cervical rib underlies the true neurogenic thoracic outlet syndrome. The compression site frequently involves the lower trunk or medial cord, which form the median, ulnar, and medial cutaneous nerves of arm, and medial cutaneous nerve of forearm. (From Rosati LM, Lord JW, *Neurovascular Compression Syndromes of the Shoulder Girdle.* New York, Grune and Stratton, 1961, with permission.)

usually the fibers from the C8 and T1 roots and the lower trunk. Symptoms include an intermittent ache and numbness in the ulnar aspect of the arm and forearm, and chronic or slowly progressive weakness of the intrinsic hand muscles. Wasting of the hand muscles, most prominently the thenar muscles at the base of the thumb, appears in those significantly affected. Provocative maneuvers such as Adson's test are unreliable, perhaps revealing the vascular type of TOS, but otherwise serving only to distract from the neurologic features. Diagnosis by EMG and nerve conduction studies is quite subtle. One reported electrodiagnostic trick has been proven fraudulent.[21]

Surgical treatment of TOS should be reserved for those with significant disability. The supraclavicular approach is preferred. First rib resection by transaxillary approach has been seriously challenged. Operative brachial plexus injuries are the basis of a number of recent law suits and the subject of damning medical reviews.[4] Other varieties of TOS are controversial, and caution should be exercised in forwarding this diagnosis; effort should be directed instead to excluding other more common and remediable conditions.

Another condition causing diagnostic confusion is *reflex sympathetic dystrophy* (RSD). Reflex sympathetic dystrophy may follow a nerve injury in the arm, forearm, or hand, or even a minor limb trauma, by days or weeks. Clinical features include severe burning pain that is not well demarcated, joint stiffness and tenderness, change in appearance of the skin, hair and nails, and vasomotor changes, usually manifest by swelling and discoloration.[19] The pain usually occurs near the location of the injury but may lag in onset for several days or a few weeks and, along with the other features, evolves over weeks or months with variable severity. Muscle wasting, frozen shoulder, and flexion contractures are common features in the full-blown syndrome. The pathogenesis is obscure. Treatments are speculative and the results are often disappointing, but sympathetic blockade (by injection into the sympathetic ganglia of the neck, regional infusion, or systemic medication) shows promise.

NEUROLOGIC LOCALIZATION

Ignorance or neglect of peripheral nerve anatomy leads to iatrogenic injuries, a distressingly common cause of referral to our peripheral nerve injury center and the topic of a recent review.[5] Laceration, cautery, or suture injury occurs if the presence of a nerve is not expected and respected. Also, careless clinical localization may direct the surgeon to operate at the wrong site (e.g., cervical laminectomy for suspected disc herniation when carpal tunnel syndrome is the true source of symptoms). In contrast, the impressive success of judicious entrapment release, careful laceration repair, and nerve grafting when indicated underscores the importance of accurate lesion localization. The general concepts of localization apply simple pattern recognition: does the patient's signs/symptoms complex agree with known anatomy?

Upper Extremity Neurologic Evaluation

For neurologic disorders of the upper extremity, signs generally hide behind symptoms. In other words, the patient comes to the physician with pain or sensory loss, but careful examination reveals focal weakness, often to the patient's surprise.

Patients are annoyed by questions about the quality of pain or sensory paresthesias because their experience may not be simple burning, aching, or stabbing, but rather a sensation beyond common human experience and lacking a lexicon. Some terms have been defined:[16]

Hyperesthesia: increased sensitivity to stimulation.

Allodynia: pain experienced in response to non-noxious stimuli

Hyperpathia: painful response to a noxious stimulus with increased threshold, overreaction, and persistence.

Causalgia: burning, severe, persistent pain following nerve injury, usually radiating beyond the territory of the injured nerve.[19]

A symptom review should include questions about onset and time course: Are the symptoms fixed, intermittent, or progressive, and what, if anything, brings relief? Ask what makes the symptoms worse and what, if anything, brings relief. A classic symptom complex is that of carpal tunnel syndrome, worse with elevation of the hands (reading a newspaper, driving a car) or at night, and relieved by shaking the

hands or sleeping with the arm draped over the side of the bed. In contrast, pain due to nerve root disease typically radiates down the arm with coughing, sneezing, or straining; worsens with lifting or stress; and is relieved by rest or traction.

Motor symptoms are less frequently volunteered, but questions regarding function may be revealing. Ask about difficulty turning doorknobs or keys, buttoning clothes, or using dinner utensils. Twitches or cramps suggest a more proximal disorder such as nerve root or anterior horn cell disease.

The objective approach begins with a general examination, including a close look at the skin and checking for asymmetries of temperature or hue. Check the pulses and examine the shoulder and joints for mobility and tenderness. Look for signs of old fracture (carpal tunnel syndrome is common with prior Colles' fracture) and examine the fingers for signs of arthritis. Next is a general neurologic examination. If cranial nerve abnormalities or leg abnormalities accompany upper extremity findings, then a CNS process is revealed and the patient should be referred to a neurologist.

Specific attention is first paid to the neck, with inspection and range of motion. The foramenal compression test (gentle downward pressure on the head with the neck extended and rotated) may trigger radicular pain revealing cervical nerve root irritation. Muscular testing is an essential tool in the examination of the PNS and is detailed in a concise atlas that is available from the Editorial Committee of *Brain*.[1] Inspection for focal wasting is done with the limbs held side by side.

Motor Examination. Motor weakness should fit a pattern, e.g., thenar muscle weakness in carpal tunnel syndrome, sparing the other 15 intrinsic hand muscles. When limb weakness is found, is it an *upper motor neuron pattern* of weakness causing greater involvement of extensor muscles and with increased tone and spastic reflexes, or is it a *lower motor neuron pattern* in line with root, plexus, or nerve anatomy and with decreased tone, muscle wasting, and reflex loss? Lastly, if a focus of weakness is found, test a muscle or muscles bearing the same nerve root supply as the weakened muscle, but in the territory of a different nerve. Some helpful general rules of localization are shown in Table 2.

    Example. George is a roofer. He is having trouble with his right (dominant) hand, noting a drop

TABLE 2. General Rules of Nerve Root Localization

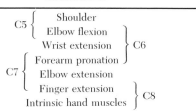

in the grip strength and an ache of the forearm and shoulder. Examination shows loss of bulk and weakness of the thenar muscles. Sensory testing is patchy, thought to reflect his thick palmar skin. Careful testing shows weakness beyond the thenar muscles affecting the thumb adductor, interosseous muscles, hypothenar group, and, to pin it down exactly, weakness in the index extensor, thumb extensors, and the long flexor of the thumb. These muscles have but one thing in common: they all take their nerve supply from the C8 nerve root. He has an EMG test (*vide infra*) showing denervation in these same muscles as well as in the lower cervical paraspinal muscles. So George has an eighth cervical nerve root lesion. X-ray study shows C7–T1 disc disease and neural foramenal narrowing at that level as well. Careful examination in this case helps to distinguish the problem from simple carpal tunnel syndrome or ulnar neuropathy, both in the differential diagnosis of hand weakness.

Reflexes. Upper extremity reflexes are enhanced if tested with the patient standing: biceps and brachioradialis (C5 and C6 roots) with the forearm held slightly flexed; triceps (C7 root) with the hand on the hips. A heavy rubber reflex hammer is essential; jaw clenching reinforces the response.

Sensory Examination. Sensory testing is the *bete noir* of the neurologic examiner, and a rule of thumb is that an exam exceeding 5 minutes will be useless. Accuracy demands subtlety. For example, regions of sensory loss due to distal lesions (carpal tunnel syndrome) are well marginated, but proximal lesions such as nerve root impingement lack a discrete perimeter due to dermatomal overlap. Light touch is tested with a cotton swab. Break the stick to make a sharp end for pinprick testing. The flat side of a metal tuning fork is adequate for temperature testing. Note that sensory testing will yield a different margin if the edge is approached from within the zone of sensory loss compared to moving from without to within. Also, vibratory sense does not respect the midline if tested over bony structures such as the

skull or sternum. These are points of value in distinguishing the malingerer or hysteric. More formal sensory testing is possible with Semmes-Weinstein monofilaments, commercial vibrameters, and current perception and thermal sensitivity equipment, often available at hand rehabilitation centers.

CLINICAL NEUROPHYSIOLOGY

The powerful tools of neurologic localization are amplified by clinical neurophysiologic testing, which can be used to confirm the clinical findings. The term *electromyography* (EMG) refers in the broad sense to a set of diagnostic tests employing neurophysiologic techniques that are performed on nerves and muscles. In the more specific sense, EMG refers to one of these tests in which a small needle is used to probe selected muscles, recording electrical potentials from the muscle fibers. This double meaning causes confusion. The label *clinical neurophysiology* is a favored term encompassing EMG, nerve conduction velocity (NCV), and somatosensory evoked potential (SEP) testing. An EMG machine, used for all these tests, is simply an oscilloscope with biologic amplifiers and electronics tailored for special test protocols. Clinical neurophysiology is a medical subspecialty practiced primarily by neurologists and physiatrists, requiring written and oral examinations for certification.[2] Below, we will describe the spectrum of available tests, emphasizing that clinical neurophysiology seldom stands alone and should serve as an extension of the practitioners diagnostic tools of history-taking and physical examination.

Electromyography

A motor neuron has a cell body in the spinal cord and extends into the nerve root, an axon that exits the spine, traverses the plexus, travels within a nerve, and then forms many distal branches. A *motor unit* consists of one such cell and the several muscle fibers that it innervates. A muscle contains many motor units with its fibers that are intermixed like colored pencils in a bundle (Fig. 13A). Muscle force is generated by activation of increasing numbers of motor units under command from the brain via the spinal cord. As a motor unit fires, a small electrical signal is generated and can be recorded by placing a small needle electrode,

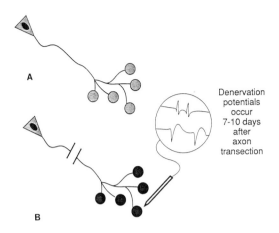

Denervation
potentials
occur
7-10 days
after
axon
transection

FIGURE 13. *A*, The motor unit. *B*, Fibrillations and positive waves.

acting as a tiny antenna, through the skin and into the muscle near the motor unit fibers. The signal is amplified, filtered, digitized, and displayed on the screen of the oscilloscope.

Single *motor unit potentials* (Fig. 14A) are sampled. Their amplitude in millivolts, duration in milliseconds, and number of phases are noted and recorded. The motor unit potentials begin to fire repetitively at about 5 per second, with *recruitment* of more units and increase in the firing rate as greater force is generated.

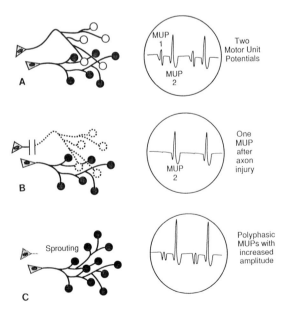

MUP 1
MUP 2
Two
Motor Unit
Potentials

One
MUP
after
axon
injury
MUP 2

Sprouting
Polyphasic
MUPs with
increased
amplitude

FIGURE 14. *A*, Two motor unit potentials in a simplified muscle. *B*, Axon injury. The remaining motor unit fires rapidly. *C*, Sprouting and reinnervation creates a high amplitude polyphasic motor unit potential.

Will full force, the screen fills with these signals, which is an appearance called the *full interference pattern*. The amplifier output is also fed to a loudspeaker, allowing recognition of characteristic sounds and patterns, a powerful tool for the experienced electromyographer. In primary diseases of muscle such as *muscular dystrophy* or *myositis*, the motor unit potentials become low in amplitude and brief in duration, and the interference pattern is full even with minimal force of contraction. Should nerve injury cause axonal breakage, the distal axon degenerates (*Wallerian degeneration*) and the muscle fibers of the motor unit become electrically irritable. Needle movement then generates *denervation potentials* called *fibrillations* and *positive waves*, which have a recognizable appearance on the oscilloscope screen (Fig. 13B) and a characteristic sound from the loudspeaker. The advent of these denervation potentials is delayed for about 10 days even after complete nerve transection. The motor unit potentials in chronic *neuropathic* processes (due to nerve disease or injury) develop high amplitude and long duration, an effect due to sprouting of intact axons and enlargement of the motor unit (Fig. 14C). *Fasciculations* occur with proximal lesions such as nerve root impingement and with diseases of the neuron cell body in the spinal cord, such as *amyotrophic lateral sclerosis*.

EMG allows direct quantitation of motor unit function and thus enables the electromyographer to differentiate neuropathic from *myopathic* (due to muscle disease) causes of weakness. Also, anatomical localization is made possible by finding a pattern of denervation confined to muscles in the distribution of a particular nerve or nerve root. A table such as Table 1 is kept close at hand in the EMG lab. EMG is also useful for following the recovery from nerve or muscle disease and the results of treatment, but is usually adjunctive to physical examination.

Newer techniques include *single fiber EMG*, whereby a specialized needle with a microscopic side port is used to record potentials from small groups of muscle cells, a technique of greatest utility in diagnosing diseases of the neuromuscular junction such as myasthenia gravis. *Macro EMG* employs a needle with an unshielded barrel to record gross motor unit activity and is more specific in differentiating neuropathic from myopathic processes. EMG can also be used for kinesiologic studies and in the assessment of tremors.

Nerve Conduction Studies

EMG machines are also fitted with a nerve stimulator that is used to apply an electrical shock to the skin surface at accessible points along a nerve, depolarizing a segment of the nerve and generating a nerve action potential that travels outward in both directions from the point of stimulation. If applied to a sensory nerve, the nerve action potential can be recorded from skin surface electrodes or finger-ring electrodes at a distal point (Fig. 15A). The distance from stimulus to recording site is measured with a cloth tape. The time of flight, called *latency*, and action potential *amplitude* are determined from the oscilloscope tracing. Distance is divided by time to yield a sensory nerve conduction velocity (or *sensory NCV*), usually about 50–60 meters per second in normal adults. *Motor NCVs* are recorded from surface electrodes taped over muscles distally in the limb, often on the thenar or hypothenar muscle groups for median or ulnar nerve studies.

Compound motor action potentials (Fig. 15B)

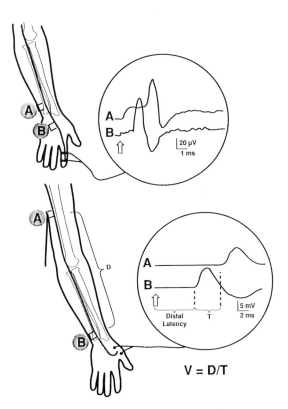

FIGURE 15. Sensory and motor nerve conduction velocity tests.

are recorded when the nerve is stimulated at two or more sites proximally. Distances are measured, latencies and amplitudes are recorded, and NCVs are calculated segment by segment, also in the range of 50–60 meters per second. In the absence of nerve disease, NCVs are remarkably constant, remaining uniform from age 3 through adulthood; mild slowing begins after age 55. Limb temperature has a dramatic effect on NCV, slowing 5% for each degree below 34°C, and should be recorded on any complete report. If limb temperature is below 30°C, the extremity should be warmed before testing. Segmental slowing (for example in the ulnar nerve around the elbow) suggests the presence of a chronic lesion, i.e., an entrapment or nerve compression. Loss of action potential amplitude implies a focal conduction block, usually associated with a more acute process, which can be localized by "inching" up the nerve with the stimulator probe. Motor and sensory NCVs should be recorded below, above, and around a suspected lesion, and other uninvolved nerves should be sampled to screen for an underlying generalized neuropathic process such as diabetes or uremia. Abnormalities should be compared to the same nerve in the other limb. NCVs can also be used to sort generalized neuropathies into myelinopathic (with generalized slowing of conduction) and axonopathic (with low amplitude) categories.

Special Techniques

The *f-wave* is of small amplitude, occurring with a significant delay after the compound motor action potential. Stimulation of the nerve discharges a pulse in both directions. The proximally travelling pulse enters the spinal cord where some of the motor neurons backfire, sending another pulse distally to elicit this small *late response*. Another response is the *H-reflex*, a true reflex analogous to the Achilles tendon reflex and serving mainly as an indictor of S-1 nerve root integrity. Initiated by stimulation of the tibial nerve at the knee, the H-reflex is recorded from surface electrodes over the soleus muscle. Repetitive nerve stimulation studies are used as a test for neuromuscular junction diseases such as myasthenia gravis, organophosphate poisoning, or botulism; in these disorders the compound motor action potential loses amplitude in response to successive nerve stimulations at about 3 per second.

Somatosensory Evoked Potentials

Following nerve stimulation, an afferent pulse of large fiber sensory activity travels proximally, enters the spinal cord, ascends in the posterior columns, and synapses in the brainstem. Post-synaptic activity reaches the thalamus and eventually the parietal cortex of the brain. Although the CNS pathways are complex, a small brain wave occurs at a fixed time following nerve stimulation and is recordable from electrodes on the scalp surface. The signal is small and buried in the higher voltage EEG, but the technique of *signal averaging* is used to extract the signal from the background noise. Multichannel equipment allows recording of these *somatosensory evoked potentials* (SEPs or SSEPs) simultaneously from several points along the course of the impulse journey; e.g., from above the clavicle at *Erb's point*, which overlies the brachial plexus, over the cervical spine, and from the scalp overlying the parietal lobe of the brain. Median SEPs (Fig. 16) and ulnar SEPs are the most commonly studied in the upper extremity.

SEPs are useful in a manner analogous to NCVs, with the advantage that central as well as peripheral pathways are tested. However, the test is less specific and technical difficulties leave room for error. Their use for diagnosis of nerve root disease is questionable at present; due to the multisegmental contribution to most major nerves, the SEP may remain normal even in the face of a complete single nerve root lesion. A more practical application involves spinal cord monitoring during spine surgery, but stimulation is usually applied to the lower extremities. Upper extremity SEPs, however, are a useful check during brachial plexus surgery.

Dermatomal SEPs (DSEPs) represent an attempt to make these techniques more localizing of nerve root lesions. Digital or cutaneous nerves are stimulated with recording from Erb's point, cervical spine, and scalp. Poor correlation and difficult reproducibility have cooled the initial enthusiasm for DSEPs.

The Report

EMG, NCV, and SEP reports should never stand alone, but always be interpreted in light of the physician's clinical assessment. These tests are technical, and the report may be difficult to interpret due to the use of unfamiliar phrases and physiologic jargon. The EMG/NCV report (Fig. 17) should display the raw data, including the distal latencies (prolonged in carpal tunnel syndrome), the NCVs, and the action potential amplitudes, allowing identification of an underlying generalized neuropathy such as occurs in diabetes. Normal and abnor-

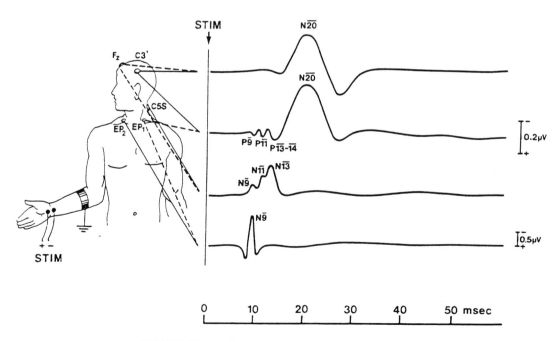

FIGURE 16.   Median nerve somatosensory evoked potentials.

UCSD EMG/NCV Studies... REPORT:

Patient Identification:

John Doe

Requested by:	Source:
	Request date: 1/1/99

Examination Requested:

Clinical Diagnosis:

Date:			Right				Left			
			Amp mV/μV	**Lat'y** mS	**Dist** mm	**CV** m/S	**Amp** mV/μV	**Lat'y** mS	**Dist** mm	**CV** m/S
Nerve		**Stim**	**Rec**							
Median	M	Wrist	APB	10.0	5.1	70		9.0	4.0	70	
"	M	Elbow	APB	10.0	9.1	220	55.0	9.0	8.1	225	54.9
"	M	Axilla	APB	10.0	12.1	180	60.0	9.0	11.0	175	60.3
"	S	Wrist	Digit II	20	4.0	140	35.0	22	3.0	140	46.7
"	S	Palm	Wrist	50	2.3	80	34.8	44	2.0	80	40.0
Ulnar	M	Wrist	ADM	12.0	2.3	70				70	
"	M	Bel Elb	ADM	12.0	6.3	205	51.3				
"	M	Ab Elb	ADM	12.0	8.3	100	50.0			100	
"	M	Axilla	ADM	12.0	10.5	110	50.0				
"	S	Wrist	Digit V	15	2.5	140	56.0			140	

Note: Amp column header: mV/μV; Lat'y: mS; Dist: mm; CV: m/S

Muscle: R L	Spontan. Activity				Motor Unit Potentials			
	Fibs	**PW**	**Fasc**	**CRD**	**Amp**	**Dur**	**Poly**	**Recr/Interf**
Abductor Policis Brevis	2+	3+	0	0	2–4	10	30%	decreased # / rapid firing
1st Dorsal Interosseus	0	0	0	0	2–4	10	0	normal # / normal rate

Report: Right carpal tunnel syndrome with thenar denervation. Mild left carpal tunnel syndrome. Normal right ulnar NCVs.

Joe Physician, M.D.

FIGURE 17.   Sample EMG report form.

mal muscles found on needle EMG should be listed and a pattern of denervation should be evident. Lastly, a phone call to the physician performing the test for a discussion of the results is very advisable, especially before forming decisions regarding surgery.

REFERENCES

1. Aids to the Examination of the Peripheral Nervous System. London, Bailliere Tindall, 1986.
2. American Board of Electrodiagnostic Medicine, Rochester, Minnesota.
3. Asbury AK, Johnson PC: Pathology of Peripheral Nerve. Philadelphia, WB Saunders, 1978, pp 28–31.
4. Cherington M, Happer I, Mechanic B, Parry L: Surgery for thoracic outlet syndrome may be hazardous to your health. Muscle Nerve 9:632–634, 1986.
5. Dawson DM, Krarup C: Perioperative nerve lesions. Arch Neurol 46:1355–1360, 1989.
6. England JD, Summer AJ: Neuralgic amyotrophy: an increasingly diverse entity. Muscle Nerve 10:60–68, 1987.
7. Gilliatt RW: Thoracic outlet syndromes. In Dyck PJ, Thomas PK, Lambert EH, et al (eds): Peripheral Neuropathy. Philadelphia, WB Saunders, 1984, pp 1409–1420.
8. Gilliatt RW, LeQuesne PM, Logue V, et al: Wasting of the hand associated with a cervical rib or band. J Neurol Neurosurg Psychiatry 33:615–624, 1970.
9. Gilliatt RW, Sears TA: Sensory nerve action potentials in patients with peripheral nerve lesions. J Neurol Neurosurg Psychiatry 17:104, 1958.
10. Gilliatt RW, Willison RG, Dietz V, et al: Peripheral nerve conductions in patients with a cervical rib and band. Ann Neurol 4:124–129, 1979.
11. Hembree D: Warning: computing can be hazardous to your health. MacWorld, Jan 1990.
12. Howell CM: A consideration of some symptoms produced by seventh cervical ribs. Lancet i:1702–1707, 1907.
13. Kimura J: Assessment of individual nerves. In Kimura

J: Electrodiagnosis in Diseases of Nerve and Muscle: Principles and Practice. Philadelphia, FA Davis, 1986, pp 111–112.

14. LA Times Sunday Magazine, March 12, 1989.
15. Lederman RJ, Breuer AC, Hanson MR, et al: Peripheral nervous system complications of coronary artery bypass graft surgery. Ann Neurol 12:297–301, 1982.
16. Merskey H, Albe-Fessard DG, Bonica JJ, et al: Pain terms: a list with definitions and notes on usage. Pain 6:249, 1979.
17. Mitchell SW: Injuries of Nerves and Their Consequences. Philadelphia, JB Lippincott, 1872.
18. Mitchell SW, Morehouse GR, Keen WW: Gunshot Wounds and Other Injuries to Nerves. Philadelphia, JB Lippincott, 1864.
19. Schwartzman RJ, McLellan TL: Reflex sympathetic dystrophy: a review. Arch Neurol 44:555–561, 1987.
20. Thomas PK: Clinical features and differential diagnosis. In Dyck PJ, Thomas PK, Lambert EH, et al (eds): Peripheral Neuropathy. Philadelphia, WB Saunders, 1984.
21. Wilbourn AJ: Evidence for conduction delay in thoracic outlet syndrome is challenged. N Engl J Med 310:1052–1053; 1984.
22. Wilbourn AJ: True neurogenic thoracic outlet syndrome: case report #7. Rochester, MN, American Assn of EMG and Electrodiagnosis, 1982.

Chapter 9

FIRST AID FOR HAND INJURIES

L. Scott Levin, MD

First aid is immediate assistance given in the case of injury or sudden illness by a bystander or other layperson before a physician's care can be obtained. Most large industrial plants have trained personnel available to provide basic medical care. Even the most minor and innocuous-appearing hand injury can cause severe disability if not treated properly. Recognition of disease, familiarity with potential problems associated with certain injuries, and prompt referral to physicians who concentrate on surgery and rehabilitation of the injured hand are essential. This chapter provides information helpful in the first line of treatment for common hand injuries. A hand surgeon should provide definitive care and follow-up of most industrial injuries to the hand.

HAND INJURIES IN THE WORKPLACE

Approximately one-third of all traumatic injuries for which people seek medical attention involve the hand or the upper extremity.[5] Injuries to the fingers and thumb alone account for up to 14% of total disabling injuries occurring at the workplace and for 6% of worker's compensation paid. From personal experience with minor cuts or abrasions, most of us can appreciate that the manual laborer may be incapacitated by injury to just one fingertip, which may result in time lost from work, labor shortage, and compromised productivity. Despite improvement in industrial, government, and union regulations, ignorance or neglect of worker safety specifications may lead to industrial accidents (Fig. 1).

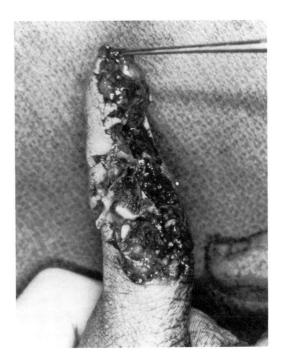

FIGURE 1. A grinding injury to the digit. Note destruction of soft tissue. The distal and proximal phalangeal joints are exposed, and there is skeletal instability. The wound was debrided, and the digit covered by a volar flap.

A wide range of injuries can occur in the workplace. The worker may regard simple lacerations or abrasions as occupational hazards that can be self-treated and not reported. Welders sometimes sustain penetrating burns to the forearm from molten metal and do not seek treatment. At the other extreme are mu-

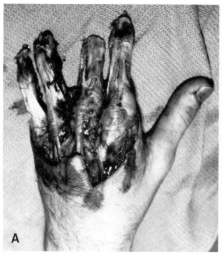 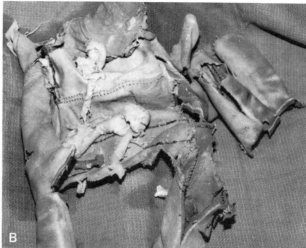

FIGURE 2. *A,* Soft tissue avulsion caused by a textile machine injury. *B,* The patient's glove and soft tissue.

tilating hand injuries or limb amputations at the elbow from textile plant machinery (Fig. 2). These are potentially life-threatening injuries that must be managed expeditiously by plant personnel.

APPROACH TO THE PATIENT

While the majority of injuries to the hand are not life threatening, sometimes the first line of treatment involves basic life support. Examples include electrical burns accompanied by cardiac arrhythmia; hemorrhagic shock due to laceration of major arteries; metabolic abnormalities that cause seizure or diabetic coma; and injuries brought about by cardiac arrest, which may cause the worker to fall into a machine and injure the upper extremity. Injury as a result of an explosion or fall requires evaluation of all systems—not just the hand. Cardiopulmonary resuscitation (CPR) may be required to save a worker's life. In these instances, hand injuries are secondary problems.

History

Once it has been determined that the injury is confined to the upper extremity, a careful history is taken and physical examination is made. Whenever an acute hand injury is evaluated, rings, watches, and jewelry should be removed from the extremity. The history should be thorough; it often aids the treatment plan.

For example, if a digit is amputated and the patient is referred for replantation, the type of machinery involved may influence the decision to replant. If information indicating, for example, that the finger was crushed by rollers rather than sharply amputated is not transmit-

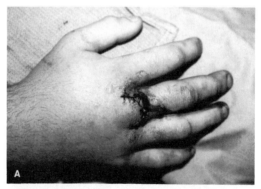

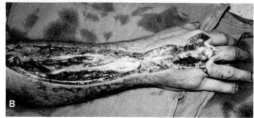

FIGURE 3. *A,* A 2-cm laceration sustained when a cinder block fell on the patient's hand while he was working as a mechanic. The wound was closed primarily. The patient presented 48 hours later with clostridium tetanus, destruction of the extensor tendons of the hand, and gangrene of the forearm. *B,* Hyperbaric oxygen and extensive debridement were necessary.

ted to the accepting physician, much time and effort may be wasted in attempting to replant a digit that is beyond salvage. The history should include the patient's age, occupation, hand dominance, time of injury, mechanism of injury, whether the hand had been previously injured (such as by fracture or nerve injury), systemic medical problems, medications, drug allergies, and tetanus status (Fig. 3). The time when the patient last ate or drank is important if general anesthesia is considered. Concentrated effort should be spent on mechanism with reference to type of machinery, force produced, and length of time between injury and presentation (was the hand trapped in a machine for several hours?) If the hand was lacerated, how deep and at what angle is the cut? Was the surrounding environment clean or dirty? What position was the hand in when it was injured? This is helpful information particularly in tendon injuries.[11]

Physical Examination

Physical examination is important in terms of being able to describe the injury to a hand surgeon if referral is necessary. Integument, tendons, nerves, blood vessels, and bony architecture may be involved in any combination. Systematic review of each system enables the health care worker to diagnose the injury so that appropriate treatment can be planned.

Skin. Examination of the traumatized hand should begin with the skin. Identify where the skin is broken. Is the laceration ragged or sharp (Fig. 4)? It is sometimes helpful to sketch the injury. Is there active bleeding? Are recognizable structures such as bone or tendon in the wound? No attempt should be made to probe or explore the wound at initial evaluation. Furthermore, if an object such as a nail or knife is impaled in the hand, it should not be removed (Fig. 5).

Vascular Supply. The next system that should be evaluated is the vascular supply to the hand. Often grease and dirt on the hand make assessment of capillary refill difficult (Fig. 6). A small alcohol swab is helpful in clearing an area of the pulp on digits suspected of being ischemic. Remember that even simple punctures at the level of the proximal phalanx can render a digit avascular and that early assessment of vascularity is essential to correct intervention (Fig. 7). Testing capillary refill involves depression of the skin 1–2 mm with an object such as a cotton-tipped applicator and

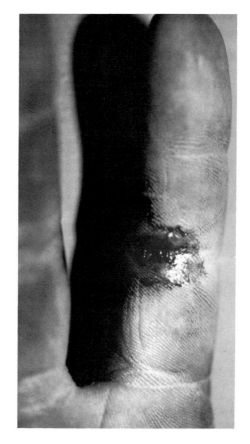

FIGURE 4. Laceration at the level of the proximal interphalangeal joint. Injury to the neurovascular bundle is not uncommon in soft tissue injuries such as these.

observation of the blanching and capillary refill. If more than 2–3 seconds are needed, there is reason to suspect vascular injury. Depressing the nail plate and observing return of blood under the nail is not an accurate method of testing blood supply. A more reliable test is to blanch the skin adjacent to the nail plate (eponychial fold) on either the radial or the ulnar order of the nail plate. If rapid refill is seen here, blood supply is assured. A digit with venous insufficiency should be noted. The skin appears purple or blue. A classic instance of a seemingly trivial injury that can result in disastrous complications is the ring avulsion injury (Fig. 8). The skin may remain intact even though arteries or veins are disrupted.[12] The Allen test can be performed if damage to the radial or ulnar artery is suspected.[13] Open injuries and pain sometimes make this test difficult to perform. The main object of assessing blood supply in the first aid evaluation is to make sure that all digits are perfusing.

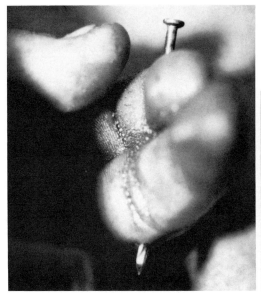

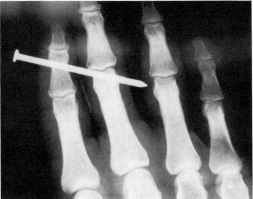

FIGURE 5. A nail-gun injury to the index and long fingers. *A,* Photograph. *B,* X-ray. The nail should not be removed at the workplace. It may be removed in the operating room, where both wounds are explored. The ulnar vascular bundle of the index finger was injured.

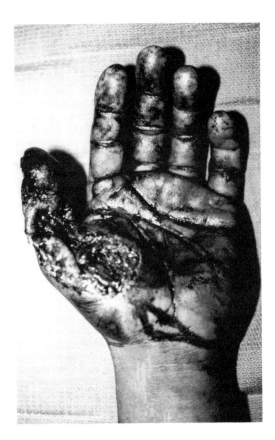

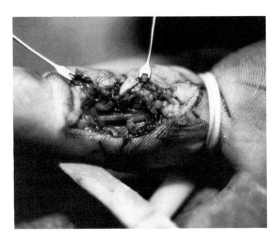

FIGURE 7. Proximity of the neurovascular bundle to the skin surface that was contused.

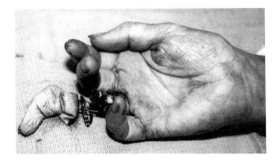

FIGURE 6. A grinding injury. Gross contamination is seen with these injuries. Cleaning the skin helps in the assessment of vascularity of the thumb.

FIGURE 8. A ring avulsion injury. Note the stretched blood vessel enclosed by the ring.

Peripheral Nerves. Peripheral nerves accompany the arterial supply to the hand and digits. Testing sensibility of the hand after injury can be done quickly and thoroughly according to the following sequence. Two-point discrimination may be tested for each digit. This test is sometimes time consuming, and stress can alter the results. The most important sensory information is whether the affected digit has perception of light touch similar to either the adjacent digits or the opposite hand. Stroke the palmar pad of the distal phalanx on the radial or ulnar side with a cotton-tipped applicator and ask the patient, "Do you feel this?" Perform the same maneuver on the remote digit or, better yet, on the opposite hand. Then ask, "Are the two sensations the same or different?" If the patient says they are different, chances are the nerve is lacerated or contused. Exploration is indicated, and the sensory examination can stop there. For injuries across the wrist or in the palm, the sensory distribution of the median, ulnar, and radial nerves should be checked (Fig. 9). For lacerations across the back of the hand, the superficial radial and dorsal sensory branch of the ulnar nerve should be checked. Ulnar intrinsic muscles can be checked by having the patient cross the index and long finger. The motor branch of the median nerve can be checked by having the patient oppose the thumb to the little finger or by abducting the thumb from the palm.

Tendons. Determination of tendon injury can be made in some instances by simple observation of the attitude of the digits. The naturally occurring arcade of each digit when the hand is supinated is lost when the profundus or sublimis tendon is lacerated (Figs. 10 and

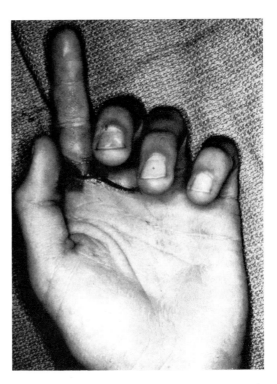

FIGURE 10. The attitude of the hand in a patient with a flexor tendon injury. The laceration is at the level of the metacarpophalangeal joint. Note that the digits of the second, third, and fourth fingers are held in flexion. The patient is unable to flex the index finger at either the distal or the proximal interphalangeal joint.

11). Block all adjacent digits and ask the patient to flex the proximal interphalangeal (PIP) joint. If the joint will not flex, injury to the sublimis tendon is indicated. Because the ring and little fingers may have a common tendon origin, these digits should be allowed to flex together. An-

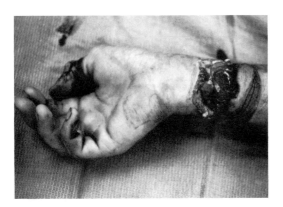

FIGURE 9. A laceration at the level of the volar wrist crease with injury to the ulnar nerve, artery, and flexor tendons.

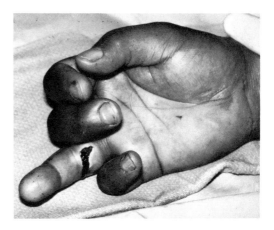

FIGURE 11. Another digital tendon laceration. The hand is lying in a relaxed position with the ring finger extended. This position indicates a flexor tendon injury.

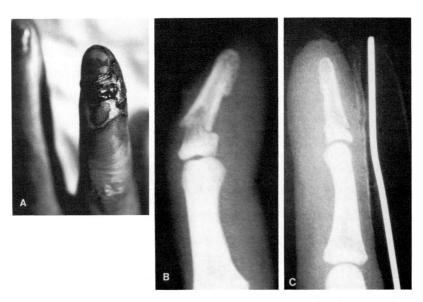

FIGURE 12. *A* and *B*, Transverse distal phalangeal fracture associated with injury to the nail bed. The nail was removed and the nail bed repaired. The fracture was reduced and held with a splint (*C*).

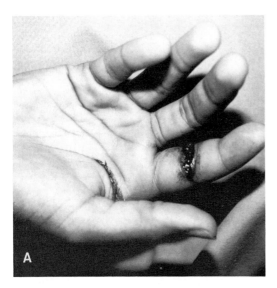
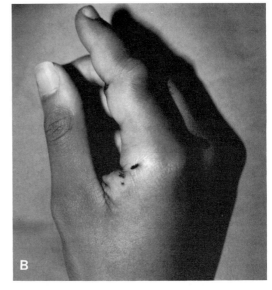

FIGURE 13. *A* and *B*, Compound dislocation of the proximal interphalangeal joint.

other way to examine the integrity of the flexor system is to ask the patient to flex the digits into the palm. If the profundus tendon is lacerated, the distal joints will not flex. To examine the extensor tendon system ask the patient to place the hand flat on the examining table, palm down. If the patient can lift the digit off the table, the extensor mechanism is intact. This method eliminates extension by the intrinsic system, but it does not rule out a partial tendon laceration.

Fractures. Diagnosis of fractures is based on clinical suspicion, localized point tenderness, swelling, and deformity. Fractures or dislocations of the phalanges or metacarpals can be open or closed; an open fracture, even if it occurs over the distal phalanx, is referred for surgery owing to the risk of infection and osteomyelitis (see Fig. 12). Any wound over a fracture should be considered an open fracture until proven otherwise. Displaced or rotated fractures of the phalanges and metacarpals may cause malalignment and scissoring of digits on flexion if they are not adequately reduced and stabilized. Fractures of the carpal bones are often unrecognized and must be suspected after a fall on the outstretched hand. In addition, ligamentous injury of the wrist carries high morbidity and should be suspected. No wrist injury should be assumed to be a simple sprain. Any click or clunk should be thoroughly investigated with detailed examination and radiography directed by a hand surgeon.

Distal radius fractures also accompany falls on the outstretched hand; a "dinner fork" deformity indicates such a fracture. Dislocations are often obvious, particularly at the PIP joint (Fig. 13). The digit appears shortened and deformed, and pain prevents the patient from flexing or extending it. As long as capillary refill is present, reduction should not be attempted at the scene without appropriate x-rays and analgesia.

Now that the diagnosis of injury has been made, we must determine what first aid is given for specific injuries.

FIRST AID FOR SPECIFIC HAND INJURIES

Simple Lacerations

By definition, simple lacerations are injuries that involve the skin only. The most important principle in the care of these wounds is to avoid infection and to stabilize the wound.[1] Appropriate prophylaxis against tetanus is required, regardless of the wound size. Guidelines are listed in Tables 1 and 2. First aid requires covering the wound with a sponge soaked in sterile saline solution and then dressing the hand with a sterile compression bandage. Pouring alcohol or iodine on the wound is painful and toxic to exposed tissue; it is not indicated.

Hand Splinting

Very few of the multitude of textbooks describing care of the hand indicate how to place a dressing on the operated or injured hand. It is agreed that the hand should be held in a position of anatomic function, but the exact sequence and choice of dressing materials remain nebulous concepts. The emergency bandage may remain with the patient for several hours before secondary care can be reached. Protection of the injured extremity and the patient's comfort are both important considerations, even before definitive surgical therapy is done. Elevation, which is essential, can prevent significant edema. The ideal position for the hand is with the wrist in 20–30 degrees of extension, the metacarpophalangeal (MCP) joints flexed at 70 degrees, and the interphalangeal joints in slight flexion.[10] The hand should appear to be holding a magazine. The wrist should be supported with a volar plaster splint that extends to the level of the proximal palmar

TABLE 1. Clinical Features of Wounds That Are Prone to Develop Tetanus

Clinical Feature	Non-Tetanus–prone Wounds	Tetanus-prone Wounds
Age of wound	≤6 hours	>6 hours
Configuration	Linear wound	Stellate wound, avulsion, abrasion
Depth	≤1 cm	>1 cm
Mechanics of injury	Sharp surface (e.g., knife, glass)	Missile, crush burn, frostbite
Signs of infection	Absent	Present
Devitalized tissue	Absent	Present
Contaminants (dirt, feces, soil, saliva, etc.)	Absent	Present
Denervated or ischemic tissue	Absent	Present

Source: American College of Surgeons Committee on Trauma: A Guide to Prophylaxis against Tetanus in Wound Management, 1987 revision. Chicago, IL, ACS, 1987. Reprinted with permission.

TABLE 2. A Summary Guide to Tetanus Prophylaxis of the Wounded Patient

History of Adsorbed Tetanus Toxoid (doses)	Non-Tetanus–prone Wounds		Tetanus-prone Wounds	
	DT*	TIg†	DT*	TIg†
Unknown or <three	Yes	No	Yes	Yes
≥Three‡	No§	No	No‖	No

* DT, diphtheria-tetanus toxoid. For children under 7 years diphtheria-tetanus-pertussis toxoid (DTP), or DT if pertussis vaccine is contraindicated, is preferred to tetanus toxoid alone. For persons 7 years old and older, DT is preferred to tetanus toxoid alone.

† Human tetanus immune globulin.

‡ If only three doses of fluid toxoid have been received, a fourth dose, preferably an adsorbed toxoid, should be given.

§ Yes, if more than 10 years have passed since last dose.

‖ Yes, if more than 5 years since last dose. (More frequent boosters are not needed and can accentuate side effects).

Source: American College of Surgeons Committee on Trauma: A Guide to Prophylaxis against Tetanus in Wound Management, 1987 revision. Chicago, IL, ACS, 1987. Reprinted with permission.

crease, or beyond if the digits require support. A moist sterile dressing should be placed over the wound to prevent tissue desiccation. Gauze sponges are added to the palm for bulk, and cotton gauze is loosely wrapped around the hand. Next the splint is applied and is secured by a nonelastic bandage. To avoid ischemia and excessive compression, use elastic bandages only with caution for acute wounds. Studies by Levin and Hnat using a mechanical hand model and different dressing sequences have demonstrated that stiff materials (such as elastic bandages) prevent edema and do not allow the normal physiological mechanism to take place.[8] Translated into the clinical setting, dressings that are too tightly applied and not split cause more harm than good. The most beneficial treatment the hand can receive after injury is a proper splint.

Abrasions

By definition, abrasions do not involve full-thickness skin loss. The epithelium is violated, but the dermis remains intact. These minor injuries can be treated by gentle wound cleansing and topical care with antibiotic ointment or vaseline gauze to keep the wound environment moist. An eschar forms and is followed by re-epithelialization. The hand should be bandaged and elevated to control swelling.

Fingertip Injuries

Machinery accounts for many fingertip injuries. These are often untidy lacerations that may involve injury to the nail plate, nail bed, and distal phalanx (Fig. 14). If they are not managed appropriately, permanent deformity of the nail as well as distal phalanx osteomyelitis can occur. Crushed fingertips should be referred to a hand specialist for treatment. The nail plate is usually removed, and the nail bed and germinal matrix repaired.

Hematoma under the nail plate indicates the possibility of an open fracture with probable laceration of the nail bed. These injuries are often ignored, but they are exquisitely painful. They respond to drainage of the hematoma and, if necessary, repair of the nail bed. Fingertip injuries involving amputation distal to the base of the nail plate should also be referred to a hand surgeon. If possible, the amputated part should be located and sent with the patient. The tissue, though it is avascular, may be used as a composite graft.

Amputations of digits and hands require special first aid (Fig. 15). Success in replanting digits and hands exceeds 80% in some centers.

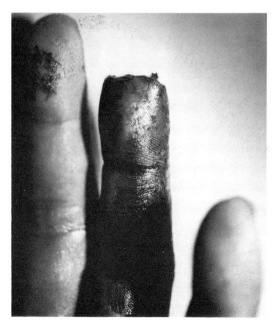

FIGURE 14. Transverse amputation of the fingertip. The fingertip was saved and put back on as a composite graft.

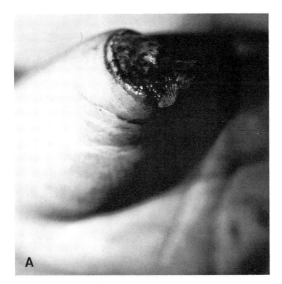

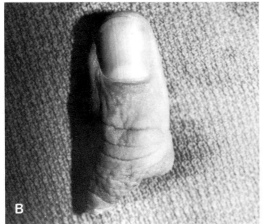

FIGURE 15.   *A* and *B*, Amputation at the level of the thumb interphalangeal joint.

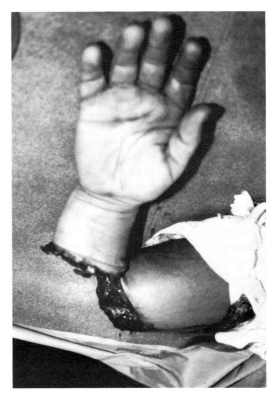

FIGURE 16.   Amputation of the forearm. The patient presented to the emergency room in shock due to blood loss. After appropriate resuscitation, the patient was taken to the operating room and underwent replantation of the limb.

Particularly if the amputation is clean and distal to the level of the sublimis insertion (middle joint), results can be good functionally and aesthetically. Major limb and hand amputations can also be replanted (Fig. 16). In these instances, the patient may have a life-threatening injury that requires immediate care. The amputated part should be wrapped in a moist saline gauze and placed in a container such as a medicine cup or specimen jar. The package is placed in a larger container that contains ice and water (a slurry or slush) so that the part can be stored at approximately 4°C. The amputated part should not be placed directly on ice and should not be frozen.[7] Bleeding from the extremity is controlled by compressive dressings and elevation. If persistent bleeding

is encountered, a blood pressure cuff can be applied and inflated above the patient's systolic pressure for up to 2 hours. Clamping exposed vessels is to be avoided. If there is no evidence of other significant injury and the vital signs are stable, the patient and the part should be transported as rapidly as possible to a replantation center. The decision to replant the part is never made at the scene of the accident. The patient should be kept calm and assured. All amputated parts, regardless of how mutilated, should be sent with the patient. Spare parts, such as vessels, nerves, skin, and bone can be harvested from nonreplantable digits and used to repair other salvageable digits.

Fractures

Treatment of fractures of the hand varies from simple buddy taping to open reduction and internal fixation. Mallet finger results from fracture of the distal phalanx at the level of the extensor tendon insertion (Fig. 17). It is due

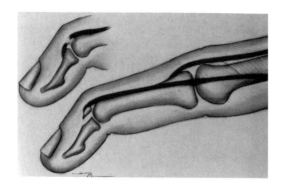

FIGURE 17. Schematic diagram of a mallet finger. This can be caused by either bony avulsion of the insertion of the extensor tendon apparatus or rupture of the extensor tendon itself.

to avulsion or direct trauma. If it is unrecognized, ability to extend the distal phalanx is permanently impaired. One way to assess metacarpal or phalangeal injuries is to look at the pattern of the nails next to one another when the hand is cupped. All suspected fractures should be x-rayed. Another problem associated with apparently minor fractures is injury to the volar plate with PIP hyperextension. A fleck of bone from the middle phalanx is avulsed with the volar plate. Special extension block splinting is necessary to regain motion of this joint.[2] Any injury to the PIP joint should be x-rayed. Similarly, injury to the ulnar collateral ligament of the thumb may produce avulsion of bone or no fracture at all. However, stress x-rays of the thumb MCP joint should be obtained to rule out injury to the ligament. All suspected fractures should be x-rayed, regardless of how trivial the injury. Regardless of the fracture pattern, it is imperative that splinting and immobilization be supervised by a physician. Simply strapping a tongue blade on the hand with circumferential tape is to be condemned. An important rule in bone injuries of the hand and digits is that seemingly insignificant injuries can result in extensive morbidity. These include injuries to the collateral ligaments with or without avulsion and the so-called game keeper's thumb or ulnar collateral ligament avulsion.

The most important first aid for tendon injuries is recognition. Often lacerated flexor tendons are accompanied by artery and nerve injuries that may be difficult to diagnose owing to pain and swelling. If the capillary refill is normal in the lacerated hand suspected of a flexor or extensor tendon injury, time is less

critical than if the digit is avascular. The hand should be wrapped in a sterile saline-soaked gauze and a bulky hand dressing. The patient should then be referred to a surgeon for appropriate intervention.

Injuries caused by high pressure injection guns may appear to be trivial, but foreign materials such as grease or paint forced into tissues cause significant necrosis. These injuries are surgical emergencies and should be referred to a hand surgeon (see Chapter 16).

Burns

Burns can be caused by chemical agents, electricity, friction, and fire.

First-degree burns appear as erythema. These burns are usually painful because they leave sensory elements intact. First aid consists of washing the hand in cold water and mild soap.

The burned hand can be covered with 1% sulfadiazine and wrapped in sterile gauze. The hallmark of first aid here is to keep the hand elevated and clean.

Second-degree burns involve partial loss of the skin, particularly the dermis. Deep palmar burns are unusual. With second-degree burns, there is erythema and blistering. Blisters should not be ruptured. The hand should be splinted in an intrinsic plus position, and 1% sulfadiazine should be applied.

Third-degree burns have essentially no sensation. Skin does not have normal capillary refill and may be white or black. If the burn is circumferential—for example, around the forearm—release of skin burn eschar to avoid a compartment syndrome may be necessary.

Fourth-degree burns are a continuation of third-degree burns that irreversibly damage underlying structures such as tendons. They should be referred to a hand surgeon.

Acid Injuries

The severity of chemical burns of the hand is a function of the concentration and volume of the chemical and the duration of exposure.[3] Acid burns are usually painful. The worker's symptoms are more severe than the objective findings. Flooding the involved areas with water is the best first aid and minimizes the depth of injury from hydrogen-ion–induced coagulation necrosis. Solutions of sodium bicarbonate can be used to neutralize the acid. The patient should be referred. Hydrofluoric acid is quite virulent upon contact with the skin, though onset of symptoms may be delayed for several hours. The hand burn should be irrigated with cool water for at least 15 minutes. Following this 2.5% calcium gluconate gel should be massaged into the injured skin to neutralize the fluoride ions. If need be, 10% calcium gluconate solution can be injected locally.

Alkaline burns should also be treated with water dilution. Topical acid should be used sparingly because acid can also cause contact injuries and an exothermic reaction to the acid-alkaline mixture can be damaging to the skin. Phosphorus burns should be treated by removing any embedded phosphorus from the skin and washing the hand in dilute copper sulfate solution. All contact injuries require careful documentation and close follow-up. Hand function can be severely impaired if the burns are not treated appropriately.

Electrical Injuries

The tissue planes of least resistance to electricity are blood vessels and nerves, which conduct electrical energy through the upper extremity, where it causes extensive tissue damage away from its point of entrance.

Electrically injured patients should be immediately taken to an emergency room, where their cardiac systems should be evaluated. Necrosis accompanying these wounds usually requires extensive debridement, fasciotomy, and sometimes amputation.[9]

Infection

Most infections occur within 12–24 hours of injury. Organisms such as the atypical mycobacteria may linger for several weeks.[14] Patients with recalcitrant infections should be referred to a hand surgeon for incision and drainage. A potentially devastating infection of the hand is acute flexor tenosynovitis, which usually follows by a day or so a penetrating injury of a tendon sheath. The four hallmarks that characterize flexor tenosynovitis are fusiform swelling, tenderness along the flexor sheath, a semiflexed posture of the digit, and pain on passive extension of the distal interphalangeal joint.[4] The pain with passive stretching is the most pathognomonic sign and should alert the plant health care personnel.

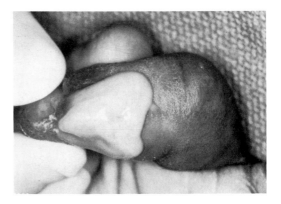

FIGURE 18. Distal phalangeal joint pyarthrosis. The patient was punctured by a splinter 48 hours before admission and presented with a hot, painful joint and purulence.

This infection cannot be treated with oral antibiotics or elevation; it needs surgical intervention.

Another emergent problem the health care worker may see is joint immobility after injury or puncture in the area of the joint (Fig. 18). Untreated septic arthritis leads to destruction of cartilage and osteomyelitis. If motion of a joint is limited, infection should be suspected and the patient should be referred.

Foreign Bodies

Particles of metal from heavy machinery can become embedded in the soft tissue of the hand and digits. They may be seen on x-ray. Some embedded particles become walled off and give rise to no reaction; others cause a local infection in the soft tissue. Patients with foreign bodies should be referred for adequate x-rays and removal of the object if removal is surgically feasible. Foreign bodies include splinters of wood and other materials.

Conclusion

This chapter has described some of the basic hand injuries that may occur in the workplace in order to alert the health care worker to the importance of proper evaluation and initial treatment of hand injuries. In the majority of instances, these patients should be referred to a hand surgeon for management. When in doubt, contacting the local hand surgery consultant saves time and ultimately benefits the patient.

REFERENCES

1. Brown PW: Open injuries of the hand. In Green, DP (ed): Operative Hand Surgery. New York, Churchill Livingstone, 1988, pp 1619–1653.
2. Eaton RG: Joint Injuries of the Hand. Springfield, IL, C. C. Thomas, 1971.
3. Hankin F: Contact injuries to the hand. Occup State Art Rev 4:473–483, 1989.
4. Knavel AB: Infections of the Hand. A Guide to the Surgical Treatment of Acute and Chronic Suppurative Processes in the Fingers, Hand, and Forearm, 7th ed. Philadelphia, Lea & Febiger, 1943.
5. Kasdan ML (ed): Occupational Hand Injuries. Occup Med State Art Rev 4:393–574, 1989.
6. Lamb DW, Hooper G: Hand Conditions. New York, Churchill Livingston, 1984.
7. Levin LS: Replantation. In: Surgical Residents of the Duke University Medical Center: Manual of Surgical Intensive Care Practices. Chicago, Yearbook Medical Publishers, 1988.
8. Levin LS, Breidenbach WC, Hnat B, Goldner JL: Engineering analysis of hand dressings and edema. Paper presented to the American Association of Hand Surgery, San Francisco, October 27, 1989.
9. Mubarak SJ, Hargens AR: Compartment Syndromes and Volkmann's Contracture. Philadelphia, W.B. Saunders. 1981.
10. Newmeyer WL: The Hand: Primary Care of Common Problems. Aurora, CO, American Society for Surgery of the Hand, 1985.
11. Strickland JW: Management of flexor tendon injuries. Orthop Clin North Am 14:827–846, 1983.
12. Urbaniak JR, Evans JR, Bright DS: Microvascular management of ring avulsion injuries. J Hand Surg 6:25–30, 1981.
13. Wilgis, EFS: Vascular Injuries and Diseases of the Upper Limb. Boston, Little, Brown, 1983.
14. Williams CS, Riordan DC: *Mycobacterium marinum* (atypical acid-fast bacillus) infections of the hand: A report of six cases. J Bone Joint Surg 55A:1042–1050, 1973.

Chapter 10

LOCAL AND REGIONAL BLOCK ANESTHESIA FOR THE UPPER EXTREMITY

Donald M. Ditmars, Jr, MD

The use of local and regional anesthesia allows most hand operations to be performed in an outpatient setting, which enhances the patient's safety and convenience. The duration and extent of the planned procedure determine the type of anesthesia chosen for a particular situation. Many hand operations are localized to a small area. The anatomy of the nerves of the upper extremity is ideal for the administration of effective regional blocks.

Administration of the injectable agents used for these blocks can be done with a high degree of safety if toxic doses are known and not exceeded and if the lowest effective dose in the smallest possible concentration is used. The use of the most distal block possible for a given task allows the smallest amount of anesthetic agent to be used and minimizes the risk of peripheral nerve damage. The tourniquet position and time required for its use are important factors in determining the level of block required.[11] Digital tourniquets can be easily tolerated for 30 minute with only a digital block. Forearm tourniquets involve muscle compression and ischemia and can be tolerated for only 15–20 minutes without significant sedation; tourniquets above the elbow are even less well tolerated. Thus, the more distal the placement of the tourniquet, the smaller the amount of agent needed and the more localized the area blocked.

Because the time of onset, effectiveness, duration, and complications of the many available

agents vary significantly, the surgeon should become familiar with only a few agents to ensure safe usage. Stocking only an intermediate- and a long-acting agent in an office setting avoids accidents due to ignorance or mishandling.

The level of monitoring is based upon the health of the patient, the level of block required by the operation, and the administration of sedation.[13] The patient's health can be estimated by the Dripps American Society of Anesthesiology method of classification:

Grade 1—no disease other than the surgical pathology and no systemic disease
Grade 2—moderate systemic disturbance due to general disease or surgical condition
Grade 3—severe systemic disturbance
Grade 4—systemic disorder with imminent threat to life
Grade 5—moribund.

All patients require constant observation for 15–20 minutes immediately after instillation of local anesthetic agents. Grades 2–5 require full monitoring with immediate availability of resuscitation delivery systems. When a risk of intravascular injection is associated with the block, an intravenous line should be inserted before injection. Since tourniquets are used in much hand surgery, blood loss is rarely a systemic threat. However, the risks of anesthesia, even without sedation, are just great enough that only small cutaneous local infiltrations and blocks at and distal to the wrist can be safely performed without an intravenous line and continuous monitoring.

Standard texts should be consulted before new procedures or agents are used.[2,10]

PHARMACOLOGY OF LOCAL ANESTHETIC AGENTS

Stimulation of a nerve results in depolarization of the nerve membrane to the threshold potential followed by spontaneous progressive depolarization or conduction. Repolarization occurs until the resting potential of -60 to -90 mv is reached.[1,6,7] Local anesthetic agents act at the nerve cell membrane to decrease the rate of depolarization, thus blocking conduction. Blockade begins with displacement of calcium ions from receptor sites, which blocks sodium channels, inhibiting sodium flux across the membrane. The rate of depolarization is depressed, the threshold potential is not attained, the action potential is not propagated, and conduction is blocked. Pain, temperature, and touch sensations are blocked before proprioception and skeletal muscle tone. The available drugs vary in potency, time of onset, and duration of blockade.

All agents are dissolved in acid solutions that must be neutralized by the tissues before diffusion can occur. This accounts for the decreased potency of agents locally infiltrated into abscesses that are acidic. Acidic solutions are painful when injected, but pain can be reduced by first buffering with a sodium bicarbonate solution.[5]

Other physicochemical properties that are important in determining the action of local anesthetic agents are lipid solubility and protein binding.[7] Drugs that are highly lipid soluble are more potent and can be used in relatively dilute solutions. Procaine is an example of a poorly soluble agent that requires concentrations of 2% to be effective. By contrast, bupivacaine is effective in a 0.25% concentration. Lidocaine, which has intermediate lipid solubility, can be effective at 0.5–1%. The duration of anesthesia is related to the degree of binding to the proteins in the nerve membrane; the longer-acting drugs are more highly bound. Bupivacaine lasts up to three times longer than lidocaine.

Of the many drugs that have some local anesthetic properties, two groups have been commonly used: amino esters (procaine) and amino amides (lidocaine, mepivacaine, bupivacaine). The esters are more rapidly diffused and poorly bound than the amides. They reach the plasma, where they are hydrolyzed primarily into para-aminobenzoic acid, which is excreted in the urine. The amide group undergoes enzymatic degradation in the liver before urinary excretion. This process, which is very noticeable with bupivacaine, is slow in infants and patients with liver disease. Lidocaine after subcutaneous infiltration reaches peak blood levels in 30 minutes, then tails off over 2 hours. The addition of epinephrine for its vasoconstrictive effect decreases the rate of absorption so that the peak blood level for the same injected dose is delayed and lower.

The effectiveness of a particular agent for a given operation is related to the time of onset, depth, and duration of effective anesthesia.[7] The time of onset is a factor of the intrinsic potency of the drug, the concentration used, the use of epinephrine, the location of the block, and the mode of administration. Proximal nerve blocks involve large mixed nerve trunks and take a longer time to become effective. Highly bound drugs such as bupivacaine develop a profound effect for a longer time than agents that are rapidly diffused, such as procaine. Lidocaine and mepivacaine are intermediate in both respects (Table 1).

All local anesthetics except cocaine are smooth muscle relaxants and cause vasodilation. The vasoconstrictive effect of epinephrine delays the onset of anesthesia and the diffusion of the drug into the blood stream. Local anesthetic agents, when mixed with epinephrine, are held locally at the site of injection, resulting in more profound and longer-lasting anesthesia. Although epinephrine is supplied commercially with local anesthetics in dilutions of 1/100,000 and 1/200,000, vasoconstrictive effects are good at 1/400,000 and the anesthetic effect is prolonged with dilutions of 1/800,000, which cause almost no tachycardia.

TABLE 1. Drug Effectiveness

Agent	Onset	Duration
Amides		
Lidocaine (Xylocaine)	10 min	$\frac{1}{2}$–1 hr
Lidocaine with epinephrine	20 min	2 hrs
Bupivacaine (Marcaine)	30 min	2–3 hr
Bupivacaine with epinephrine	45 min	4 hr
Mepivacaine (Carbocaine)	20 min	$1\frac{1}{2}$ hr
Ester		
Procaine	5 min	30 min

The recommended maximum single dose is related to the potency of the drug and the presence of epinephrine (Table 2). Procaine is rapidly diffused and metabolized and is thus the least toxic and least potent. Bupivacaine, the most potent and long-lasting agent, rarely has to be repeated.

TOXIC REACTIONS

Causes

Toxic reactions to local anesthetic agents are due to vasovagal anxiety reactions, properties of the agent, and epinephrine effects.

The anxiety reaction is manifested by a pale, cold, clammy appearance, which may progress to dizziness, nausea, vomiting, and syncope with hypotension and bradycardia.[1]

The drug-related major reactions are dose-related with the amide group and true allergic/hypersensitive reactions with the ester drugs. Methemoglobinemia is a known dose-related complication of prilocaine. Procaine, the least potent local anesthetic, is the least toxic after rapid absorption. The dose-related symptoms of brief excitation followed by depression, lightheadedness, nervousness, apprehension, euphoria, confusion, nausea and vomiting,

drowsiness, and shivering precede convulsions, unconsciousness, respiratory arrest, hypotension, and cardiac arrest. These effects are due to rapid absorption of an excessive dose. The most potent agents, including bupivacaine, are associated with the most dramatic progression of toxic effects and a rapid onset of cardiovascular collapse. The allergic reactions of urticaria and anaphylactic shock, usually provoked by members of the ester group, commonly occur at a repeat exposure. The ester family compounds are derivatives of para-aminobenzoic acid, as is methylparaben, a preservative in multidose vials of amide anesthetics.

The epinephrine effects of jitteriness, nervousness, tachycardia, and a "pounding heart" were common with some older dental preparations using a 1/50,000 dilution and can be confused with an anxiety reaction.

Malignant hyperthermia is a smooth muscle hypermetabolic state triggered by anesthetics and succinylcholine.[14] The syndrome, which is inherited and has a high mortality, involves the development of intracellular hypercalcemia resulting in tachycardia, rapid temperature elevation, muscular rigidity, and arrhythmias. Although in the acute phase the creatinine phosphokinase (CPK) can be elevated to more than 20,000 units in association with marked

TABLE 2. Maximum Dosage

Agent	Concentration (%)	Recommended Maximum Single Adult Dose (mg)	mg/% max. dose in 10-ml of solution
Amides			
Lidocaine (Xylocaine)	0.5	300	50 mg/17%
	1	300	100 mg/33%
	2	300	200 mg/67%
Children	1	75	7.5 ml = 100%
Lidocaine with epinephrine	0.5	500	50 mg/10%
	1	500	100 mg/20%
	2	500	200 mg/40%
Bupivacaine (Marcaine)	0.25	175	25 mg/14%
	0.5	175	50 mg/29%
(Not recommended for children under 12 years old)			
Bupivacaine with epinephrine	0.25	225	25 mg/11%
	0.5	225	50 mg/22%
Mepivacaine (Carbocaine)	1	400	100 mg/25%
	1.5	400	150 mg/38%
	2	400	200 mg/50%
Ester			
Procaine	1	1000	100 mg/10%

elevation of the enzymes of muscle damage, all studies may be normal in an asymptomatic but susceptible person. Amide local anesthetic agents have been implicated, however, some studies show that neither group of local anesthetics triggers malignant hyperthermia in susceptible swine or humans. Because of the current controversy, during an acute crisis procaine is recommended for management of arrhythmias.

Prevention

As with most medical situations, an accurate history of reactions to local anesthetics is most important and easy to elicit. Many "allergic reactions" are described as a pounding heart, actually an epinephrine effect, or extreme nervousness and fainting. Because a true allergy to an amide drug is rare, the single-dose vial, which does not have the preservative, can be used. If an allergic reaction has indeed occurred, a nonrelated compound such as dibucaine can be tried or general anesthesia used. If there remains any question, then even a very minor procedure should be done in an ambulatory surgery unit with full monitoring and resuscitative equipment available for immediate use.

A history of malignant hyperthermia, muscle disorder, or anesthetic death in a patient or his family is highly significant because no practical laboratory test can predict an acute reaction to anesthetics.[15] If the history is positive, pretreatment with dantrolene (4–8 mg/kg/day) for 2 days before the operation is recommended.[14]

Vasovagal and anxiety reactions can be minimized by placing the patient in a supine position for all injections, no matter how small. This positioning should be accompanied by reassurance, diversionary discussion, and accurate information about the proceedings.[12] Reducing the pain of infiltration by using 27- or 30-gauge needles increases the patient's confidence. A block should be skillfully done and should be effective before the operation is begun. Any pain beyond the predicted traction sensations decreases confidence. Even mild toxic effects, which may add to the patient's apprehension, can be prevented by avoiding intravascular injections and keeping well below the toxic doses. Preoperative sedation does not replace human contact with the patient and increases monitoring and support requirements.

Intraoperative sedation always requires anesthesia monitoring.[13]

Dose-related toxic effects are avoided by not exceeding the maximum recommended dose (Table 2). The least amount of the most dilute solution that will do the required block or local infiltration should be used. By allowing time for the blockade to develop, less volume and concentration are required. Ten minutes is sufficient for 1% lidocaine without epinephrine. Twenty minutes should be allowed when 1% lidocaine with epinephrine is used with local infiltration or wrist blocks. Axillary blocks may take 45 minutes to become effective. Thus, patience is a virtue in a surgeon who uses local anesthetics. A large intravascular bolus injection can be avoided by advancing a small-gauge needle slowly while infiltrating or aspirating before injecting more than 1 ml at one site, especially when the site is adjacent to a major vessel.

The level of monitoring is related to the agent selected, the health and age of the patient, the use of sedation, and the planned operation. The minimum monitoring after any injection is constant observation for several minutes or until the patient relaxes from the injections. Electrocardiograph (EKG) monitors are recommended for patients who receive perioperative sedation, require the maximum doses of local anesthetics, have heart disease, or are more than 50 years old. The pulse oximeter provides a continuous, noninvasive measurement of oxygen saturation, which recently has been shown to be reliable for patients of all ages and is being used more often.[2]

An intravenous line is recommended when more than small amounts of local anesthetic agent are used, for patients with medical problems (Dripps Grade 3–5), and for all sedated patients.

Treatment

The mainstay of the treatment program is oxygen, which is used at the first clinical sign of toxicity. The pulse/oxygen saturation monitor can indicate the onset of a problem before unmistakable signs develop, allowing timely delivery of oxygen. Restlessness and agitation in a previously calm patient are early symptoms that are often completely relieved after several minutes of 50% oxygen by mask. Oxygen should be given before (more) intravenous sedation.

Oxygen also stops nausea remarkably well, allowing operations to proceed without upsetting both the patient and the surgeon. Immediate oxygen is required with bupivacaine overdose because of the known rapid onset of myocardial depression. At the first sign of malignant hyperthermia, 100% oxygen is started and dantrolene follows.

Vasovagal reactions can be helped by elevating the feet to treat postural hypotension and using smelling salts.[4] The patient should be positioned with the head to the side to clear the airway if vomiting occurs. If this reaction occurs, discharge from the medical facility should be delayed until the patient is fully recovered and is accompanied, even if the procedure was minimal.

Epinephrine excitement usually lasts only several minutes and resolves if the operation is delayed until the patient calms.

If the reaction progresses beyond mild symptoms, diazepam (Valium), 5–10 mg intravenously, raises the threshold for convulsions. Convulsions can be treated with the ultra-short-acting barbiturate, thiopental (Pentothal), given intravenously as a 10–100 mg bolus.

Airway control must be immediately at hand during predictable problem periods, such as tourniquet release after intravenous regional blockade (Bier block).

CHOICE OF AGENT

Although procaine is safe at relatively high dosages, its weak, short-acting analgesic effect is associated with frequent allergic reactions. It is rarely used today.

Lidocaine, of intermediate potency and duration, is the most versatile of all the available agents.[6,7] Without epinephrine, the effective anesthesia wears off in under 1 hour. The absence of hemostatic effect is less of a problem in the upper extremity because a tourniquet can be used. The fast onset with a small volume makes it ideal for fingers distal to the distal palmar crease, where epinephrine is contraindicated. Lidocaine with epinephrine can be used from the mid-palm proximally for procedures lasting up to 2 hours. Locally infiltrated, the hemostasis effect reduces the requirement for a tourniquet for excision of skin lesions, carpal tunnel releases, and dorsal wrist ganglion excisions.

Bupivacaine is indicated for long procedures or, when injected into the wound at the end of an operation, for postoperative pain relief. Epinephrine is not needed to prolong the effect, but it increases the maximum safe dose and localizes more of the drug to the area of infiltration. Because of bupivacaine's severe and rapid toxic myocardial effect, it is not to be used for intravenous regional blocks (Bier block). Prilocaine, the least toxic of the amide group to the central nervous and cardiovascular systems, has been recommended for Bier blocks.[8] It has not been universally accepted due to methemoglobinemia causing cyanosis, usually at total doses of more than 600 mg.[7,8] Mepivacaine has a more profound blockade than lidocaine and is preferred for the axillary block.

TECHNIQUES OF ADMINISTRATION

The nerve anatomy of the upper extremity is particularly suited for nerve blocks at various levels. The risk of systemic effects of general anesthesia are reduced when only an isolated area of sensory or motor blockade is required. Often, the desires of the patient and the skill and experiences of the surgeon and anesthesiologist determine the selection of anesthetic.[3] Although the brachial plexus at the truncal level is anatomically easily located, the complications of pneumothorax, postoperative neuralgias (paresthesias are obtained in the performance of this block), and intravascular injection, along with the frequent occurrence of phrenic nerve block and Horner's syndrome, make me favor the axillary block when anesthesia of both the hand and forearm is required. At the intersection of the borders of the pectoralis major and the coracobrachialis muscles, the ulnar, median, and radial nerves lie on the axillary artery within the axillary sheath of the brachial plexus, where they can be blocked by instillation of anesthetic solution. The musculocutaneous nerve has taken off proximal to this site; thus a supplementary field block is required for the radial side of the forearm and thenar eminence. The nerves at the axillary, elbow, and volar wrist are mixed motor and sensory. The dorsal hand and digital nerves are sensory only.

The methods of administration of local anesthetic agents in the upper extremity fall into the categories of local infiltration (small skin lesions, carpal tunnel releases), digital nerve blocks (distal and middle phalanges), wrist block (mid-palm and distally), major nerve blocks at elbow (no real advantage to alternatives), intravenous blockade (mid-forearm and distally), and axillary block (distal to elbow with supplementation). Since distal injuries are more common, most emphasis is placed on the performance of digital and wrist blocks.

Effective administration of local anesthetic agents requires patient cooperation. This is achieved with a thorough preoperative assessment of a particular patient's ability to tolerate the anesthetic and operation. Discussion of the procedure in detail, even with children who are mature enough to listen and understand, results in less anxiety and a more pleasant experience for both the patient and the surgeon.[10] Adequate premedication may be required after consideration of the block's capabilities and the requirements of the operation.[11] Gentleness, concern, and patience by all medical personnel in contact with the patient greatly enhance the experience, which may be routine for the medical staff but is weird, even frightening, for patients. Friendly conversation by the nurse, technician, or anesthesiology frees the surgeon to concentrate on the technical aspect. All injections are given with the patient lying down. Small-caliber needles cause less pain on insertion and on infiltration because they limit the speed of injection. A 30-gauge needle is used for skin wheals and a 27-gauge needle for subcutaneous infiltration. A 25-gauge needle is helpful to feel the transverse carpal ligament during the block of the median nerve at the wrist (see Fig. 3, below). Slow incremental injection with forward motion reduces pain and the risk of a bolus intravascular injection. The lidocaine with epinephrine as commercially supplied can be diluted with plain lidocaine to inject dilutions of 1/200,000 or 1/400,000, which prolong the duration and produce minimal systemic effect in hypertensive or cardiac patients. Mixing bupivacaine with the lidocaine prolongs pain relief well into the post operative period.

Local infiltration of 1% lidocaine with epinephrine into the distal 5 cm of the forearm and proximal interthenar palm, using a total of 10 ml, results in excellent anesthesia with hemostasis for carpal tunnel releases. Division of the transverse carpal ligament is rendered nonpainful if it is infiltrated with 2 or 3 ml using four or five perpendicular punctures along its course in the midpalm and wrist as part of the initial infiltration. A median nerve block is avoided to reduce postoperative paresthesias. A useful mixture for carpal tunnel releases is 2.5 ml of 1% lidocaine with epinephrine, 1.5 ml of 0.25% bupivacaine, and 6.5 ml of 1% plain lidocaine, which results in fast onset, relatively long duration, and a final epinephrine dilution of 1/400,000.

The intermetacarpal digital block anesthetizes the finger more proximally and reduces the risk of pressure ischemia (Figs. 1 and 2). Epinephrine is avoided in all digital blocks. If a procedure is likely to take longer than 30 minutes, then a wrist block using an anesthetic solution containing epinephrine should be considered. The wrist block (Fig. 3) is the mainstay for simple procedures in the hand.[8] Addition of a field block of palmar cutaneous branch of the median nerve in the palm allows safe, effective performance of most procedures localized to the hand. A tourniquet placed low on the forearm and inflated to 80–100 mm Hg more than the systolic pressure will be tolerated 15–20 minutes without sedation, allowing rapid procedures to be comfortably performed with minimal or no premedication. The tourniquet can be inflated for the crucial dissection (e.g., finding the cut ends of nerves) and then deflated when hemostasis is less of a problem (e.g., the actual nerve repair and wound closure). Flexor tendon repairs in no-man's-land (the area of flexor tendon excursion beneath the retinacular pulley system) and proximally

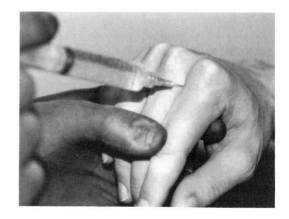

FIGURE 1. Digital nerve block—intermetacarpal approach. With the metacarpophalangeal joints flexed, the fingers are grasped between the operator's thumb and index finger. The operator controls the entire hand. The radial side of the index lies in the patient's distal palmar crease. A 1½-inch, 25- or 27-gauge needle is inserted into the relatively less sensitive dorsal web space and advanced until its tip can be felt under the palmar skin. As the needle in withdrawn, 3 ml of 1% plain lidocaine are injected.

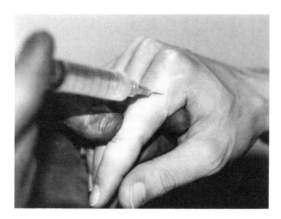

FIGURE 2. **Digital nerve block—intermetacarpal approach.** The procedure in Figure 1 is repeated on the opposite side of the digit. The radial digital nerve of the index and the ulnar digital nerve of the little finger course more centrally across the distal palm and require more angulation of the needle toward the middle of the palm.

The solution remaining in the 10-ml syringe is injected dorsally in the subcutaneous layer over the metacarpophyalangeal joint to block radial or ulnar sensory branches. This block is excellent for procedures lasting less than 30 minutes on the distal and middle phalanges when a digital tourniquet is used.

usually require a block that includes the forearm. Extensor tendon repairs distal to the distal third of the metacarpals can be done with a wrist block, except for repairs of the extensor pollicus longus in which the proximal end has retracted into the forearm. Ulnar blocks at the elbow, although easy to do, are commonly followed by annoyingly persistent paresthesias. Axillary or intravenous regional (Bier) blocks are therefore used when wrist blocks are not appropriate.

Intravenous regional blockade is performed by injecting a volume of local anesthetic solution into a vein of an exsanguinated extremity distal to a tourniquet. This solution is carried to the cores of the nerve trunks, partly diffusing into the nerve bundles and causing blockade.[9] The duration of anesthesia is related to the tourniquet inflation time and not particularly to the anesthetic agent. This technique is recommended for operations in the distal forearm and wrist that can be done within the tolerance time for the tourniquet. Although the procedure is easy and can be accomplished with a reliable onset of functional analgesia within 5–10 minutes, there are enough variables so that constant competent monitoring with resuscitation equipment at hand is required. The chance of leakage of anesthetic solution into the general circulation or even total tourniquet

deflation is great enough so that prilocaine, the least toxic amide agent, is recommended by a recent text.[9] Bupivacaine, which can cause disastrous cardiovascular collapse when injected as a bolus, is contraindicated for this method. The reported fatalities have been due to bupivacaine.

An intravenous line is inserted in the opposite arm, EKG and O_2 saturation monitoring are installed, and availability of oxygen is assured. Then a double tourniquet is applied to the arm above the elbow, and a butterfly needle is inserted into a dorsal hand vein and temporarily taped. The extremity distal to the tourniquet is exsanguinated with an Esmarch bandage, and the proximal tourniquet is inflated to 250 mm Hg. Forty milliliters of 0.5% lidocaine without epinephrine, drawn from a single-dose vial to be free of additives, are injected slowly. After analgesia and muscle relaxation have developed (usually within 5 minutes), the needle is removed and the extremity is prepped for surgery. To minimize the tourniquet pain after the onset of anesthesia, the distal tourniquet is inflated, checked, and secured. The proximal tourniquet is then deflated, thus effectively placing the tourniquet pressure at an anesthetized level while relieving the painful pressure at the original, more proximal site. This maneuver adds 15–20 minutes of comfortable tourniquet time for the operation, although it does not remove tourniquet pain as a factor limiting the time allowed.

Close monitoring during the entire procedure is mandatory because anesthetic solution can leak into the general circulation via intraosseous veins with the tourniquet inflated and via peripheral veins owing to a malfunctioning tourniquet. At the conclusion of the operation the tourniquet is released for a few seconds at a time at 5-minute intervals to slowly wash out the anesthetic solution in three or four small doses. Transient toxic reactions of paresthesias, tinnitus, and dizziness can be expected at this time. Although a significant amount of solution remains intravenously for the entire time that the tourniquet is inflated, the recommended minimum cuff inflation time is 15 minutes to avoid rapid infusion of the whole dose.

In contrast to the Bier block, the success of an axillary block is related to the skill and experience of the anesthesiologist. The perivascular axillary block has become one of the proven mainstays for blocking the nerves of the arm.[3] The patient, while lying supine, has his arm

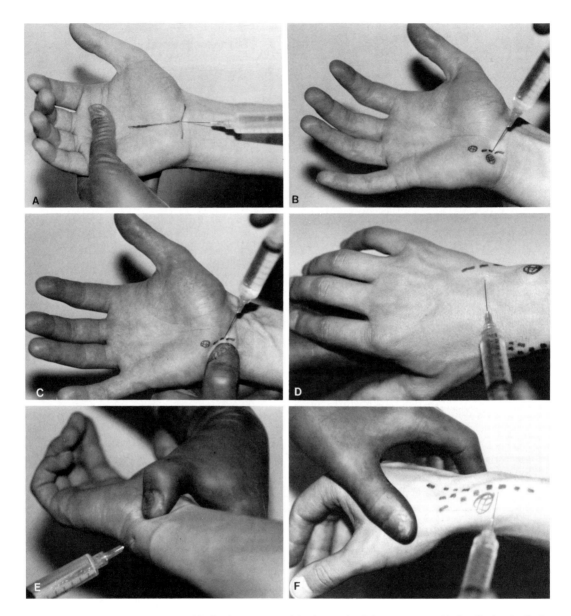

FIGURE 3. *A,* **Median nerve wrist block.** The junction of the longitudinal thenar crease with the distal wrist flexion crease lies at the proximal end of the thick transverse carpal ligament and just to the ulnar side of the median nerve. The needle is angled distally with the hand held firmly in slight hyperextension. Gently advanced, the needle is felt to pop through the tough transverse carpal ligament. Two milliliters of 1% lidocaine with epinephrine are injected into the carpal tunnel. Paresthesias are not required to obtain a good block after a 20-minute wait. If paresthesias are encountered, the injection is limited to 0.5 ml and the needle is withdrawn to just under the skin and redirected slightly more ulnarly for injection of the remaining 1.5 ml. Firm support of the patient's hand by the operator's nondominant hand during needle insertion prevents injury and enhances perception of needle position.

B, **Ulnar nerve wrist block.** The ulnar nerve can be blocked where it obliquely traverses the space between the pisiform proximally and the hook of the hamate distally. This level of block is preferred to a block in the olecranon groove because of annoying paresthesias that commonly persist for weeks if this nerve is traumatized at the elbow level. Some authors prefer the block at the elbow because of its reliability and ease of performance.[11]

C, **Ulnar nerve wrist block.** The block is given by inserting the needle just radial to the palpated pisiform down to the bone, injecting 2 ml at that point. The injection can be divided into two or three insertions of the needle at slightly different radial angles. This blocks only the palmar aspect of the ulnar one-and-one-half digits. In this situation, as with the median nerve block, notice the support by the operator's hand.

D, **Dorsal ulnar nerve wrist block.** The dorsal branch of the ulnar nerve must be blocked in the subcutaneous tissue distal to the ulnar styloid as it courses around the wrist.

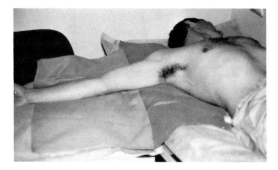

FIGURE 4. **Axillary block.** The arm of the supine patient is abducted in the body plane, avoiding hyperextension and forced external rotation of the shoulder. This position allows identification of anatomic landmarks and rotates the humeral head so that it does not block the proximal flow of the anesthetic solution within the axillary sheath.

abducted to 90° in the plane of the body. The hyperextended position is avoided (Fig. 4).[8] The axilla is swabbed with an antiseptic skin preparation. The axillary artery is palpated with the index finger, and a blunt, 22-gauge needle on an intravenous extension tube/closed syringe system is inserted through the skin over the fingernail toward the apex of the axilla (Fig. 5). The light touch required to feel the needle pop through the axillary sheath is facilitated by using the short intravenous extension tube connected to the needle.

Paresthesias are not required, but they indicate that the needle tip is positioned within the sheath. An assistant aspirates the syringe. Blood return in the tubing indicates that repositioning is required. A negative aspiration is mandatory before injection of several ml of the anesthetic solution as a test dose. Tachycardia, if epinephrine is used, indicates intravenous placement, and the needle can be repositioned. If there are no systemic effects from the test dose, the remainder of the 40 ml of anesthetic solution is injected as a single dose.

The needle is withdrawn and the arm adducted to the patient's side. A gauze is placed in the axilla.

Since the onset of blockade is slow, taking up to 45 minutes, it should be instilled well ahead of time (see Table 1). Solutions should be calculated to keep the total dose of anesthetic agent under the toxic limit (Table 2). About 2 hours of anesthesia can be expected with 1% lidocaine with 1/200,000 epinephrine. Up to 3 hours of useful anesthesia can be expected if mepivacaine is substituted to obtain a more profound motor block. Some increase in reliability has been experienced by using 30 ml of 1.25% mepivacaine (a mixture of 1% and 1.5%). Bupivacaine 0.25% with epinephrine can be substituted if the procedure is expected to last longer than 3 hours. If the operation should last beyond 4–6 hours, a continuous infusion can be done through an indwelling catheter inserted initially into the sheath.[11]

CONCLUSION

Local and regional block anesthesia has allowed a large number of upper extremity operations to be safely and comfortably performed in an outpatient setting, saving both time and money. The selection of the site for the operation—office, ambulatory surgery unit, or hospital operating room—is usually related to the expectation of problems requiring monitoring and support. The patient's age and health in relation to the extent and duration of the operation determine the choice of anesthetic. The available modes of delivery of local anesthetic agents at different levels in the upper extremity are adequate to allow painless performance of procedures distal to the elbow without exceeding maximum recommended drug doses. Overdosage, the most common

E, **Alternative ulnar nerve wrist block.** The needle is inserted laterally, deep to the flexor carpi ulnaris. The ulnar border of this muscle can be defined by initially instructing the patient to flex the wrist ulnarly. The radial border of the flexor carpi ulnaris is firmly depressed, pushing the ulnar nerve into the course of the needle as it is advanced toward the palpating thumb tip. Two ml of 1% lidocaine with epinephrine are all that is usually required. If paresthesias are encountered, the needle is withdrawn very slightly before injecting. Both the mixed motor and sensory volar and dorsal sensory branches are blocked at this site.

F, **Radial nerve wrist block.** The dorsal sensory branch of the radial nerve is reliably blocked at the radial styloid in the subcutaneous tissue deep to the cephalic vein. Two ml of 1% lidocaine with epinephrine will result in a good block for 1½–2 hours.

Ten ml of 1% lidocaine with epinephrine (20% of maximum recommended adult single dose) will be sufficient to perform a complete wrist block.

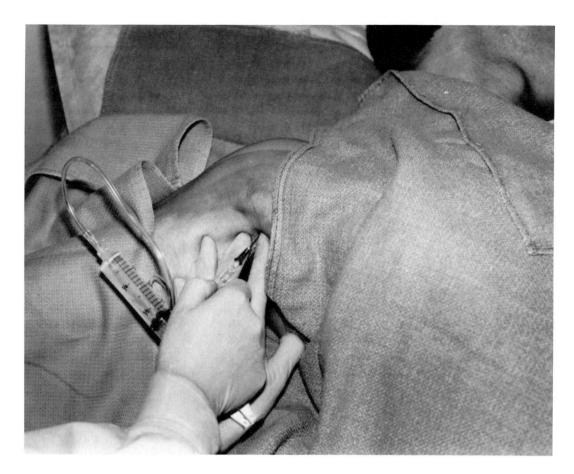

FIGURE 5. **Axillary block.** The axillary artery is palpated, and a needle connected to a short intravenous extension tubing is inserted toward the apex of the axilla using a light touch. After a pop through the axillary sheath is felt, 30–40 ml of anesthetic solution are injected. Accurate dosage calculation is required, because higher concentrations are used to obtain a more profound blockade (see Table 2). The maximum recommended dose is required when mepivacaine is used. A lag time of 45 minutes is common for onset of effective anesthesia. Supplemental local infiltration is frequently required at the beginning of an operation.

cause of serious toxic reactions with the most commonly used agents, can be prevented by using the least amount and the lowest concentration that are effective. The maximum single dose for each drug preparation used should be known and not exceeded. Tourniquets are better tolerated if they are placed as distal as possible, thus reducing the amount of anesthetic and sedation required. Resuscitation measures should be available. When intravenous regional blockade or axillary blocks are used, it is advisable to have complete constant monitoring, with cardiorespiratory support systems and medications immediately available.

Local and regional anesthesia techniques can provide excellent, safe anesthesia for most hand operations, especially for those done in emergency situations.

REFERENCES

1. Baker JD, Blackmon BB Jr: Local anesthesia. Clin Plast Surg 12:25–31, 1985.
2. Barash PG, Cullen BF, Stoelting RK (eds): Clinical Anesthesia. Philadelphia, J. B. Lippincott, 1989.
3. Bridenbaugh LD: The extremity: Somatic blockade. In Cousins MJ, Bridenbaugh PO (eds): Neural Blockade in Clinical Anesthesia and Management of Pain, 2nd ed. Philadelphia, J. B. Lippincott, 1988, pp 387–416.
4. Brown LL: Anesthesia in the geriatric patient. Clin Plast Surg 12:51–60, 1985.
5. Christoph RA, Buchanan L, Begalia K, Schwartz S: Pain reduction in local anesthetic administration through pH buffering. Ann Emerg Med 17:117–120, 1988.
6. Covino BG: Pharmacology of local anesthetic agents. Surg Rounds July 44–51, 1978.
7. Covino BG: Clinical pharmacology of local anesthetic agents. In Cousins MJ, Bridenbaugh PO (eds): Neural Blockade in Clinical Anesthesia and Management of

Pain, 2nd ed. Philadelphia, J. B. Lippincott, 1988, pp 111–122.

8. Earle AS, Blanchard JM: Regional anesthesia in the upper extremity. Clin Plast Surg 12:97–114, 1985.

9. Holmes CM: Intravenous regional blockade: In Cousins MJ, Bridenbaugh PO (eds): Neutral Blockade in Clinical Anesthesia and Management of Pain, 2nd ed. Philadelphia, J. B. Lippincott, 1988, pp 433–459.

10. Miller RD: Anesthesia, 2nd ed. New York, Churchill Livingstone, 1986.

11. Miller SH, Graham WP: Anesthesia. In Kilgore ES, Graham WP (eds): The Hand: Surgical and Non-surgical Management. Philadelphia, Lea & Febiger, 1977, pp 437–444.

12. Pratt JM Jr: Analgesics and sedation in plastic surgery. Clin Plast Surg 12:73–81, 1985.

13. Reines HD: Monitoring the plastic surgical patient. Clin Plast Surg 12:3–16, 1985.

14. Rosenberg H, Seitman D: Pharmacogenetics. In Barash PG, Cullen BF, Stoelting RK (eds): Clinical Anesthesia. Philadelphia, J. B. Lippincott, 1989.

15. Stromberg BV: Complications in plastic surgical anesthesia. Clin Plast Surg 12:91–95, 1985.

Chapter 11

PREOPERATIVE CARE OF THE SURGICAL PATIENT

Ann S. Kasdan, R.N.

The occupational health nurse is very often the first responder in trauma. The purpose of this chapter is to examine the various hand injuries that are frequently seen and to outline for the nurse how best to handle them. The role of the nurse in the preoperative care of the employee scheduled for elective surgery is also discussed.

A knowledge of the basic anatomy of the hand is recommended. The primary concern when a patient has a hand injury is to make sure no other serious, life-threatening problems must be taken care of first.[1,6] Bleeding must be controlled. Direct pressure and elevation of the hand will stop bleeding in almost all cases. It is important to make the patient comfortable and to ensure that vital signs are stable. An accurate description of the accident in the patient's own words, as well as a detailed medical history, should be obtained. The nurse should note any unusual behavior that might indicate drug or alcohol abuse as a contributing factor. The patient should be instructed to take nothing by mouth until the need for surgery is assessed. Included in the history should be drug allergies, daily medications, tetanus immunizations, dominant hand, previous injuries to the injured extremity, and systemic diseases that might influence treatment.

It is important to examine the hand in order to establish what structures have been injured.[6] The position of the hand at the time of injury should be established. The area of the hand that is injured must be described in de-

tail. The nurse should be familiar with hand terminology.

Often the information obtained from the patient by the nurse and physician at the initial visit or time of injury becomes crucial. Sometimes in a compensation claim it is the decisive evidence of the cause of the patient's disability.[7]

Many minor hand injuries can be cared for in the plant medical department. If the severity of the injury or a lack of equipment necessitates transferring the patient, as much information as possible should accompany the patient.

Accurate records kept in the plant medical department should include tetanus immunization history as well as prior injuries, current medications, and systemic diseases.

In the case of emergency transfers, the key points to remember are:

DO:
Hold direct pressure on the wound to stop bleeding. Elevate the injured part (Fig. 1). Apply a clean dressing.
Save *any* amputated tissue or part. If necessary, send someone back to the site of the injury to retrieve the missing skin or tissue. Place the amputated tissue in a moist cloth or gauze pad. Then place the cloth in a clean plastic bag or cup. Put the closed bag or cup in water and ice (Fig. 2).
Splint the hand if fingers are deformed (Fig. 3).
DO NOT:
Use dry ice.

Put antiseptic in the wound or on the amputated tissue.

Permit the patient to eat or drink anything.

In the case of a burn to the hand or upper extremity, specific information about the nature of the burn should be obtained, such as direct handling of a burning object, flash burns, electrical burn, or caustic chemical burn. Establish whether the burn occurred in a closed

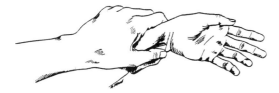

FIGURE 1. The safest way to stop bleeding is to apply direct pressure to the wound.

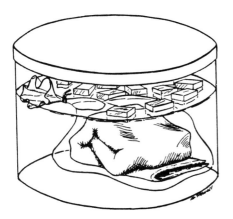

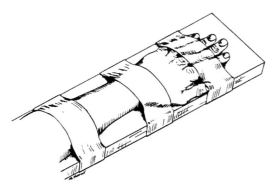

FIGURE 2. Amputated tissue should be placed in a moist clean or sterile cloth in a clean plastic bag or container. The closed bag or container should be placed in water and ice. Do *not* use dry ice.

FIGURE 3. If the hand or fingers are deformed and the bones appear to be unstable, the patient will be more comfortable with the hand splinted for support.

space—i.e., a closet or small room. The extent and depth of a burn can vary from a superficial-partial to a full-thickness injury. A superficial-partial burn (first degree) involves the outer layer of the epidermis. Erythema (redness) is characteristic of this burn. In deep, partial-thickness injury (second degree) the epidermis and dermis are affected, and blisters form. A full-thickness injury (third degree) destroys the epidermis and all of the dermis; sensibility and bleeding are absent.[2,3] The immediate treatment for all burns of the hand is submersion in cold water.

When an employee is scheduled for an operative procedure for a condition related to work it may be cost effective to do the preoperative tests in the medical department. The most common tests are a complete blood count, a urinalysis, an electrocardiogram, blood chemistries, and an x-ray of the involved area. The purpose of the preoperative laboratory tests is to assess surgical risk, detect any coexistent disease, and provide a baseline for comparison in the event of postoperative complications.[5] It is recommended that the testing be done at least 1 week before the scheduled surgery so that any abnormalities can be addressed before surgery. In the case of an emergency hand trauma, if time permits the hand can be x-rayed and blood drawn for laboratory tests in the medical department. The x-ray should accompany the patient to the place of treatment, but the laboratory can be called by telephone after the patient is in transit.

An important point to remember and convey to the treating physician is the availability of light or limited duty for the injured employee. The patient who leaves the workplace knowing he will be expected to return as soon as possible and that light duty will be provided during recovery has a much more secure attitude going into the surgical procedure. Employees who do not return to work as soon as possible following an injury—i.e., the next day—have a more difficult time getting back to work, and often their physical recovery is impaired.[5]

Cooperation and communication between the occupational nurse and physician and the specialist caring for the injured employee are essential. In the case of a severe injury, a member of the management team should accompany the employee to the hospital if possible. This person can notify the family and remain with the employee until the family arrives. This gesture conveys to the patient and family that the company cares. Our system of workers' compensation rewards the patient monetarily for not getting well. The patient soon learns this, but if a good relationship is established between employer and employee, an optimum recovery will occur in spite of workers' compensation.

REFERENCES

1. ASSH: The Hand: Primary Care of Common Problems. Aurora, CO, The American Society for Surgery of the Hand, 1985, p. 1.

2. ASSH: The Hand: Primary Care of Common Problems. Aurora, Co, The American Society for Surgery of the Hand, 1985, pp 62–67.

3. Kaiser TL, Bradley DE, Boswick JA: What can nurses do? Burns of the hand. Today's OR Nurse 5(4):14–23, 1983.

4. Kasdan AS, McElwain NP: Return-to-work programs following occupational hand injuries. Occup Med State Art Rev 4:539–545, 1989.

5. Kasdan ML, Kasdan AS, Romm S: Laboratory screening prior to hand surgery. Surg Clin North Am 64:743–746, 1984.

6. Lister G: The Hand: Diagnosis and Indications, 2nd ed. Edinburgh, Churchill Livingstone, 1984, p 1.

7. Steinberg F: The law of workers' compensation as it applies to hand injuries. Occup Med State Art Rev 4:559–571, 1989.

Chapter 12

FINGERTIP AND NAIL BED INJURIES

Donald M. Ditmars, Jr., M.D.

Because the hands are used in most mechanical activities, it is not surprising that they are so frequently injured. As disabling work injuries, thumb and finger injuries are second only to trunk injuries; they account for 11–14% of disabling work injuries and 6% of total compensation paid.[26] These statistics do not include first-aid cases, which account for many more hours off work. Lacerations and tissue loss injuries account for the majority of compensable fingertip injuries. In the manufacturing sector, where more than half of occupational finger injuries occur, job experience is inversely related to the frequency of injury, and the highest concentration of injuries is in the 21- to 25-year age group. The number of compensable finger injuries in Michigan has been declining for several years, from 12.0% of the total in 1979 to 10.6% in 1985 (from 9,596 to 6,861 cases).[24] Safety programs structured on an accumulating body of research are given most of the credit for this change.

PREVENTION

Occupational Safety and Health Administration (OSHA) requirements for machine guarding have been proved to be effective in reducing injuries. Enforcement is a management responsibility and requires commitment to safety at all stages of production. The design of production processes incorporating ergonomic considerations involves the plant safety engineer and the union health and safety representative. Thus, a team representing both management and labor is responsible for ongoing job safety analysis. Workers found some methods tried in the past impractical and refused to use them. An example is cable restraints, which were bypassed because they were "dehumanizing" and cumbersome. Tool loading of machines and the use of two buttons instead of one are more effective means of removing hands from danger zones.

Some processes are inherently dangerous, and protective gloves cannot always be used. Gloves can become entangled in rotating machinery, and they can decrease dexterity, making them unusable where palpation of fit and finish is required. In the automotive industry, small lacerations and minor skin amputations are most commonly due to sheet metal injuries.

Safety awareness programs for machinery workers include training sessions with trained leaders using videotapes and printed handouts. "An Energy Control and Power Lockout Training Program" is a joint venture with management and unions to ensure that employees do not function in an unsafe manner.[37] Safety professionals lead small groups of production, repair, and supervisory personnel in sequential hourly sessions to progressively recognize and use safety procedures for the equipment they encounter in their own work place. The goal of these sessions is work habit modification for safe use of tools and machinery. Those who complete the program receive some form of recognition. Although these company safety programs cover many areas, their use is associated with a reduced number of finger injuries.

Injury investigations, including employee and

witness interviews, determine the mechanisms of injury. Procedures are evaluated so that corrective measures can be taken.

Because drugs and alcohol are facts of life in the modern workplace, supervisors need training in the recognition and removal of employees with impaired coordination.

ANATOMY

The fingertip is composed of skin, subcutaneous tissues, nail and nail bed, and bone. Each component has unique qualities. The skin is thick and relatively inelastic; its softness is related to use[38,39] (Fig. 1). The subcutaneous tissues contain fat, terminal blood vessels, nerves, tactile corpuscles of Meissner, and flat corpuscles of Ruffini and Golgi-Mazzoni.[4,13] These structures are held in place by cutaneous retinacular septa to the periosteum. These septa limit the shearing motion of the skin on the bone. The nerves originate from the median nerve (thumb, index and middle fingers, and half of the ring finger) or the ulnar nerve (half of the ring finger and the little finger).

The nail lies in a bed surrounded by the curled lateral nail folds and the proximal nail fold, which covers some of the soft, forming nail. The nail plate is produced by the germinal matrix starting under the proximal nail fold and extending into the visible, pale, proximal lunula, with a covering sheen provided by the deep surface of the proximal nail fold.[40,41] The softer, more flexible proximal nail can be easily avulsed from the germinal matrix, which usually remains in anatomic position. The cuticle (eponychium) is firmly attached to the nail plate at the proximal end of the exposed surface. Of more importance is the firm attachment of the deep surface of the nail plate to the distal nail bed (sterile matrix), which bleeds when the nail plate is avulsed. This attachment limits the mobility of the nail because the nail bed lies directly on the periosteum of the distal terminal phalanx. Normal nail growth is approximately 1 mm/week.[11] There is an interconnecting arterial blood supply in the distal phalanx, which is anatomically described as three arcades: superficial, proximal subungual, and distal subungual. These arcades transmit sufficient blood to allow retrograde flow in a severed digital artery, even if the tuft is amputated.[16]

FUNCTION

Normal fine touch requires intact skin and nerves of normal anatomic configuration. The usual two-point discrimination of 3–4 mm can be widened by thick, hyperkeratotic skin or by nerves that have been damaged or moved in a flap from another location.

End-to-end pinch between the finger and thumb tips is best with normal digit length, distal interphalangeal joint motion, and sensation. Key pinch is the approximation of the flat portion of the pulp of the terminal phalanx of the thumb to the radial side of the middle phalanx of the index finger. Power in this case is derived from the flexor pollicis longus with the stabilization of the intrinsic thenar muscles. The thumb is buttressed against all four fingers in parallel, which are supported by the radial dorsal interosseous muscles and the taunt collateral ligaments of the flexed metacarpophalangeal joints.

Grasp and power grip require flexion of the

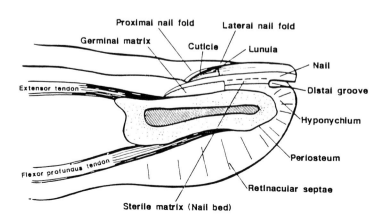

FIGURE 1. Anatomy of the distal phalanx.

Proximal nail fold
Germinal matrix
Cuticle
Lateral nail fold
Lunula
Nail
Extensor tendon
Distal groove
Hyponychium
Flexor profundus tendon
Periosteum
Retinacular septae
Sterile matrix (Nail bed)

distal interphalangeal joint and the length of the distal phalanx for a hooking effect. Scratching and picking use a stable nail of normal length that is firmly attached to the distal nail bed.[32,40] The tuft of the distal phalanx supports the nail plate for normal longitudinal growth so that it projects straight off the end of the finger.

INJURIES

Most injuries are minor cuts, scratches, abrasions, or contusions that are easily treated.[33] Amputations of areas of tip skin and subcutaneous tissue of less than 1 sq cm most often fall into the above category.[11] Lacerations can involve any of the tip structures, including the nail. Composite traumatic flaps involving combinations of tissues can retain enough vascularity for viability or survive as grafts.[40,41]

Nail plate avulsions can be complete or partial. Compared with distal elevations of the nail from the nail bed, which are usually isolated simple injuries, proximal avulsions frequently are associated with fractures of the waist or tuft of the distal phalanx. Tears of the germinal and sterile matrices are to be expected with proximal avulsion injuries. The nail plate, which easily separates from the germinal matrix, may remain attached distally. This will control the position of a distal fracture fragment.[38] A common result of a palmar distal crush is a combination of proximal nail elevation, oblique lacerations of the sides of the proximal nail fold, laceration of the nail matrices, and an angled, displaced shaft fracture. The intact nail plate in this case remains attached to the distal fracture fragment (Fig. 2).

Contusions cause interstitial and subungual hematomas, which are painful because of tension developed in limited spaces. The relatively inelastic volar retinacular septa limit expansion causing distal ischemia that might lead to tip pulp necrosis. The irregular bursting lacerations that commonly occur can actually relieve this tension; however, they are associated with significant edema.

Fractures of the distal phalanx are defined in the usual manner with descriptions of angulation, displacement, and comminution. Because of the firm attachment of the bone to the matrices, angulation and displacement of bone fragments result in lacerations of the germinal and sterile matrices. Therefore, fractures with elevations of the nail are considered open. As-

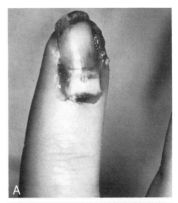
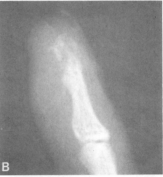
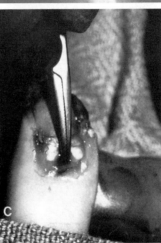

FIGURE 2. Typical proximal elevation of the nail from the germinal matrix associated with a fracture and matrix laceration. *A,* Proximal nail rests on the proximal nail fold. *B,* Tuft fracture is controlled by the attached distal nail. *C,* Displaced soft proximal nail is gently "shoehorned" into anatomic position beneath the proximal nail fold.

sociated injuries of the adjacent structures increase the importance of these fractures. Painful pulp hematomas occur with tuft fractures. Subungual hematomas can occur with any fracture of the distal phalanx.

Tip amputations are described according to

level and direction of bevel. The level is identified by naming the structures involved: skin, subcutaneous tissue, bone, nail, and matrix. Laterally beveled amputations can remove the lateral nail folds. The vertical bevel description is based upon the amount of valuable sensate pulp loss. A favorable defect faces dorsally and distally. An unfavorable defect faces volarly[2,20] (Fig. 3). Some distal nail bed with a small chip of tuft bone is commonly lost with favorable angle amputations.

TREATMENT

Initial treatment follows the basic principles of wound care. The entire hand is surgically prepared with a germicidal soap. The open wound is irrigated with sterile saline, and a sterile field is set up. Gloves and mask are used. A digital block without epinephrine allows sufficient time for the initial treatment of minor injuries. Wrist blocks using epinephrine give added time for longer procedures. A broad

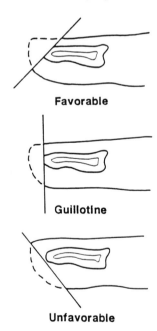

Favorable

Guillotine

Unfavorable

FIGURE 3. Amputation classification based on the amount of remaining sensate volar skin. Although the favorably angulated amputation commonly removes some nail and bone, the volar skin is available for easy coverage. This amputation type is "favorable" for treatment by dressings only, allowing wound repair by contraction and epithelialization. The volarly angulated amputation angle is "unfavorable" for conservative management and usually requires a reconstructive procedure.

tourniquet, such as clamped thyroid drain or a finger cut from a sterile glove, is preferred to a rubber band in order to minimize local tissue crushing. Magnification (2×) is recommended for debridement to preserve as much viable nail matrix as possible. The patient should be specifically instructed to maintain the hand above heart level at all times postoperatively. A sling is not routinely used.

Minor injuries are treated with basic wound care, antibiotic ointment, and nonconstrictive gauze dressings. Nondistracted lacerations can be taped or supported by a grease gauze. Skin lacerations, including small traumatic flaps, are loosely sutured with 6-0 nylon. Sutures should be tied very loosely when the tip is contused, and swelling can be expected. Lacerations of attached nails can be sutured with 5-0 nylon through drill holes; during nail regrowth, they can be supported with reinforced nail polish.

A distal nail elevation is taped for several weeks to prevent snagging while the nail bed heals. The typical proximal nail elevation with a fracture may not require removal of the nail plate. The soft, proximal part of the nail is anatomically replaced under the proximal nail fold, the distal fracture fragment being controlled by the attached nail. The matrix laceration is stented by the replaced nail[38] (Fig. 2). An avulsed nail plate should be surgically cleansed and saved for use as a stent after repair.

When the nail is gone, any matrix laceration is sutured, using magnification, with 6-0, 7-0, or 8-0 absorbable sutures.[30] A prosthetic nail stent to prevent adhesions between the germinal matrix and the proximal nail fold can be cut from the sterile suture pack, remembering that the proximal nail has square corners. The stent remains in place for several weeks between the proximal nail fold and the germinal matrix to prevent adhesions while an intact nail forms. It usually falls out during a dressing change (Fig. 4). A commercially available substitute nail has been proven to be an effective splint.[27] Untreated lacerations of the germinal matrix can result in permanent synechia with the proximal nail fold, resulting in a split nail (Fig. 4C). Distal sterile matrix deficiencies result in nonadherent, elevated nails. Partial thickness grafts from the same sterile matrix, if the defect is small enough, or from another digit, may be used primarily or as a delayed procedure.[22]

A painful, ballotable subungual hematoma is relieved by melting holes in the proximal nail

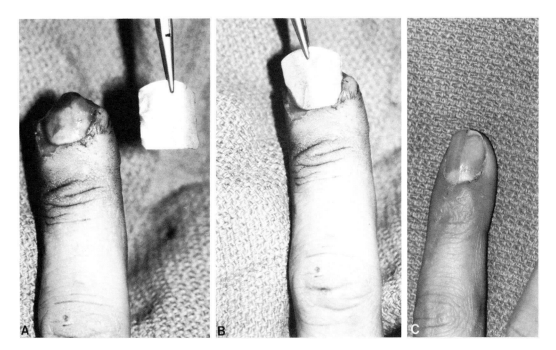

FIGURE 4. Stent for missing nail. *A*, An aluminum suture packet is cut to the size and shape of the missing nail and (*B*) inserted between the germinal matrix and the proximal nail fold. *C*, The healed nail after nail bed laceration demonstrates a split nail plate; the halves have grown at different rates.

with a paper clip held with a needleholder and heated red hot with an alcohol burner. An ophthalmic, battery-powered coagulator can also be used in this manner. This procedure can be done quickly without anesthesia; however a digital block is required for alternative hole-drilling methods using a number 11 scalpel blade, small drill, or Kirschner wire.

Uncomplicated tuft and unangulated or undisplaced shaft fractures can be protected with a splint until they are asymptomatic, usually within 4–6 weeks. Unstable fractures not controlled by an attached nail plate require internal fixation with a fine, longitudinal Kirschner wire that controls the major fragments. Additional tiny fragments in comminuted fractures can be secured in position by suturing their soft tissue attachments (Fig. 5). Short-term antibiotics (cefazolin, 1–2 gm, intravenously during the operation or cephradine, 500 mg, every 6 hours for six doses) are suggested for open fractures and internal fixation. Because of the thin dorsal covering, most angulated shaft fractures are considered open. Heavily contaminated and crushed digits may need antibiotics longer.

Sharply amputated tips that have not been shredded or crushed may be transported in a saline-moistened gauze inside a sterile container placed on ice, but not frozen. Small, thin tips may be considered composite grafts, which after thorough irrigation with saline and surgical preparation of the finger, can be sutured accurately with 6-0 nylon and dressed with a bulky, loose dressing. Clean but ragged amputated tips should be sharply revised in a guillotine fashion because piecemeal defatting leaves a concave dead space that diminishes chances for graft vascularization.[8] The amputation stump should be conservatively sharply debrided to smooth major irregularities.[11] Even when a small piece of the tuft is in the tip requiring a small Kirschner wire, an approximately 50% success rate can be expected (Fig. 6). An even higher success rate has been reported for removal of the bone fragment in the amputated tip, creating a hole. The soft tissues are shortened circumferentially on the proximal stump the length of the distal discarded bone, saving a minimum 2 mm of germinal matrix. The proximal exposed bone is pushed into the hole in the tip, and the skin is accurately sutured.[31]

When the amputated part is unavailable or unacceptable for graft application, various options are available, depending on the size, location, and position of the amputation. Rarely

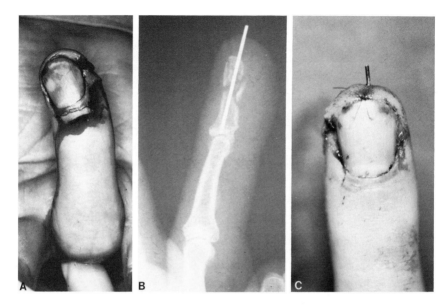

FIGURE 5. Comminuted fracture not controlled by the nail. *A,* A subungual hematoma under the entire nail indicates separation of the nail from the distal matrix. *B,* A small wire stabilizes the major fragments. The smaller attached fragments are supported by the soft tissue closure. *C,* A single suture stabilizes the nail in position after suture of the matrices.

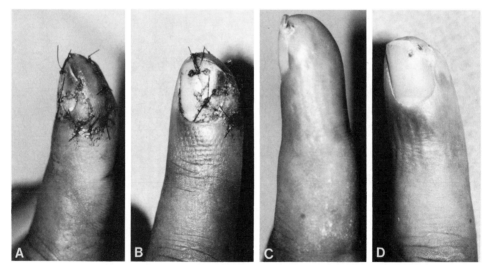

FIGURE 6. Lateral oblique tip amputation including part of nail and tuft. *A,* Sutured en bloc. *B,* Small holes burned into nail prior to very gentle suture placement. *C,* Complete survival of the amputated part as a composite graft. *D,* The growing nail has almost covered the replaced bed. The sutured distal nail fragment that was used as a splint has fallen off.

is bone shortening required unless an amputation of the entire distal phalanx is required. Amputations that are superficial, under 1 cm, or in a favorable angle may be simply sutured to the remaining nail or allowed to close over several weeks by wound contraction and epithelialization. In many cases only a small dressing is required, allowing the patient to return to work[1,3,7,10,18] (Fig. 7). Guillotine or unfavorable angle amputations may be initially skingrafted. Most cases have some degree of contamination and demonstrate improved graft "take" if application is delayed 3–5 days after injury and initial wound care.[23] The hypothenar eminence provides excellent skin for the fingertip, is easily available in the same

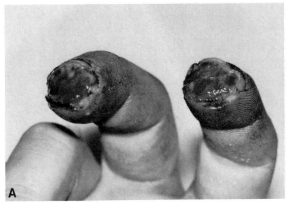

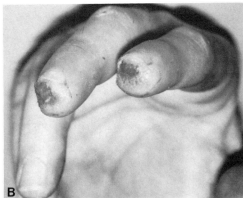

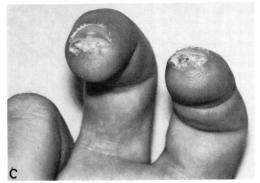

FIGURE 7. Healing by wound contraction and epithelialization. *A,* After surgical wound preparation, the initial wound is covered with antibiotic ointment and a dry sterile dressing. *B,* After 2½ weeks, wound contraction has pulled the volar skin over the tip. *C,* At 7 weeks, the small residual crust covers the scar, which will be protected by the growing nail.

sterile field, and heals well, even in elderly patients (Fig. 8). After a closed wound has been obtained, a definitive flap procedure can be undertaken, if needed, with minimal risk of infection. This also allows time for the patient to use the hand to see if the graft will be stable. We have found that less than half of their procedures require revision because of tip tenderness, weakness of the thin graft, or unacceptable appearance. Our preferred reconstructive flap is the volar finger flap, which maintains anatomic sensation and can be advanced with or without distal folding, depending on the degree of the unfavorable angle. This procedure is performed when ideal surgical skin preparation can be done. Dissection is done in clear anatomic planes to the extent necessary to advance the flap without tension. In unfavorable angle amputations, the "wings" of skin on either side are sutured together for added length and contour.[35] Flexion of the interphalangeal joints allows the flap to reach the end of the finger. The finger is progressively straightened by dynamic traction splints after the wound heals. This flap leaves fewer scars on the tip[12,32,35] (Fig. 9).

Secondary nail bed repairs for residual nail deformities have inconsistent results. Removal of deformed nails with linear excision of scars in the germinal and sterile matrices and elevation and suture approximation of the fragile flaps is prone to recurrences and to formation of a visible longitudinal ridge in the new nail. Full thickness germinal matrix losses result in nail absences or markedly irregular spicules of nail, which grow from remnants of matrix in the scar. The offending pieces of nail can be excised with the underlying matrix to produce a fingertip that, though without a nail, is nontender and does not catch on clothing. Reconstitution of a full-thickness germinal matrix loss requires a full-thickness germinal matrix graft from usually the second toe, which destroys the nail in the donor digit.[40] Nails formed from these grafts have been inconsistently functional (Fig. 10).[28] Recent advances in technique have led to reports of success with free microsurgical transfers of the proximal nail fold, nail, and matrices, anastomosing dorsal toe vessels, to totally reconstruct missing nails.[14,28] For the present, a reliable reconstruction of cosmetically pleasing nails remains an elusive goal.

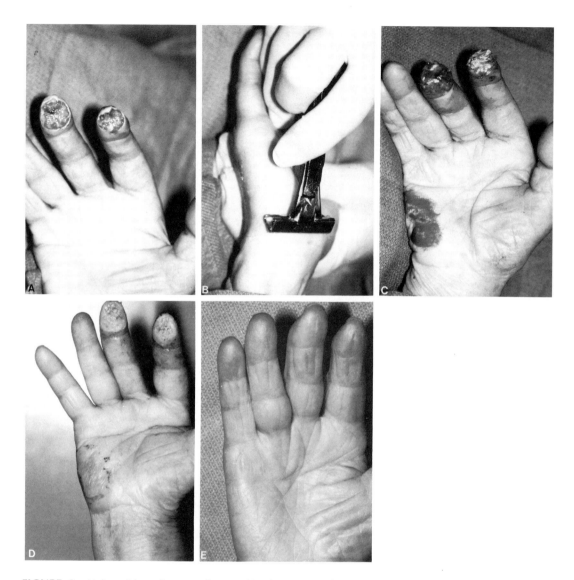

FIGURE 8.   Unfavorable angle amputations resulting from a rotary lawn mower injury in an elderly patient. *A*, There is a good amount of subcutaneous tissue remaining. The exposed bone is localized to just under the nail. *B*, After infiltration of a local anesthetic, the 0.0014-inch split-thickness skin graft is taken freehand from the hypothenar eminence with a guarded blade such as a Weck or, in this case, a Schick razor. *C*, The grafts are loosely sutured into position and, along with the donor site, dressed with nonadherent and dry sterile dressings. *D*, One month later, the donor site has epithelialized. The superficial epithelium of the grafts has separated. *E*, Three months later, there is very little graft hyperpigmentation, the donor site has completely healed, and the patient has little functional deficit or cosmetic problem to show for her injury.

DISCUSSION

The goal of treatment is to maximize function and appearance by the anatomic restoration of as many structures as possible. Methods employed should be the most simple and direct to achieve the best possible result.[34] Wound care for the initial treatment of the injury should be complete in order to minimize subsequent problems with wound infection and delayed healing, which can transform a minor problem into a major one causing permanent disability of the entire hand.

As with most reconstructive procedures, the initial definitive tip repair is the most important operation; yields from subsequent ones will diminish. A major complication can destroy the best chance to achieve an optimal result and can even convert a fingertip injury

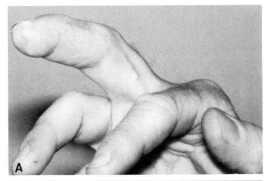

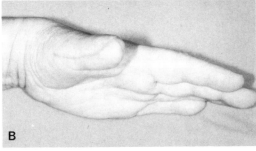

FIGURE 9. Volar advancement flap. *A*, The original unfavorable angle amputation was skin grafted. The tender graft was excised later and the total volar flap advanced with cupping of the distal end. *B*, A similar procedure demonstrates good contour and bulk of the distal thumb. The original amputation was not shortened.

into loss of function of other digits. I do not like to submit a reconstructive procedure to an increased risk of infection by performing it primarily in the emergency room. When there is contamination, the concept of delayed closure of the primary wound should be used. All definitive repairs should be done as soon as pos-

sible after bacteriological control of the wound has been achieved.

Permanent functional changes can result from changes in fingertip shape, length, sensation, or motion. Alteration of the shape of the distal thumb pad changes pinch and therefore the total pattern of hand use, making some activities difficult or impossible. Although thumb and one-finger pinch may be possible with a single, shortened distal phalanx, the same deficit causes a change in balance in thumb and two-finger ("chuck") pinch, which frequently changes finger use. An example of the latter situation is an amputation of more than half of the distal phalanx of the index finger. In this case, the index finger function is commonly transferred to the middle finger. An insensate radial tip of the index causes the same effect. A single, tender fingertip weakens grip because an attempt to extend the digit to get it out of the way tethers the rest of the flexor profundus tendons, limiting their excursions. Distant flaps (e.g. cross-finger or palmar) or flaps that are nonanatomically innervated may have altered sensation that may result in changed patterns of use for years (Fig. 11).[29]

Procedures that are appropriate for children cannot be assumed to be effective for adults.[7] Tip amputation healing by secondary intention is faster in children. After several years, bone can regrow, leaving very little deformity. Amputated tips and nail bed grafts survive routinely in children, but total nail bed grafts have only about a 50% chance of satisfactory take in adults. Central relearning following nerve repairs and transfer is far superior in children and produces better results.

FIGURE 10. Free nail grafts from toes to fingers for traumatic losses of nails. *A*, The scars remaining in the healed fingertips make poor recipient beds for the composite germinal/sterile matrix grafts. *B*, Composite grafts in place.

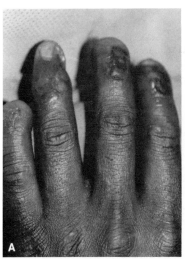

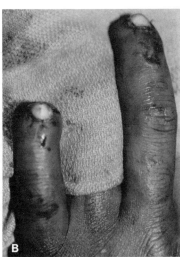

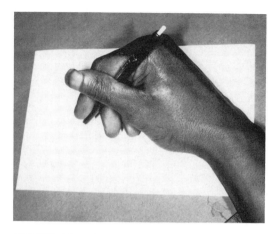

FIGURE 11. Altered configuration of the three-point chuck. A radially innervated cross-finger flap from the index to the thumb gave good bulk and stable skin and also maintained length; however, the patient had only protective sensation for 2 years. Here the pen is held so that the normal, sensate skin of the thumb is used.

Some surgeons recommend removal of attached nails to suture matrix lacerations.[23] A reason given for this is that soft tissue retained in a fracture line might lead to a nonunion, which would require a bone graft later. Another reason proposed is that accurate approximation of the matrices is required to reduce the possibility of growth of deformed and split nails, which are difficult to repair later. We recommend gentle handling of the fragments to minimally disrupt remaining attachments of the nail plate to the distal matrix. The nail then acts as an anatomic support for both the matrix and the bone and also separates the germinal matrix from the proximal nail fold. We have seen very few instances of nonunion or permanent nail deformities in these cases. The new nail grows in during the next several months with a ridge growing distally or by pushing the old nail ahead. The old nail plate protects the distal bed during this regrowth phase.

The plethora of procedures recommended for tip amputation reconstruction indicates the magnitude of the problem in this tiny area of the body and the ingenuity of many hand surgeons.[2,12,15,19,21,36] Thirty years ago, a clinical study indicated that the morbidity for such wounds could be extended from 1 month to as long as 3 months as the complexity of repair increased.[5] Although flaps intrinsically have better skin and subcutaneous tissue from the start, split-thickness skin grafts adapt over time to meet the demands of the recipient site. Over half of the skin grafts applied to pulp ampu-

tations never require a subsequent procedure. Other donor sites commonly used are the volar/ulnar forearm in the Caucasian male and the anterior hairless high thigh in others. Although skin from these sites yields satisfactory grafts initially, it tends eventually to become hyperpigmented in blacks and orientals.

Full-thickness skin grafts are supposed to supply better quality skin and even support for the nail when the tuft has been amputated. But because they yield much poorer initial take and the return of sensation is delayed, this technique is reserved for ideal cases. Full-thickness grafts are very useful, however, to close donor defects in local flap advancements when the grafts are applied to noncritical areas and to cover distal spots where the flaps cannot reach.[21] A donor site that can be primarily closed is the ulnar side of the hand.[17]

The designs of local tip flaps are variations of island pedicle flaps based on one or both digital neurovascular bundles, which are advanced over the tip amputation stump.[2,15,30] Those with limited dissection have limited excursions and result in tight closures or small remaining defects. They are most easily performed in favorable angle amputations when the donor sites can be closed in a "V–Y" manner. In more extensive amputations, the flap donor sites and areas not reached by the flaps can be skin-grafted or allowed to heal by secondary intention. Each incision line leaves a scar with a propensity for long-term tenderness. A long volar flap based on one neurovascular pedicle can be dissected and advanced to cover an amputated tip.[9] The problems of extending a proximally based pedicle to the end of the finger are solved by the distally based "reverse digital artery flap," which is pivoted on a single digital artery with a cuff of perivascular tissue at a point 5 mm proximal to the proximal interphalangeal joint.[16] This flap, which does not include the nerve, survives on the reverse flow in the digital artery from the three vascular arcades in the distal phalanx. The total volar advancement finger flap, which includes both digital arteries and nerves, has been very reliable for me and results in a tip with fewer tender scars. Because it derives sensation from normal nerve distribution, it results in superior function.

CONCLUSION

Damage to any of the anatomic structures of the fingertip can result in a change in the use of the hand and can even make some tasks impossible. Prevention of injuries is naturally most important; however, when an injury occurs, anatomic restoration should be the goal. Treatment should be as direct and simple as possible to reach the optimal structural and functional result. Caveats of treatment are: (1) save nails; (2) reapproximate nail matrix lacerations; (3) use wound contraction and epithelialization to advantage; (4) restore pulp when necessary with volar innervated flaps from the same finger; (5) reduce fracture angulation and displacement; (6) use skin grafts when subcutaneous tissue is sufficient; and (7) replace small, noncrushed skin-pulp amputations and traumatic flaps.

REFERENCES

1. Allen MJ: Conservative management of fingertip injuries in adults. Hand 12:257–265, 1980.
2. Atasoy E, Ioakimidis E, Kasdan ML, et al: Reconstruction of the amputated fingertip with a triangular volar flap. J Bone Joint Surg 52A:921–926, 1970.
3. Bojsen-Moller J, Pers M, Schmidt A: Fingertip injuries: Late results. Acta Chir Scand 122:177–183, 1961.
4. Boyd JD: Peripheral nervous system. In Hamilton WJ (ed): Textbook of Human Anatomy. London, Macmillan, 1957, pp 827–831.
5. Clifford RH: Evaluation of three methods for fingertip injuries. Arch Surg 65:464–466, 1952.
6. Ditmars, DM: Fingertip and nail bed injuries. Occup Med State Art Rev 4:449–461, 1989.
7. Douglas BS: Conservative management of guillotine amputation of the finger in children. Aust Paediatr J 8:86–89, 1972.
8. Elsahy NI: When to replant a fingertip after its complete amputation. J Plast Reconstruct Surg 60:15–21, 1977.
9. Evans DM, Martin DL: Step-advancement island flap for fingertip reconstruction. Br J Plast Surg 41:105–111, 1988.
10. Farrell RG, Disher WA, Nesland RS, et al: Conservative management of fingertip amputations. J Am Coll Emerg Phys 6:243–246, 1977.
11. Flatt AE: The Care of Minor Hand Injuries, 4th ed. St. Louis, C. V. Mosby, 1979, pp 122–157.
12. Furlow LT: V–Y "cup" flap for volar oblique amputations of fingers. J Hand Surg 9B:253–256, 1984.
13. Goss CM (ed): Gray's Anatomy of the Human Body, 26th ed. Philadelphia, Lea & Febiger, 1955, pp 1177–1179.
14. Koshima I, Soeda S, Takase T, Yamasaki M: Free vascularized nail grafts. J Hand Surg 13A:29–32, 1988.
15. Kutler W: A new method for fingertip amputation. JAMA 133:29–30, 1947.
16. Lai CS, Lin SD, Yang CC: The reverse digital artery flap for fingertip reconstruction. Ann Plast Surg 22:495–500, 1989.
17. Lie KK, Magargle RK, Posch JL: Free full-thickness skin grafts from the palm to cover defects of the fingers. J Bone Joint Surg 52A:559–561, 1970.
18. Louis DL, Palmer AK, Burney RE: Open treatment of digital tip injuries. JAMA 244:297–298, 1980.
19. Ma GFY, Cheng JCY, Chan KT, et al. Fingertip injuries—A prospective study on seven methods of treatment on 200 cases. Ann Acad Med 11:207–213, 1982.
20. Markley JM: Fingertip injuries, amputations, and infections of the hand and upper extremity. In Grabb WC, Smith WC (eds): Plastic Surgery, 3rd ed. Boston, Little, Brown, 1979, pp 569–585.
21. Massart P, Saucier TH, Bezes H: Restoration of the pulp with a homodigital neurovascular flap. Ann Chir Main 4:219–225, 1985.
22. Matsusba HM, Spear SL: Delayed primary reconstruction of subtotal nail bed loss using a split-thickness nail bed graft on decorticated bone. J Plast Reconstruct Surg 81:440–443, 1988.
23. Melone CP, Isani A: Fingertip injuries: A rational approach to management. Orthop Rev 14:83–93, 1985.
24. Michigan Department of Labor: Compensable Occupational Finger Injury and Illness Report, Michigan, 1985. Reference #184064, September 1987, pp 13–14.
25. Nakayama Y, Iino T, Uchida A, et al: Vascularized free nail grafts nourished by arterial inflow from the venous system. J Plast Reconstruct Surg 85:239–245, 1990.
26. National Safety Council: Accident Facts, 1986 ed, pp 24–27.
27. Ogunro EO: External fixation of injured nail bed with the INRO surgical nail splint. J Hand Surg 14A:236–241, 1989.
28. Pribaz JJ: Discussion of Nakayama Y, et al: Vascularized free nail grafts nourished by arterial inflow from the venous system (J Plast Reconstruct Surg 85:239–245, 1990.) J Plast Reconstruct Surg 85:246–247, 1990.
29. Robbins TH: The "jam roll" flap for fingertip reconstruction. J Plast Reconstruct Surg 81:109–111, 1988.
30. Romm S, Kasdan ML, Spear SL: Management of fingertip injuries. Tech Orthop 1:61–67, 1986.
31. Rose EH, Norris MS, Kowalski TA, et al: The "cap" technique: Nonmicrosurgical reattachment of fingertip amputations. J Hand Surg 14A:513–518, 1989.
32. Rosenthal EA: Treatment of fingertip and nail bed injuries. Orthop Clin North Am 14:675–697, 1983.
33. Russell RC, Casas L: Management of fingertip injuries. Clin Plast Surg 16:405–425, 1989.
34. Sandzen SC: Treating acute fingertip injuries. Am Fam Physician 5:68–79, 1972.
35. Snow JW: The use of a volar flap for repair of fingertip amputations: A preliminary report. J Plast Reconstruct Surg 40:163–168, 1967.
36. Sturman MJ, Duran RJ: Late results of finger-tip injuries. J Bone Joint Surg 45A:289–298, 1963.
37. UAW-Ford National Joint Committee on Health and Safety: An Energy Control and Power Lockout Program, 1987.
38. Verdan CE, Egloff DV: Fingertip injuries. Surg Clin North Am 61:237–266, 1981.
39. Zook EG, Van Beek AL, Russell RC, Beatty ME: Anatomy and physiology of the perionychium: A review of the literature and anatomic study. J Hand Surg 5:528–536, 1980.
40. Zook EG: Injuries of the fingernail. In Green DP (ed): Operative Hand Surgery. New York, Churchill Livingstone, 1982, pp 895–914.
41. Zook EG: The perionychium. In Green DP (ed): Operative Hand Surgery, 2nd ed. New York, Churchill Livingstone, 1988, pp 1331–1371.

Chapter 13

TENDON INJURIES OF THE HAND

Mark R. Wilson, M.D.
Fred M. Hankin, M.D.

Tendon injuries of the hand and forearm are common. In the workplace, mechanisms of injury include hand-intensive repetitive tasks and press-induced crush injuries. Sharp metal, glass, and ceramic objects may produce penetrating injuries with concomitant tendon disruption. Innocuous looking wounds and trivial injuries may be associated with significant tendon problems and subsequent long-term impairment.

Tendon injuries provide the examiner a unique opportunity to correlate anatomy and functional loss. The prehensile and reaching functions of the hand make it vulnerable to the laceration and crush injuries that may disrupt tendons. In the hand, complete disruption of a tendon results in a distinct deficit of finger motion, and patients usually refer themselves for medical care.

The initial treatment of upper extremity tendon injuries is critical.[12] A prompt and thorough evaluation is the key initial step toward optimal recovery. The evaluation should include a thorough history, including the specific mechanism of injury. The clinical assessment should include the status of the wound, tissue viability, associated functional deficits, and other accompanying problems such as vascular and nerve injuries. Radiographs often help in assessing the presence of fractures and foreign bodies.

Partial tendon lacerations can be difficult to diagnose. Pain with active motion and pain or weakness with gentle, resisted active motion of the tendon unit suggest such an injury. The mechanism of injury—whether a penetrating stab wound or a blunt crush injury—can also corroborate the clinical impression. Associated nerve or vessel injuries can be indicators of laceration depth. Unrecognized or untreated partial tendon injuries can predispose the patient to future tendon rupture or triggering. If such an injury is suspected, appropriate splinting and serial re-examination is warranted. Surgical exploration may be necessary.

The need for oral antibiotics after lacerations to the hand varies. Contaminated injuries and those with significant soft-tissue trauma warrant antibiotic coverage. Closed tendon injuries do not require antibiotic treatment. Whether clean, simple lacerations need antibiotic coverage is controversial. Treatment should be based on the injury mechanism, co-existing systemic illnesses, and existing standards of care.

After a significant injury, hand therapy plays an important role in the patient's recovery. The therapy program needs to be individualized according to the exact nature of the injury and the specific treatment provided. The postoperative rehabilitation after a tendon injury should be done by skilled personnel.[8,9]

Flexor and extensor tendon injuries should be treated with the same respect. The treatment of a tendon injury should not be considered a simple exercise. Combinations of injuries may occur, but to facilitate discussion we will consider each category separately.

EXTENSOR TENDON INJURIES

The dorsal aspect of the hand and wrist has been divided into five zones to facilitate communication among medical personnel. Generalized treatment recommendations are made for each zone.

Zone I Injuries

Zone I of the extensor mechanism extends from the portion distal to the insertion of the central slip into the proximal portion of the middle phalanx to the insertion of the terminal portion of the extensor tendon into the proximal portion of the distal phalanx. This terminal insertion of the extensor mechanism into the dorsal aspect of the original epiphysis is very narrow.[5] The extensor mechanism in zone I is flat and includes the oblique retinacular ligaments and the triangular ligament.[6,16] Injuries in this zone result from forced flexion of the extended distal interphalangeal (DIP) joint, completely rupturing the tendon, or from lacerations. Clinically, with a complete zone I tendon interruption, the DIP joint is flexed and cannot be actively extended. The clinical deformity has been described as a mallet finger — one resembling the hammers striking piano strings.

An acute mallet finger may not be particularly painful, but the characteristic clinical deformity is diagnostic.[1] With partial zone I extensor lacerations, the patient can still completely extend the DIP joint, especially if the digit has been anesthetized with a digital block. After a laceration, a partial zone I tendon injury can be diagnosed with certainty only by inspection of the wound. Further evaluation should include radiographs of the involved finger, which may reveal an avulsed intra-articular fragment from the dorsal base of the distal phalanx (Fig. 1). Other findings may include subluxation of the distal phalanx volarly on the middle phalanx (Fig. 2).

The primary treatment of all zone I tendon injuries is by closed methods.[2,3,11] Occasionally, if a wound is open and large enough to require formal debridement, open repair of the tendon may be indicated. The operating physician must be cautioned against placing too many sutures (foreign material) into a traumatized region that has only a thin skin layer available for coverage. Immobilization of the DIP joint in a neutral position by a splint for 4–8 weeks continuously and for an additional 4–6 weeks during activities provides adequate treatment for zone I injuries.[2,17] If an extension

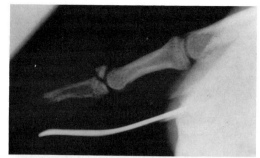

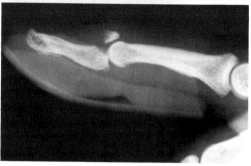

FIGURE 1. Mallet fracture with avulsed fragment. A volar aluminum splint immobilizes the DIP joint in a neutral position.

FIGURE 2. Avulsion of the extensor tendon from the distal phalanx has resulted in volar subluxation of the DIP joint. Splinting may not provide effective treatment of this particular mallet finger, and surgery may be indicated.

lag is present after a 3-month splinting program, treatment may be continued for several more weeks. When satisfactory active DIP joint extension is present, the splinting may be discontinued.

A hairpin splint fabricated from a thermoplastic material is very suitable for these injuries because it can be tightened or loosened to accommodate changes in digit swelling (Fig. 3A). The proximal interphalangeal (PIP) joint does not need to be included with the immobilization (Fig. 3B). Volar or dorsal aluminum or commercially available plastic splints also provide effective immobilization for these injuries. Placing the splint dorsally on the digit permits the use of the volar fingertip for tactile tasks. The splints can be removed for showers, but the patient must hold the digit in passive extension during this time in order to avoid attenuation of the repair process.

As the DIP joint is brought into extension, the skin on the dorsum of the joint must be carefully monitored. Skin necrosis can occur in this region if extension is pursued too vigorously in a swollen, stiff joint by a tight splint.[13]

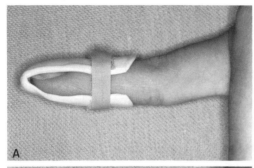

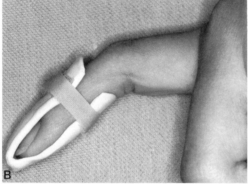

FIGURE 3.   A, A hairpin splint fabricated from a thermoplastic material can be used to treat mallet fingers. B, PIP joint flexion is permitted and encouraged with the hairpin splint treatment of a mallet finger.

Pressure necrosis can be avoided by monitoring the condition of the dorsal skin and serially bringing the DIP joint into further extension over the course of the first 2 weeks as the swelling subsides.

Mallet fractures can often be treated by closed (splinting) methods. Radiographs of the splinted digit are obtained to evaluate the fracture reduction. If the joint surfaces are congruous and the fracture is satisfactorily reduced, then splinting is continued. Serial radiographs are obtained on a weekly or biweekly basis in order to reassess fracture position and joint alignment. Should joint subluxation or excessive distraction of the fragment occur, then some authors recommend open reduction and internal fixation of the displaced fragment.[3] Postsurgical therapy is often indicated in order to regain DIP joint motion. Some authors recommend closed treatment with splinting even in the face of a displaced fragment or subluxation of the joint.[17] Good functional recovery and clinical appearance have been reported by advocates of each of these treatment methods.

Proximal interphalangeal joint hyperextension may occasionally occur with the mallet deformity, especially if the injury is untreated. This produces the typical swan-neck deformity with hyperextension of the proximal interphalangeal joint and flexion at the distal interphalangeal joint (Fig. 4). The loss of active extension across the DIP joint (DIP joint flexion) results in increasing extensor forces acting across the PIP joint (PIP joint hyperextension) and the resultant swan-neck posture.[6,16] Patients exhibiting a swan-neck deformity of a digit following a DIP joint mallet injury usually have concomitant PIP joint volar plate laxity. If the cause of the swan-neck deformity is an isolated DIP joint mallet injury, splinting of the DIP in extension may be the only treatment required. Several other mechanisms can lead to the development of such deformities, including intrinsic muscle tightness, PIP joint volar plate laxity, and volar subluxation of the metacarpophalangeal joint.[3,6,16] Reconstructive techniques are available that can balance the complicated extensor mechanism in such cases.

Zone II Injuries

The zone II extensor mechanism extends from the metacarpal neck to the proximal aspect of the middle phalanx. This region includes the central tendon, the lateral band components from the intrinsic muscles, the sagittal bands, and transverse retinacular ligament portions of the extensor hood.[6,16] The extensor mechanism

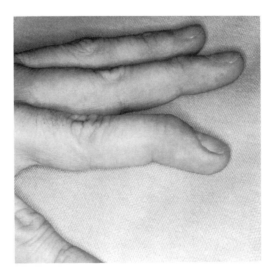

FIGURE 4.   Disruption of the extensor mechanism over the DIP joint results in a mallet deformity. The extensor tendon imbalance resulting from the mallet deformity results in a mild swan-neck posture of the digit.

in this zone is relatively flat and has been described as a hood or shroud. The insertion of the central slip into the dorsal aspect of the original middle phalanx epiphysis is very narrow.[5] Injuries to this zone result from forced flexion of the extended PIP or metacarpophalangeal joint and from lacerations.

Disruption of the terminal central slip insertion into the middle phalanx, with associated volar subluxation of the lateral bands beneath the PIP joint flexion axis results in a boutonnière deformity.[1,3] Clinically, this presents with hyperextension of the DIP joint and flexion of the PIP joint (Fig. 5). Because the dorsal structures are no longer present over the PIP joint, the proximal phalanx head can buttonhole (or boutonnière) through the extensor mechanism. While both central slip disruption and lateral band subluxation are required for the clinical deformity, an untreated central slip injury can promote later lateral band migration and an eventual boutonnière digit.

Recognition of these actual and potential boutonnière extensor tendon injuries can be difficult in the acute postinjury period. Clinical findings include the specific site of postinjury tenderness (dorsal PIP joint), limitation of active PIP extension, and hyperextension deformity of the DIP joint. The initial clinical picture may consist only of PIP joint swelling, dorsal tenderness, and a slight extensor lag across the PIP joint.

PIP joint volar plate injuries can result in flexion contractures of the PIP joint that can be confused with boutonnière deformities (Fig. 6). These injuries can be differentiated by checking the active flexion of the DIP joint, which should be severely restricted with a boutonnière deformity and unimpeded by a PIP joint volar plate injury (Fig. 7). Also, careful palpation of the PIP joint reveals whether the patient is tender dorsally (boutonnière) or volarly (volar plate injury). A careful history also helps to elucidate the mechanism of injury and

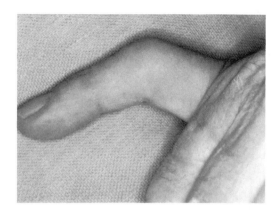

FIGURE 6. PIP joint volar plate injury has resulted in a flexion contracture. The DIP joint is not involved in this injury pattern.

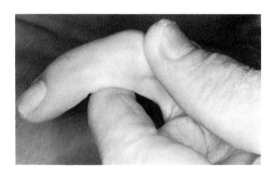

FIGURE 7. In the evaluation of a PIP joint flexion deformity, the ability to actively flex the DIP joint favors the diagnosis of a PIP joint volar plate injury over a boutonnière deformity.

to define the anatomic derangements present. Standard radiograms can help delineate the pathology if a fracture fragment is present volarly or dorsally about the PIP joint (Fig. 8A). If a boutonnière deformity is suspected, the digit should be splinted in extension (Fig. 8B). The metacarpophalangeal (MCP) joint usually does not need to be included in the splint. Similarly, the DIP joint can be excluded from the splint and active DIP joint motion can be encouraged to minimize stiffness at that joint and to maintain the normal length relationships of the lateral bands. Active DIP joint extension can promote dorsal positioning of the lateral bands (Fig. 9).

Usually, isolated PIP joint immobilization is difficult and impractical because the length of digit available for splint purchase is small. Incorporating the DIP joint into the splint is usually required, and if the digit is especially short, inclusion of the MCP joint may aid in effecting and maintaining an extended posture of the

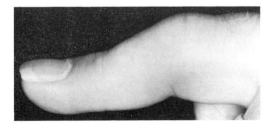

FIGURE 5. Boutonnière deformity of this digit demonstrates DIP joint hyperextension and PIP joint flexion.

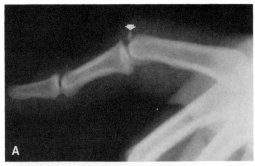

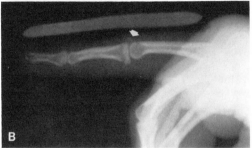

FIGURE 8. A, Avulsion of the extensor tendon central slip insertion (arrow) from the middle phalanx combined with disruption of the triangular ligament (over the middle phalanx) results in this boutonnière deformity. B, The small bone fragment (arrow) is associated with a central slip tendon avulsion in this boutonnière deformity. The tendon injury is treated by extension splinting of the digit.

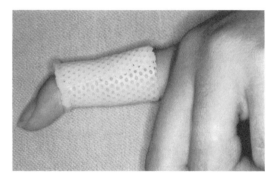

FIGURE 9. DIP joint flexion is permitted and encouraged with this particular cylinder splint used in the treatment of a boutonnière deformity. The splint is fabricated from a thermoplastic material.

PIP joint. If a flexion contracture of the PIP joint has developed, then serial casting or dynamic extension splinting may be needed to help achieve full extension at the PIP joint. Once full extension is accomplished, then splinting is maintained in full extension on a continuous basis for 6–8 weeks. Splinting is then used during activities for another 4–6 weeks. A therapy program is frequently required to regain PIP joint flexion.

Boutonnière injuries are difficult to treat, and postinjury functional results are not predictable. Acute injuries with lateral bands that cannot be held dorsally by active extension of the digit may require different management from injuries in which the PIP joint can be held in active extension.[3] Chronic injuries require different treatment from acute injuries because secondary PIP joint changes frequently complicate matters. Once the boutonnière deformity has been diagnosed or is suspected, referral to a hand surgeon is prudent.

Lacerations to or forced flexion of an extended MCP joint can result in disruption of the extensor mechanism. The clinical appearance of such digits may include no deficit, an extensor lag (inability to fully extend) across the MCP joint, or a laterally subluxing (translocating) tendon across the metacarpal head. Significant tears in the central tendon portion of the hood may result in the extensor lag, whereas rents in the sagittal bands can lead to snapping subluxation of the central tendon across the metacarpal head during active motion of the digit. Sagittal band injury may not be evident while the finger is held in extension at the MCP joint level but may manifest in radial or ulnar dislocation of the extensor mechanism during MCP joint flexion.

Acute injuries of these types can often be managed by closed means, although surgery is frequently recommended.[7,14] Nonoperative treatment involves splinting the joint in extension for 4–6 weeks. The MCP joints of the ulnar four digits must all be held in neutral during this time as the active pull of juncturae and common muscle bellies can separate the opposing tendon edges. The PIP joints can be left free in the splint. Isolated injuries to the MCP joint of the thumb do not require immobilization of the other digits.

Operative management of these zone II MCP joint injuries is frequently recommended in order to assess the exact nature and extent of the injury.[3,7] Surgical repair can then be performed and the anatomy restored. A postoperative splinting program similar to that described for the closed treatment method is pursued. The particular treatment rendered depends on the mechanism of injury, concomitant hand problems, and patient preference.

Puncture wounds of the MCP joint can be difficult to diagnose. These include human bites sustained when a clenched fist strikes a foe's teeth. The normal tendon and skin excursion over the joint makes difficult the clinical diagnosis of penetrating joint wounds. The exact alignment of skin, tendon, and joint capsule present during the puncture may be difficult to duplicate during a superficial exploration of the hand. If the hand was in a fist formation when the laceration occurred, the examiner needs to recognize that the level of tendon laceration is different from the skin laceration when the hand is examined with the fingers extended. The wound should be extended proximally or distally as needed for complete and thorough inspection and treatment. Probing the puncture wound in an effort to determine whether the joint has been violated is not beneficial. Radiographs may disclose an associated fracture or foreign body. Air present in the joint, as revealed by a radiograph, also indicates the depth of the contamination. Injuries that penetrate the MCP joint must be suspected and frequently require surgical exploration. Human bite wounds should not be closed.

Injuries to the intrinsic muscle tendons are difficult to diagnose because these structures often have dual insertions. Clinical suspicion is raised when absence of, or pain with, an attempted specific digit motion is noted.[6,16] Functional deficits of such injuries may be minimal, but referral to a hand specialist is warranted.

Zone III Injuries

Zone III of the extensor tendons extends from the portion distal to the extensor retinaculum to the metacarpal necks. The tendons in this zone are oval, and they can usually be visualized beneath the intact dorsal skin of the hand. Juncturae connecting the extensor digitorum communis (EDC) tendons in this zone can mask lacerations of the inidividual tendons. Extensor lags across the MCP joints or pain with resisted extension of an MCP joint corroborates the diagnosis of such an injury. Lacerations of the extensor indicis proprius (EIP), extensor digiti quinti (EDQ), abductor pollicis longus (APL), extensor pollicis brevis (EPB), and extensor pollicis longus (EPL) can be difficult to diagnose. Functional deficits must be carefully sought. An inability to extend the MCP joints of the index and small fingers when the middle and ring finger MCP joints are held flexed would suggest injuries to EIP and EDQ. Difficulty

abducting the thumb metacarpal (APL) or extending the thumb MCP joint (EPB) suggests an injury to these tendon units. The APL can also have multiple tendon slips. Extension of the thumb interphalangeal (IP) joint to neutral is possible by the action of the thenar intrinsic muscles. Hyperextension of the thumb IP joint and extension of the thumb dorsally away from the hand are not possible without the action of EPL. As EPL, APL, and EPB do not have any juncturae attachments to adjacent tendons, lacerations of these units in zone III usually result in proximal retraction of the tendons. Palpation of the hand and wrist in these situations often demonstrates a deficit where the tendon formerly resided. Surgical repair of tendon disruptions in zone III is warranted. Postoperative immobilization for 4–6 weeks is usually required.

Zone IV and V Injuries

The portion of the extensor tendons beneath the dorsal wrist retinaculum is termed zone IV, and the portion proximal to the retinaculum is considered zone V. Disruption of the extensor tendons in these zones results in functional deficits similar to those described for zone III. Surgical intervention is recommended.

Attritional ruptures of the extensor tendons frequently occur in patients with rheumatoid arthritis. Sharp bone surfaces, especially the distal ulna, can lacerate the digital extensor tendons. Distal radius fractures can also predispose patients to future rupture of extensor tendons because repetitive excursion across a sharp osteophyte or fracture surface can lead to tendon disruption. The EPL tendon is frequently subjected to this attritional process.

FLEXOR TENDON INJURIES

The digital flexor tendons act in concert to permit prehensile movements of the worker's hand. Deficits in these structures can result in significant impairment of grip strength and fine motor control.

The resting hand normally exhibits mild flexion (the normal cascade) of all digits. Loss of these tendons causes the injured digit to be postured in extension owing to the unopposed pull of the EDC tendon (Fig. 10). Similarly, in the normal hand, passive flexion and exten-

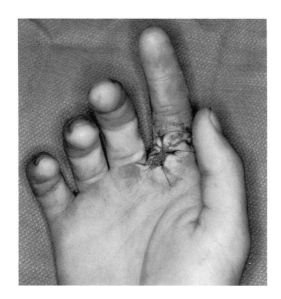

FIGURE 10. Laceration of the index finger FDS and FDP tendons results in an extension posture of the digit and loss of the normal resting appearance of the hand (flexion tone).

sion of the wrist results in, respectively, passive extension and flexion of the fingers owing to the tenodesis effect (passive pull) of the digital tendons. An injured finger without a flexor tendon does not exhibit this check-rein tenodesis response.

Specific testing of the flexor tendons involves selectively blocking the motion of the adjacent finger joints so that only the unit being examined can function. The flexor digitorum profundus (FDP) and the flexor pollicis longus (FPL) tendons function to flex the terminal joints of the digits. These units are tested by blocking all other joints of the finger and asking the patient to flex the isolated DIP or thumb IP joint. Documentation of flexor digitorum sublimis (FDS) tendon function is accomplished by holding the adjacent digits in full extension in order to block the digital flexion effect of the FDP tendons and asking the patient to selectively flex the PIP joint of interest.

Complete flexor tendon disruption cannot be treated by nonoperative methods. Once an injury is recognized, referral to a hand surgeon is prudent. Suspected partial flexor tendon injuries should also be referred. Unrecognized or untreated partial lacerations can result in rupture, adhesions, or triggering. Patients with partial flexor tendon lacerations may exhibit pain with active motion and pain or weakness with gentle, resisted active motion. Surgical

exploration is advocated to restore the anatomy.

Flexor tendon injuries can also be divided into zones to permit more accurate medical record documentation. The zone implicated should describe the location of the tendon injury rather than the skin laceration and should be determined with the wrist and fingers held in neutral (zero degree) positions.[15] For example, a patient clenching his fist (pulling his flexor tendons proximally) around a sharp blade may have skin lacerations in the palm (apparent zone III) but may actually have zone II tendon lacerations when the hand is held in neutral. His injury would be designated as a zone II flexor tendon injury.

Zone I

Zone I extends from the middle phalanx (distal to the flexor sublimis tendon insertion) to the end of the flexor profundus tendon onto the distal phalanx. This region represents the terminal portion of the FDP tendon. The FDP and FPL tendons have broad attachments along the volar metaphyseal surfaces of the distal phalanges.[5]

Flexor tendon injuries in Zone I result from lacerations and ruptures. Jersey finger is a term used to describe rupture of the FDP tendon, most frequently seen in the ring finger, from the distal phalanx.[10] This results from an active flexion by the FDP against a passively extended DIP joint, as might happen in an attempt to grab the jersey of an opposing football player. Clinical examination reveals the loss of active flexion of the individual DIP or IP joint (Fig. 11A). Tenderness may be present and ecchymosis may be visible along the flexor sheath. Radiographs can help confirm this injury, as frequently a small piece of bone is avulsed off the distal phalanx and is attached to the FDP tendon (Fig. 11B). The examiner must be cautious to avoid diagnosing this injury as a "jammed finger" in the face of normal radiographs.

Zone II

Zone II, or no-man's-land, is the area of flexor tendon excursion beneath the retinacular pulley system. This corresponds to the area from the distal palmar flexion crease to the midportion of the middle phalanx. In various segments

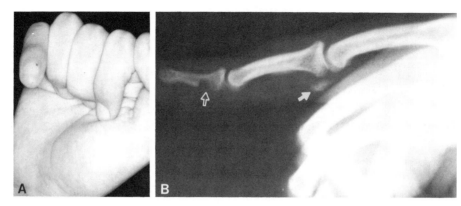

FIGURE 11. *A,* Rupture of the FDP tendon from its insertion into the distal phalanx of the small finger results in the inability to completely flex the digit into the palm. *B,* Radiographs can help corroborate the diagnosis of the FDP avulsion injury. The bone fragment (solid arrow) is attached to the avulsed flexor tendon. The original insertion site is noted in the distal phalanx (open arrow).

of this confined region, both FDS and FDP tendons glide alongside each other, FDS splits into two tails, FDP passes through the bifurcation, and the FDS tails insert onto the middle phalanx. The FDS tendon insertion is also broad and extends onto the proximal volar metaphyseal surface of the middle phalanx.[5]

The term no-man's-land reflects the poor surgical results historically noted after lacerations and subsequent repair of the structures in this busy area. During the past decade, research has improved our understanding of flexor tendon anatomy, nutrition, and healing to the point that primary repair of all structures in zone II is recommended.[4,15]

Zone III

Zone III extends from the distal margin of the transverse carpal ligament to the distal palmar flexion crease (start of the digital pulley system). The lumbrical muscles that take origin from the FDP tendons are located in this region. The significance of this is twofold. Usually, the lacerated FDP tendon in zones I, II, and III will not retract proximally to the palm because they are tethered by the lumbricals. A lacerated FDP tendon no longer exerts a pull on the digit but can continue to pull on the attached lumbrical muscle. This can result in a "lumbrical plus" (flexion of the MCP joint and extension of the PIP and DIP joints) when the FDP muscles are contracting.[16] Surgical repair can help to rebalance this network.

Zones IV and V

Zone IV covers the territory in the carpal tunnel, and zone V the tendon portions proximal to the transverse carpal ligament. Lacerations in these zones can result in proximal retraction of the tendon into the forearm. Attritional ruptures of the tendons can occur as they rub against sharp osteophytes on the wrist carpal bones. These spurs occur in osteoarthritic and rheumatoid arthritic patients. Similarly, patients with previous distal radius fractures and sharp cortical margins can present with secondary attritional ruptures of flexor tendons.

CONCLUSION

After surgical repair of a tendon injury, the patient's ultimate function cannot be accurately predicted. Factors that directly influence the result include the zone of tendon injury, postoperative therapy, patient compliance, and wound-healing characteristics. This last factor may be the most crucial, as some patients seem more prone to developing adhesions, scar, and contractures, despite the surgeon's and therapist's best efforts. The early controlled motion techniques used in postoperative therapy programs help to maximize the patient's potential outcome and improve the overall prognosis.[8,9]

The long-term prognosis regarding any tendon injury should remain guarded. While optimism may be expressed by the medical staff regarding a specific injury, the patient must be adequately informed of the various complications inherently associated with these injuries. While management efforts must always be exact and appropriate, the patient must understand from the outset that the end result may depend more on the nature of the specific injury than the treatment rendered.

Acknowledgment

The authors wish to thank Ms. Helen Prussian for her expert help in the preparation of this manuscript.

REFERENCES

1. American Society for Surgery of the Hand: The Hand: Examination and Diagnosis, 2nd ed. New York, Churchill Livingstone, 1983.
2. American Society for Surgery of the Hand: The Hand: Primary Care of Common Problems. Aurora, CO, American Society for Surgery of the Hand, 1985.
3. Doyle JR: Extensor tendons—Acute injuries. In Green, DP (ed.): Operative Hand Surgery, 2nd ed. New York, Churchill Livingstone, 1988, pp 2045–2072.
4. Gelberman RH, Manske PR, Akeson WH, et al: Flexor tendon repair. J Orthop Res 4:119–128, 1986.
5. Hankin, FM, Janda, DH: Tendon and ligament attachments in relationship to growth plates in a child's hand. J Hand Surg 14B:315–318, 1989.
6. Harris C, Rutledge GL: The functional anatomy of the extensor mechanism of the finger. J Bone Joint Surg 54A:713–726, 1972.
7. Harvey FJ, Hume KF: Spontaneous recurrent ulnar dislocation of the long extensor tendons of the fingers. J Hand Surg 5:492–494, 1980.
8. Hunter J, Schneider L, Mackin E, Callahan A: Rehabilitation of the Hand, 3rd ed. St. Louis, C.V. Mosby, 1990.
9. Lane, C: Therapy for occupationally injured hand. Hand Clin. 2:593–602, 1986.
10. Leddy JP: Avulsions of the flexor digitorum profundus. Hand Clin 1:77–84, 1985.
11. Patel MR, Lipsen LB, Desai SS: Conservative treatment of mallet thumb. J Hand Surg 11A:45–47, 1986.
12. Peters CR: Emergency care of the injured hand. Hand Clin 2:507–511, 1986.
13. Rayan G, Mullins P: Skin necrosis complicating mallet finger splinting and vascularity of the distal interphalangeal joint overlying skin. J Hand Surg 12A:548–552, 1987.
14. Ritts GD, Wood MB, Engber WD: Nonoperative treatment of traumatic dislocations of the extensor digitorum tendons in patients without rheumatoid disorders. J Hand Surg 10A:714–716, 1985.
15. Schneider LH: Flexor Tendon Injuries. Boston, Little, Brown, 1985.
16. Smith RJ: Balance and kinetics of the fingers under normal and pathologic conditions. Clin Orthop 104:92–111, 1974.
17. Wehbe MA, Schneider LH: Mallet fractures. J Bone Joint Surg 66A:658–669, 1984.

Chapter 14

OCCUPATIONAL HAND FRACTURES AND DISLOCATIONS

David P. Falconer, MD, Paul J. Donahue, MD,
Melissa L. Barton, MD, Charles J. MacDonald, MD,
and Steven R. Sonkowsky, OPA-C, RPA

Fracture of the bones of the hand is an everyday occupational injury. The initial assessment of these injuries is frequently the role of the first-aid team, industrial nurse, or occupational physician. A proper understanding of the nature and variety of these fractures is essential to ensure good triage, initial care, and end result.

The hand is unique in the human body in its complex interrelationship of soft tissues, neurovascular structures, muscles, tendons, and underlying skeleton. Harmonious interaction between the stable skeletal structure and the closely apposed gliding and mobile soft tissues is disrupted whenever injury or immobilization occurs. These special anatomic and functional considerations require that the assessment of hand injuries in general, and fractures in particular, take into account the fact that treatment of one component, such as bone or joint structures, may actually detract from the needs or goals of another, such as tendon gliding. Delay in initiating the most appropriate mode of treatment may not just prolong, but actually worsen, the overall outcome of a particular injury.

In this context, the goal of the occupational health professional should be to distinguish those injuries that are amenable to the traditional treatments of rest and immobilization from those that need a specialist's attention, which if neglected or delayed, may multiply in complexity of treatment. Appropriate referral is an important consideration so that specific therapy, whether surgical or other, may be initiated promptly.

FRACTURE CONCEPTS AND TERMINOLOGY

Although the concepts and terminology of emergency evaluation are connected by a common thread that is familiar to all medical workers, some special considerations apply to the orderly analysis and discussion of skeletal injury, whether in the hand or elsewhere. The question commonly asked by patients in the early stages of orthopedic evaluation, "Doctor, is it fractured or just broken?" highlights the need for a common terminology for the analysis, discussion, and comparison of injuries. A universally used terminology can clarify the anatomy, severity, and treatment of an injury, as well as provide a basis for predicting the final result.

The static or stabilizing structures of the hand, the bones, are commonly described as having a middle, tubular structure, the **diaphysis**; flared or expanding ends consisting of thinning cortical bone and increasing spongy or cancellous bone, the **metaphysis**; and cartilage-lined ends proximally or distally, or at both ends, the **epiphysis**. Because the term *epiphysis* also designates the secondary growth areas of tubular long bones, the terms **articular bone** and **subchondral bone** are often substituted to designate areas at the ends of bones where the bones overlap with joint surfaces.

Fractures. An injury that disrupts the integrity of the bone substance is a **fracture**. Displacement of bones between the joint surfaces is **subluxation**, if partial, and **dislocation**, if complete (Fig. 1). These terms are not mutually exclusive. An injury causing disruption of the joint with associated fracture of the articular bone of one joint surface may be termed a **fracture-dislocation**.

Directional terms are also used, and certain assumptions are made in orthopedic description. The terms *medial* and *lateral* are discouraged because pronation or supination of the forearm changes the location of a more distally injured part. Direction is described in terms of anatomic constants such as **dorsal** or **palmar, radial** or **ulnar**, and **distal** or **proximal**. The assumption is made that the more proximal part, either a fracture fragment or a joint surface, is in its "normal" anatomic position, and the distal injured "part" is thought of as displaced or angulated relative to the proximal normal.

Fractures are **complete** when the bone is broken into two distinct fragments, and **incom-**

plete when one cortex of bone is damaged but the other is not and the likelihood of displacement is limited. If there are more than just two fracture fragments, the fracture is described as **comminuted**, implying that a relatively large force was absorbed and a relatively severe injury was sustained. Distinct fracture fragments that maintain the same anatomic shape and position as they had in the pre-injury state are termed **nondisplaced fractures**. Fragments that have shifted out of anatomic position are termed **displaced** or **angulated**, or both. The degree and extent of angulation and displacement reflect the degree of injury and frequently imply associated soft tissue damage to the surrounding periosteal sleeve, the overlying muscles, and supporting ligaments.

Displacement is described in terms of direction, such as palmar or dorsal, or radial or ulnar, and is measured in terms of distance. A fragment may be described as being "dorsally displaced" by, say, 10 mm.

The descriptive terminology of fracture angulation is a bit more arbitrary, and the accepted convention often confuses newcomers to orthopedic description. Angulation results in displacement of the distal end of the fractured bone relative to its normal position; the convention, however, describes angulation in terms of displacement of the apex of the angle formed by the angulated fracture fragments relative to the anatomic position of the unfractured bone (Fig. 2). This means that, when a bone is fractured so that the distal end is displaced palmarly relative to the nonfractured bone, the apex is dorsal and the fracture is described as dorsally angulated, or often (for clarification's sake) as "apex-dorsally" angulated.

Finally, a fracture needs to be analyzed for **rotational malalignment** along the long axis of the bone. This is especially important in the hand and digits, where multiple parallel structures hinge in unison. Rotational malalignment is often the most subtle form of fracture displacement and is frequently a clinical diagnosis not evident on the x-ray film. Failure to detect or anticipate it is frequently the cause of later surgical correction and legal action (Fig. 3).

Once a fracture has been characterized as displaced, angulated, or comminuted, an overall assessment of its nature or anticipated behavior pattern may be made. It is often important to take into account associated ligament or other soft tissue injury in this characterization because ultimately the decision must be

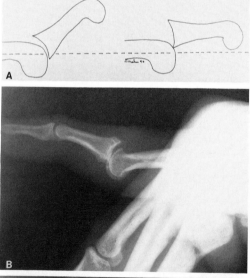

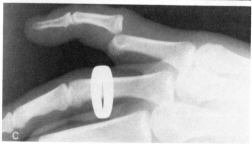

FIGURE 1.   *A*, Dorsal subluxation of a joint (left); dislocation with loss of joint contact (right). *B*, Dorsal subluxation of an arthritic PIP joint. *C*, Dorsal dislocation of a fifth finger PIP joint.

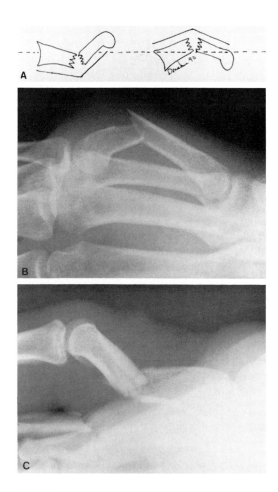

FIGURE 2. *A*, When the apex of an angulated fracture is palmar to its normal alignment, it is said to be (apex-) palmarly angulated (left); when the apex is dorsal, the fracture is said to be (apex-) dorsally angulated. *B*, A fractured fifth metacarpal with dorsal angulation. *C*, A fractured proximal phalanx with palmar angulation.

made whether a fracture is **stable** or **unstable**. Stability has important implications for treatment; an unstable fracture usually requires operative fixation in one form or another, whereas a stable fracture does not.

Dislocation. Disruption and displacement of joint surfaces are termed **subluxation**, if partial, and **dislocation**, if complete. By convention, the direction of dislocation is designated in terms of displacement of the most distal of the two joint surfaces. A joint that easily redisplaces after dislocation has been reduced is termed **unstable**, whereas a joint that maintains its normal alignment during joint motion is termed **stable**. A further concept regarding the description of joint injury is that of **simple** versus **complex**. A simple dislocation is one that can be reduced back into position by ap-

propriate manipulation (see discussion below); in a complex dislocation, interposed soft tissue structures are trapped in the joint, causing a mechanical block to reduction (Fig. 4). Because soft tissues are usually not seen on x-ray, it's important to know where they are located and when to suspect a complex fracture.

HISTORY AND PHYSICAL EXAMINATION

The patient who has sustained a hand injury or fracture, especially in an occupational setting, should be initially evaluated as any other trauma patient would be. An immediate brief history should be obtained, and the patient as a whole should be inspected so as to establish what other injuries are present and a hierarchy of treatment urgency. When appropriate, establish and maintain an airway, and stabilize the patient's vital signs by appropriate treatment measures. Even isolated hand or finger injuries can cause shock from profound blood loss or loss of consciousness owing to vasovagal hypotension.

In evaluating the hand injury per se, details

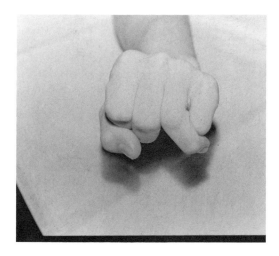

FIGURE 3. Rotational malalignment can result in severe overlap of the flexed fingers.

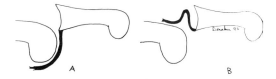

FIGURE 4. *A*, A simple dislocation; no interposed soft tissue blocks closed reduction. *B*, The volar plate has become entrapped in the joint. Surgical removal of the volar plate is required to achieve reduction.

of the patient's injury, including direct or indirect trauma, direction of hand or finger position and motion, and chemical or thermal exposure should be documented. Any pre-existing injury or disability should especially be documented in the occupational injury.

Prior to any anesthetic intervention, physical examination should carefully characterize and depict the location of a laceration, the presence or absence of swelling, ecchymosis, and deformity, and when possible, the specific anatomic levels of joint motion, tendon function, and nerve sensation. Open wounds should be gently irrigated and covered with moist saline dressings, and profound or pulsatile bleeding should be dressed with additional firm compressive materials. **Use of formal tourniquets and emergency placement of hemostats or suture ligatures are to be avoided.** They can cause extremity ischemia or damage to nerve structures adjacent to lacerated arteries and are unnecessary when direct pressure can be applied.

A temporary splint, especially one made of radiolucent cardboard or plastic, may be applied for temporary immobilization of severe hand injuries while the patient is sent for x-rays. The splint must not obscure or interfere with the x-ray studies. Frequently the splint must be removed to obtain clear and meaningful films.

A frequent, and well-intentioned, action on the part of many emergency staffs is to begin an intravenous antibiotic, usually a cephalosporin, in a patient with an open wound associated with a fracture. Far more important

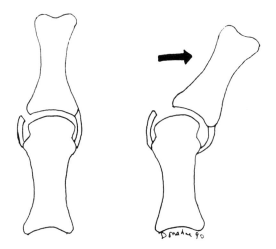

FIGURE 5. When one collateral ligament is torn, stress along that side of the joint opens up the joint. Clinical exam arouses suspicion, which is confirmed by stress x-ray.

is a proper assessment of the wound, if any, and a history of the injury.[5] The tetanus immunization status should be determined and updated with hyperimmune globulin and tetanus toxoid as necessary.[2] Wounds characterized as tidy, or clean, especially when sustained on sharp or clean-cutting surfaces, benefit more from proper wound irrigation and repair than from any immediate use of an antibiotic. Alternatively, in contaminated or crush-type injuries with significant soft tissue devitalization or damage overlying fracture, serial wound cultures, proper wound debridement, and initial broad-spectrum antibiotics followed by culture-specific antibiotics (based on positive wound cultures) should be used. Primary or emergency use of inappropriate antibiotics may interfere with later analysis of wound cultures and may cloud the picture.

RADIOGRAPHIC EXAMINATION

All acute hand injuries should be x-rayed in the initial evaluation phase of occupational or other trauma. X-rays should be clearly and properly exposed. It is important to obtain clear and visible views in two planes 90 degrees apart (usually posteroanterior [PA] and lateral planes) and to x-ray widely enough to demonstrate clearly the joints proximal and distal to the site of injury. Too often x-ray studies return with inadequate technique, multiple oblique views, or multiple fingers overlapped, making interpretation impossible. The treating professional must insist on, or repeat, studies until the injured part has been thoroughly and adequately visualized in two planes.

In some cases, the awareness of special views may facilitate visualization of problem fractures. While scaphoid or navicular views[38,51] of the carpus are commonly requested in the assessment of traumatic wrist pain (see Fig. 9), **Robert's view** of the trapeziometacarpal joint of the thumb (see Fig. 17)[45] and the **Brewerton view** of the metacarpal head and collateral ligament recess (see Fig. 21)[35] are less well known. Other special views include the carpal tunnel view (Fig. 12A),[24] the "reverse-oblique" or Norgaard view,[54] and the 15-degree–pronated lateral view of the base of the thumb metacarpal.[3]

Ligament structures may be injured in the course of metacarpophalangeal (MCP) joint and proximal interphalangeal (PIP) joint dislocations. These structures can often be assessed by examination, although local anesthesia may be required to relieve pain related to stress applied to the suspect structure. It is often helpful to obtain a **stress x-ray** of the injured part while it is numb. This is done by taking a regular (usually) PA view of the injured joint while the patient or an assistant applies angular bending forces to the collateral ligaments (Fig. 5). Stress x-rays are particularly useful when making surgical decisions regarding the ulnar collateral ligament of the thumb MCP joint, the so-called gamekeeper's (or skier's) thumb.

In the presence of persistent bone or joint pain after injury, x-rays may need to be repeated in 14 days. In some instances, fracture-site resorption in the healing process permits x-ray confirmation of a fracture not initially revealed. When x-rays continue to appear normal, yet history and examination demonstrate bone pain with palpation or stress, specialized radiographic techniques must be considered.

Special Studies. Technetium-99m bone scan, with magnified and pinhole collimated views, is an extremely sensitive technique; a negative scan categorically rules out an occult fracture. A scan may be positive, however, when significant joint or ligament injury, or an inflammatory condition (acute or chronic), is present. Underlying arthritis, synovitis, or infection may cause a scan to be positive. In the absence of these clinically obvious findings, a positive scan with focal uptake in the area of recent trauma may be an indicator of hidden fracture. Additional studies such as tomography, arthrography, computerized tomography (CT), and magnetic resonance imaging (MRI) of the area of focal uptake may be necessary to make a specific diagnosis.

Tomography, either **polytomography, trispiral tomography**, or, rarely, **computed tomography**, may be necessary to visualize a fracture or, more commonly, to clearly define the extent of the underlying injury, especially for surgical decision making. By comparison with regular polytomography, trispiral tomography equipment is less widely available and more expensive to use, but it allows thinner tomographic sections. Computed tomography allows axial images in serial cross-section, and more recently, high-resolution, thin-cut views, in the AP, lateral, and oblique planes using computed reconstruction of images generated by x-ray absorption. The particular features and abilities of this technique depend in part on the particular machine and software available.

Magnetic resonance imaging uses computed reconstruction to yield images based on the electromagnetic response of hydrogen atoms in a strong magnetic field. The uses and limitations of this technology are evolving daily, especially in the evaluation of musculoskeletal injury. At present, it is exquisitely sensitive for such otherwise obscure diagnoses as early avascular necrosis of the lunate (Kienböck's disease) and may prove useful in evaluation of soft tissue tumors or even metastatic disease to bone, but it has relatively little use currently in the diagnosis of occult fracture.

GENERAL PRINCIPLES OF FRACTURE TREATMENT

With an understanding of the assessment techniques and a grasp of the terminology, one can quickly develop a rational basis for an approach to fracture treatment. As a general principle, if a fracture can be described as stable and nondisplaced, it can be expected to heal in a reasonable period of time with an excellent result. Immobilization of the injured part is generally recommended, both for the patient's comfort and to protect the weakened part from adverse forces. The immobilization device recommended, its application, and the length of time it is needed depend to some extent on the particular area of injury and are discussed below in the sections on specific fractures.

If, however, a fracture cannot be characterized as both stable and nondisplaced, specific intervention is necessary. How much displacement of a particular fracture can be accepted varies from fracture to fracture. Displacement of a few millimeters may be considered negligible in a fracture of the distal radius, yet may be unacceptable in an intra-articular fracture involving the proximal interphalangeal (PIP) joint of a finger. Apex-dorsal angulation up to 40 degrees may be considered acceptable in an otherwise stable fracture of the fifth finger metacarpal neck, whereas no more than 5–10 degrees should be accepted in a fracture of the index finger metacarpal shaft (Fig. 6). The specific functional demands of the fractured part must be considered before deciding whether displacement is acceptable or not.

Fractures that are not in anatomic position must, of necessity, be manipulated into proper, or at least acceptable, reduction before splint or cast immobilization can be initiated. Some degree of anesthesia, whether local, regional,

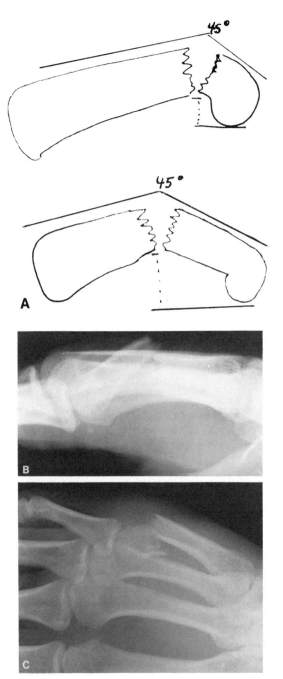

likely to displace. In the same way that unsatisfactory position mandates fracture reduction, instability usually requires direct or "internal" fixation. Recognition of these increasing levels of complexity, as manifested in standard terminology, is often then the basis for a decision regarding treatment or referral to an appropriate specialist.

FRACTURE HEALING: PRINCIPLES AND ASSESSMENT

Once a fracture has been judged acceptable, either before or as the result of reduction or fixation, a period of immobilization must generally take place before functional or even limited use of the injured hand can be begun. The exact period of time depends again on a judgment of fracture stability. Stability can be increased by fixation, and so, often, a fracture that has been internally secured with a sturdy fixation device, such as a plate and screws (Fig. 7), may be allowed some limited degree of function almost immediately. The generally observed time guidelines for fracture healing, as opposed to stability, however, are not dramatically changed by any particular method of fixation, in the hand at least, and so must be observed before full heavy-duty or functional use of the injured hand can begin.

Fractures of the diaphyseal, or midshaft, parts of the bones usually take longer to heal than the more vascular and spongy metaphyseal ends. As a result, a general guideline of 6–8 weeks' healing time is recommended in these fractures. Metaphyseal fractures often have a greater degree of inherent stability, as well as improved vascularity and a larger surface area for fracture healing, and often require only 3–4

FIGURE 6. *A*, Different metacarpal fractures with equal angulation. The more proximal the fracture, the greater the palmar displacement. More angulation can be tolerated in a more distal fracture. *B*, A midshaft metacarpal fracture showing more palmar displacement than the similarly angulated boxer's fracture in *C*.

or general, and special "tricks of the trade" often facilitate fracture reposition. At this same time, fracture stability should be assessed. There is little point in manipulating a fracture that is

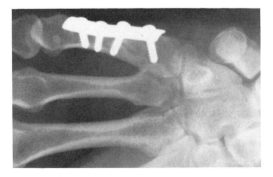

FIGURE 7. An open "internal fixation" with a plate and screws.

weeks of immobilization before functional use can begin. Local conditions that decrease stability, or decrease vascularity, such as a small articular fragment with a destabilizing tendon insertion attached to it, may dramatically increase the time needed for healing to occur.

During the healing interval, it is common to make new x-rays of a fracture. The physician is often asked, "Is it healing OK?" In general, fracture healing is not evident on early x-rays; it often lags behind clinical healing by weeks to months. The principal purpose of repeat x-rays is to verify that no loss of fracture position has occurred during the recovery process, so that the conditions of acceptable displacement and stability can be maintained and documented. Fracture healing is often largely an educated guess based on recommended time guidelines, combined with clinical assessment. Firm palpation directly over a fracture site, combined with gentle torsional stress, should not cause pain in a healed fracture, and persistence of pain with palpation or stress is an indication for additional immobilization time. The presence of healing callus on x-ray films does not necessarily signal fracture union, nor does its absence indicate lack of healing. Very slight motion is required to generate fracture callus, and diaphyseal fractures that are rigidly fixed internally, or metaphyseal fractures that are inherently stable and rapidly healing may never manifest any callus, not even long after fracture union has occurred.

TREATMENT OF SPECIFIC FRACTURES

Table 1 summarizes the treatments of specific fractures.

Fracture of the Scaphoid

The scaphoid fracture is the most frequent carpal bone fracture in young adults. It often occurs without other signs of injury and is dismissed as a "sprain." Untreated, it can result in persistent wrist pain and disability.

Diagnosis. A history of wrist pain, swelling, and tenderness localized to the "anatomic snuffbox" (Fig. 8) suggests a scaphoid fracture and demands radiographic confirmation. Four wrist films should be obtained, including PA, lateral, and two oblique projections. A PA film with ulnar deviation of the wrist may improve visualization of the fracture (the "scaphoid view,"

Fig. 9).[38,51] If the initial studies are normal, the wrist and thumb should be immobilized for 2–3 weeks, at which time repeat x-rays are obtained. If a fracture has occurred, bone will be resorbed along the fracture site, making delayed visualization possible.[30] Other diagnostic tests include a bone scan of the wrist area, which, if negative, virtually rules out a scaphoid fracture.

Treatment. The majority of undisplaced scaphoid fractures will unite if adequate immobilization is begun immediately. Delaying treatment for 2–3 weeks until the fracture is visualized on x-rays increases the risk of fracture displacement and nonunion or malunion.

For cast immobilization to be successful, the cast must remain effective throughout the course of treatment. Synthetic cast material is preferred as it is lighter and stronger and allows x-rays to be taken through the cast. The wrist should be maintained in a position of function, with the thumb immobilized in a position of opposition (a thumb spica cast, Fig. 10). A long-arm cast eliminates rotational motion of the forearm, which could increase motion at the fracture site. A long-arm thumb spica cast may be used for up to 4 weeks; it is followed by a short-arm thumb spica cast until union is complete. Accurate cast immobilization of the stable scaphoid fracture should result in a 95% rate of healing.[53]

The vast majority of acute scaphoid fractures heal if immobilized properly for a sufficient length of time. Unstable fractures, however, can be difficult and may require surgery. Unstable fractures are those with more than 1 mm of displacement between fragments, or with angulation of fragments and abnormal carpal alignment. Findings of displacement and angulation are subtle; although they may be suspected from regular x-rays, trispiral tomography may be required to determine clearly actual fracture position. Unstable fractures are best treated with open reduction and frequently with bone grafting as well to obtain anatomic union.

Fracture of the middle third of the scaphoid is the most common type of fracture. The majority of these heal in approximately 12 weeks if nondisplaced and immobilized properly. Fractures of the proximal third of the scaphoid are more prone to delayed union and nonunion because the fracture may interfere with the vascular supply to the proximal fragment. Avascular necrosis of the proximal pole fragment may result in nonunion and risk of future joint degeneration. These fractures may take

TABLE 1.   Treatment Summary

Location	Fracture Type	Treatment/Comments
Scaphoid	Distal/tubercle	Heal easily with 6 weeks' immobilization in a thumb spica cast.
	Waist	Nondisplaced fractures usually heal if immobilized immediately and casted 4–6 weeks in long-arm thumb spica cast, followed by short-arm thumb spica until healed. Displaced fractures require open reduction to prevent secondary carpal collapse and later arthritis; evaluation with tomograms, referral if displacement persists.
	Proximal pole	High likelihood of nonunion and avascular necrosis. Refer all.
Lunate	Transverse	Prolonged immobilization if nondisplaced; open reduction if displaced. Refer all; high likelihood of secondary arthritis if joint is involved.
	Kienböck's	Treatment depends upon stage at the time of diagnosis; most treatment is surgical. Refer.
Triquetrum	Dorsal chip	Wrist support splint for 3–4 weeks; many are asymptomatic despite nonunion.
	Comminuted	Rare; usually involve significant other carpal trauma; may require either partial excision or surgical fixation.
Pisiform	Articular	Surgical excision if symptomatic joint degeneration is expected or results. Refer.
	Nonarticular	Splint immobilization for 4–6 weeks.
Trapezium	Nondisplaced	Thumb spica cast for 6 weeks.
	Displaced/articular	Usually associated with fractures of the thumb metacarpal or radius; may require surgical reduction or fixation; likely to cause painful arthritis that may require future surgery. Refer.
Capitate	Body	Splint nonarticular fractures for 6 weeks in wrist splint or cast.
	Proximal pole	Associated with other carpal fractures and dislocations. Treatment is usually surgical; avascular necrosis and later joint degeneration may result. Refer.
Hamate	Hamulus (hook)	Associated with handle rebound injuries in the base of the palm. Difficult to see on x-ray; carpal tunnel view or axial CT shows it. Acute fractures may heal with splint of wrist and ulnar fingers. Symptomatic nonunions treated with surgical excision.
Hamate	Body	6 weeks' wrist immobilization. Fractures that involve the joint of the fifth metacarpal base may become arthritic; refer.
Metacarpal	Base	Generally stable; can be splinted for 3–6 weeks, except fracture involving articular surface of base of fifth with subluxation of shaft (reverse Bennett's), which should be referred.
	Shaft/transverse	Tend to be unstable and angulate into dorsiflexion. If more than 10–15 degrees of angulation, refer for surgical fixation. Otherwise, splint 6–8 weeks with frequent x-ray.
	Shaft/spiral	May shorten or malrotate. Can accept 2–3 mm of shortening if no rotational overlap. Splint for 4–6 weeks in safe hand position including fingers. If any overlap, refer.
	Neck (boxer's)	Closed reduction; splint in safe hand position including adjacent fingers for 3 weeks. Up to 45 degrees of angulation in ulnar fingers acceptable.
	Head/articular surface	Brewerton view helpful. Articular surface fractures require surgical replacement, except in "human bite" injuries. Small ligament avulsion fractures treated in safe hand position.
MCP joint	Subluxation	Reduce by flexion; splint in safe hand position 4–6 weeks. Do not reduce with hyperextension, which may convert to complex dislocation and require surgery.
	Dislocation	Index, small fingers mainly involved; may be complex with entrapment of soft tissue. Refer if not easily reduced on first try. Splint after reduction as for subluxation.
Proximal phalanx	Base	Avulsion fractures about bases generally stable; can treat for 3–4 weeks in safe hand position splint. Angulated, impacted fractures should be reduced to minimize finger overlap.

TABLE 1. Continued

Location	Fracture Type	Treatment/Comments
	Shaft/transverse	Often unstable; angulate into palmar flexion. Reduce in flexion at MCP and PIP joints. Splint in safe hand position; x-ray frequently. Unstable fractures should be referred; stable fractures heal in 6 weeks.
	Shaft/spiral	Frequently displaced and rotated. Many require operative fixation; risk of malrotation is high even in splint. Refer all.
	Condylar	Usually require surgical stabilization. Refer all.
PIP joint	Dislocation/dorsal	Closed reduction with local anesthesia. Check stability of joint in extension; of unstable, refer. If stable, splint PIP joint slightly flexed for 7–10 days, then begin gentle motion with buddy tapes.
	Dislocation/lateral	Closed reduction with local anesthesia. Check stability of radial collateral ligaments. If unstable, repair may be required; consider referral. Otherwise, similar to dorsal dislocation.
	Dislocation/palmar	Surgical repair of damage to central extensor tendon; refer all.
	Fracture/dislocation	Small chip fractures from the base of the middle phalanx can be treated as simple dorsal dislocation. Refer more complex fractures; stiffness and disability high; special therapy, often surgery, required.
Middle phalanx	Shaft	Fractures associated with open crush injury require referral for surgical treatment of soft tissues and fracture.
	Spiral	Evaluate with 3 x-ray views and careful clinical evaluation for malrotation. Nondisplaced fractures can be treated in finger splint with frequent x-ray. Refer if displaced or rotated.
Middle phalanx	Condylar	Treatment is usually surgical. Refer.
Distal phalanx	Dorsal (mallet)	Check lateral x-ray for joint subluxation and size of fragment. If no subluxation and fragment is less than 30% of joint surface, reduce in hyperextension finger splint of the DIP joint. Repeat lateral x-ray. If reduced or <2 mm displaced, accept (may have dorsal bump). If joint subluxed, fragment >30%, or >2 mm displaced when splinted, refer. Splint must be used for 6 weeks.
Palmar	Base (flexor tendon)	Check for flexor tendon function; check lateral x-ray along course of tendon sheath. Refer all for surgical repair.
	Shaft	Usually associated with significant soft tissue trauma; refer for surgical repair of soft tissue and fracture.
	Tuft	Stable fracture that is supported by soft tissue. Repair soft tissue (nail bed); splint for comfort.
Thumb	Distal phalanx	Similar to fingers.
	Proximal phalanx	Similar to fingers, although more rotation accepted for spiral fractures— overlap not a problem.
	Ulnar base	Avulsion fracture of the ulnar collateral ligament causes instability of the thumb MCP joint. If displaced, refer for surgical repair; if nondisplaced, cast in thumb spica for 6 weeks.
	Metacarpals	Similar to fingers, except fractures of thumb metacarpal base.
	Bennett's	Refer for closed pinning and cast or open fixation and early protected motion.
	Rolando's	Some controversy about treatment; most receive open reduction. High likelihood of symptomatic degenerative arthritis; refer.
	Nonarticular base	Angulates dorsally. Closed reduction and thumb spica splint or cast for 6 weeks.

6–11 weeks longer to heal than fractures of the midportion of the scaphoid.[47]

Fractures of the distal third of the scaphoid are infrequent. They are usually of a transverse type and stable. They unite rapidly, usually in 4–8 weeks. The tuberosity of the scaphoid may also fracture, usually as an avulsion injury by the inserting ligaments. These extra-articular fractures heal promptly with 6 weeks of immobilization.

Scaphoid nonunion is more common in the fractures of the proximal third of the scaphoid, or in fractures in which avascular necrosis of the proximal pole fragment occurs (Fig. 11). Delay in diagnosis and treatment greatly increases the risk of nonunion. Untreated nonunion inevitably leads to disabling periscaphoid arthritis.[46] If the scaphoid fracture has not healed after appropriate immobilization, further invasive treatment must be considered. Russe advocates bone grafting,[47] which is indicated for all established nonunions and symptomatic delayed unions in which no osteoarthritis has developed. Electrical stimulation of fracture healing may be considered as an alternative to surgery in some cases; success rates are up to 80%.[18] Further immobilization in casts incorporating an external electrical stimulator is required. Recently, open reduction and internal fixation with a specially designed screw device has also been advocated.[25]

Fracture of the Trapezium

Isolated fracture of the trapezium is rare. Simultaneous fracture of the thumb metacarpal is the most frequently associated injury, and fractures of the distal radius are next most common. Multiple oblique x-ray views and a Robert's view may be necessary to visualize the nondisplaced fracture. Nondisplaced fractures may be treated with a short-arm thumb-spica cast or splinted for 4–6 weeks. Displaced fractures, especially the vertical intra-articular shear fracture, require open reduction and internal fixation to restore displaced joint surfaces. Secondary degenerative arthritis is common even after accurate joint realignment and may require secondary reconstructive procedures such as arthrodesis or arthroplasty.

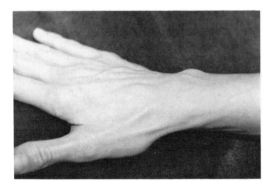

FIGURE 8. The "anatomic snuffbox" is clearly seen here bordered by the raised tendons of the extensor pollicis longus and brevis muscles.

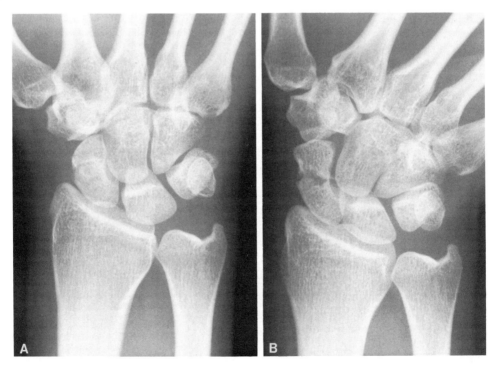

FIGURE 9. *A,* A regular PA view of the wrist fails to demonstrate clearly the fracture of the scaphoid. *B,* The "scaphoid" view with the forearm supinated and the wrist ulnarly deviated allows easy visualization of the fracture.

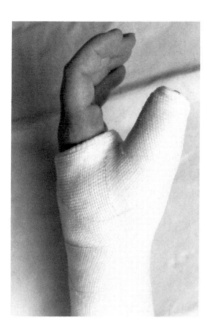

FIGURE 10. A proper thumb spica cast should be snug, positioning the thumb in opposition and the wrist in neutral position or slight dorsiflexion. The thumb should be immobilized to beyond the IP joint, and the cast should not hinder flexion of the finger MCP joints by extending beyond the palmar crease. Synthetic cast material is often used.

Fracture of the Capitate

Fracture of the capitate may occur in association with scaphoid fracture or, less commonly, as an isolated injury. The diagnosis is made with careful x-ray evaluation; the fracture can be easily missed. Tomograms and bone scan studies may be helpful. Treatment of the nondisplaced capitate fracture consists of 6 weeks of splint or cast immobilization.

The very rare scaphocapitate syndrome is a fracture of the neck of the capitate with rotation of the displaced proximal fragment associated with fracture of the waist of the scaphoid. Careful open reduction of the capitate fracture and internal fixation of both scaphoid and capitate fractures are required. Avascular necrosis of the proximal pole of the capitate can develop despite optimal treatment.

Fracture of the Hamate

Fractures of the hamate may involve the body of the bone or the hamulus, the hooklike process extending palmarly. These injuries cause pain, swelling, and tenderness over the ulnar

half of the wrist, either dorsally (hamate body fracture) or palmarly (hamulus fracture). Fractures of the body of the hamate are produced by a shearing injury involving a sudden isolated torque. Fracture of the hamulus is caused by a sudden forceful blow to the ulnar border of the palm, such as from a fall. Typically, however, the force is transmitted from a clenched handle or tool such as a golf club, racquet, or hammer that strikes an unexpectedly resistant object.[41]

As with other carpal bones, multiple oblique views or tomography of the body of the hamate may be necessary to demonstrate fracture clearly. Fracture of the hook of the hamate can be easily missed. It should be suspected when a deep, ill-defined pain is present in the ulnar half of the palm. A special x-ray view, the carpal tunnel view (Fig. 12A), and oblique views of the hand with the forearm in 30–45 degrees of supination (the Norgaard view) are useful to visualize this injury, but it can be seen best of all with an axial CT study of the wrist (Fig. 12B).

Treatment of fractures to the body of the hamate generally require splint immobilization

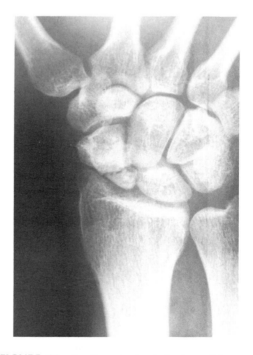

FIGURE 11. Small proximal pole fractures of the scaphoid can develop avascular necrosis and nonunion, both demonstrated here. These difficult fractures often fail to heal despite ideal treatment from the outset; they frequently require surgery. Degenerative wrist arthritis, pain, stiffness, and disability often result.

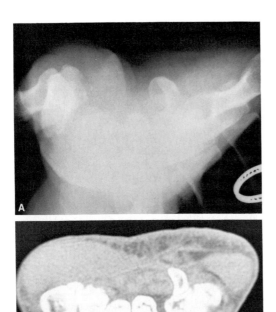

FIGURE 12. *A,* A "carpal tunnel" x-ray may demonstrate fracture of the hook of the hamate, although overlap with the pisiform and soft tissues may obscure the image. *B,* Axial CT cuts through the wrist clearly show the fracture at the base of the hamulus.

for 6 weeks. Involvement of the articular surface may require open reduction. Acute fracture of the hook of the hamate may be treated with splint or cast immobilization, including the wrist and ulnar fingers, for 6–8 weeks. Persistent pain in this area, or nonunion resulting from a missed diagnosis, is common and can be treated by surgical excision of the hamulus process. Other symptoms, including ulnar neuropathy at the wrist and rupture of the fifth finger flexor tendon, may be unusual presenting symptoms that result from nonunion of the hamulus at the boundary between the ulnar nerve tunnel of Guyon and the flexor tendon sheath through the carpal tunnel.

Fracture of the Lunate

Occasionally, the lunate is fractured after significant trauma. These fractures are aligned along the frontal plane of the lunate. They produce two large fragments of roughly equal size and, if nondisplaced, may heal with prolonged immobilization. Displacement of any amount

requires open reduction. This type of fracture should not be confused with collapse fracture of the lunate secondary to avascular necrosis, or Kienböck's disease.

Kienböck described avascular necrosis of the lunate in 1910.[34] The etiology has remained elusive. The condition leads to internal structural weakness of the lunate with resultant collapse and fracture formation. It may result from ischemia after wrist ligament trauma, although frequently a history of specific injury is not present. Alternatively, the fracture may rep-

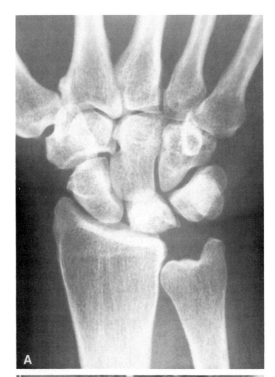

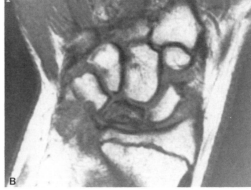

FIGURE 13. *A,* x-ray demonstrating sclerosis and early collapse fracture in the lunate bone with Kienböck's disease. Also note the discrepancy in length of the ulna, the ulnar minus. *B,* MRI image shows avascular condition of the lunate in comparison with the other carpal bones.

resent internal stress due to mechanical over-load in the anatomically predisposed person with a short ulna or ulnar-minus variant.[20] In these people stress fracture may leave a portion of the bone avascular owing to anatomical watershed areas in the circulation to the lunate.

The diagnosis of Kienböck's disease may be suspected in young adults with wrist pain and stiffness and swelling and tenderness localized dorsally over the lunate. The history often reveals a minor injury but usually not a specific or severe event. X-rays early in this condition may be normal. As the condition progresses, sclerosis of the lunate, followed by cleavage fracture, collapse, and secondary degenerative change, may be detected (Fig. 13A). Bone scans show intense focal uptake in the early phases before regular x-ray change is evident. MRI studies are specific for this condition (Fig. 13B) and can differentiate avascularity from inflammatory, traumatic, or degenerative changes that may cause a bone scan to be hot.

Kienböck's disease has been treated with prolonged immobilization, excisional and/or silicone arthroplasty, intercarpal fusion, and revascularization procedures. Attempts to revascularize the lunate with bone grafts and vascular implants have produced inconclusive results. Silicone arthroplasty has been abandoned because of long-term complications related to silicone particle breakdown and reactive synovitis.[7] Recently, joint-leveling procedures to align the radius and ulna appear to offer benefit by reducing internal stresses within the substance of the lunate.[43]*

Fracture of the Triquetrum and Pisiform

Fracture of the triquetrum is uncommon, with the exception of the dorsal chip fracture, which is frequently seen after a minor fall on the outstretched hand. It is suspected with tenderness directly over the proximal ulnar carpus. X-ray in the lateral view shows a small avulsion chip fracture usually displaced 1–2 mm above the overlapping carpal bones. The fracture is the result of stress along the heavy radiotriquetral ligament, the most robust of the dorsal wrist ligaments. Treatment is by splint support of the wrist in 30 degrees of dorsiflex-ion for 3–4 weeks, until discomfort resolves. Frequently, the chip fracture remains nonunited without long-term symptoms.

Fracture of the pisiform bone may occur after either a direct blow or forced wrist dorsiflexion in a fall. The pisiform bone lies embedded in the tendon insertion of the flexor carpi ulnaris tendon, acting much as the patella does for the quadriceps mechanism of the knee. Fracture that involves the articular surface with the triquetrum may lead to arthritic degeneration of this joint and pain. When this occurs, or can be anticipated, treatment by surgical excision of the pisiform is recommended. Fractures not involving the joint surface can be treated with supportive wrist splinting for 4–6 weeks.

Fractures and Dislocations of the Thumb

The thumb is a unique digit in its position, function, and anatomy and is prone to injuries distinct from those of the fingers. The special functions of the thumb account for up to 50% of overall hand use. Injury is especially disabling, and careful attention to proper treatment is paramount.

Trapeziometacarpal Joint

The special anatomy of the trapeziometacarpal (TMC) joint allows the thumb the wide range of rotational and angular motion away from fingers and palm that makes the thumb unique. A broad, flat saddle joint, the metacarpal is firmly secured to the trapezium by means of heavy ligaments, especially a palmar, ulnar thickening of the joint capsule. As a result, isolated dislocations of this joint are relatively infrequent;[13] they occur in a dorsiradial direction when force is sufficient to rupture the ligament. Much more commonly, the base of the first metacarpal is fractured. The injury may be an avulsion fracture of the articular base of the metacarpal by the strong palmar ligament, termed a Bennett's fracture (Fig. 14), with subluxation of the remaining metacarpal joint surface due to muscular pull of the adductor pollicis brevis muscle and the abductor pollicis longus tendon. In older people, comminuted fracture of the articular surface without joint subluxation is more common and is known as a Rolando's fracture (Fig. 15). In skeletally immature people and young adults, an extra-articular fracture of the base of the metacarpal immediately distal to the joint surface

---

* Editor's comment: Dr. Kirk Watson has reported good results treating Kienböck's disease with fusion of the scaphoid, trapezium, and trapezoid.[55]—MLK.

is the most common pattern of injury (Fig. 16). In all of these injuries, the usual mechanism is a forceful axial load along the metacarpal when the thumb is flexed, as in a first position.

Although most injuries to the area of the TMC joint are demonstrated adequately with routine PA and lateral x-ray views, a Robert's view[45]—a hyperpronated, true AP view of the joint—removes the overlap of the trapezoid and index metacarpal base and gives the best assessment of the joint surface (Fig. 17).

When the relatively rare pure dislocation of the TMC joint is diagnosed, closed reduction and immobilization in a thumb spica cast or splint is usually adequate. This injury, when neglected or missed, may be satisfactorily treated with open reduction and stabilization, with the use of local tendon material to reconstruct the ligament damage if treatment is done in the first few months after injury.[12] Prolonged dislocation or instability in this joint, however, leads to degenerative joint damage that may necessitate arthrodesis in the younger manual worker or arthroplasty in the older or more sedentary person.

Treatment of intra-articular fractures of the metacarpal base depends on fracture type. Bennett's fracture is really a dislocation of most of the joint surface when it loses the support

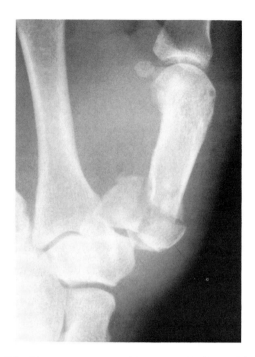

FIGURE 15. Comminuted fracture at the base of the thumb metacarpal is known as Rolando's fracture.

of the stabilizing palmar ligaments. Reduction of the dislocation is the principal consideration in this case. It may be accomplished with closed reduction and manipulation while the thumb is held in a snugly molded thumb-spica cast in a position of abduction and pronation relative to the palm. However, as edema resolves and gentle use of the hand is begun, this fracture frequently displaces despite good initial reduction. As a result, some degree of internal fixation using pins, wires, or a screw is almost always necessary and is frequently recommended at the time of initial treatment.[19,26] Six weeks of splint or cast immobilization are usually recommended after all but the most secure direct screw fixation, which permits some limited early motion.[9,31]

When the joint surface is comminuted into multiple articular fragments, as in Rolando's fracture, the joint may not be dislocated and yet direct internal stabilization of the pieces may be technically impossible. Older treatment techniques emphasized short-term immobilization with bulky dressing for edema control and initial discomfort, followed by relatively early motion exercises from a removable splint, to allow the pieces to mold into some semblance of their original structure.[17] This reportedly led to an x-ray study showing severe joint disruption but relatively acceptable mo-

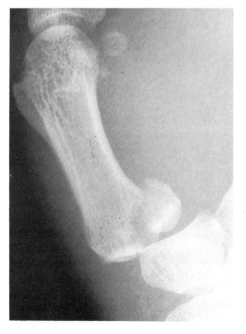

FIGURE 14. Bennett's fracture of the base of the thumb shows avulsion fracture of the palmar-ulnar rim of the metacarpal base with subluxation of the remainder of the metacarpal on the trapezium.

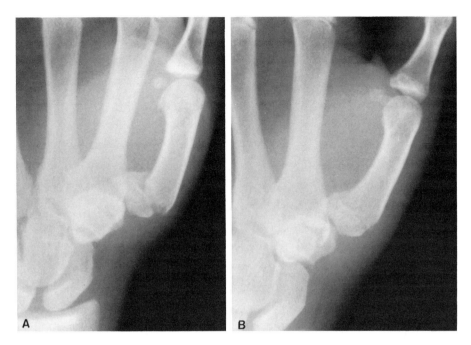

FIGURE 16. *A*, A nonarticular fracture of the base of the thumb. Because the joint surface is intact, these fractures seldom cause chronic disability. *B*, Closed reduction of the fracture in *A* by means of longitudinal traction and pressure over the fracture site results in nearly anatomic position.

tion and function. More recently, the use of distraction via ligamentous insertions onto the various fracture fragments, termed "ligamentotaxis," has been made possible by miniature external fixation devices. This technique, in addition to percutaneous wire fixation guided by image-intensifier x-ray equipment, has led to more frequent surgical treatment of Rolando's fractures. Despite this, secondary degenerative arthritis is a fairly common end result; when symptomatic, it may require arthrodesis or arthroplasty.

Fractures of the base of the metacarpal adjacent to the joint surface are generally stable impacted fractures with some degree of apex-dorsal angulation. Because of the large amount of flexion-extension and rotation in the TMC joint, a moderate degree of fracture site deformity does not affect thumb function and can be tolerated, although an attempt at closed reduction to restore the normal alignment is always warranted (see Fig. 16). Fractures of this sort can be splinted or casted for 3–6 weeks, after which hand rehabilitation is begun.

Thumb Metacarpal Shaft

Fractures of the thumb metacarpal shaft are relatively uncommon and are usually related to concomitant severe soft tissue injury such as is seen in severe crush or laceration injuries. They are usually treated surgically with internal fixation at the time of soft tissue repair.

Thumb Metacarpophalangeal Joint

The thumb MCP joint is stabilized by collateral ligaments and a fibrocartilaginous volar plate, as are the MCP and PIP joints of the fingers. The significant differences relate to the special demands placed upon this joint, especially during pinch and grasp. These demands subject the thumb MCP joint to strong radial deviating forces that are counteracted by the ulnar collateral ligament, along with the dorsal joint capsule, volar plate, and hand intrinsic muscles, mainly the adductor pollicis brevis and first dorsal interosseus muscles. The ulnar collateral ligament in particular has a close approximation with the adductor tendon insertion about the base of the thumb proximal phalanx, and this relationship has special significance in treatment of ligament ruptures, known as gamekeeper's (or skier's) thumb, as discussed elsewhere. The normal range of motion of the thumb MCP joint is extremely variable and can be assessed by examining the uninjured hand.[8]

The MCP joint of the thumb can be dislo-

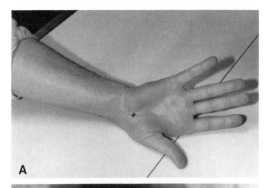

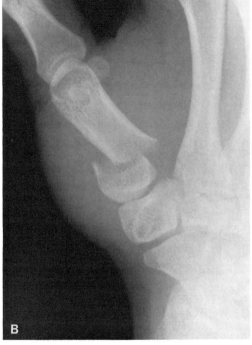

FIGURE 17. *A*, Robert's view of the TMC joint is positioned by hyperpronating the forearm (with the elbow extended). The x-ray beam is aimed at the base of the thumb in the area marked with an *X*. *B*, The poor articulation of the trapezium and the alignment of the TMC joint are demonstrated in Robert's view in a patient with fracture of the base of the thumb metacarpal.

cated in dorsal hyperextension injuries and indeed is the most frequently dislocated of the MCP joints of the hand.[13] Dislocation may draw either the volar plate or the flexor tendon into the joint to create a soft tissue block to reduction (see Fig. 4). In this case, closed reduction may not be possible, although flexion of the wrist and flexion-adduction of the metacarpal may relax these entrapped structures enough to achieve closed reduction with longitudinal traction. Splint immobilization with MCP joint flexion is used for a period of 4–6 weeks. Fail-

ure to successfully reduce the joint closed may necessitate open reduction, after which similar splinting is used.

Fractures about the thumb MCP joint include avulsion fractures of the collateral ligament insertion about the bases of the proximal phalanx. Often rotations of 90–180 degrees create joint instability similar in nature to a pure ligamentous gamekeeper's thumb injury. Because of the size of the fracture fragment, displacement outside the adductor insertion is less likely to happen. If the fracture fragment is nondisplaced, a short-arm thumb spica cast with slight ulnar deviation of the thumb is used for 6 weeks. Displacement or rotation of this fragment should be corrected by open reduction and internal fixation, with postoperative casting for 6 weeks (Fig. 18).

Fractures of the sesamoid bones, which lie within the substance of the volar plate, are uncommon and represent a variation of volar plate tear usually seen with MCP joint dislocation. These fractures rarely displace and heal with cast treatment for the dislocation injury. They should be differentiated clinically from bipartite sesamoids, which are nontraumatic, pain-free results of abnormalities of ossification during growth.

Fracture of the Proximal and Distal Phalanges of the Thumb

The shaft of either phalanx of the thumb can fracture; proximal phalanx injuries exceed distal phalanx injuries and are more frequently the result of twisting or bending forces on the shaft of the thumb. As a result, they are more often spiral or oblique fractures, whereas distal phalanx fractures, which are more often the result of crush injuries to the end of the thumb, are often transverse and communicate with an overlying wound (Fig. 19). Repair of the overlying soft tissue injury, especially the nail bed, may stabilize these fractures of the distal phalanx, although larger fragments are often pinned in position. As mentioned above, the thumb, with its greater arc of rotation, can tolerate more rotational deformity than the fingers can; therefore, some degree of shortening or rotation can be accepted in oblique fractures, which, when the joint surfaces are not involved, can usually be treated in a thumb spica splint or cast for a period of 3 weeks.

Intra-articular fractures of the interphalangeal (IP) joint may involve one or both condyles

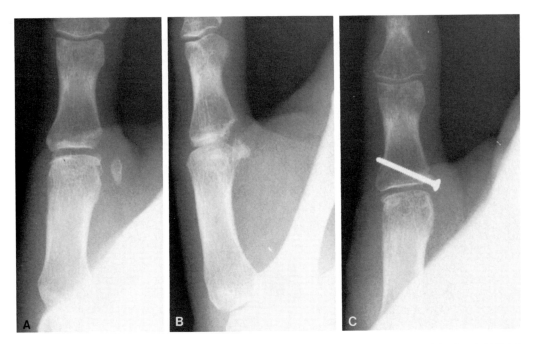

FIGURE 18. *A,* Displaced avulsion fracture of the insertion of the ulnar collateral ligament of the thumb MCP joint. *B,* Same fracture as in *A,* oblique view. *C,* Same fracture after screw fixation.

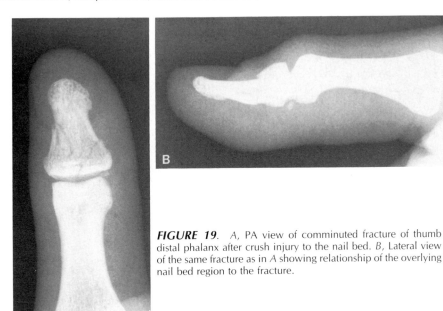

FIGURE 19. *A,* PA view of comminuted fracture of thumb distal phalanx after crush injury to the nail bed. *B,* Lateral view of the same fracture as in *A* showing relationship of the overlying nail bed region to the fracture.

of the head of the proximal phalanx. Internal fixation is required because displacement occurs easily, and both joint degeneration and deformity can result from poor initial position. Avulsion fracture of the extensor tendon insertion on the dorsal base of the thumb distal phalanx (Fig. 20), although not as common as

in the fingers, can occur after a direct blow to the thumb IP joint or after forcible flexion of the extended thumb. Small or nondisplaced fractures can be treated with extension splinting for 6 weeks; larger fragments should be reduced and pinned. Avulsion of the flexor tendon insertion on the volar base of the distal

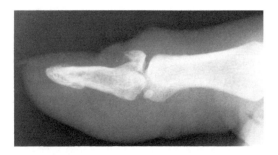

FIGURE 20. Displaced fracture of the dorsal rim of the thumb distal phalanx containing the insertion of the thumb extensor tendon.

phalanx, because of the strong pull of the flexor tendon, usually requires surgical reinsertion of the tendon into the base of the digit.

Fractures and Dislocations of the Hand Metacarpals

Fractures of the Metacarpal Neck

Axial loading of the metacarpal neck area occurs frequently, causing fracture that invariably angulates apex-dorsally because of the muscle forces of the hand intrinsic muscles. Because the axial load frequently occurs in the clenched fist struck in anger, it is often known as boxer's or fighter's fracture (see Fig. 6B). Injury to the fourth and fifth fingers is most common, and multiple fingers may be involved. Acute swelling often masks the degree of bony deformity, which is usually clearly evident on lateral x-ray views. Because of the relative mobility of the fourth and fifth carpometacarpal joints, combined with the great degree of mobility of the MCP joints in these fingers, fairly normal function can accommodate a great deal of angular deformity. Most authors accept up to 45–50 degrees of apex-dorsal angulation before recommending open reduction,[15] and satisfactory function has been reported with up to 70 degrees.[27] Others, however, point out that the knuckle may be prominently displaced into the palm and the affected finger clawed from as little as 20–30 degrees of residual angulation.[49] There is good agreement that much less deformity is tolerated in the less mobile index and long fingers, and operative correction is recommended if more than 10–15 degrees of dorsal angulation exist after manipulation.[44]

Although the significance of fracture deform-

ity, especially in the ulnar digits, is controversial, an attempt at closed reduction under local or regional anesthesia is always appropriate. Flexion of the MCP joint is combined with firm, dorsally directed pressure over the head of the proximal phalanx. A forearm-based cast or splint is then applied with the MCP joints flexed and the IP joints extended. Taping of the injured digit to adjacent fingers helps ensure rotational stability. Immobilization lasts 3–4 weeks.

Fractures of the Metacarpal Head

The head of the metacarpal fractures less commonly than the neck. A head fracture may be caused by direct or penetrating injury to the articular surface, or may be a result of angular torsion on the flexed fingers, which causes avulsion fractures by traction in the collateral ligaments. These fractures, if small, are not always seen because the metacarpal neck area is tapered. A special x-ray position, the Brewerton view,[35] allows visualization of this area (Fig. 21). Articular surface injuries must be surgically opened to achieve restoration of the joint surface, but most small- to moderate-sized ligament avulsion injuries of the collateral lig-

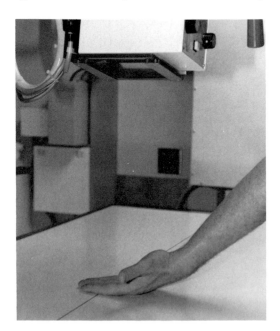

FIGURE 21. The Brewerton view of the metacarpal head ligament recesses is positioned by laying the fingers flat on the x-ray table, flexing the MCP joints 60–80 degrees, and angling the x-ray beam 15 degrees from the ulnar side.

ament origin resolve with 3 weeks of splinting with the MCP joints flexed.

Fractures of the Metacarpal Shaft

Metacarpal shaft fractures are usually transverse if they result from a direct or axial blow (Fig. 22A) or spiral oblique if they occur after a twisting injury to the finger (Fig. 22B). These fractures are unlikely to shorten significantly because metacarpals are splinted by each other through strong ligamentous support at both ends. Transverse and short oblique fractures can angulate dorsally as a result of interosseous muscle pull. The more proximally along the shaft this fracture occurs, the less well tolerated is the angulation.

Oblique fractures tend not to angulate because of their length and soft tissue attachments, but even slight shortening may be accompanied by rotation along the inclined plane of the fracture face that is virtually impossible to detect on x-rays (Fig. 23A).[42] Because of this, clinical examination of the alignment and rotation of the fingers is critical. The patient should be asked to open and close the fingers, and the axial alignment should be checked by examining the parallel alignment of the nail plates of the fingers (Fig. 23B, C). The fingers should

close without overlap (Fig. 23D) and should converge pointing toward the scaphoid tubercle at the base of the thumb (Fig. 23E). When rotational deformity is even suspected, referral is warranted because the deformity is frequently the source of malpractice allegations.

When angulation and rotation are believed acceptable, these fractures are treated in a short-arm splint or cast extended to include the involved finger but leaving the other fingers free. Fractures of the midshaft, especially transverse fractures, take 6–8 weeks to unite, whereas oblique fractures, with their greater stability and fracture area, unite in as little as 3 weeks.

Fractures and Dislocations of the Metacarpal Bases

Fractures of the base of the index and long finger metacarpals are uncommon because of the dense supporting ligaments that secure and stabilize these joints. Even when fracture occurs, it is usually stable and often requires little in the way of treatment except splinting for comfort. The fifth finger carpometacarpal (CMC) joint is the most mobile and, because of its border position, the most frequently injured. Fractures that do not involve the joint can be splinted in position for 3–4 weeks. Fractures

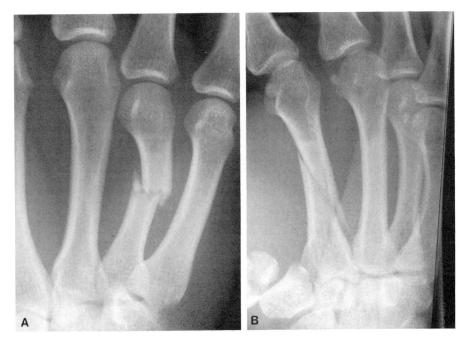

FIGURE 22. *A*, A transverse fracture of the metacarpal shaft results from an axial or direct blow to the metacarpal. *B*, A spiral fracture of the metacarpal shaft results from a twisting injury to the finger. Malrotation may not be evident except by clinical examination.

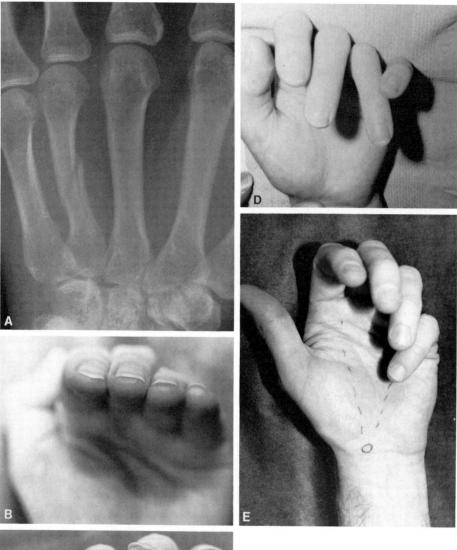

FIGURE 23.   *A*, A short spiral fracture of the fourth finger metacarpal does not appear badly out of position. *B*, Rotational alignment of the fingers can be checked by inspecting the alignment of the nail plates while the fingers are flexed. *C*, In this patient, the long finger is malaligned. *D*, Clinically severe finger overlap in the patient in *A. E*, The fingers should taper in a cascade and point toward the scaphoid tubercle.

that extend into the joint, however, may behave like a Bennett's fracture of the thumb and have been termed reverse Bennett's injuries.[33] The ulnar wrist flexor and extensor tendons can act on the base of the metacarpal to displace the alignment of the joint, and if the joint is displaced, closed reduction and pinning or open reduction may be required to maintain congruity of the joint surface. Delay in treatment or chronic malunion can lead to symptomatic painful joint degeneration that may require later arthrodesis.[22]

Dislocations of the Metacarpophalangeal Joint

Direct hyperextension displaces the MCP joint, for all practical purposes, in only the index and small fingers, besides the thumb (Fig. 24).[1] Stabilization from adjacent metacarpal supporting ligaments makes these injuries rare in the long and ring fingers. During hyperextension, the volar plate proximal margin tears, allowing the joint first to hyperextend while maintaining bone-to-bone congruity. If this process continues with further hyperextension, the volar plate displaces into the joint, the joint completely dislocates, and reduction is blocked by the combination of entrapped volar plate and encircling flexor tendons and intrinsic muscles, which hold the head of the metacarpal trapped like the strands of a Chinese finger trap (Fig. 25).[32] Neurovascular structures may be excessively stretched, and numbness in the digital nerve distribution is occasionally seen.

When hyperextended MCP joint subluxation is seen with the joint surfaces still in contact, reduction is accomplished by simply flexing the joint passively and holding it flexed in a splint for 3–4 weeks. Attempts to reduce by distraction or increasing hyperextension usu-ally convert the simple subluxation to the more complex entrapped dislocation.[10] In most instances this dislocation, when complete, requires open reduction to manually remove the volar plate via either a palmar or a dorsal incision in the operating room. After surgery, the MCP is again splinted in flexion for 4–6 weeks.

Fractures of the Proximal Phalanx

Fractures of the proximal phalanx may be transverse, oblique, spiral, or comminuted. They are usually palmarly angulated owing to flexion of the proximal fracture fragment by the interosseous muscles and flexion of the PIP joint by the flexor tendon.[40] Accurate reduction is necessary to reduce the incidence of flexion contractures of the PIP joint and rotational abnormalities. Rotation of the fracture site needs to be precisely reduced and usually requires pinning; as few as 5 degrees of rotational malalignment can cause a functional disability.

Closed reduction of the transverse or oblique proximal phalanx fracture can frequently be performed with digital block anesthesia, manipulating the MCP and PIP joints into full

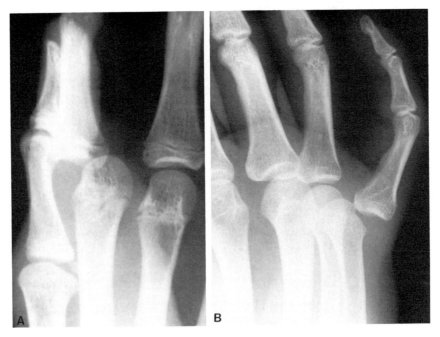

FIGURE 24. *A,* Dorsal dislocations of the MCP joints mainly occur in the border fingers—the index and small fingers—besides the thumb. An index finger MCP joint dislocation is shown here. *B,* The MCP joints of the long and ring fingers are stabilized by heavy intermetacarpal ligaments from either side, and isolated dislocation is very rare. A fifth finger MCP dislocation is shown here.

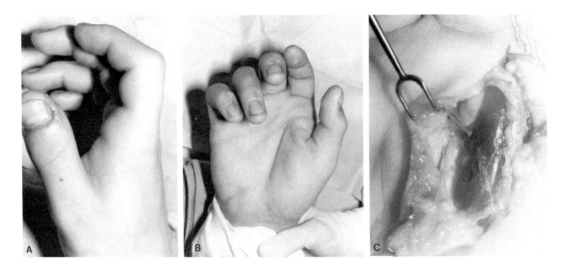

FIGURE 25. *A,* A lateral view of a complex MCP joint dislocation of the index finger. *B,* A palmar view of a complex MCP joint dislocation of the index finger. Note the characteristic pucker of the palmar skin anterior to the MCP joint. This is a clinical sign of displacement of the volar plate into the joint, blocking closed joint reduction. *C,* At surgery, the hand is opened through a palmar approach. The metacarpal head is caught in the "Chinese finger-trap" effect between the displaced flexor tendons on the ulnar side and the lumbrical muscle on the radial side.

flexion to reduce the angulated fracture (Fig. 26).[28] The reduction should be checked for rotational alignment by fully flexing all digits. No overlap of the digits should occur in flexion.

A stable fracture that is noncomminuted and has minimal soft tissue injury should be immobilized for 3–4 weeks. The wrist and involved digit should be encased in a plaster cast in the safe or intrinsic-plus position (MCP joints flexed and IP joints extended; Fig. 27).[29] The position of reduction (Fig. 26) should not be maintained because it causes a severe contracture of the PIP joint. After reduction, a splint or cast with aluminum splint extension to the involved finger is applied (Fig. 28). X-rays are obtained in the splint or cast at weekly intervals until clinical union has occurred.

Clinical healing of midshaft proximal phalanx fractures takes 4–7 weeks on average and up to 10–14 weeks for transverse fractures through the hard cortical portion of the proximal phalanx.[48] Immobilization should continue until clinical signs of union—no further tenderness to palpation and no motion at the fracture site—have occurred.

Treatment after immobilization consists of buddy taping the digits, warm soaks, active range of motion exercises, and strengthening exercises. Molded plastic splints should be used for protecting the digit on the job. Radiographic union is usually complete by 5 months, and clinical union occurs in about one-fourth of this time.

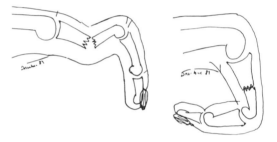

FIGURE 26. Transverse fractures of the proximal phalanx invariably angulate palmarly owing to the interosseous muscle pull. Reduction is accomplished by flexion at both the MCP and PIP joints.

Percutaneous Pinning. Frequently, transverse fractures of the proximal phalanx are unstable, angulated, or rotated after reduction. In crush injuries, they are frequently accompanied by varying degrees of soft tissue injury. The fractures can be stabilized by limited internal fixation with percutaneous pins if satisfactory reduction can be achieved (Fig. 29). If unreducible, the fracture may require direct open reduction and internal fixation.[14,21]

Closed pin fixation has the advantage of avoiding an incision; however early motion is usually not possible because the pins pass through the extensor mechanism and limit motion. Cast or splint immobilization is necessary for 4–6 weeks in conjunction with pinning techniques. Following pin removal, gentle active range of motion exercises are begun as outlined above.

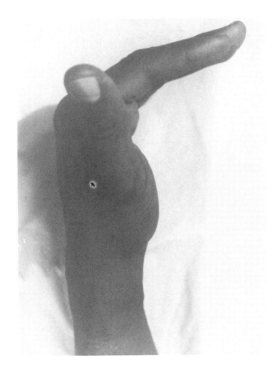

FIGURE 27. The safe position of hand immobilization, with mild wrist dorsiflexion, MCP joint flexion, and PIP and DIP joint extension, is the best posture to use to minimize postimmobilization stiffness.

Phalangeal Fractures Likely to Require Internal Fixation

Spiral Oblique Fractures. Spiral oblique fractures of the proximal phalanx occur from torsion injuries to the digits with a minimum of soft tissue injury. They are seldom markedly displaced but are frequently malrotated and are best treated with internal fixation when reduction cannot be maintained reliably, as is often the case. Percutaneous pinning is most easily performed within several days of the injury. Open reduction may be required if delay beyond 1 week has occurred. Because the fracture involves a large surface area, clinical union occurs within 4–5 weeks.

Articular Fractures of the Proximal Phalanx. Condylar fractures of the proximal phalanx are frequent and tend to be missed because the involved digit moves quite well. Oblique x-rays help visualize the fracture and show any displacement. As with all articular fractures, only minimal displacement can be accepted. Condylar fractures are usually treated with closed reduction and percutaneous pins if the patient is seen within the first week of injury (Fig. 30). If untreated, a late loss of re-

duction will most likely occur, and displacement and angulation are the rule.

Articular Fractures of the Base of the Middle Phalanx. Avulsion fractures of the dorsal base of the middle phalanx occur with displacement of a piece of bone containing the extensor tendon insertion site. Displacement of more than 2 mm results in loss of PIP joint extension and can lead to secondary deformity. Anatomic replacement of the bone is essential; it is followed by splinting in extension for 6 weeks.

Comminuted fractures of the articular surface are difficult to repair and frequently result in stiffness. Treatment may consist of reduction of joint alignment and transarticular pin stabilization with the joint in extension (Fig. 31). For the severely comminuted fracture, treatment in traction with early motion may preserve some functional range of motion while maintaining fracture alignment.

Dislocations and Fracture-Dislocations of the Proximal Interphalangeal Joint

Injuries to the PIP joint are the most common ligament injuries in the hand. The majority are incomplete disruptions of the liga-

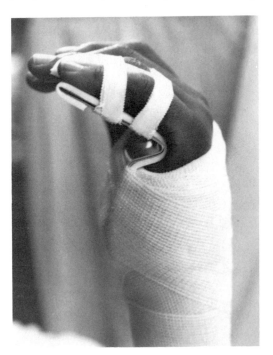

FIGURE 28. Use of a cast with incorporated splint extension of the fourth and fifth fingers in the safe hand position. This device might be used to treat a boxer's fracture or a stable proximal phalanx fracture.

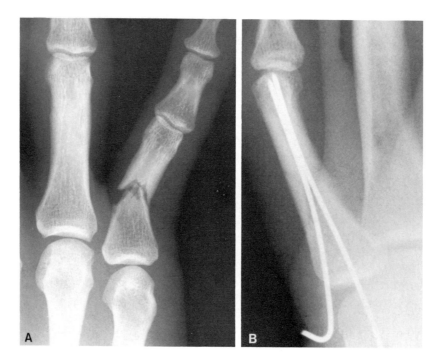

FIGURE 29. *A,* This angulated fracture of the proximal phalanx could be reduced but was unstable. Percutaneous wire fixation was used after a closed reduction was performed. After 4 weeks of splint immobilization, the wires were removed and hand rehabilitation was begun. Full function was recovered. *B,* The fracture illustrated in *A* after percutaneous wire stabilization.

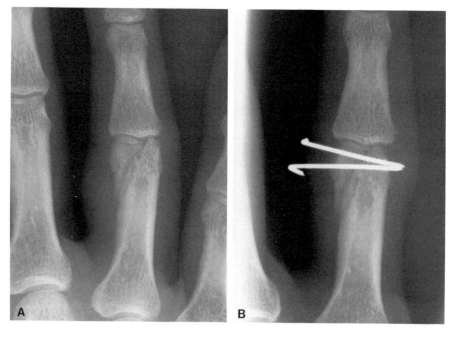

FIGURE 30. *A,* Although this condyle fracture of the head of the proximal phalanx appears nondisplaced, these fractures are notoriously unstable. Surgical treatment is usually recommended. *B,* This fracture was easily reduced closed and percutaneously pinned with the use of local anesthesia.

ments that cause swelling and pain but no instability or joint disruption (the so-called jammed finger). Dislocations and fracture-dislocations however, may result in significant stiffness and disability. Optimal treatment is based on an accurate diagnosis and an understanding of the pathology of the injury.

Evaluation. Initial PA and lateral x-rays of the involved digit should be made to determine if the joint is dislocated. Films obtained before reduction often better demonstrate the nature of articular damage.

Often, the patient reduces simple dislocations immediately after injury and seeks medical attention only when pain and swelling occur over the next several hours. If x-rays show the joint to be reduced, stability to both active and passive range of motion should be assessed with the use of digital block anesthesia if necessary. Gentle stress testing of the collateral ligaments and volar plate should also be done, and the results should be compared to those for a noninjured digit (see Fig. 5).[13]

Treatment of the stable joint with incomplete ligament injury consists of splinting for 10–14 days followed by joint mobilization and buddy taping. Complete mobility should be obtained by 6 weeks. Chronic joint swelling frequently results.

Dorsal PIP Joint Dislocation

Type 1 (Hyperextension).[11] Dorsal hyperextension deformities of a PIP joint result in avulsion of the volar plate from the base of the middle phalanx and a minor tear of the collateral ligaments (Fig. 32). These dislocations are usually spontaneously reduced and may be treated with 2 weeks of splinting and buddy taping.

Type 2 (Dorsal Dislocation). This injury results in a complete avulsion of the volar plate and a major tear in both collateral ligaments (Fig. 33). Reduction requires digital block anesthesia. Longitudinal traction and gentle hyperextension are followed by flexion. The joint should be felt to snap into place. X-rays are obtained, and the joint is splinted in slight flexion for 2–4 weeks. Active motion and buddy taping follow.

Type 3 (Fracture-Dislocation). These injuries result in avulsion fractures through the volar base of the middle phalanx and dorsal subluxation of the remainder of the phalanx (Fig. 34A). If the fracture fragment is less than 40% of the joint surface, as viewed on the lateral x-ray, the joint can usually be reduced and maintained in 30 or more degrees of flexion.[39]

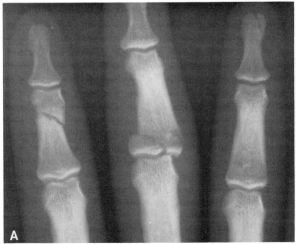

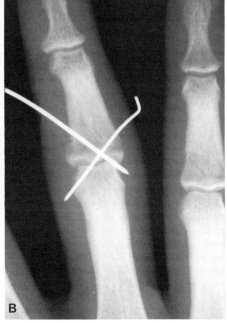

FIGURE 31. *A*, Comminuted fractures of the base of the middle phalanx involving the PIP joint often require fixation across the PIP joint surface to secure the fragments. *B*, The fracture in *A* after open reduction and multiple wire fixation.

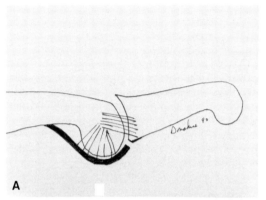

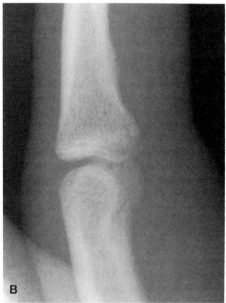

FIGURE 32. *A,* Type 1 hyperextension injury of the PIP joint causes damage to the insertion of the volar plate at the base of the middle phalanx. *B,* Frequently, a small avulsion chip fracture may be seen at the base of the middle phalanx. The joint does not displace.

The joint is then gradually extended to full extension by means of a series of extension-block splints over 3 weeks or so. Active motion between 30 and 90 degrees of joint flexion may be allowed in the extension block splint; it helps decrease joint stiffness.

Fractures of more than 40% of the joint surface or comminution of a large segment of the articular surface of the middle phalanx results in an unstable fracture-dislocation. Accurate closed reduction is rarely possible. Open reduction is usually necessary (Fig. 34B, C). Impaction of the articular surface frequently makes accurate joint repair difficult. Volar plate advancement is sometimes necessary. These in-

juries result in significant finger function disability.

Lateral PIP Joint Dislocation

Lateral dislocation of the PIP joint causes rupture of one collateral ligament and a partial avulsion of the volar plate (Fig. 35). Closed reduction and splinting for up to 3 weeks result in adequate joint stability. Open ligament repair is infrequently necessary.

Palmar PIP Joint Dislocation

Palmar dislocation of the PIP joint is rarely seen. This injury represents the rupture of a collateral ligament, partial avulsion of the volar plate, and rupture of the joint capsule and extensor insertion. While closed reduction may be possible, open repair of the associated ligament and tendon insertions is at times advised; it is followed by transarticular pin fixation of the joint in extension for 4–8 weeks. Some degree of stiffness invariably results.[50]

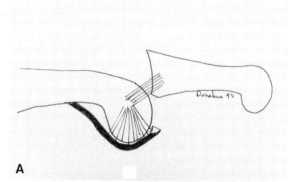

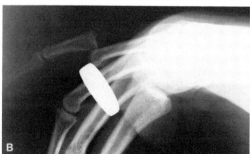

FIGURE 33. *A,* Type 2 hyperextension injury of the PIP joint results in tearing of the volar plate insertion and portions of the collateral ligaments sufficient to let the joint dislocate dorsally. *B,* An example of a type 2 hyperextension injury, dorsal dislocation of the PIP joint.

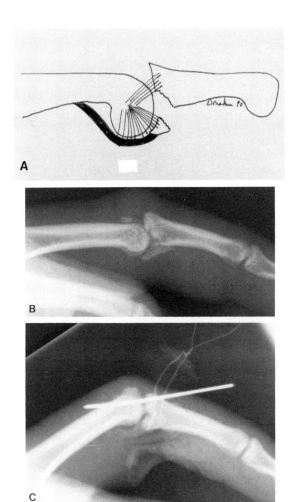

reduction is obtained, splint immobilization is used for 4–6 weeks, and the position is verified with follow-up x-rays. Significant comminution or displacement should be referred to a hand specialist. This pattern of fracture is usually associated with crush injury, and careful attention to splinting and therapy for range of motion is indicated (Fig. 36).

Small chip avulsion fractures are often seen along the proximal palmar base of the middle phalanx in the area of insertion of the PIP joint volar plate (see Fig. 32B). If the joint is otherwise stable to stress testing, especially in hyperextension, these fractures can be splinted for 1–4 weeks. Then active range of motion exercises with buddy-tape support to an adjacent finger can begin.

Displaced intra-articular fractures in this area, as in others, have a significant risk of stiffness, deformity, and traumatic arthritis (Fig. 37). Referral to a hand specialist is often appropriate because surgery is usually necessary to restore joint congruity. Even nondisplaced condylar fractures (Fig. 38) about the distal interphal-

FIGURE 34. *A,* Type 3 hyperextension injury of the PIP joint. This injury involves fracture of more than 40% of the joint surface and is unstable. *B,* This type 3 hyperextension injury is subluxed dorsally. An accurate lateral x-ray is required to diagnose this injury because the PA can look almost normal. *C,* This fracture requires accurate open reduction and frequently results in chronic stiffness and disability.

Fractures of the Middle and Distal Phalanx

Middle Phalanx

Many fractures of the middle phalanx are shaft, or diaphyseal, fractures. They should be assessed with three views on x-ray: PA, lateral, and oblique. The degree of displacement varies with the mechanism of fracture and also with the flexor and extensor tendon pull on the fragments. Twisting injuries usually cause a long, oblique spiral fracture; transverse fractures result from an axial load or direct blow. If closed

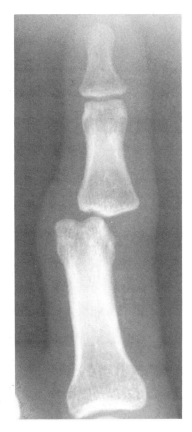

FIGURE 35. An example of a lateral PIP joint dislocation.

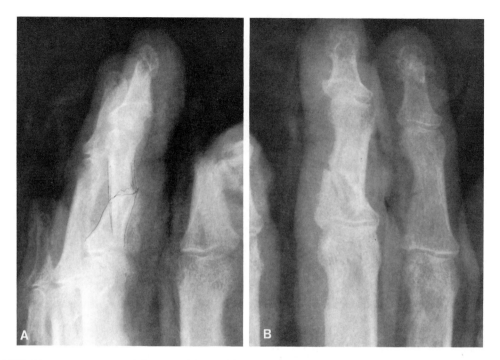

FIGURE 36. *A*, A comminuted fracture of the middle phalanx sustained in a crush injury, with associated open wounds. *B*, Multiple views demonstrate the intra-articular involvement of this fracture.

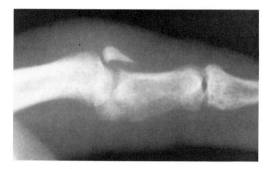

FIGURE 37. Crush injury of the middle phalanx with severe displacement and comminution.

angeal (DIP) joint are likely to lose position and are usually stabilized by internal fixation.[4] Spiral oblique fractures that extend to one corner of the joint may shorten, causing distortion or disruption of the joint collateral ligaments, and are best reduced and pinned (or wired) in anatomic position.

Distal Phalanx

The fingertip is subject to multiple injuries. Most are crushing injuries associated with fractures of the distal end of the distal phalanx, the tuft, and with nail bed lacerations (Fig. 39). Most often, soft tissue repair of the skin and

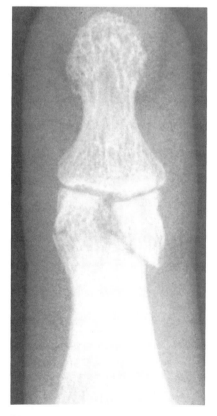

FIGURE 38. This nondisplaced fracture involving the DIP joint is quite unstable; it may be pinned in place.

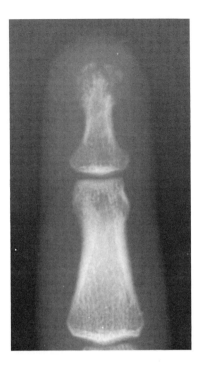

FIGURE 39. Fracture of the distal tuft of the distal phalanx after a fingertip crush injury. Even though this is an "open" fracture, treatment consists of repair of the nail bed and fingertip lacerations. The fracture is stabilized by its soft tissue attachments.

nail bed is all that is needed to treat this type of fracture.[6] More proximal injury can result in fracture of the short diaphyseal portion of the distal phalanx, and if displaced, these fractures are best stabilized with pins at the time of soft tissue repair (Fig. 40). Fracture of the palmar lip of the base of the distal phalanx is usually caused by avulsion of the insertion of the profundus flexor tendon, which may be displaced proximally along the tendon sheath (Fig. 41). Operative repair to reinsert the tendon is necessary.[37]

Fractures of the dorsal lip of the base of the distal phalanx are known as "mallet" or "baseball" fractures (Fig. 42) because they are often associated with either a direct blow or an axial blow on the fingertip held extended as in catching a ball.[23] Either mechanism may disrupt the terminal portion of the extensor tendon or avulse off the corner of the joint, leaving the extensor tendon attached to the displaced fragment. Loss of extensor function causes a severe droop in the DIP joint because of the strong, unbalanced pull of the intact flexor tendon.

Treatment of this common fracture is initially to correct the "droop" by passively splinting the DIP joint in full extension or slight hyperextension. A dorsal aluminum-foam fin-

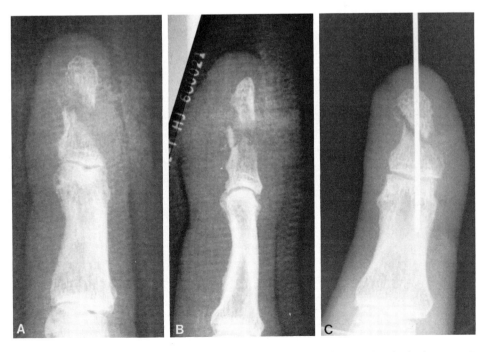

FIGURE 40. A, Crush injury to the midportion or shaft area of the distal phalanx, with wide displacement. B, Lateral view of the fracture in A, demonstrating comminution. C, Because of the hard cortical bone, which heals slowly, in the midportion of the distal phalanx, wire stabilization is used at the time of soft tissue repair.

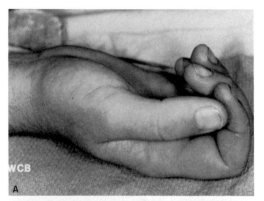

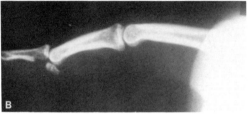

FIGURE 41. *A*, A fracture with avulsion of the profundus flexor tendon insertion. Note loss of the normal flexion cascade in the slightly extended ring finger. *B*, An x-ray showing the fracture of the insertion of the flexor tendon. This fragment can retract proximally along the course of the tendon sheath quite a distance; the fracture can be missed if the x-ray field is not wide enough. The PA x-ray appears normal. Photographs courtesy of Dr. Warren C. Breidenbach, Louisville, KY.

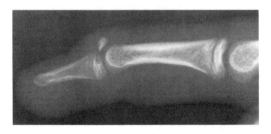

FIGURE 42. This fracture is the result of sudden forced flexion of the extended finger, causing avulsion of the dorsal rim of the base of the distal phalanx. The extensor tendon of the DIP joint remains attached to the fragment and can displace the fragment proximally. Note the "droop" of the end of the finger and the dorsal swelling.

ger splint or special Stack finger splint may be used (Fig. 43A, B). Lateral x-rays should be taken to assess the fracture position (Fig. 43C). If the fracture is seen to be reduced, extension splinting is continued for 6–8 weeks.

When anatomic position of this fracture cannot be obtained by extension splinting, treatment is controversial. Fractures of less than 30% of the joint surface, as viewed from the side, may be allowed to heal in a displaced

position with recovery of DIP joint extension if less than 2 mm of fracture gap remain, although a prominent dorsal mass will persist and may cause symptoms of local tenderness (Fig. 44). Surgery may prevent the dorsal prominence but may increase stiffness in the final range of motion. Fractures of more than 30% of the joint surface usually result in some palmar subluxation of the remainder of the distal phalanx and DIP joint (Fig. 45A). Open reduction of the joint subluxation and replacement of the dorsal fragment is sometimes recommended (Fig. 45B),[23,52] although even this is a matter of some dispute.[56]

IMMOBILIZATION TECHNIQUES

Adequate splinting of hand fractures, as of other fractures, generally requires that the joints proximal and distal to the site of fracture be

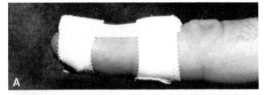

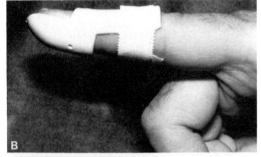

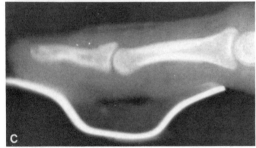

FIGURE 43. *A*, A dorsal aluminum-foam splint of the DIP joint. *B*, A Stack finger splint of the DIP joint. Note that the PIP joint is not restricted and should be allowed to move to prevent stiffness. *C*, A lateral x-ray showing excellent reduction of the mallet fracture fragment. Note the bending of the palmar surface aluminum-foam splint used here.

immobilized and that any displacing muscle forces be reduced by flexion of the injured part. Because of the close proximity of gliding tendon surfaces and delicate joint structures to many hand fractures, treatment must consider the detrimental effects of immobilization to these tissues. The PIP joints, especially, suffer from prolonged disuse, particularly when in the position of flexion; the MCP joints, although less sensitive, are prone to develop dorsal adhesion and ligament tightness when immobilized in the extended position.

It is often assumed that immobilization of the hand or fingers in the "position of function" (wrist dorsiflexed, MCP and PIP joints moderately flexed) maintains or protects function, but this in fact is not the case. The "safe" po-

sition is that of full MCP joint flexion and full PIP joint extension, known as the intrinsic-plus position after the isolated action of the hand intrinsic muscles (see Fig. 27).[29] Injuries that cannot be adequately splinted or casted in this position may require operative treatment to achieve fracture stability so as to avoid the need for a "malignant" position of immobilization. Alternatively, special splints that allow partial

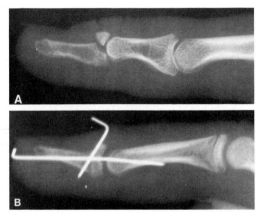

FIGURE 45. *A,* Mild subluxation of the DIP joint and more than 30% of the joint surface involved in the fragment. *B,* Open reduction and wire fixation of both the joint subluxation and the fracture displacement.

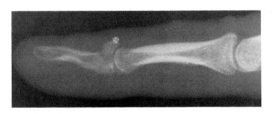

FIGURE 44. This fracture reduction position was accepted and healed with recovery of full extension, but with a palpable dorsal bump.

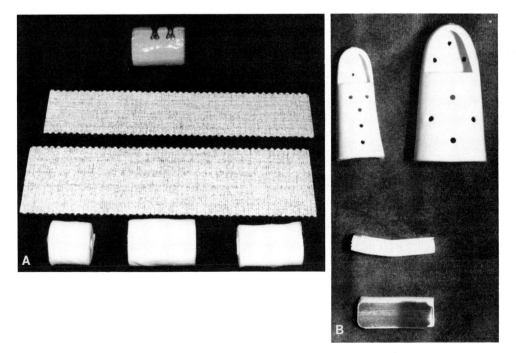

FIGURE 46. *A,* Plaster splinting materials commonly used for wrist, hand, and some finger splint applications. *B,* Aluminum-foam material can be cut to size as required. Care should be taken not to splint the PIP joint if possible. Various sizes of the Stack finger splint are available.

range of motion, such as extension block splints that prevent motion beyond a certain point, may be necessary.

Splinting materials available to treat hand fractures abound, and a variety of special splints have been created to meet special situations. Unfortunately, some ready-made materials do not incorporate the "safe" hand position. These devices either inadequately immobilize, improperly position, or excessively splint non-injured parts. In general, conventional padded plaster splints or casts for immobilization of the wrist and hand, and aluminum-foam and tape splints for isolated finger injuries, are adequate to treat all injuries (Fig. 46). Use of synthetic casting material is generally necessary only in special circumstances, such as in the treatment of scaphoid fracture. The treating physician must at all times remember the specific demands of the particular injury, while allowing the maximum reasonable motion of noninvolved parts.

REHABILITATION OF HAND FRACTURES

Injury and immobilization almost always cause some degree of temporary hand dysfunction, usually in the form of stiffness and weakness in the injured part. Time and treatment should be provided so that hand function can be regained before full occupational use is allowed. Treatment may take the form of simple soaks and gentle motion exercises carried out by the patient on his own, or it may involve formal hand therapy and special treatment to reduce swelling, adhesion, and scar tenderness and regain joint motion and strength.

Modern thermoplastic splinting materials allow the custom fabrication of splints that may be easily removed and reapplied.[16] After initial fracture healing, such splints often provide sufficient protection to allow some partial functional or occupational hand use.*

CONCLUSION

Hand fractures include a challenging array of injuries, from the simple to the complex. Even straightforward, minor injuries alter the manner in which the hand is used, and treatment must at all times be directed toward preservation and restoration of function. Knowledge of orthopedic terminology of fracture conditions allows intelligent communication among physicians. In many instances, orthopedically correct analysis points in the direction of necessary treatment. Thus, a fracture that can be described as stable and nondisplaced can be treated with proper immobilization in a safe position. Such injuries, including most metacarpal fractures and some phalangeal fractures, can be treated by primary caregivers. A fracture that is displaced or angulated must be manipulated into an acceptable position before immobilization can begin. Such fractures include significantly angulated metacarpal shaft and neck fractures and rotated or angulated phalangeal fractures. They are often treated by manipulation and splinting under local anesthesia and do not require hospitalization or prolonged time off work. Fractures that are unstable, intra-articular, or compound with associated soft tissue trauma usually require surgical fixation. These include complex dislocations, metacarpal fractures involving the joint, such as Bennett's fracture, and fracture-dislocations of the PIP and DIP joint surfaces, as well as the more complex scaphoid and carpal fractures. These are best referred to hand specialists who can anticipate the pitfalls and vagaries of these problem injuries.

REFERENCES

1. Adler GA, Light TR: Simultaneous complex dislocation of the metacarpophalangeal joints of the long and index fingers. A case report. J Bone Joint Surg 63A:1007–1009, 1981.
2. American College of Surgeons, Committee on Trauma: Early Care of the Injured Patient, 2nd ed. Philadelphia, W.B. Saunders, 1976.
3. Billing L, Gedda KQ: Roentgen examination of Bennett's fracture. Acta Radiol 38:471–476, 1952.
4. Bloem JJAM: The treatment and prognosis of uncomplicated dislocated fractures of the metacarpals and phalanges. Arch Chir Neerl 23:55–65, 1971.
5. Brown PW: Open injuries of the hand. In Green DP (ed): Operative Hand Surgery. New York, Churchill Livingstone, 1988, pp 1631–1636.
6. Burton RI, Eaton RG: Common hand injuries in the athlete. Orthop Clin North Am 4:809–838, 1973.
7. Carter PR, Benton LJ: Late osseous complications of carpal silastic implants. Paper presented at the 40th annual meeting, American Society for Surgery of the Hand, Las Vegas, January 1985.
8. Coonrad RW, Goldner JL: A study of the pathological findings and treatment in soft tissue injury of the thumb metacarpophalangeal joint. J Bone Joint Surg 50A:439, 1968.

---

* Editor's comment: Patient motivation and cooperation are essential to a good result. —MLK.

9. Crawford GP: Screw fixation for certain fractures of the phalanges and metacarpals. J Bone Joint Surg 58A:487–492, 1976.

10. Cunningham DM, Schwarz G: Dorsal dislocation of the index metacarpophalangeal joint. Plast Reconstr Surg 56:654–659, 1975.

11. Dray GS, Eaton RG: Dislocations and ligament injuries in the digits. In Green DP (ed): Operative Hand Surgery. New York, Churchill Livingstone, 1988, p 779.

12. Eaton RG, Littler JW: Ligament reconstruction for the painful thumb carpometacarpal joint. J Bone Joint Surg 55A:1655, 1973.

13. Eaton RG, Littler JW: Joint injuries and their sequelae. Clin Plast Surg 3:85, 1976.

14. Edwards GS, O'Brien ET, Hechman MM: Retrograde cross pinning of transverse metacarpal and phalangeal shaft fractures. Hand 14:141–145, 1982.

15. Eichenholtz SN, Rizzo PC: Fracture of the neck of the fifth metacarpal. Is overtreatment justified? JAMA 178:425–426, 1961.

16. Fess EE, Gettle KS, Strickland JW: Hand Splinting, Principles and Methods. St Louis, C.V. Mosby, 1981.

17. Flatt AE: Fractures. In Care of Minor Hand Injuries, 3rd ed. St Louis, C.V. Mosby, 1972.

18. Frykman GK, Taleisnik J, Peters G, et al: Treatment of non-united scaphoid fractures by pulsed electromagnetic field and cast. J Hand Surg 11A:344–349, 1986.

19. Gedda KO: Studies on Bennett's fracture: Anatomy, roentgenology, and therapy. Acta Chir Scand Suppl 193, 1954.

20. Gelberman RH, Salamon PB, Jurist JM, Posch JL: Ulnar variance in Kienbock's disease. J Bone Joint Surg 57A:674–676, 1975.

21. Green DP, Anderson JR: Closed reduction and percutaneous pin fixation of fractures of the phalanges. J Bone Joint Surg 55A:1651–1653, 1973.

22. Hagstrom P: Fracture-dislocation in the ulnar carpometacarpal joints: Open reduction and pinning. A case report. Scand J Plast Reconstr Surg 9:249–251, 1975.

23. Hamas RS, Horrell ED, Pierret GP: Treatment of mallet finger due to intra-articular fracture of the distal phalanx. J Hand Surg 3:361–363, 1978.

24. Hart VL, Gaynor V: Roentgenographic study of carpal canal. J Bone Joint Surg 23:382, 1941.

25. Herbert TJ, Fisher WE: Management of the fractured scaphoid using a new bone screw. J Bone Joint Surg 66B:114–123, 1984.

26. Howard, FM: Fractures of the basal joint of thumb. J Hand Surg 12A:26, 1987.

27. Hunter JM, Cowen NJ: Fifth metacarpal fractures in a compensation clinic population. J Bone Joint Surg 52A:1159–1165, 1970.

28. Jahss SA: Fractures of the proximal phalanges: Alignment and immobilization. J Bone Joint Surg 18:726–731, 1936.

29. James JIP: Fractures of proximal and middle phalanges of the fingers. Acta Orthop Scand 32:401–412, 1962.

30. Jorgensen TM, Andresen JG, Thommesen P, Hansen HH: Scanning and radiology of the carpal scaphoid bone. Acta Orthop Scand 50:663–665, 1979.

31. Jupiter JB, et al: Intra-articular fractures of the basilar joint of the thumb. Hand Clin 4:491, 1980.

32. Kaplan EB: Dorsal dislocation of the metacarpophal-angeal joint of the index finger. J Bone Joint Surg 39A:1081–1086, 1957.

33. Ker HR: Dislocation of the fifth carpometacarpal joint. J Bone Joint Surg 37B:254–256, 1955.

34. Kienböck R: Uber Traumatische Malazie des Mond-biens und Kompression Fracturen. Fortschr Roent-genstralen 16:77–103, 1910–1911.

35. Lane CS: Detecting occult fractures of the metacarpal head: The Brewerton view. J Hand Surg 2:131–133, 1977.

36. Lange RH, Engber WD: Hyperextension mallet finger. Orthopedics 6:1426–1431, 1983.

37. Leddy JP, Packer JW: Avulsion of the profundus tendon insertion in athletes. J Hand Surg 2:66, 1977.

38. Mazet R, Hohl M: Conservative treatment of old fractures of the carpal scaphoid. J Trauma 1:115–127, 1961.

39. McElfresh EC, Dobyns JH, O'Brien ET: Management of fracture-dislocation of the proximal interphalangeal joints by extension-block splinting. J Bone Joint Surg 54A:1705–1711, 1972.

40. McNealy RW, Lichtenstein ME: Fractures of the metacarpals and phalanges. West J Surg Obstet Gynecol 43:156–161, 1935.

41. Nisenfield FG, Neviaser Rj: Fracture of the hook of the hamate: A diagnosis easily missed. J Trauma 14:612–616, 1974.

42. Opgrande JD, Westphal SA: Fractures of the hand. Orthop Clin North Am 14:779–792, 1983.

43. Ovesen J: Shortening of the radius in the treatment of lunatomalacia. J Bone Joint Surg 63B:231–232, 1981.

44. Posner MA: Injuries to the hand and wrist in athletes. Orthop Clin North Am 8:593–618, 1977.

45. Robert P: Bull Mem Soc Radiol Med France 24:687–690, 1936.

46. Ruby LK, Stinson J, Belsky MR: The natural history of scaphoid non-union. A review of fifty-five cases. J Bone Joint Surg 67A:428–432, 1985.

47. Russe O: Fracture of the carpal navicular. Diagnosis, nonoperative treatment and operative treatment. J Bone Joint Surg 42A:759–765, 1960.

48. Smith FL, Rider DL: A study of the healing of one hundred consecutive phalangeal fractures. J Bone Joint Surg 17:91–109, 1935.

49. Smith RJ, Peimer CA: Injuries to the metacarpal bones and joints. Adv Surg 2:341–374, 1977.

50. Spinner M, Choi BY: Anterior dislocations of the proximal interphalangeal joint. A cause of rupture of the central slip of the extensor mechanism. J Bone Joint Surg 52A:1329–1336, 1970.

51. Sprauge B, Justis EJ: Non-union of the carpal navicular: Modes of treatment. Arch Surg 108:692–697, 1974.

52. Stark HH, Boyes JH, Wilson JN: Mallet finger. J Bone Joint Surg 44A:1061–1068, 1962.

53. Stewart MJ: Fractures of the carpal navicular (scaphoid): A report of 436 cases. J Bone Joint Surg 36A:998–1006, 1954.

54. Vaslas A, Grieco RV, Bartone NF: Roentgen aspects of injuries to the pisiform bone and pisotriquetral joint. J Bone Joint Surg 62A:271–276, 1980.

55. Watson HK, Ryu J, DiBella A: J Hand Surg 10A:179–187, 1987.

56. Wehbe MA, Schneider LH: Mallet fractures. J Bone Joint Surg 66A:658–669, 1984.

Chapter 15

REPLANTATIONS AND AMPUTATIONS OF THE UPPER EXTREMITY

Luis R. Scheker, M.D., and David T. Netscher, M.D.

REPLANTATION

The feasibility of limb replantation was demonstrated experimentally as early as 1902, by Carrel,[6] even though his heterotransplant of a kidney from one dog to another ultimately failed. A pioneer of replantation research in the United States, Carrel reported on the replantation of hind legs in dogs and described the triangulation method for connecting small blood vessels.[7] His work was forgotten until 1954, when Lapchinsky in Russia started replanting hind legs of dogs.[28] Snyder, who brought this research to the U.S., outlined indications for replantation in humans.[47]

Further advances awaited new technological developments. In 1956, Barraquer[4] described the use of the microscope in ocular surgery, and by the mid-1960s neurosurgeons were using the dissecting microscope to perform intracranial vascular surgery.

Restoration of circulation to a nonviable upper extremity was first reported by Kleinert and Kasdan[24] in 1963. Shortly thereafter, Malt and McKhann reported successful replantation of a completely amputated arm in a 12-year-old boy.[31] Next, clinical anastomosis (connection) of even smaller vessels was reported, with successful digit revascularization.[25] In 1968, Komatsu and Tamai reported the first successful replantation of an amputated digit by microvascular technique.[26]

Subsequent progress was rapid. Development of precision instruments, microcaliber needles, and nonreactive suture materials paved the way to improved rates of successful replantation.[1,2,40] In a 7-year span reported by Weiland et al.,[62] survival of replanted limbs rose from 32% in 1970 to 74% in 1975 and to more than 90% in 1976. Many centers now report excellent rates of survival for replants (Table 1).

Now that survival of replanted parts can be assured, emphasis has shifted to the important consideration of long-term functional results. Restoration of optimal function requires improved methods of postoperative rehabilitation and judicious use of secondary surgical procedures. Patient selection criteria for replantation also must be more closely scrutinized.

DEFINITIONS

Replantation is reattachment of a part that has been completely amputated. **Revascularization** requires reconstructing vessels in a limb that has been severely injured or incompletely amputated such that vascular repair is necessary to prevent distal necrosis, but some soft tissue (skin, nerves, or tendons) is intact. Revascularization has a generally better success rate than replantation because some of the venous and lymphatic drainage may be intact. However, some revascularizations, such as those

215

TABLE 1. Review of Clinical Survival of Replants

Author	No. Replants (% viable)
Sixth People's Hospital,[46] 1975	320 (54%)
Weiland,[62] 1976	50 (90%)
Tamai,[50] 1978	102 (86%)
Urbaniak,[55] 1979	107 (82%)
Hamilton,[17] 1980	83 (65%)
Schlenker,[44] 1980	51 (71%)
Kleinert,[23] 1980 (upper and lower extremity)	347 (70%)
May,[33] 1982	24 (96%)
Urbaniak,[60] 1985	59 (86%)

involving ring avulsion injuries in which the finger is torn away when a ring is caught on an object, may be extremely difficult and tedious for several reasons: individual teams cannot prepare the parts simultaneously as with complete amputations; both arteries and veins may be severely crushed; and one may be unable to shorten bone, which necessitates interposition of long vein grafts and results in significant problems with soft tissue cover.

Minor replantation is replantation of the wrist, hand, and digits, whereas **major replantation** is that performed proximal to the wrist. This clinical distinction exists because, in the case of major replantations, ischemic time is crucial to functional outcome and viability of muscle. Ischemic muscle may result in myonecrosis, myoglobinemia, and infection, which may threaten the patient's life as well as limb.

Amputation can be classified into three types—guillotine, crush, and avulsion—according to the mechanism of injury. In **guillotine amputations** the tissue is cut by a sharp object and is minimally damaged. Blood vessels and nerve ends can be approximated without using interposition grafts, and the survival rate is greater than 90%.

Crush amputations are of two types—local and diffuse—depending on the size of the contact surface of the compressing object. A crush amputation of the local type can be converted to a guillotine injury simply by debriding back edges of the wound and bone.

Avulsion amputations are the most unfavorable for replanting. Structures are injured at different levels. Extensor tendons are shredded, and flexor tendons often are avulsed at the musculotendinous junctions. Nerves are stretched and may be ripped from end organs. Avulsion injury is often combined with some crushing to the distal amputated part (Fig. 1).

FUNCTIONAL OUTCOME

Measures of Functional Recovery

Sensory recovery has been used as an indication of functional return and is often measured with two-point discrimination, which denotes the distance between two points required for the patient to discern that he is being touched at more than one point. Gelberman et al.[12] found that two-point discrimination in a replanted digit reached normal levels only when pulse pressure in the digit was greater than 85% of pulse pressure in the opposite normal digit. Two-point discrimination was generally worse in replanted digits than in digits with isolated nerve injuries. Schlenker et al.[44] found two-point discrimination of less than 10 mm in only 9 of 20 replanted thumbs.

Evaluation of grip and range of motion also has been used to assess function. Matsuda et al.[32] reported effective recovery of pinch, grip, and sensation in 60% of their replants. Evaluation of thumb replants by Schlenker et al.[44] revealed that average active range of motion for the interphalangeal (IP) joint was 24% of normal, and for the metacarpophalangeal (MCP) joint, 29% of normal.

Numerous standards are used to evaluate functional recovery after replantation. One of the more exhaustive tests of upper extremity function is Carroll's comprehensive quantitative test,[8] which he calls the upper extremity function test. This test uses a series of 33 tasks to measure the patient's ability to perform the general activities of daily living that involve the hand and arm.

Zhong-Wei et al.[65] categorized various levels of functional return following replantation into 4 grades, with grade I representing complete or nearly complete recovery and grade IV representing almost no function (Table 2). Using these grades to classify results of replantation following amputations at different levels, they found that recovery for 32% of patients fell in grade I, 37% in grade II, 28% in grade III, and 3% in grade IV.

Amputation Level and Functional Outcome

It is important to interpret outcome in the context of amputation level. In assessing results of 293 upper extremity replants performed over 20 years, Tamai[51] found that the

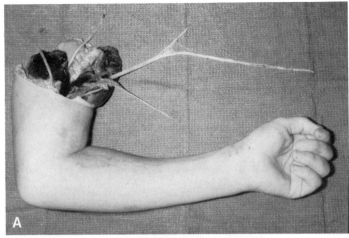

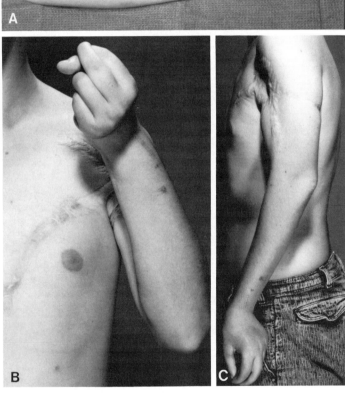

FIGURE 1. *A*, This young man's upper arm was amputated in an agricultural machine resulting in crushed biceps, brachialis, and triceps muscles and extensive nerve avulsion. *B*, Significant shortening of the humerus was needed to achieve direct skin closure and direct contact between vessels and nerves. The nerves present proximally were matched by expected function to those present distally. *C*, A pectoralis muscle transfer was needed to provide elbow flexion because the biceps and brachialis muscles were completely lost. The arm is used as a helper only, but the patient is happy having his own arm.

more distal (farther from the trunk of the body) the replant, the better the functional recovery. In his series, overall good to excellent recovery was achieved in 72% of cases. Percentages of excellent and good recovery respectively were as follows for each anatomic site: arm—0%, 20%; forearm—20%, 30%; hand—20%, 43%; digit—39%, 36%. Russell et al.[43] found a higher percentage (42%) to have good or excellent functional results following major upper limb replantation. All these were guillotine amputations; avulsion and crush amputations of the arm had poor outcomes.

Amputation at the transmetacarpal level can markedly affect function of the hand; however, replantation of transmetacarpal amputations has consistently shown poor functional outcome. For example, transmetacarpal amputation of the index finger has been found to reduce grip strength by 20% and pronation strength by 50%.[38] Usually, intrinsic muscles do not regain function after replantation of a transmetacarpal amputation. Using Carroll's comprehensive quantitative test, Russell et al.[43] reported a series of eight cases in which only three results were fair or better.

Unlike transmetacarpal amputations, amputations of the hand proximal to (closer to the

TABLE 2.   Criteria for Functional Return after Replantation

Grade	Function
I	Able to resume original work, ROM* above 60% of normal, complete or nearly complete recovery of sensation, muscle power grade 4 or 5 on a scale of 1–5.
II	Able to resume some suitable work, ROM above 40% of normal, nearly complete recovery of sensation, muscle power grade 3 or 4.
III	Able to carry on activities of daily life, ROM above 30% of normal, poor but useful recovery of sensation, muscle power grade 3.
IV	Almost no function of viable limb.

Adapted from Zhong-Wei et al.[65]
* ROM, range of motion.

trunk of the body) but near the wrist joint do well (Fig. 2). A retrospective analysis of 49 hand amputations demonstrated that 80% had excellent or good results, falling in Zhong-Wei grades I or II.[34]

Thumb replants usually have good functional outcome because a mobile carpometacarpal joint usually compensates for any lack of motion in the MCP or IP joint.[9] Furthermore, smooth gliding of the flexor pollicis longus tendon is not as crucial to thumb function as is smooth gliding of the long flexor tendons of the finger.

Digital replantations distal to the proximal interphalangeal (PIP) joint also do well. In a series of 24 digits replanted distal to the PIP joint, May et al.[33] found mean active range of motion at the PIP joint of 95 degrees and two-

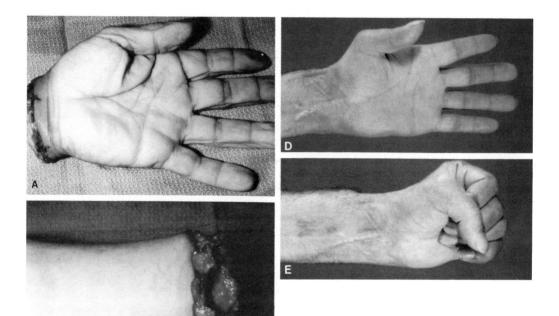

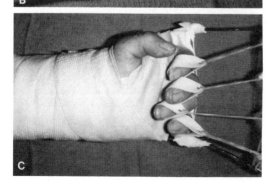

FIGURE 2. *A* and *B*, The left hand of a 41-year-old man was amputated at wrist level by a chain saw used at work. There was very little crush and no avulsion. Minimal bone shortening was required to create a clean amputation. Rigid internal fixation allowed early motion. *C*, An extension block to the MCP joints to prevent clawing and an extensor outrigger to prevent rupture of the extensor tendons were required in the immediate postoperative period. *D* and *E*, Skin closure intercalating a Z-plasty on the volar and dorsal aspects produces a good closure without creating a constriction band. The patient demonstrates excellent range of active motion.

point sensory discrimination of 11 mm. Of 59 single digit replants, Urbaniak et al.[60] found the average range of motion at the PIP joint to be 82 degrees if the amputation was distal to that joint and only 35 degrees if amputation was proximal to it.

In adults as well as children, above-elbow replantation must be considered if there is a reasonable possibility of salvaging a functioning elbow. The functional difference between above-elbow and below-elbow prostheses justifies an attempt at salvage.[53]

Age and Functional Outcome

Children generally have better functional outcome than adults who undergo replantation.[24,25,58,61] Furthermore, in most cases the epiphysis continues to grow after replantation. In children below the age of 8 years, the average increase in bone length achieved during follow-up was 92% of normal.[39]

Comparison of Replantation to Amputation as a Measure of Success

Although the goal of replantation is to return the severed part to normality, it is rarely achieved. The results of replantation should perhaps be judged by comparison with an equivalent level of amputation rather than with the opposite normal extremity. In a study contrasting amputation and replantation, groups of amputation and replantation patients had intensive functional analysis.[21] Patients in the replantation group were unable to work for an average of 104 days after surgery compared to 151 days for patients with amputations. For thumb and multiple finger injuries, grip strength was much greater after replantation than after amputation, but this difference was only marginal in the group with single digit amputations. Functional dexterity scores were much better for thumb replantations than for thumb amputations. Functionally, multiple digit (two or three fingers) and single digit replantations had only a small advantage over amputations in the same categories.

Amputation sometimes carries a risk of specific sequelae that might be avoided with replantation. For example, hyperesthesia or painful sensitivity in the thumb–middle finger web space, which was experienced by 59% of patients, was the most disabling complication of index finger amputation.[38]

INDICATIONS AND CONTRAINDICATIONS FOR REPLANTATION

The viability of a replantation—its ability to survive—must not be construed as a measure of its success and useful function. Replantation may endanger the patient's life in certain circumstances. Replantation has both absolute and relative contraindications.

Absolute Contraindications

The following are strong contraindications to replant surgery at any level of amputation.

Significant concomitant life-threatening injury. Life-threatening injury is more commonly associated with major limb amputations than with more distal injuries.[65]

Severe chronic illness that precludes transportation or prolonged surgery. Chronic illness is not as critical in replantation of digits because ischemia time, which is the length of time without blood supply, is less crucial and surgery can be performed with the use of local or regional anesthesia.

Extensive injury to the affected limb or amputated part. Extensive injury includes multiple level amputations, widespread crush, severely mangled injuries, and amputation of a poorly functioning, previously injured digit. In a badly mutilated digit, the distal pulp may be replanted on the stump, even though the rest of the digit is discarded. This provides adequate soft tissue cover and prevents formation of painful neuromas (tumors largely composed of nerve cells and fibers) by repairing the digital nerves. Replantation of soft tissue that ordinarily would have been discarded also salvages length and provides good protective cover of the stump following major limb amputation.

Other Factors

Other factors must be considered, including ischemia, the part affected, and patient considerations.

Ischemic Time. For amputated digits, more than 12 hours of warm ischemia is a relative contraindication for replantation.[23] Promptly cooling the part to 4–10°C dramatically alters the ischemia factor so that even ischemia exceeding 24 hours does not preclude successful replantation. Ischemic time is more crucial for replants above the proximal forearm. Increasing leakage of muscle enzymes (creatine phosphokinase, serum glutamate oxaloacetate transaminase) has been noted after 6 hours of ischemia in the replanted dog hind limb, even with cooling.[37] Extensive cellular damage also was noted on routine histological examination and this correlated with serum enzyme levels. Replantation of upper extremities amputated proximal to the midforearm has been said to be contraindicated if warm ischemia time exceeds 6 hours.[64] However, in our experience, parts with a mean ischemic time of 10 hours have survived with favorable outcome in more than 30 major replantations.

Affected Parts. Good candidates for replantation are amputations of the thumb, amputations of multiple digits, and amputations through the palm, wrist, and individual fingers distal to the insertion of the flexor digitorum superficialis tendon. Because function of the thumb accounts for 40% of total hand function, almost all amputated thumbs should be replanted, with care taken to preserve the length of the thumb (Fig. 3). Replantation should be considered in cases involving even the most distal thumb amputations.

Controversy surrounds replantation of single digits and of complete ring avulsion injuries. We believe that reattachment of a single amputated finger should not be universally condemned. As indicated previously, excellent functional potential is possible for replants distal to the flexor digitorum superficialis tendon. To achieve good functional outcome, a reasonable flexion arc is required for the middle, ring, and little fingers, which are involved in power grasp. Working against the palm, they form the basic unit of power grasp. In contrast, the index finger functions primarily in conjunction with the thumb pad to achieve precision pinch; therefore, good flexion arc is much less critical in the index finger. Thus, replantation of an index finger proximal to the insertion of the flexor digitorum superficialis tendon results in a more functional hand than amputation.

When all four fingers are amputated proximally to the insertion of the flexor digitorum superficialis tendon, at least two fingers should be reattached, usually at the index and middle positions. If only one of four amputated fingers can be replanted, it is probably best to place

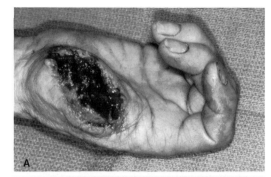

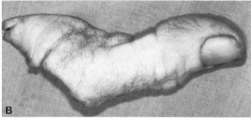

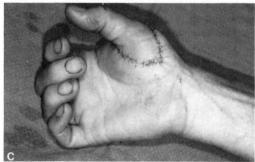

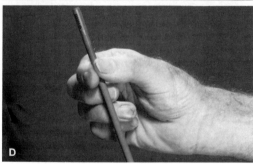

FIGURE 3. *A* and *B*, A 51-year-old man sustained an amputation of his right thumb by a table saw in a work-related injury. Replantation of an amputated thumb should always be attempted because of the importance of the digit. *C*, The MCP joint was destroyed, and primary fusion was necessary. Primary repair of all involved structures was obtained. *D*, In spite of a fused MCP joint, the patient recovered excellent function in his dominant hand.

it in the middle finger position. This will provide some depth to the first web space. Because recovery of a functional flexion arc is not assured, replantation in a position ulnar to the middle finger may not permit contact with the thumb. It is not unusual to transpose replanted digits. For example, it may be functionally prudent to replant an amputated fingertip on a partially amputated thumb to restore length to the thumb.

Replantation of complete ring avulsion degloving injuries, in which the skin is torn from the amputated digit, is controversial.[5] These are class III injuries according to the classification of Urbaniak et al.[59] We have had favorable functional results with replantation of such injuries.[53] Usually the skin injury is at the PIP joint level, and bony amputation is at the distal interphalangeal (DIP) joint level. If the bony amputation is distal to the PIP joint and the flexor digitorum superficialis tendon is functional, microsurgical repair is the treatment of choice. If the PIP joint is damaged, completion of the amputation is performed.

Patient Considerations.   The decision to replant a single digit proximal to the insertion of the flexor digitorum superficialis tendon is influenced by special circumstances, such as a patient who is a young woman, a violinist, or a pianist. Not only are occupation and sex important considerations, but so are the patient's age, mental health, and even nationality. In a child, an attempt should be made to replant almost any amputated body part because useful function usually can be anticipated. Because the child's eventual vocation is unknown and may require all the digits that can be saved, even single digit replantation proximal to insertion of the flexor digitorum superficialis tendon must be undertaken. Old age is usually not a barrier to replantation, provided the vessels are not seen to be atherosclerotic when examined under the microscope and the patient is in good health.

Replantation in mentally unstable patients is usually not undertaken, although mental stability is frequently difficult to assess in the limited time available for preoperative evaluation. Patients who are mentally unstable often are unable to follow through with the therapy required after replantation.

Concerning issues of culture, Tamai,[50] working with Japanese patients, generally replants single digits when wound conditions are favorable and if the patient desires, because absence of a single digit in Japanese patients may label them as gangsters.

PERTINENT ANATOMY

Vessel Size

Comparative vessel diameters for adults and children are shown in Table 3. Although it has been stated that replantation in children is less frequently successful than in adults (largely owing to the small caliber of vessels),[56] with current instrumentation there is probably very little difference in survival rates of replants in children and adults. Kleinert and his group[20] achieved 100% survival of replants at the middle phalangeal level and 80% survival of replants at DIP joint level in children under 16 years of age.

The Palm

The anatomy of the palm creates problems in replantation. If the superficial palmar arch is destroyed by the injury, its reconstruction may require a vein graft with multiple side branches, for which the dorsal venous arch of the foot is ideally suited. Revascularization of the common digital vessels may create retrograde flow in the volar metacarpal vessels, which should be ligated to prevent bleeding into the palm and formation of postoperative hematoma.[30]

The metabolic requirement of intrinsic muscles at this level limit the period of warm ischemia that can be tolerated. Necrosis of these muscles due to ischemia or direct trauma necessitates debridement that further limits muscle function. As a result, a hand replanted at this level frequently maintains the intrinsic minus posture.

In the unusual circumstances in which hemodynamic instability of the patient or prolonged anesthesia precludes formal reconstruction of the superficial palmar vascular arch, establishing circulation through a single common digital vessel may provide blood flow to all fingers.[52] Transverse commissural vessels connect ulnar and radial digital vessels just proximal to the PIP and DIP joints. Retrograde

TABLE 3.   Comparative Diameter (mm) at Different Levels of Digital Artery in a 4-Year-Old Child and an Adult

	Child	Adult
MCP joint	0.7	1.0
PIP joint	0.4	0.7
DIP joint	0.2	0.4

blood flow to adjacent common digital vessels then revascularizes adjacent digits.

Venous Anatomy

Reestablishing venous outflow is frequently difficult, partly because of problems in locating suitable veins. An excellent anatomical study of the venous system of the hand[36] shows three dorsal digital venous arches, each connected by longitudinal veins. Valves direct flow from distal to proximal, from radial to ulnar, within the dorsal arches, and from palmar to dorsal surfaces at the level of the MCP joints. In addition, in the distal part of the digit, veins are located principally in the volar pulp.

Arterial Anatomy of the Thumb

Locating vessels for anastomosis may be confusing in thumb replants. In 20% of thumbs, the superficial palmar vessels contribute significantly to circulation. However, in no case do arteries of the thumb originate exclusively from the superficial arch.[42] In 15% of thumbs, the first dorsal metacarpal artery is the main artery to the thumb rather than the princeps pollicis artery, which is the first palmar metacarpal artery given off as the radial artery emerges in the palm. In 90% of hands, the ulnopalmar digital artery is larger than the radial side and is the more important of the two for anastomosis.[11]

TECHNIQUE OF REPLANTATION

Many factors affect the treatment options available to a patient with a traumatic amputation affecting the upper extremity. The first aid the person receives immediately following injury, the care given the amputated part, and the timing of treatment are critical.

First Aid after Traumatic Amputation

Care of the Injured Person. The affected extremity should be cleaned as much as possible, and a compressive dressing should be applied to the wound. While waiting for transport to the facility that will evaluate the patient for replantation, the patient should be treated according to the general principles of wound management. Tetanus toxoid should be administered, and the patient's body fluids should be replenished with intravenous injection of lactated Ringer's solution. If a large vessel has been damaged in the injury, a 16-gauge intravenous cannula should be placed in the noninjured extremity to permit rapid replacement of fluids if required later. If possible, an x-ray of the injured extremity and amputated part should be taken and sent with the patient.

The referring physician should provide the following information to the staff at the facility where the patient will be evaluated for replantation: the level of amputation (parts affected), the mechanism of injury, the condition of the part, the patient's age (both chronological and physical), diseases or conditions, any medications the patient is taking, general health, occupation, and smoking history. The latter is especially important since smoking is the leading cause of thrombosis in the replanted part in the second to third week after replantation. Patients are asked to quit smoking for 6 weeks after replantation; if the patient is unwilling to agree to this, replantation may not be advisable.

Care of the Amputated Part. Before transportation, the amputated part should be placed inside a clean, dry plastic bag that is sealed and placed on top of melting ice in a container, preferably a styrofoam cooler (Fig. 4). This keeps the part sufficiently cool at the optimal temperature (4–10°C) without freezing. The part should not touch the ice directly. Dry ice should *not* be used. The amount of ice should be increased for larger parts (such as a hand or arm) so that the temperature of the part can be lowered quickly.

Timing is one of the most important factors in the success of replantation. Timing is especially crucial for more proximal amputations because the larger the muscle mass in the amputated part, the shorter the period of ischemia it can tolerate. Occupational physicians and other medical personnel can save valuable time by acquainting themselves with the closest medical facilities that can perform replantations before the need to refer a patient with a traumatic amputation arises.

After Arrival at the Hospital. The patient's time in the emergency room should be as short as possible, only long enough to evaluate vital signs and determine whether the patient is fit for surgery. The amputated part should be sent immediately to the operating room for preparation. The patient should be taken to the operating room as quickly as possible.

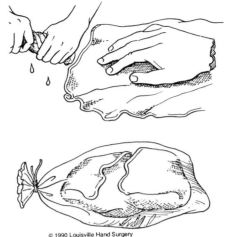

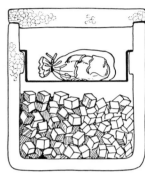

FIGURE 4. An amputated part should be placed in moistened clean gauze and sealed inside a clean plastic bag, which is placed in a styrofoam cooler, not in direct contact with ice.

© 1990 Louisville Hand Surgery

To save time and thus minimize the period of ischemia for the amputated part, replantation typically uses two teams of surgeons. One team evaluates the condition of the part and identifies vessels, tendons, and other structures; the second team evaluates the patient's condition and prepares the stump.

After considering the condition of the part, the patient's condition and wishes, and the likelihood of functional recovery, the decision whether to replant the part or revise the amputation is made. Functional recovery—rather than survival—is the key consideration. The expense of replantation surgery and the time required for the patient to recover are pointless concerns if the replanted part will not regain a useful degree of function.

Surgical Procedures

Microsurgical Instruments. A variety of new and expensive microinstruments are on the market. However, the instrumentation can be kept quite simple. Our small instrument set consists of four jeweler's forceps, one pair of microadventitia scissors, one pair of microsuture scissors, one spring-loaded needle driver, a double clamp, and various sizes of single microclamps.

A hand or microsurgery microscope is used. These differ from an ear, nose, and throat microscope in that the field is viewed at a 90-degree angle (Fig. 5). To allow ample space to use surgical instruments, the lower part of the lens should be no closer than 20 cm to the part undergoing surgery. Microscopes that allow the surgeon to adjust position and change the field of vision quickly, without assistance, are best.

Order of and Procedures for Repair. The order in which structures are repaired depends on circumstances. Usually, two teams identify neurovascular structures in both the amputation stump and the distal part. Next, bone shortening allows skin to be debrided back to where it is free of contusion and where direct tension-free closure can be achieved. In the thumb, bone shortening should be minimized to less than 10 mm[15] and to removal of only the amount of bone necessary to achieve skin closure and allow direct nerve repair.[15] Vein grafts are preferable to excessive bone shortening when repairing vessel damage in the thumb.[9]

It has been suggested that neurovascular structures be exposed through midlateral incisions. However, we use Bruner incisions. Subsequent skin closure can be done as a Z-plasty, which prevents cicatricial narrowing (scarring) at the site of skin closure.

The order of repair is usually bone, tendons and muscle units, arteries, nerves, and finally veins. Our favored methods of bony fixation are either by an oblique Kirschner wire and an intraosseous wire[29] or by 90-90 intraosseous wires.[66] Single or double longitudinal Kirschner wires may be more suitable for bony fixation in more distal replants.

In replanting the proximal portion of a digit, preplacing the sutures in the free tendon ends may help speed up the tendon repair because the surgeon only needs to knot the ends of the sutures. Once neurovascular repairs are completed, tendon ends are coapted by the Tajima method[48] (Fig. 6). In this way, the digit is easily held in extension to expose neurovascular structures on the volar surface.

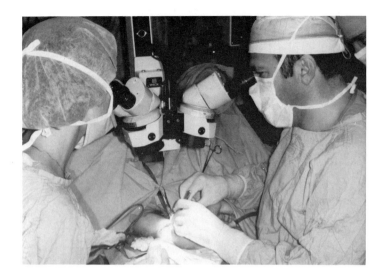

FIGURE 5. The operating microscope used in hand surgery requires ample space between the operative field and the lens. The eyepiece needs to be in a 90-degree angle with the lens and the operative field.

Establishing arterial flow before venous flow clears lactic acid from the replanted part. In addition, this procedure more clearly outlines the venous network. The most functional veins can be detected by their spurting backflow. With this approach, however, blood loss must be closely monitored, especially in children and patients undergoing multidigit replants. Tension-free repair is essential to maintain patency of venous anastomoses. Ligation of the side branches of veins may be necessary to increase mobility of the vessel and achieve extra length (Fig. 7). Should this maneuver fail to provide sufficient length to obtain tension-free anastomosis, vein grafts must be harvested for use in the replanted part.[57]

The order of repair of structures is altered for replants at the distal phalanx. In these cases, a longitudinal Kirschner wire is first driven antegrade through the distal part. Skin closure along the volar aspect enables the two parts to be held open like a book. Artery and nerve repairs are then performed, followed by completion of retrograde Kirschner wire placement. Venous repair may be difficult in these distal replants. Veins are located on the volar aspect of the digit. Failure to locate veins may necessitate recourse to one of three alternatives: (1) anastomosis of one distal artery (which has back flow) to a proximal vein, (2) use of medical grade leeches, or (3) removal of the nail plate and subsequent scraping of the raw nail bed with a heparin-soaked cotton pledget every 2 hours.[15]

In thumb replantation, preliminary anastomosis of vein grafts to the distal digital vessels of an amputated thumb greatly simplifies po-

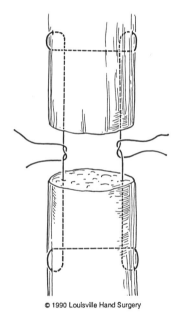

© 1990 Louisville Hand Surgery

FIGURE 6. Use of the Tajima suture saves time in tendon repair during finger replantation. Half of the suture is placed in the recipient tendon and the other half in the amputated part. Tying the knots is the only step required for repair of the tendon(s).

sitioning of the hand under the microscope.[45] Osteosynthesis is then performed, followed by anastomosis of the proximal end of the vein graft in an end-to-side fashion into the radial artery at the "anatomic snuff-box."

Occasionally, in addition to replantation of an amputated part, soft tissue cover is needed, which may require a free tissue transfer. The free tissue transfer may even be used as a conduit to supply vessels to the distal replanted

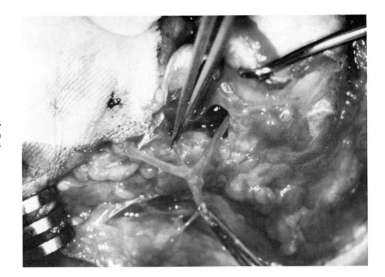

FIGURE 7. Ligation of side branches of arteries or veins allows mobilization of these vessels, which are relatively lengthened.

structures. The lateral arm flap is ideally suited because its large-diameter through-flow artery traverses the full length of the flap. Soft tissue cover also may be required to salvage more distal replants. With ring avulsion injuries, the ring frequently gouges into the dorsal skin. A reverse cross-finger flap[3] may solve the problem, providing both soft tissue cover and dorsal veins for outflow. Venous flaps may be used to salvage replants either in the acute situation, where swelling prevents dorsal skin closure, or in the subacute situation, when the patient with a failing replant is returned to the operating room for reexploration.[19,54]

For major replantation, reestablishing arterial circulation as rapidly as possible is crucial to limiting ischemia time.[41] Insertion of a shunt between the arterial ends enables circulation to be reestablished and lactic acid to be washed out while debridement continues. A Scrivner dialysis shunt or Javid carotid shunt is ideally suited. Blood loss must be closely monitored, and intermittent clamping of the shunt may be necessary. In the upper extremity, bone shortening can be aggressive to achieve primary skin closure and primary nerve repair.

In unusual situations, ectopic implantation of undamaged parts may be required. An example would be a bilateral amputation where the distal part of only one limb is well preserved but the proximal stump is so mutilated as to preclude ipsilateral replantation. In such circumstances, replantation to the opposite side is indicated. Temporary ectopic implantation of a hand in the axilla while the proximal stump is prepared for receipt of the distal undamaged part has also been described.[13]

Intravenous Fluids and Irrigation Solutions. It is our practice to administer an intravenous solution of low molecular weight dextran (LMD) and heparin (5000 units of heparin mixed with 500 cc of LMD). A bolus dose of 100 ml is given before completing the first arterial anastomosis and then maintenance of 30 ml per hour is continued into the postoperative period. We believe this regimen minimizes clotting problems and allows judicious use of tourniquets for ease of microvascular anastomoses and reduction of blood loss. Topical application of 2% lidocaine or papaverine may help relieve vasospasm.

Dressing. The postoperative dressing serves three purposes: (1) absorption of drainage, (2) protection, and (3) palliation of pain.[27] Longitudinal strips of nonadherent fine-mesh gauze are applied over suture lines to avoid constriction from a circular dressing. Loose fluff gauze or sterile dacron batting is placed around the hand, and replanted parts are left exposed for clinical examination. The entire extremity is then surrounded by foam sponge sheeting, over which plaster is applied extending from above the elbow to beyond the fingertips. This cast usually remains in place for 5–10 days (Fig. 8).

POSTOPERATIVE MANAGEMENT

Immediate Postoperative Care

Extremity Elevation and Ancillary Precautions. Postoperative elevation is important in minimizing edema and venous congestion.

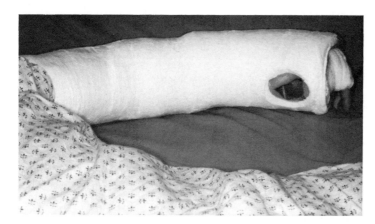

FIGURE 8. Replantation dressings require immobilization of the elbow and should cover the amputated part, allowing access for monitoring.

However, excessive elevation may decrease tissue perfusion and tissue oxygen levels. The patient must be kept well hydrated. We also keep the patient's room comfortably warm and permit no use of caffeine or tobacco. Smoking, particularly, has been shown to have a deleterious effect on replant survival.[18]

Postoperative Medications. Perioperative antibiotics (usually cephazolin or cephamandol) are used as an adjunct to surgical debridement.[16] Narcotic analgesics are titrated to a dose that keeps the patient comfortable. This helps eliminate pain-induced anxiety that may led to vasospasm. Chlorpromazine (10 mg orally, three times per day) helps alleviate anxiety and also causes vasodilation.[57]

For our replant patients, the intravenous solution of LMD and heparin is continued for 5 days and then tapered off. We usually also give one baby aspirin (80 mg) per day. Acetylsalicylic acid in this dose retards synthesis of thromboxane A_2, resulting in inhibition of platelet aggregation.[63] Aspirin should be continued for at least 5 days—the length of time required for smooth endothelium to line the vessel anastomosis.

Postoperative Monitoring. A key to survival of replants is early recognition of vascular compromise and reexploration. The replant is observed hourly for the first 24 hours. Color, pulp turgor, and capillary refill are the most helpful signs, although these are difficult to observe in patients with dark skin. We have found skin temperature to be a reliable and inexpensive method of monitoring replants.[48] If digital temperature remains higher than 31°C, problems are rarely encountered. Abrupt decrease in temperature of more than 2.5°C usually is associated with arterial compromise. Replants with sustained temperatures below 30°C have a poor prognosis.

Reexploration. Of replantations that fail, 50% fail within 72 hours and the remainder within 10 days.[23] If vascular problems are encountered in the first 3 or 4 days, reexploration is likely to be helpful. After that time, operative intervention is disappointing. For the first 24 hours after replantation surgery, patients are usually given nothing or only clear liquids by mouth, in case reexploration is required. A salvage rate of 60–70% usually can be achieved with the use of vein grafts if the vascular problem is detected early enough.[35]

Management after Discharge

The patient is usually discharged on postoperative day 5 after minor replantation. The need for continued elevation and avoidance of cold, caffeine, and nicotine is reinforced. The first dressing change is usually done between 5 and 10 days after injury. A volar plaster slab is used to maintain the hand in the safe, intrinsic plus position. With rigid internal fixation, we have more recently started protected rubber band mobilization at a progressively earlier time—sometimes as early as 2 days after surgery. If the MCP joints are held in flexion, dynamic extension traction occurs at the PIP joint and is not transmitted directly to the flexor tendon.

Physical Therapy. Physical therapy usually starts 48–72 hours after replantation. The first 3 weeks of physical therapy focus on controlling edema and initiating motion[22] to keep the joint supple. Passive range of motion exercises and early assisted active muscle contraction can usually be started after the first week.

After 3 weeks, once wounds are healed and vascularity is assured, edema can be more effectively controlled by retrograde massage and wrapping the amputated part in Coban, an elastic wrap used to control edema. Active range of motion exercises can be performed more vigorously at this stage. Static splinting is continued at night for protection and joint positioning. Later, if the patient reports development of paresthesias (abnormal sensations), a sensory re-education program is instituted.[10]

From 6 weeks on, physical therapy focuses on regaining range of motion and strength. After 8 weeks, progressive resistive exercises may begin.

Secondary Surgical Procedures. After 4 months, the rate of collagen deposition starts to decrease. At this stage the surgeon can start to determine if further surgical intervention is necessary. If progress with physical therapy reaches a plateau that still falls short of anticipated outcome, surgery is performed. The most common procedures required are surgery to tendons (tenolysis, tendon grafting, or tendon transfers), joints (capsulotomy, capsulodesis, joint replacement or fusion), skin (scar contracture revision), bone (fixation or grafting for malunion or nonunion), and nerves (neurolysis, nerve grafting).

Thumb Reconstruction. Because of the thumb's importance to hand function, in cases where the thumb cannot be replanted because of damage to the part, reconstruction should be considered. A number of methods are available to reconstruct the thumb including pollicization of another digit, osteoplastic thumb reconstruction, and toe-to-thumb transfer.

Pollicization entails moving another digit, often the index finger, to the thumb position. Although it is not indicated in heavy laborers because it narrows the span of the hand and reduces power grip, pollicization works well for other workers and for children.

With osteoplastic reconstruction of the thumb, a bone graft covered with a tube of skin is used to reconstruct the thumb. Usually a neurovascular island flap from the ring finger or the ulnar side of the long finger is used to provide sensation. The reconstructed thumb lacks a nail. This method of reconstruction is not considered cosmetically acceptable for some patients.

A more accepted method of reconstruction involves transfer of a big toe or second toe to the thumb position. For heavy laborers, transfer of the big toe provides greater grip and pinch strength (Fig. 9). The disadvantage is that the donor site is more noticeable than with transfer of the second toe. Also, care must be

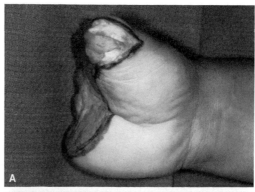

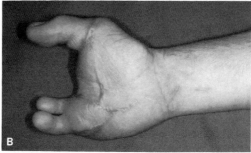

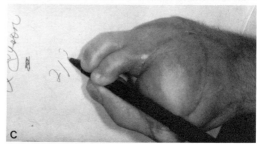

FIGURE 9. *A,* When amputated parts are not replantable, severe disability occurs, especially when the amputation is transmetacarpal. In the dominant hand, reconstruction is mandatory and can be achieved by multiple toe transfers. *B,* A big toe is transferred from one foot and two toes from the other foot to allow pinch and a limited grasp. *C,* After sensation is recovered, the patient is able to write with the reconstructed hand.

taken to avoid transferring too much skin from the base of the big toe. Insufficient skin coverage can cause breakdown at the donor site.

Transfer of the second toe (Fig. 10) is less traumatic at the donor site, but pinch and grip are not as strong as with big toe transfer. This option may be a good choice for workers who do not perform heavy labor.

Another procedure uses a wrap-around flap of skin and nail from the big toe to cover the existing bone or a bone graft taken from the iliac crest or from the second toe. The vascularized flap can be tailored surgically to look very much like the normal thumb. Sensation

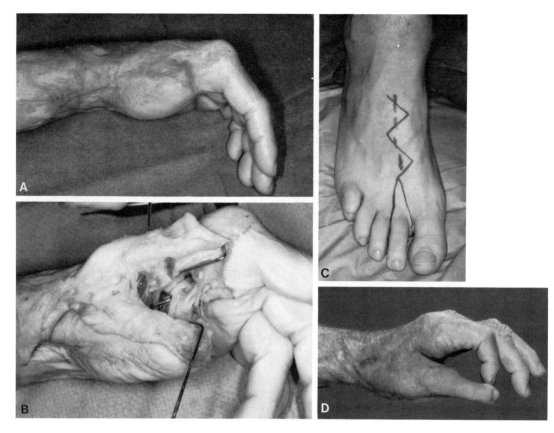

FIGURE 10. A, This is the only hand of a 42-year-old man who was involved in a fire accident. He lost his right arm and sustained severe burns over 60% of his body. The web space is narrow and lacks adequate skin cover to allow toe transfer. B, The first web space was opened, and a lateral arm flap was performed to cover the defect. The space was kept open by a W-shaped wire. C and D, The second toe from his right foot was transferred with a satisfactory result.

is as good as with toe-to-hand transfer, and deformity in the donor site is minimal.

Some of these procedures for thumb reconstruction are not recommended for certain patients. For people who are concerned about the appearance of the foot, a second toe transfer is likely to be a better option than big toe transfer or a wrap-around flap from the big toe. Patients with diabetes mellitus are not good candidates for toe-to-thumb transfer—especially transfer of the big toe—because of difficulty in healing at the donor site.

Possible Long-Term Sequelae. After successful replantation, some long-term problems include stiffness, cold intolerance, dysesthesia, hyperesthesia, and pain. In some cases, stiffness is hard to overcome even with the most intensive physical therapy. The difficulty may stem from the patient's lack of compliance with early stages of the therapy regimen, or it may relate to the injury. In the latter circumstances, although the muscle unit survived, dense fibrosis may contract the muscle so that it does not slide well. In this case, the hand may be used as a sensate post, or if the hand has crude pinch or grip, it can serve as a "helping hand."

With cold intolerance, the patient experiences pain when the replanted part is exposed, unprotected, to cold. The condition results from the process of reinnervation as much as from vascular insufficiency. This sensitivity usually disappears in the first 2 years following replantation.

Problems with sensation may include dysesthesia, which is abnormal sensation produced by normal stimuli, and hyperesthesia, which is increased sensitivity. Both conditions can be treated with a physical therapy program of sensory re-education, which is most effective when begun before sensation reaches the most distal portion of the replanted part.

When intractable pain persists following replantation, it often can be attributed to the mechanism of injury that has damaged the nerve proximal to the replanted part. If use of a trans-cutaneous electrical nerve stimulation (TENS) unit, which uses electrical impulses to block pain, is not sufficient, the patient should be referred to a pain clinic. In cases where the pain stems from nerve injury proximal to the replanted part, even reamputation is not likely to alleviate the pain.

AMPUTATION

Amputation should not be considered an old-fashioned operation. Rather, it is a necessary procedure in cases where replantation is not indicated because of the condition of the part, the functional prognosis, or the patient's inability or unwillingness to follow through with the treatment and therapy required after replantation.

SURGICAL PROCEDURE

When primary amputation is performed, the stump should be preserved with as much length as possible. With amputations below the elbow, preservation of a functioning elbow joint and stump distal to the elbow permits the use of a below-the-elbow prosthesis, which is more functional than an above-the-elbow prosthesis. Free flaps from the amputated part can be used to cover the stump adequately.

The ends of cut nerves should be buried deep in the muscle at the midshaft level to help reduce the likelihood of painful neuromas. Because these nonmalignant tumors that form at the ends of cut nerves are mainly painful with pressure or contact, placing nerve ends in positions of least contact or pressure can prevent problems with pain. Placing the cut nerve end close to a joint or at the end of the stump virtually guarantees pain from neuromas.

The stump should be surgically shaped in a cone so that it fits a prosthesis.

POSTOPERATIVE MANAGEMENT

Immediate Care. The affected limb is elevated, and a compressive dressing is applied to minimize edema in the stump and to help shape the stump into a cone that will fit a prosthesis after the stump heals. The patient must be kept well hydrated. If flaps have been used

to cover the stump, they must be monitored by photoplethysmography every hour for the first 48 hours for signs of vascular compromise due to venous or arterial thrombosis. The interval for monitoring is gradually increased until day 5–7 after surgery.

Perioperative antibiotics are used, and narcotic analgesics are titrated to a dose that keeps the patient comfortable.

Prostheses. To help prepare the patient for a prosthesis, a cast shaped to fit the stump may be worn after the patient leaves the hospital. Some prostheses are functional, others are primarily cosmetic. Functional prostheses include a simple hook, a cable-powered prosthesis operated by movement of the shoulder and/or elbow, and the myoelectric arm (Fig. 11). The latter is not widely used because it requires frequent repairs. Patients can be fitted with one of these prostheses once all wounds are healed and swelling has settled. Depending on the patient's age and the type of prosthesis, the time required to learn to use the device can range from 3 weeks to 2 months. Cosmetic prostheses have no function other than hiding the amputation, which is important to some patients, especially if their work demands frequent contact with people.

Possible Long-Term Sequelae. Problems with pain may follow amputation, including phantom pain and painful neuromas. The origin of phantom pain, which is pain perceived as originating in an absent limb, is poorly understood.

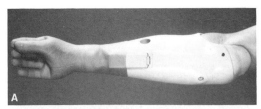
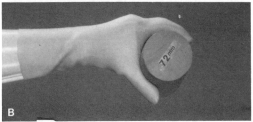

FIGURE 11. A and B, Myoelectric prostheses are functional and cosmetically pleasing. Some of the disadvantages are a high breakage rate, high cost, and small number of servicing facilities. The patient must use sight to compensate for the lack of sensation.

Prevention of painful neuromas is far preferable to available treatment. As discussed under "Surgical Procedure" above, placement of the cut nerve end deep in the muscle can prevent pain from neuromas. There are multiple forms of treatment for painful neuromas. In our experience, the only effective treatment is neuroma transposition.

CONCLUSION

Considerable progress has been made in the 27 years since Malt and colleagues performed the first successful replantation. Improved instrumentation has led to better survival. We can now also anticipate better functional results as a consequence of improved postoperative management, institution of early protected motion, and more rational patient selection criteria. Judicious use of free tissue transfers in association with replantation as well as late reconstructive surgery also have led to overall functional improvement.

Editor's Comment

This chapter by Drs. Scheker and Netscher is excellent. They paint an optimistic picture for replantation. The reader is cautioned, however, that their optimism is not universally accepted. Other views worth reading are those of Paul W. Brown in "Detachment about Reattachment" in *Controversies in Hand Surgery*, edited by R. T. Neviaser, published in 1990 by Churchill Livingstone, and William L. White, in "Why I Hate the Index Finger" *Orthopaedic Review* 9:23–29, 1980. Replantation should not be just a technical exercise. The entire patient must be considered. — MLK

REFERENCES

1. Acland R: A new needle for microvascular surgery. Surgery 71:130, 1972.
2. Acland R: A flat-bodied needle for microvascular surgery. Plast Reconstr Surg 61:793, 1978.
3. Atasoy E: Reversed cross-finger subcutaneous flap. J Hand Surg 7:481, 1982.
4. Barraquer JI: The microscope in ocular surgery. Am J Ophthalmol 43:6, 1956.
5. Burkhalter WE: Ring avulsion injuries: Care of amputated parts, replants and revascularization. Emerg Med Clin North Am 3:365, 1985.
6. Carrel A: The operative technique of vascular anastomosis and the transplantation of viscera. Med Lyon 98:859, 1902 (Engl. tr. in Clin Orthop 29:3, 1963).
7. Carrel A, Guthrie CC: Results of a replantation of a thigh. Science 23:393, 1906.
8. Carroll D: A quantitative test for upper extremity function. J Chronic Dis 18:479, 1965.
9. Chow JA, Bilos ZJ, Chunprapaph B: Thirty thumb replantations. Indications and results. Plast Reconstr Surg 64:626, 1979.
10. Dellon AL, Curtis RM, Edgerton MT: Re-education of sensation in the hand after nerve injury and repair. Plast Reconstr Surg 53:297, 1974.
11. Earley MJ: Blood supply of the thumb. J Hand Surg 11B:163, 1986.
12. Gelberman RH, Urbaniak JR, Bright DS, et al: Digital sensibility following replantation. J Hand Surg 3:313, 1978.
13. Godina M, Bajec J, Baraga A: Salvage of the mutilated upper extremity with temporary ectopic implantation of the undamaged part. Plast Reconstr Surg 78:295, 1986.
14. Gordan L: Microsurgical Reconstruction of the Extremities: Indications, Technique and Postoperative Care. New York, Springer-Verlag, 1988, ch 5.
15. Gordan L, Leitner DW, Buncke HK, et al: Partial nail plate removal after digital replantation as an alternative method of venous drainage. J Hand Surg 10A:360, 1985.
16. Gustilo RB, Anderson JT: Prevention of infection in the treatment of one thousand and twenty five open fractures of long bones. J Bone Joint Surg 58A:453, 1976.
17. Hamilton RB, O'Brien BM: Replantation and revascularization of digits. Surg Gynecol Obstet 151:508, 1980.
18. Harris GD, Finseth F, Buncke HJ: The hazard of cigarette smoking following digital replantation. J Microsurg 1:403, 1980.
19. Honda T, Nomura S, Tamauchi S, et al: The possible applications of a composite skin and subcutaneous vein graft in the replantation of amputated digits. Br J Plast Surg 37:607, 1984.
20. Jaeger SH, Tsai TM, Kleinert HE: Upper extremity replantation in children. Orthop Clin North Am 12:897, 1981.
21. Jones JM, Schenck RR, Chesney RB: Digital replantation and amputation—Comparison of function. J Hand Surg 7:183, 1982.
22. Kader PB: Therapist's management of the replanted hand. Hand Clin 2:179, 1986.
23. Kleinert HE, Jablon M, Tsai TM: An overview of replantation and results of 347 replants in 245 patients. J Trauma 20:390, 1980.
24. Kleinert HE, Kasdan ML: Restoration of blood flow in upper extremity injuries. J Trauma 3:461, 1963.
25. Kleinert HE, Kasdan ML: Anastomosis of digital vessels. J Ky Med Assoc 63:106, 1965.
26. Komatsu S, Tamai S: Successful replantation of a completely cut-off thumb. Plast Reconstr Surg 42:374, 1968.
27. Kutz JE, Hanel D, Scheker LR, et al: Upper extremity replantation. Orthop Clin North Am 14:873, 1983.
28. Lapchinsky AG: Recent results of experimental transplantation of preserved limbs and kidneys and possible use of this technique in clinical practice. Ann NY Acad Sci 87:539–571, 1960.
29. Lister GD: Intraosseous wiring of the digital skeleton. J Hand Surg 3:427, 1978.
30. Lister GD, Kleinert HE: Replantation. In Grabb WC, Smith JW (eds): Plastic Surgery, 3rd ed. Boston, Little Brown, 1979.

31. Malt RA, McKhann CF: Replantation of severed arms. JAMA 189:716, 1964.
32. Matsuda M, Shibahara H, Kato N: Long-term results of replantation of ten upper extremities. World J Surg 2:603, 1978.
33. May JW, Toth RA, Gardner M: Digital replantation distal to the proximal interphalangeal joint. J Hand Surg 7:161, 1982.
34. Meyer VE: Hand amputations proximal but close to the wrist joint. Prime candidates for reattachment (long-term functional results). J Hand Surg 10A:989, 1985.
35. Monteim MS, Chacon NE: Salvage of replanted parts of the upper extremity. J Bone Joint Surg 67A:880, 1985.
36. Moss SH, Schwartz KS, von Drasek-Ascher G, et al: Digital venous anatomy. J Hand Surg 10A:473, 1985.
37. Muramatsu I, Takahata N, Usui M, et al: Metabolic and histologic changes in the ischemic muscles of replanted dog legs. Clin Orthop 196:292, 1985.
38. Murray JF, Carman W, MacKenzie JK: Transmetacarpal amputation of the index finger: A clinical assessment of hand strength and complications. J Hand Surg 2:471, 1977.
39. Nunley JA, Spiegl PV, Goldner RD, et al: Longitudinal epiphyseal growth after replantation and transplantation in children. J Hand Surg 12A:274, 1987.
40. O'Brien BM, Hayhurst JW: Metallized microsutures and a new micro needle holder. Plast Reconstr Surg 52:673, 1973.
41. O'Brien BM, Macleod AM, Hayhurst JW, et al: Major replantation surgery in the upper limb. Hand 6:217, 1974.
42. Parks BJ, Arbelaez J, Horner RL: Medical and surgical importance of the arterial blood supply of the thumb. J Hand Surg 3:383, 1978.
43. Russell RC, O'Brien BM, Morrison WA, et al: The late functional results of upper limb revascularization and replantation. J Hand Surg 9A:623, 1984.
44. Schlenker JD, Kleinert HE, Tsai TM: Methods and results of replantation following traumatic amputation of the thumb in sixty-four patients. J Hand Surg 5:63, 1980.
45. Shafiroff BB, Palmer AK: Simplified technique for replantation of the thumb. J Hand Surg 6:623, 1981.
46. Sixth People's Hospital, Shanghai: Replantation of severed fingers: Clinical experience in 217 cases involving 373 severed fingers. Chin Med J [Engl] 1:184, 1975.
47. Snyder CC, Knowles RP, Mayer PW, Hobbs JC: Extremity replantation. Plast Reconstr Surg 26:251–263, 1960.
48. Stirrat CR, Seaber AV, Urbaniak JR, et al: Temperature monitoring in digital replantation. J Hand Surg 3:342, 1978.
49. Tajima T: History, current status, and aspects of hand surgery in Japan. Clin Orthop 184:41, 1984.
50. Tamai S: Digital replantation. Clin Plast Surg 5:195, 1978.
51. Tamai S: Twenty years experience of limb replantation: Review of 293 upper extremity replants. J Hand Surg 7:549, 1982.
52. Tonkin MA, Ames EL, Wolff TW, et al: Transmetacarpal amputations and replantation: The importance of the normal vascular anatomy. J Hand Surg 13B:204, 1988.
53. Tsai TM, Manstein C, DuBou R, et al: Primary microsurgical repair of ring avulsion amputation injuries. J Hand Surg 9A:68, 1984.
54. Tsai TM, Matiko JD, Breidenbach WC, et al: Venous flaps in digital revascularization and replantation. J Reconstr Microsurg 3:113, 1987.
55. Urbaniak JR: Replantation of amputated parts: Technique, results and indications. In AAOS Symposium on Microsurgery. St. Louis, CV Mosby, 1979, pp 64–82.
56. Urbaniak JR: Replantation in children. In Serafin D, Georgiade NG (eds): Pediatric Plastic Surgery. St. Louis, CV Mosby Co, 1984.
57. Urbaniak JR: Replantation. In Green DP (ed): Operative Hand Surgery, 2nd ed. New York, Churchill Livingstone, 1988.
58. Urbaniak JR, Bright DS: Replantation of amputated digits and hands in children. Inter-Clin Inf Bull 14:1, 1975.
59. Urbaniak JR, Evans JP, Bright DS: Microvascular management of ring avulsion injuries. J Hand Surg 6:25, 1981.
60. Urbaniak JR, Roth JH, Nunley JA, et al: The results of replantation after amputation of a single finger. J Bone Joint Surg 67A:611, 1985.
61. Van Beek AL, Wavak PW, Zook EG: Microvascular surgery in young children. Plast Reconstr Surg 63:457, 1979.
62. Weiland AJ, Villarreal-Rios A, Kleinert HE, et al: Replantation of digits and hands: Analysis of surgical techniques and functional results in 71 patients with 86 replantations. J Hand Surg 2:1, 1977.
63. Weiss HG: Platelet physiology and abnormalities of platelet function. N Engl J Med 293:531, 1975.
64. Wilson CS, Alpert BS, Buncke HJ, et al: Replantation of the upper extremity. Clin Plast Surg 10:85, 1983.
65. Zhong-Wei C, Meyer V, Kleinert HE, et al: Present indications and contraindications for replantation as reflected by long-term functional results. Orthop Clin North Am 12:849, 1981.
66. Zimmerman NB, Weiland AJ: Ninety-ninety intraosseous wiring for internal fixation of the digital skeleton. Orthopedics 12:99–104, 1989.

Chapter 16

HIGH-PRESSURE INJECTION INJURIES
Preventable and Underestimated

Morton L. Kasdan, M.D., F.A.C.S., and
Ramon O. Ryan, M.D., M.S.

One of the most innocuous appearing injuries, yet one that can be most devastating, is from high-pressure injection. The high-pressure injection injury may result in many forms of permanent impairment secondary to the scarring, as well as in amputation of the involved part. Workers using high-pressure equipment are usually unaware of its danger. Frequently, the patient does not report the injury until several hours or days have elapsed. The wound initially can appear so benign that even medical personnel may underestimate its significance. The severity of these injuries and the need for aggressive treatment have been well recognized by hand surgeons for many years.[1,3,8,11,13,14,18,19,21,24,27,29]

A frequent cause of high-pressure injury is a high-pressure hose, used to clean surfaces. Workers often check to see if the equipment is working by pointing the nozzle at the non-dominant hand and squeezing the trigger (Fig. 1). Safety guards are commonly removed from pressurized tools.

PATHOLOGIC COURSE OF INJURY

Tissue necrosis results from pressure in a closed space, toxic material, and secondary infection. Thin solutions such as paint solvents profuse rapidly through the tissue and circulation to produce systemic symptoms.[12] This injury can be likened to a massive snake bite.

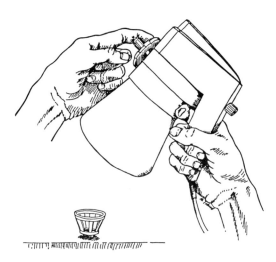

FIGURE 1. The safety guard has been removed from the airless paint gun, and the worker's index finger is placed against the nozzle.

Fever, tachycardia, and respiratory distress have been documented.

The acute stage involves an inflammatory process with swelling, leading to nerve and vascular symptoms that may advance to necrosis and infection. The pain can be severe.

The intermediate stage involves the formation of foreign-body reaction to the injected material, fibrosis, and functional loss. In late stages, soft tissue may slough and draining sinuses may develop secondary infection.

Important prognostic factors are level of pressure, type of material, and amount in-

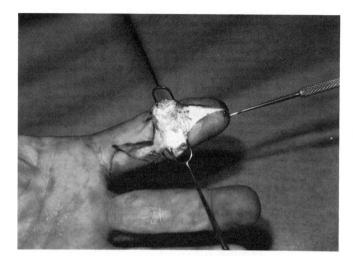

FIGURE 2.   Local infiltration of latex paint.

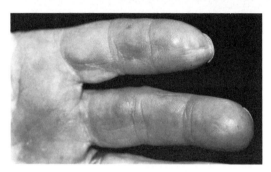

FIGURE 3.   Final result of the injury shown in Figure 2 demonstrating scar and atrophy of the distal phalanx.

jected. Body parts with small, confined areas such as fingers are affected more than larger parts such as the palm of the hand.[8] Paint solvents are highly toxic materials that cause increased systemic responses and a large number of amputations.[4,20,26] Greases and oils, although not as readily absorbed into the systemic circulation, produce extensive necrosis, fibrosis, oleomas, and draining sinuses.[4,20,23,28]

The significance of the material injected becomes apparent when the following three case reports are compared.

Case Report 1.   S.H., a 51-year-old man, was using a spray gun with latex paint. To check the equipment, he placed his index finger over the opening of the gun and fired the trigger. The paint penetrated his left index finger. Figure 2 documents the findings in the operating room. Decompression and extensive debridement were done on the day of the injury, 23 June 1986, and again on 2 July 1986. In July 1987, a third and final procedure for removal of painful scars and foreign-body granulomas was done. The material dissected proximally to the palmar digital crease.

The wound healed, but the distal phalanx of the digit atrophied (Fig. 3).

Case Report 2.   S.E., a 27-year-old man, sustained a high-pressure injury of his left index finger while testing the function of a paint gun. Initial information was that the pressure in the gun was 900 pounds per square inch. It was later learned that the pressure was actually 4,160 pounds per square inch. The solution in the gun was thought to be a paint thinner. No residual liquid was left in the tube because all of it had been injected into the patient and very rapidly dispersed throughout the soft tissue. Extensive surgical debridement and decompression extending to the elbow was done. Subsequent surgical procedures were necessary and, finally, the left index finger was amputated. Figure 4 documents the extent of damage.

Case Report 3.   S.Y., a 44-year-old man, sustained a high-pressure grease injection injury to his left, nondominant index finger. His finger was behind the object he was greasing. The gun slipped, and the grease punctured the digit (Fig. 5). The amount of pressure was 50 pounds forced through a 1/64-inch hole. The patient did not present until the next day, 3 February 1988. He was immediately taken to the operating room for decompression and extensive debridement. He did well postoperatively until several months later, when he presented with a post-traumatic tumor mass. This lesion was surgically excised on 10 August 1988 (Fig. 6). The patient's follow-up a year and a half after surgery demonstrated some lost range of motion and atrophy of the distal phalanx along with hypersensitivity of the scar.

These cases point out the differences that can be encountered according to type of ma-

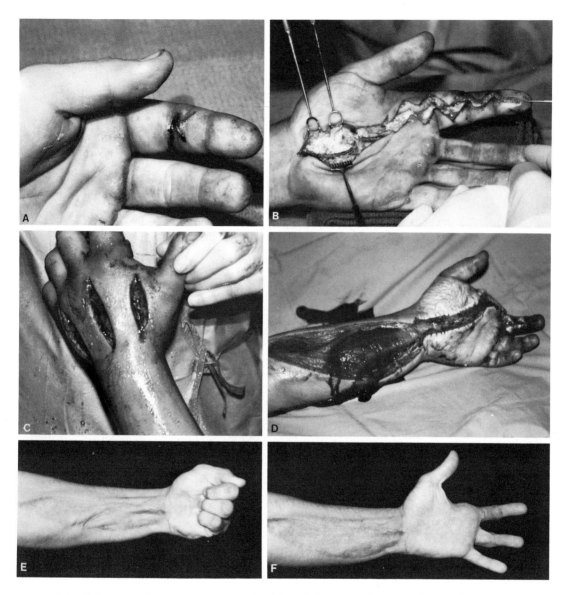

FIGURE 4. *A*, Innocuous-looking puncture wound with bloody drainage at the proximal interphalangeal joint flexion crease at the point of entry of the high-pressure injection. (Reprinted with permission from Kasdan ML: Occupational hand dysfunction. In Marsh JL (ed): Current Therapy in Plastic and Reconstructive Surgery, Vol. 2. Trunk and Extremities. Toronto, B.C. Decker, 1989.) *B*, Initial treatment consisted of extensive incision from the fingertip to the proximal palm and exploration, debridement, and fasciotomy including the carpal tunnel. *C*, As edema in the hand progressed, intrinsic fasciotomy through the dorsum of the hand was necessary. *D*, Extensive fasciotomy of the forearm with amputation of the nonviable index finger. Final result showing full flexion (*E*) and full extension (*F*) 21 months postoperatively.

terial injected. Thin materials tend to dissect further and to produce a more devastating result. Thicker materials are locally harmful, but they do not appear to produce widespread regional and systemic effects.

A careful history and physical examination are necessary. It is important to document the time of the accident, the material injected, and, if possible, the amount of pressure exerted.

The physical examination should include evaluation of the patient's general condition in an attempt to discover any systemic effects of the injected material. The regional examination should evaluate sensation and circulatory and motor function; tendon sheaths should be palpated to locate air or fluid collections. An examination of regional lymph nodes for baseline status is important.

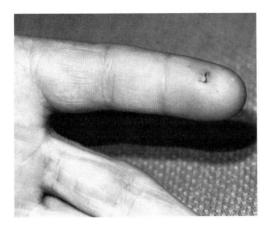

FIGURE 5. Minimal puncture site on the distal phalanx of the left index finger.

RADIOGRAPHIC EVALUATION

Radiographic evaluation can help to determine the extent of the injury in some cases. The material may disperse widely from the injected site. Injections into the fingers may spread proximally into the hand, wrist, and even the forearm.[23] Some injections may penetrate as far as the antecubital fossa.[25] Paints and many greases containing lead or graphite can be demonstrated radiographically.[6] Lucent regions may be detected on x-ray secondary to nonopaque injected materials or subcutaneous emphysema.[16]

TREATMENT

Prompt, aggressive surgical intervention is mandatory in the vast majority of high-pressure injection injuries. Decompression, exploration, and debridement are included in the process.[15] Tendon sheaths should be examined and drained if necessary.[28] Irrigation may also help in clearing injected materials.[22] Wound cultures should be taken, and the patient should be treated with appropriate antibiotics. Wounds are left open or closed very loosely. After surgery the hand should be immobilized in a conforming dressing and splinted in the safe position. The safe position is best described as the wrist in neutral or 20 degrees of extension, the metacarpophalangeal joints in 70–80 degrees of flexion, and the interphalangeal joints extended (Fig. 7). This position lessens pain

and facilitates postoperative rehabilitation. Further cleansing and debridement may be necessary. In an attempt to decrease the inflammatory response, some authors have used steroid therapy.[5,9,10,16,17,20] Patients should be observed for potential systemic effects. Fasciotomies, skin grafting, and pedicle flaps may be required later.[7,30] With severe injuries, amputation may be necessary.[29]

Conservative management has typically proved to be ineffective. Treating these injuries by expressing material from the injection site, elevating the injured site, soaking, dressing, and administering antibiotics alone leads to complications.

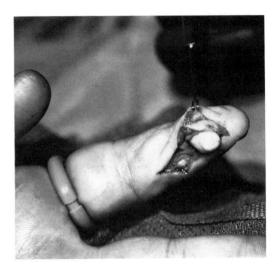

FIGURE 6. Six months after the initial injury, the patient in Figure 5 was taken to the operating room, where a post-traumatic cyst was found as a result of the grease gun injury.

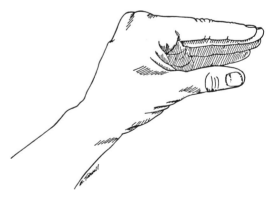

FIGURE 7. The so-called safe position with the metacarpophalangeal joints flexed and the interphalangeal joints extended.

CONCLUSION

High-pressure injection injuries are serious injuries that can lead to significant functional impairment. It seems apparent that the focus should be on prevention. Many high-pressure injection injuries are preventable through training and an understanding of the equipment. When high-pressure injection injuries occur, prompt and aggressive intervention is the appropriate course. These are true surgical emergencies that should be referred as soon as possible to an experienced hand surgeon.

REFERENCES

1. Baylor C, Samuelson C, Sinclaire H: Treatment of grease gun injuries. J Occup Med 15:799–800, 1973.
2. Bell R: Grease-gun injuries. Br J Plast Surg 5:138–145, 1959.
3. Blue A, Dirstine M: Grease gun damage. Northwest Med May:342–343, 1965.
4. Booth L: High-pressure paint gun injuries. Br Med J 2:1333–1335, 1977.
5. Bottoms R: A case of high-pressure hydraulic tool injury to the hand, its treatment aided by dexamethasone and a plea for further trial of this substance. Med J Aust 2:591–592, 1962.
6. Crabb D: The value of plain radiographs in treating grease gun injuries. Hand 13:39–42, 1981.
7. Engel J, Lin E, Tsur H: Neurovascular island flap reconstruction following high pressure injection injuries of the hand. Injury 12:181–184, 1981.
8. Gelberman R, Posch J: High-pressure injection injuries of the hand. J Bone Joint Surg 57A:935–937, 1975.
9. Gillespie C, Rodeheaver G, Smith S, et al: Airless paint gun injuries: Definition and management. Am J Surg 128:383–391, 1974.
10. Hayes C, Pan H: High-pressure injection injuries to the hand. South Med J 75:1491–1498, 1982.
11. Herrick R, Godsil R, Widener J: High-pressure injection injuries to the hand. South Med J 73:896–898, 1980.
12. Kaufman H, Williams H: Systemic absorption from high-pressure spray gun injuries. Br J Surg 53:57–58, 1966.
13. Lewis R: High-pressure injection injuries of the hand. Emerg Med Clin North Am 3:373–381, 1985.
14. Mason M, Queen F: Grease gun injuries to the hand: Pathology and treatment of injuries (oleomas) following the injection of grease under pressure. Q Bull Northwestern Med School 15:122–132, 1941.
15. O'Reilly R, Blatt G: Accidental high-pressure injection-gun injuries of the hand. J Trauma 15:24–31, 1975.
16. O'Reilly R, Blatt G: High-pressure injection injury potential hazard of "enhanced recovery." JAMA 233:533–534, 1975.
17. Phelps D, Hastings H, Boswick J: Systemic corticosteroid therapy for high-pressure injection injuries. J Trauma 17:206–210, 1977.
18. Ramos H, Psch J, Lie K: High-pressure injection injuries of the hand. Plast Reconstr Surg 45:221–226, 1970.
19. Scher C, Schuh D, Harvin J: High-pressure paint gun injuries of the hand: A report of two cases. Br J Plast Surg 26:167–171, 1973.
20. Schoo M, Scott F, Boswick J: High-pressure injection injuries of the hand. J Trauma 20:229–238, 1980.
21. Silsby J: Pressure gun injection injuries of the hand. West J Med 125:271–276, 1976.
22. Smith M: Grease gun injuries. Br Med J 2:918–920, 1964.
23. Stark H, Ashwood C, Boyes J: Paint gun injuries of the hand. J Bone Joint Surg 49A:637–647, 1967.
24. Stark H, Wilson J, Boyes J: Grease gun injuries of the hand. J Bone Joint Surg 43A:485–491, 1961.
25. Tanzer R: Grease-gun type injuries of the hand. Surg Clin North Am 43:1277–1282, 1963.
26. Walton S: Injection gun injuries of the hand with anticorrosive paint and paint solvents. Clin Orthop 74:141–145, 1971.
27. Weeks P: Airless paint gun injuries of the hand. J KY Med Assoc Nov:1086–1089, 1967.
28. Williams C, Riordan D: High velocity injuries of the hand. South Med J 67:295–302, 1974.
29. Zook E, Kinkead L: Pressure gun injection injuries of the hand. JACEP 8:264–266, 1979.

Chapter 17

EARLY REPAIR AND LATE RECONSTRUCTION OF CRUSH INJURIES

Ellen Beatty, M.D., and Robert J. Belsole, M.D.

Crush injuries in the upper extremity are frustrating problems in rehabilitation. Blunt injuries are frequently and mistakenly believed to be of much less significance than sharp injuries in which the extent of tissue destruction and loss are more evident. The majority of crush injuries are closed, or they produce such small skin loss that the patient, employer, and health care team do not recognize the extent of tissue damage and death that has occurred. The general feeling is that the patient who does not make a rapid recovery from such a minor appearing injury is probably not trying hard enough. Looking at the actual events of a crushing injury will help us to understand the forces that a patient and rehabilitation specialist are up against in their effort to regain full function. The hand is the most commonly crushed body part because of its vital role in all functions in the workplace. A crushed hand is often ignored until the edema fails to resolve and stiffness has already progressed. At this point much more effort is required for recovery than if treatment had begun soon after injury.

Tissue healing involves four major processes that proceed in an orderly manner. The length of time each process takes depends on the extent of the crush, the age and nutritional status of the patient, and the presence of metabolic diseases such as diabetes. Any deviation from an optimal physical condition at the time of injury slows and possibly prevents maximal recovery. Consideration of all the factors involved in a particular injury makes it easier for the therapist to persist in a lengthy rehabilitation.

Inflammation is the first phase in the recovery of injured tissue. Its onset is rapid. At the time of the insult a transient constriction of all blood vessels occurs in the area of injury, and possibly the rest of the extremity if the crush is circumferential. This vasoconstriction resolves and is followed by a period of dilation of the small blood and lymphatic vessels. It is during this vasodilation that the vessel walls are leaky and allow cells and other blood products to cross into the surrounding tissues. Capillaries allow blood proteins and plasma to exude, and white blood cells migrate through the walls of small veins. Small vessels that are actually lacerated at the time of the injury create pools of blood that clot and later are resorbed by the inflammatory response. Lymphatic vessels allow the very thick lymph fluid, which is high in protein, to escape into the wounded tissue. All of these fluids and cells contribute to the rapidly forming edema. The greater the crush, both in terms of force and area involved, the greater the edema that forms and, subsequently, the longer the inflammatory period. Skin defects increase the chances for bacteria to gain entrance to the area, which is now rich in an ideal culture medium of blood and protein. Infection markedly increases this response of inflammatory cells and delays recovery for months. Foreign bodies that may enter the crushed tissue also delay wound repair and increase the amount of white cells needed to clean up the area.[4]

Lymphatic vessels and venules are fragile and subject to occlusion from swelling at relatively low pressures. Once the lymphatic and smaller venous channels are blocked, the backup of lymph and blood further increases the extravasation of fluid into tissues and worsens the edema. At this time elevation and cautious compression are needed to combat the increasing pressure in the injured tissues. Immobilization also helps.

The second phase in tissue healing is epithelialization. The edges of an opening in the skin begin thickening in the first day after injury. The cells in the base of the epidermis begin to enlarge and prepare to migrate to cover any defects. The migration allows a single cell layer to cover a wound. Later it thickens and forms layers of skin as it matures. This migrated skin never is completely normal in structure and is unfortunately subject to contraction.

In the third phase, cells for the reconstruction of tissue proliferate in the injured area. This cellular phase is marked by a decrease in the number of scavenging white blood cells which remove dead tissue, and an increase in the number of fibroblasts in the wound. Fibroblasts are mobile cells that rapidly produce collagen, the fibrous tissue that makes scars. The appearance of fibroblasts precedes the development of new blood vessels.[4] Small blood vessels begin to "bud" from the preexisting vessels, probably in response to the lack of oxygen in the injured tissues. Capillary proliferation provides the essential nutrients and oxygen to rebuild tissues. The number of small blood vessels in the new tissue is greater than in normal tissue. This accounts for the pink coloration of new skin and young scars that will gradually pale back to normal coloration when some of the vessels are no longer needed.

So far what has been discussed is part of the early repair after a crushing injury. The late reconstructive phase begins about 1 month after the injury and may continue for many years as scar remodeling continues. Scars are dynamic tissue, responding to forces placed upon them. Scar tissue thins with time and most scars will be regressing by 6 months post-injury. Age and the sequelae of diseases such as rheumatoid arthritis play a role in the amount and severity of scar contraction. Tissue repair proceeds more rapidly in children than in adults. Children also have much thicker scar tissue,

which may not resolve until the hormonal changes of puberty.

SKIN AND SUBCUTANEOUS TISSUE

Skin and subcutaneous tissue are the first recipients of the crushing force in an injury. With sufficient force, the skin and underlying tissue will tear or rupture, which increases the chance of infection and delays healing. The amount of edema and the direct damage to the blood supply determine the ability of the skin to survive an insult. Demarcation of necrotic skin may take a week to be complete if it is not surgically debrided. The application of skin grafts increases the amount of scar formation on the surface of the injured tissue, because the development of blood vessels between old and new tissue requires its own inflammatory response. The skin graft contracts with age, and the amount of contraction depends on the tension the graft is under in its new location and on its thickness. A thicker skin graft contracts less owing to increased thickness of the dermis present. Full-thickness skin grafts are seldom used, however, because they can be harvested from only a very few sites on the body, they require much more blood supply to survive than thinner, partial-thickness grafts, and for optimal healing they also require immobilization, which may delay early joint motion and promote stiffness.

A flap differs from a skin graft in that it brings a blood supply with it and therefore heals faster and more reliably. Because the flap contains at least full-thickness skin and subcutaneous tissue, it also contracts less than skin grafts. The choice between a flap and a skin graft is based on the blood supply of the wound and the future needs of the tissue. Skin grafts are by nature too adherent to allow extensive reconstruction underneath them, such as tendon grafts, tendon transfers, and bone grafts (Fig. 1). Flaps are used to replace skin grafts and scars in late reconstruction to allow more mobility and in some cases a better appearance.

Contractures remain one of the hardest problems to correct after injury or surgery. Wound contraction is a vital and lifesaving force in nature. Without it, there would be no healing and the animal world might never have evolved to where it is today. The animal in the wild depends on rapid and strong contraction of wound edges to prevent infection and long-term sapping of its energy by slow wound clo-

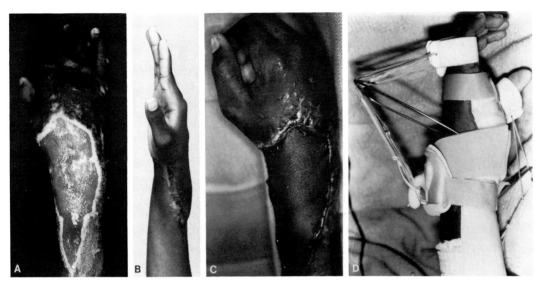

FIGURE 1. A, An avulsion injury of the dorsal soft tissues down to the level of the carpus in a 15-year-old male. B, A free flap was used to cover the exposed bone. C, Tendon grafting through the fat in the flap was performed after the flap healed. D, Result after tendon grafts and bracing.

sure. The faster its healing process, the greater the chance a species has for survival. The goal of many researchers in wound healing is to limit wound contraction to an ideal amount and to stop it abruptly before scarring occurs.[10] At present the best that can be done is to stretch the contracting tissue and maintain it at optimal length until the scar tissue is mature enough to remodel and thin itself (Fig. 2). The force needed to maintain the tissue at a desired length decreases with time. Aggressive exercise programs and splinting protocols should be implemented and continued throughout the period of scar maturation.

BLOOD VESSEL INJURIES

The blood vessels in the upper extremity are very susceptible to damage in crush injuries. Any circumferential injury presses the artery and major veins against the fascia and bone, causing spasm in the vessels. Usually the vessels begin to flow again shortly after injury, but a compression may be too great, causing a clot to form inside the vessel that permanently occludes the blood flow. Thrombosis of a major artery decreases the oxygen available distal to the injury. If the axillary, brachial, radial, or ulnar arteries are involved, the decrease in blood flow may be sufficient to cause death of the distal part. When flow remains great enough

to allow oxygenation, the smaller vessels in the limb can enlarge and carry a larger than usual proportion of blood to the distal tissue. Collateral circulation of this sort increases exercise endurance over a period of time. Thrombosed major arteries can be revascularized with vein grafts taken from the leg. Clots formed in the major veins including the axillary, brachial, basilic, and cephalic veins, lead to congestion of venous outflow and edema in the forearm and hand. Severely crushed tissue may develop the "no reflow" phenomenon.[5] Extensive damage or lengthy oxygen deprivation may make it impossible for blood vessels to resume their usual flow characteristics. Even vein grafting in these cases will not reverse the inability of small vessels to perfuse the tissue. Treatment options are to wait and see if perfusion improves spontaneously, to remove unperfused tissue, or to amputate the part.

Late reconstruction of crushed vessels is done to treat an aneurysm, which is an outgrowth of an injured artery that forms a second channel for blood to flow through. Aneurysms are pulsatile masses in the soft tissue. They may grow because the new false wall of the artery is more stretchable than the original wall. Pulsatile pressure in the aneurysm may lead to rupture and leakage of blood into surrounding tissues. The turbulent flow usually seen may also predispose the vessel to clotting. Aneurysms should be resected and vein grafted if the vessel involved is of any importance.

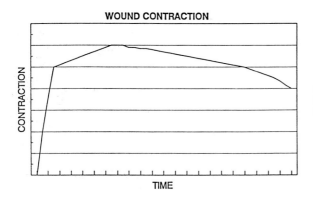

FIGURE 2. Wound contraction is rapid initially. It plateaus and then decreases slowly. The final size of the scar depends on the tension on it.

MUSCLE INJURIES

Muscle tissue is the most sensitive of all tissues to a decrease in blood supply. After 4–6 hours without blood, muscle usually does not resume normal blood flow to its fibers. Any muscle tissue not receiving enough blood supply dies. After the inflammatory response directs cells to remove the dead tissue, the area is invaded by fibroblasts, which lay down collagen. Scar tissue thus replaces portions of or entire dead muscles. The fibrotic changes seen in injured muscles decrease the motion and strength that can be expected. In crush injuries in the arm, dead and hypoxic tissue may need to be surgically removed several times to promote healing without large volumes of scar and to prevent bacteria from multiplying in the excellent culture medium that inflammation produces. A look at the tissue 24 hours after the initial surgery may reveal more tissue that is not being perfused adequately and has slowly died.

The worst complication of crush injuries is the development of high pressures from edema in the soft tissue of the extremity. The fascia around muscles and the skin can limit the expansion of tissue (Fig. 3). The swollen tissue begins to compress the blood and lymphatic vessels in the soft tissue at a pressure of about 10–30 mm Hg less than the patient's diastolic blood pressure.[10] The compartment syndrome that results from the lack of blood supply especially to the muscles and nerves can go unnoticed long enough to produce permanent damage. Any crush injury at the elbow should be followed very closely for extent of swelling and complaints of numbness and tingling in the fingers. Constrictive dressings should be avoided early in the care of all crushing injuries. Compartment syndromes may also be overlooked in the interosseous and thenar muscles of the hand.[2] Any area too swollen for active motion should be considered for surgical decompression to prevent muscle fibrosis and eventual stiffness.

The diagnosis of a compartment syndrome may be confirmed with the use of a Wick catheter,[7] which is inserted under the fascia of the arm. If the reading is above 30 mm Hg,[10] the consensus is to open the skin and fascia surgically to relieve the pressure. If the muscle was not hypoxic too long, the blood flow should improve. The skin should be left open until the swelling has subsided in order to prevent further compression in cases in which swelling actually increases after blood flow returns. Skin grafts may be placed to cover the exposed tissue and prevent introduction of bacteria. Late reconstruction of muscles that have become scarred and will not function depends on the availability of normal muscles at the same level of the extremity. If the wrist extensor muscles were not damaged in the crushing injury, they can be used as tendon transfers for forearm flexors. Hypothenar muscles can be transferred to provide thumb abduction or opposition. The muscles of the neck and back, such as the latissimus dorsi, may be transferred to replace the biceps or triceps. Muscle transfers may not always allow full strength or range of motion to be regained because of the differences in the excursion of individual muscles.[1] Attention should be paid to the tension under which a tendon or muscle transfer is sewn in.[12] The best results are obtained when the muscle is marked before being disconnected and approximated at the same resting length in its transferred position. A transfer is expected to stretch some with time and should be placed under slightly more tension. The transfer needs to be immobilized for 4–6 weeks to allow healing before the suture line is stressed.

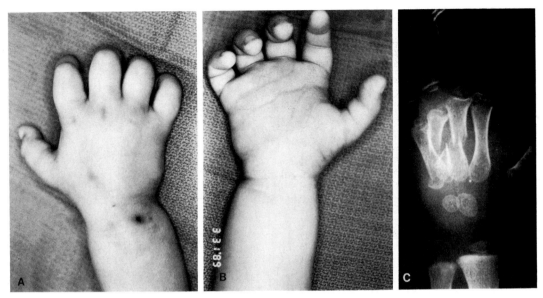

FIGURE 3. *A* and *B,* Photographs taken several hours after the crush of an 18-month-old male's right hand in a bank vault door. Swelling required dorsal and volar fasciotomies. *C,* Radiograph showing multiple metacarpal fractures.

In cases in which entire groups of muscles, such as the volar forearm flexors, are fibrosed, a muscle from the thigh or back may have to be transferred as a replacement and its nerve, artery, and vein surgically connected in the arm. These free muscle transfers require a good motor nerve to be successful and supple joints to be strong enough to power the limb. No late reconstruction should be considered unless the distal joints can be passively moved. A tenolysis and capsulotomy done separately and followed by a period of therapy may need to precede the motor transfer. It makes good sense that if the therapist is unable to mobilize a joint, then a muscle transfer will fail.

TENDON INJURIES

The damage to a tendon in a crush may be from a laceration, from avulsion of the tendon from its muscle origin or bony insertion in a rolling or grinding crush, or simply from the edema that develops. Lacerations should be repaired and care taken to cover the suture line with viable soft tissue. It is important to avoid an overlying skin graft that will adhere and limit motion of the tendon. Avulsed tendons are more difficult to treat. If it has been pulled out from its muscle belly, a tendon is useless, and there is no adequate way to reconstruct its complex connection to muscle fi-

bers. In proximal avulsions, the best result is to transfer the tendon to another tendon (side to side) that has the same function. An example is the anastomosis of the extensor tendon of the middle finger to the extensor tendon of the ring finger to allow normal excursion in unison. If there is no available adjacent synergistic tendon, an elective tendon transfer should be postponed until wounds are healed and the full extent of damage is known. Transferring a muscle with less than normal function to the avulsed tendon can then be avoided. Avulsion of the distal end of a tendon is usually treated by reinserting the tendon into the bone nearest its original position. Long-standing distal tendon avulsions usually cannot be returned to their original length and require formal tendon transfer.

The limitation of function of tendons by edema and resultant scar formation in the tendon sheath and joint capsules is best treated by prevention. Early management of edema with careful compression, elevation, and immobilization cannot be overemphasized. Motion of tendons is encouraged and dynamic bracing should be used whenever possible. The more the tendon is able to move, the less chance that fibrous scar tissue will restrict it. Active motion resists scar shortening best but may not be possible when nerve and muscle damage are involved. In those cases, passive motion should be performed several times a day. The continuous passive motion machine is useful in some instances, but it should not be depended upon.

When early motion is not possible, the late consequences of fibrosis are harder to correct and require an extended period of therapy. Swelling in the tendon sheath makes tendon gliding difficult and painful. Adhesions form very quickly in the sheath. As they thicken, they become strong enough to halt the gliding of the tendon completely. Once motion stops, shortening of the collagen may lead to permanent immobility. Surgical release of collagen scars in the tendon sheath is known as tenolysis. Once tenolysis is performed, motion must begin immediately. Both active and passive activity are essential to prevent the scar from restricting the tendon.

The joints should always be maintained in the safest position in case the return of motion is less than optimal. The ligaments of the elbow and fingers are most susceptible to shortening with time. Elbows kept flexed rapidly contract in older patients. Both the soft tissue and the joint capsules shorten. Even the median nerve and the brachial artery have shortened and limited recovery. Metacarpophalangeal joints should be flexed and interphalangeal joints extended to prevent collateral ligament shortening. Surgical release of contracted joint capsules and ligaments may be required to regain motion. Capsulotomy should be considered any time a tenolysis is required.

NERVE INJURIES

A crushing injury over a large area tends to cause fewer lacerations to the soft tissue, including the nerves, than a similar injury concentrated in a very small surface area. Roller injuries cause a higher incidence of nerve injury from the grinding force applied to the tissue at the point of the extremity where advancement into the roller is halted. A lacerated nerve should be repaired and the original alignment of motor and sensory fascicles maintained for maximal recovery of strength and sensation. Nerve grafts harvested from the sural nerve in the posterior portion of the calf are most frequently used to reconstruct gaps in lacerated or severely crushed nerves of the upper extremity. Less frequently, vascularized nerve grafts taken with their nutrient arteries are harvested and used in late reconstruction of scarred areas where the tissue would not revascularize a regular nerve graft. Repaired or crushed nerves grow from the area of injury or repair to the end plates of the nerve at a rate of 1 mm per day. Nerve growth is accomplished by the sprouting of a growth cone from the distal end of the damaged axon.[6] The growth is dependent upon the transport of nutrients from the parent stump down into the regenerating axon. Tinel's sign makes it possible to measure clinical progress in nerve regeneration. Percussion over young axons elicits the electric shock not found in nontraumatized sensory nerves. Progress in motor nerve regeneration can be followed with electromyography. The growth of some axons to the end of a nerve does not imply that the number of axons is the same as in the pre-injured nerve. Incomplete nerve regeneration is common in adults; fortunately, children often return to a normal level of function. Voluntary motor activity is monitored clinically on the basis of a scale of zero (no activity) to five (normal strength).[9]

The nerve injury in crushed extremities may not be directly related to the insult. Edema forms in the tissue, especially in the muscles bound by tight fascia or the tunnels through which nerves travel, and produces secondary nerve damage. The traumatic carpal tunnel syndrome caused by increasing swelling in the forearm and hand is a good example and is one of the most common. In an experiment using normal volunteers, Gelberman[3] measured the amount of pressure on the carpal tunnel at which function of the median nerve was impaired and the length of time to recovery of the nerve. From this study, it appears that 50 mm Hg is the pressure at which nerve survival is at risk. The recommendation for surgical tissue decompression at 40 mm Hg is a product of these results. The viability of nerves is dependent on adequate blood flow in the nutrient vessels that run along the outside wall of a nerve. The compression caused by edema is proposed to deform the branches of the veins and subsequently the arterioles entering the nerve to provide oxygen. The rigid structure of the outer covering of nerves compresses the softer blood vessel walls and decreases the amount of blood that can flow in and out of a nerve.[8] The re-

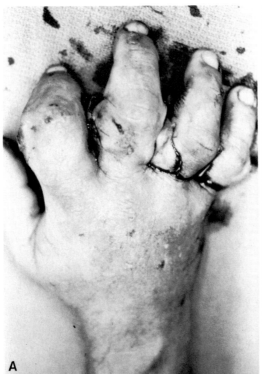

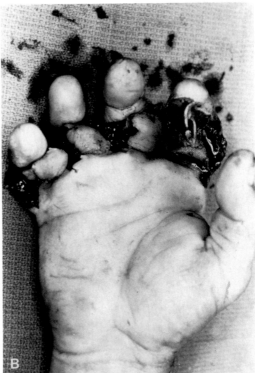

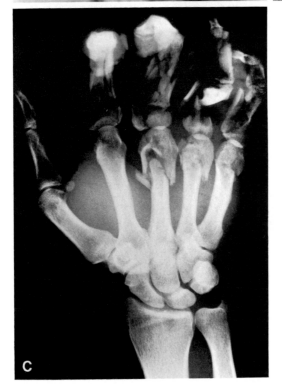

FIGURE 4. A and B, The right hand of a 35-year-old male that was compressed between two pieces of heavy machinery. The soft tissue burst under the pressure, and digits are significantly shortened. C, Radiograph of the proximal phalanges and metacarpal heads shows severe splintering, which required longitudinal pins for gross alignment and longitudinal traction in an effort to restore some of former length to bones.

tention of blood in the nerve itself when veins are compressed and the arteries remain open worsens the edema within the nerve fascicles.

Late reconstruction of nerves includes correction of nerve contusion that does not recover. If nothing can be elicited by Tinel or EMG by 3 months, surgical exploration may be warranted. A lacerated nerve or a severely crushed nerve may require nerve grafts. In some cases the nerve has simply been choked by scar that formed around it when the inflammatory process receded. Scarred nerves may regenerate when the constricting scar is incised or removed. The procedure known as neurolysis allows the nutrients in the proximal nerve to resume flow to its distal portion.

BONE INJURIES

Crush injuries are notorious for causing some of the most splintered fractures. It is quite difficult to align and fix the hundreds of tiny fragments that can be created (Fig. 4). Many such injuries require gross alignment of bones and immobilization long enough for the fragments to coalesce and heal. This is contrary to the goal of immediate rigid fixation of bones to allow early mobilization and to prevent stiffness and adhesions. The overall result in extremities with multiple fractures is greatly improved when the condition of the tissues and bone fixation allow joint motion. The larger the fracture sur-faces, the more areas there are that produce scarring to heal the tissue. If the periosteum or tendon sheaths are torn, the tendons are more likely to adhere to the bone and reduce motion; joint contracture will probably follow. When there is no loss of soft tissue, bone grafts should be done early in the treatment of bone loss to expedite fracture healing.

Long-term problems with crushed bones include failure of a fracture to heal (nonunion) (Fig. 5), bad position in a healed fracture (malunion), and retained infection in poorly vascularized healed or unhealed bone. Treatment of a nonunion requires removal of fibrous tissue that may have filled the bone gap and prevented bone from crossing the fracture. Bone graft and continued fixation are usually required to speed the union of the fragments. Malunion results in abnormal rotation and angulation of the bone, which can limit the normal arc of motion of its adjacent joints. Malunions require osteotomy (opening of the bony cortex to allow correction of angulation or rotation) with possible bone graft. Rigid internal fixation of bone is the treatment of choice to allow early motion and resumption of therapy. Infection in bone—osteomyelitis—is a long-term problem; treatment is aggressive and requires radical debridement of infected and nonviable bone. After intravenous administration of antibiotics and possibly antibiotic-impregnated beads in the remaining bone and tissue, bone graft is needed to obtain union.

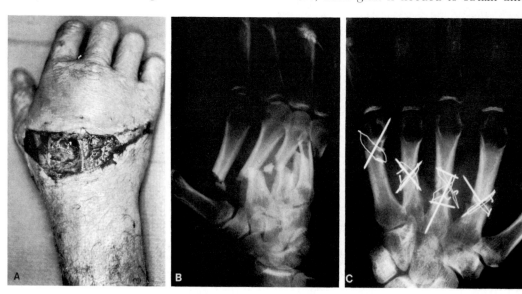

FIGURE 5. *A*, A blunt injury to dorsal hand causing death of an area of skin and subcutaneous tissue. *B*, Radiograph showing multiple displaced metacarpal fractures. *C*, Radiograph showing nonunion of metacarpals with severe scarring of extensor tendons.

Osteomyelitis may be silent and not resurface again for 10 years or more, making prevention and early treatment of infection in fractures of prime importance in every case.

CONCLUSION

After considering all of the tissue systems in the extremity to explore their individual healing characteristics, it is clear that early and aggressive treatment in crush injuries can make a difference in the time required for recovery. The control of infection and edema are vital to the overall outcome. Rigid bone fixation for early mobilization aids the therapist when it is possible. Attention to progress helps speed advancement to additional splints and exercise modalities.

REFERENCES

1. Brand PW, Beach MA, Thompson DE: Relative tension and potential excursion of muscles in the forearm and hand. J Hand Surg 6:209–219, 1981.
2. Chow SP, So YC, Pun WK, et al: Thenar crush injuries. J Bone Joint Surg 70B:135–139, 1988.
3. Gelberman RH, Szabo RM, Williamson RV, et al: Tissue pressure threshold for peripheral nerve viability. Clin Orthop 178:285–291, 1983.
4. Madden JW, Arem AJ: Wound healing: Biologic and clinical features. In Sabiston DC (ed): Textbook of Surgery, 12th ed. Philadelphia, W.B. Saunders, 1981, pp 265–286.
5. May JW, Chait LA, O'Brien BM, Hurley JV: The no-reflow phenomenon in experimental free flaps. Plast Reconstruct Surg 61:256–267, 1978.
6. McQuarrie IG, Lasek RJ: Transport of cytoskeletal elements from parent axons into regenerating daughter axons. J Neurosci 9:436–446, 1989.
7. Murbarak SJ, Hargens AR, Owen CA, et al: The Wick catheter technique for measurement of intramuscular pressure. J Bone Joint Surg 58A:1016–1019, 1976.
8. Myers RR, Murakami H, Powell HC: Reduced nerve blood flow in edematous neuropathies: A biomechanical mechanism. Microvasc Res 32:145–151, 1986.
9. Omer GE: Methods of assessment of injury and recovery of peripheral nerves. Surg Clin North Am 61:303–319, 1981.
10. Peacock EE: Wound Repair, 3rd ed. Philadelphia, W.B. Saunders, 1984, pp 102–140.
11. Smith RJ: Tendon Transfers of the Hand and Forearm. Boston, Little, Brown, 1987, pp 13–34.

Chapter 18

ELECTRICAL INJURIES

Kevin P. Yakuboff, M.D., and
Harold E. Kleinert, M.D.

The first reported fatality from commercial electricity was that of a carpenter killed in 1879 by a 250 volt alternating current dynamo.[23] Since that time electrical injuries have become an increasingly common problem in the work place.[1,10,26,33] One review identified electrical injuries as the fifth leading cause of fatal occupational injury.[33] The National Institute for Occupational Safety and Health (NIOSH) has identified five causes of electrical injury in the workplace: (1) direct contact between a worker and energized lines, (2) contact of a vehicular boom with energized power lines, (3) contact of other equipment with energized lines, (4) direct contact of a worker with energized equipment or conductors, and (5) improperly installed or broken equipment.[33] Electrical injuries most frequently involve linemen, electricians, and construction workers. In most series the majority of these injuries were sustained in the workplace rather than in nonwork-related activities.[1,10,16] It should be emphasized that the potential for electrical injury exists both at work and home, requiring active public education programs as the best means of prevention.[6,7]

In this country, electrical injuries account for approximately 3 to 5% of admissions to major burn units, with over 1,000 electricity related deaths per year.[4,10,16,17,41] In developing countries, electrical injuries account for an even greater number of admissions to burn units (18%).[15] As expected, the majority of electrical injuries involve the upper extremity, with a spectrum of injury ranging from minor burn wounds requiring minimal debridement and wound care (Fig. 1) to devastating upper extremity destruction requiring aggressive resuscitation and major limb amputation (Fig. 2). Although a significant amount of tissue damage is thermally induced, these injuries differ greatly from the flame burns.[38] Major electrical injuries are associated with more severe deep tissue damage, require larger amounts of fluid for resuscitation, and often require more complex reconstruction procedures for limb salvage.

PHYSICS OF ELECTRICITY

In electrical injuries damage occurs with the passage of electrons through tissue. The effect of electrical current in producing this injury is dependent on multiple factors, including current (amperage), voltage, resistance, the type and path of current, and the duration of contact. Current is the term used to describe the rate of flow of electrons. Voltage represents the amount of electromotive force behind the electrons. Voltage is supplied either as a continuous source (direct current—DC) with electron flow moving in one direction, or as a cyclic source (alternating current—AC) with a cyclic reversal of electron flow. Resistance is that quality of a material that impedes the flow of electrons. In biologic materials resistance varies from tissue to tissue and is influenced by factors such as skin thickness, moisture, and vascularity. The resistance of a calloused palm may reach 1,000,000 ohms/cm² while dry normal skin may have a resistance of 5,000 ohms/cm². Moist skin may have a resistance as low

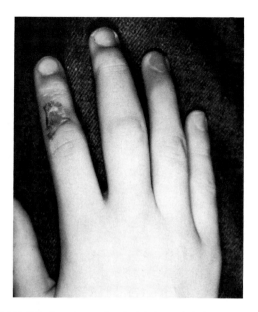

FIGURE 1. Minor electrical injury of digit requiring simple wound care.

as 1,000 ohms/cm². [4] In general, nerves and blood vessels have the least resistance and clinically sustain severe damage, whereas bone has the highest resistance and often receives little damage[11] (Table 1).

Voltage (V), resistance (R), and current (I) are related by Ohm's law: I = V/R. High voltage electrical injuries are arbitrarily defined as being 1000 volts or greater.[3,8,10,11,22,49] Since current flow is directly proportional to voltage (Ohm's law), the higher the voltage, the greater amount of tissue damage and sequelae.[32] Death may occur at much lower voltage levels with little or no tissue destruction as a result of cardiac arrhythmias or respiratory arrest.[2,4,41,49] Alternating current is particularly hazardous in this respect, producing ventricular fibrillation with current flows of 20–40 microamperes.[4,41] Sixty-cycle household current is more likely to result in lethal cardiac arrest than is higher frequency current.

PATHOPHYSIOLOGY

Considerable controversy has existed over the exact mechanism of tissue damage in electrical injury. The most commonly accepted theory is that of thermal injury resulting from the heat generated by the flow of electrons through tissue.[3,12,20,26,42] This release of heat is described by Joule's law: P = I/RT; where

P = heat, I = current, R = resistance, and T = exposure time.[4,32]

Baxter suggested that the heat generated was proportional to the resistance of the tissue through which the current is passing.[3] In this theory, heat is generated in increasing increments by nerve, vessel, muscle, skin, tendon, fat, and bone. In this model, bone would generate the most heat but because of its structure sustains minimal damage. The heat generated would damage the deep perosseous tissues, a common clinical finding in major electrical injuries. However, nerve, vessel, and muscle sustained some of the most severe damage and have relatively low electrical resistances.

Hunt proposed that living tissue acts as a volume conductor; once skin resistance is overcome, all internal tissue resistance (except bone)

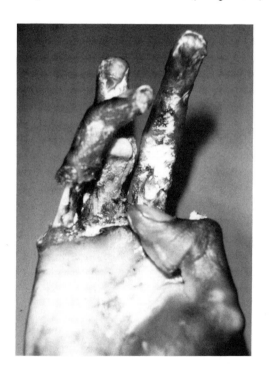

FIGURE 2. Devastating electrical injury requiring amputation of hand.

TABLE 1. Electrical Properties of Different Tissues

Conductivity	Tissue	Resistance
Lowest ↑	Bone	Highest ↑
	Fat	
	Tendon	
	Skin	
	Muscle	
	Blood vessel	
Highest ↓	Nerves	Lowest ↓

is negligible to current flow.[20] In this model, muscle and bone attain the same temperature almost simultaneously with the passage of current. Once current flow is established, the limb, trunk, and entire body act as a volume conductor. The heat generated in tissues will be a function of the voltage drop and current flow per unit of cross-sectional area (current density). This concept of current density would explain the severity of tissue damage seen clinically in extremities, as well as in entrance-exit wound sites.[42] Areas with concentrated current density sustain the most tissue damage.

In addition, the rate of heating in each tissue is not only dependent on the electrical and thermal properties of the tissue, but also on the spatial arrangement of the tissues to current flow; whether the tissue is in series or parallel determines the rate of heating.[26] This concept could explain either model proposed by Baxter (in series) or by Hunt (in parallel). In most clinical situations tissues are probably in parallel.

Earlier clinical observations developed the concept of "progressive necrosis" occurring in electrically damaged tissues.[27,29,34,36] This idea developed from the observations that apparently well-debrided wounds continued to change

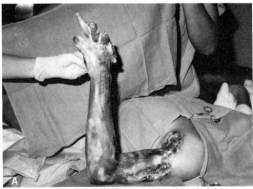
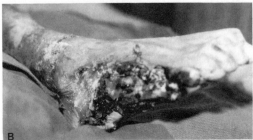

FIGURE 3. A, Entrance wound incinerating entire upper extremity. B, Exit wound on the foot of the same patient (A). Note severe tissue destruction concentrated at exit wound.

over several days or weeks, resulting in further necrosis. The concept of ongoing necrosis frequently prevented early coverage of these wounds for fear of resulting septic complications. A number of theories have been proposed to explain this apparent clinical phenomenon. These include: direct cell damage from the flow of electrons,[25] bacterial infection,[31] progressive arterial thrombosis,[27] and delayed release of inflammatory mediators (prostaglandins) from injured tissue that result in vascular compromise.[36]

In 1974 Hunt described arteriographic patterns of injury in electrically injured patients.[21] He noted that main vascular channels remained patent, but small nutrient branches to muscle were occluded. Other studies support these findings and demonstrate no evidence of progressive vascular necrosis.[5,24,50] This would indicate that "progressive necrosis" does not exist but is merely a manifestation of the original tissue injury in combination with such factors as infection, desiccation, and trauma after multiple debridement procedures.[50]

MANAGEMENT

Evaluation and Resuscitation

Resuscitation of the patient immediately following electrical injury should focus on support of the cardiorespiratory systems. Respiratory arrest and ventricular fibrillation are the principle causes of death in these injuries.[2,4,14,16,41] These victims should have cardiac monitoring in specialized care units because of the high incidence (60%) of cardiac abnormalities after electrical injury.[1,14,17] A complete assessment of the patient is mandatory to screen for associated injuries. Fractures can result from severe tetanic muscle contraction seen with exposure to alternating current.

Neurological and orthopedic injuries commonly occur after the patient is hurled from the electrical contact point. The presence and location of entrance and exit wounds should be noted. These sites sustain the most severe tissue damage (Fig. 3). The path of current through the body can be estimated by the position of these wounds. The path that electrical current takes through the body is directly related to mortality. Current coursing from hand to hand is associated with a 60% mortality rate, whereas a hand-to-foot path is associated with a 20%

mortality.[11] Hand-to-hand pathways can be expected to affect the spinal cord between C4–6 as well as the heart.

Arc injuries are common with high voltage electrical accidents. These injuries are commonly the result of current coursing external to the body. The current may arc (jump) from its source to the victim, or arc between different sites on the extremity. The flexor surface of the upper extremity is frequently the site of arcing (Fig. 4). These injuries may result in severe tissue destruction (incineration) from temperatures generated in the range of 3,000 to 20,000 C.[4]

Arcing may cause significant surface flame burns from ignition of clothing or surrounding materials. The possibility of serious intraabdominal injury should be considered with close proximity to the abdomen to current path or entrance and exit wounds.[32]

The patient with a major electrical injury will require aggressive fluid resuscitation. These injuries often require significantly more volume in comparison to the more common flame burns.[22] Using estimates based on total body surface area involvement will grossly under-estimate fluid requirements. General guidelines for fluid management recommend the use of Parkland formula as an initial aid in resuscitation.[3,16,22,32] At a minimum, resuscitation begins with Ringer's lactate at 4 cc/kg/% burn. Special attention is given to maintain the using output over 100 cc/hr. Adequate urine output must be maintained to avoid renal complications from myoglobinuria. This release of muscle pigment results from extensive muscle damage commonly seen with these injuries (Fig. 5). Persistent myoglobinuria over 6 hours' duration correlates well with massive muscle necrosis and the need for major amputation.[3] The use of mannitol (osmotic diuretic) in addition to adequate fluid administration has been recommended to promote clearance of myoglobin from the renal tubules.[3,4,22] In practice, an initial dose of 25 g is followed by hourly doses of 15 g until the urine is clear. In addition the use of sodium bicarbonate to correct acidosis and maintain an alkaline urinary pH will help prevent renal damage from myoglobinuria. The

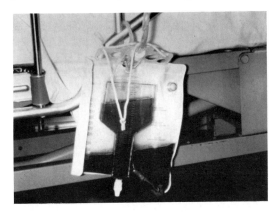

FIGURE 5. Myoglobinuria is a common finding after electrical injuries with massive muscle damage.

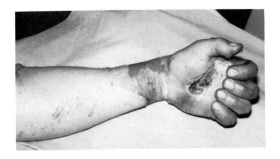

FIGURE 4. Arc injuries in electric burns commonly involve the flexor surfaces of the arm.

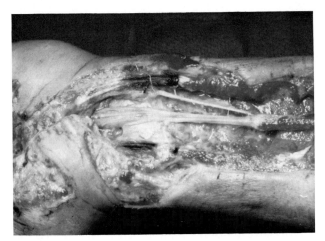

FIGURE 6. Destroyed median nerve at wrist level in a patient exposed to 7,000 volts.

incidence of renal failure in electrical injury has been reported to range from 1–7.5%.[10,38]

In addition to renal failure, numerous other sequelae may result from electrical injury.[37] Sepsis is the most common lethal complication.[3,16] Infection occurs in large necrotic muscle masses and can be prevented by early aggressive surgical debridement. Neurological sequelae represent the most common nonlethal complications seen in these injuries.[3,16] The median and ulnar nerves are the most frequently injured nerves in electrical injuries[43] (Fig. 6). Nerve injury may be the result of thermal damage, electron flow, or compartment syndrome.

Delayed neurological problems have been reported to occur as long as 2 years after injury.[11] Neurological sequelae have included seizures, headaches, causalgia, paraplegia, quadriplegia, spasticity, and peripheral neuropathy.[3,11,22,37,43] Other late complications include cataracts, cardiac abnormalities, and gastrointestinal problems.[37] The overall mortality from electrical injury is 2–26%, with higher mortality rates being reported in developing countries.[1,10,16,18,22,44]

Wound Management

A common problem in electrical injuries is the extensive limb damage that requires amputation (Fig. 7). Amputation rates reported in the literature range from 24–44%.[22,38] Early fasciotomy of all involved muscle compartments plays an important role in limiting further damage.[39] Fasciotomy is performed when the patient is stabilized but within the first 6–8 hours after injury (Fig. 8). Measurement of compartment pressures may be helpful in borderline cases, but clinical findings should dominate the decision to perform decompression.[18,40] Fasciotomy serves two roles: a therapeutic measure for relief of ischemia secondary to increased compartment pressures and a diagnostic tool to assess the amount of deep soft tissue damage. Initial debridement of obviously necrotic tissue can be performed at the time of fasciotomy. Early vascular grafting of thrombosed upper extremity arteries may be indicated in selected cases to salvage an ischemic upper limb.[48] Early and frequent trips to the operating room are necessary for proper wound care.[18] Wounds should be dressed carefully to avoid desiccation, and exposed vital structures should be covered as soon as possible. The topical antibiotic of choice for these wounds is mafenide (Sulfamylon) in consideration of its ability to penetrate tissue deeply.

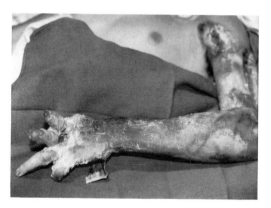
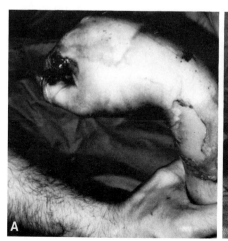

FIGURE 7. Incineration of entire upper extremity in a 5,000-volt accident.

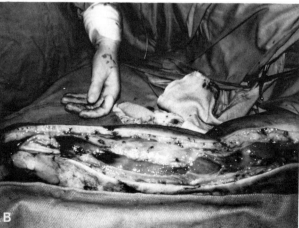

FIGURE 8. A, Major electrical injury of the upper extremity. B, Fasciotomy of the entire upper limb (same patient).

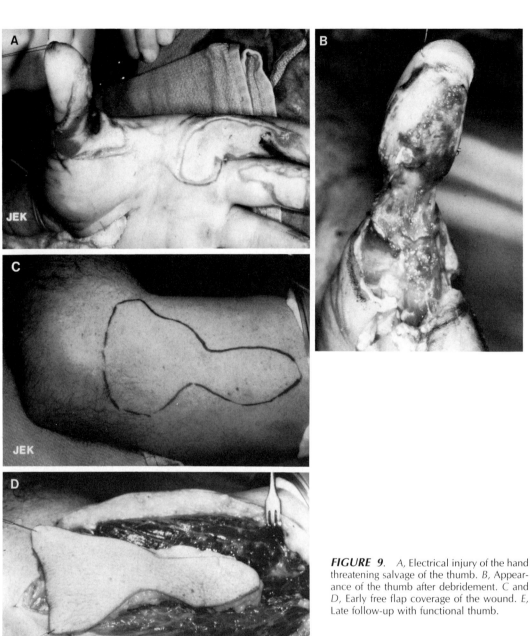

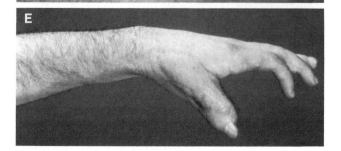

FIGURE 9. *A,* Electrical injury of the hand threatening salvage of the thumb. *B,* Appearance of the thumb after debridement. *C* and *D,* Early free flap coverage of the wound. *E,* Late follow-up with functional thumb.

Obtaining adequate debridement in electrical wounds is particularly difficult because of the pattern of injury. Muscle biopsies have demonstrated that the percentage of damaged fibers in a given muscle varies considerably, with injured and normal appearing fibers mixed together in an irregular pattern.[35] Numerous techniques have been applied as aids in the debridement of damaged muscle.[19,21,35] Initial gross appearance of the muscle is not a reliable indicator of viability. The use of fluorescein has been advocated as an indicator of muscle viability, but its interpretation is hindered by bleeding from the surrounding tissues. Arteriography has been used, but it is not a reliable indicator of the exact boundary between viable and nonviable tissue.[18] Muscle biopsy is accurate but impractical because of the large number of samples required and the time involved in processing samples. The use of technetium-99m stannous pyrophosphate scanning has been helpful in identifying injured and nonviable muscle groups in the electrically damaged area.[19]

Wound Management: Future Considerations

In the past, the concept of progressive necrosis has prevented the surgeon from attempting early definitive coverage of electrically damaged limbs for fear of covering necrotic tissue.[27,34] The clinical course in these injuries was that of multiple debridements followed by eventual amputation. Partially damaged but viable muscle, nerve, tendon, and bone left exposed by multiple debridements are subject to desiccation and infection. Prior to the development of reliable microsurgical techniques, coverage of vital structures was accomplished with the use of distant pedicled flaps such as the abdominal flap and later the groin flap. Newer pedicle flap designs have been added to this group for upper extremity coverage.[10] The pedicled flaps at some point will depend on the electrically damaged wound for survival, because these "parasitic" flaps cannot add new vascularity to an ischemic wound. This fact would explain earlier problems with flap take and subflap necrosis and sepsis. The application of free tissue transfer techniques early in the management of these difficult wounds may result in increased limb salvage and function (Fig. 9).[46,47] The free flap with its independent blood supply may be used as a nutrient flap to nourish as well as cover electrically injured vital structures. The concepts of aggressive early debridement and coverage accepted for other difficult wounds should be applied to major electrical injuries (Fig. 10).[13,28,45] Management of these injuries requires critical judgment in choosing limb salvage or ablation. Absolute in-

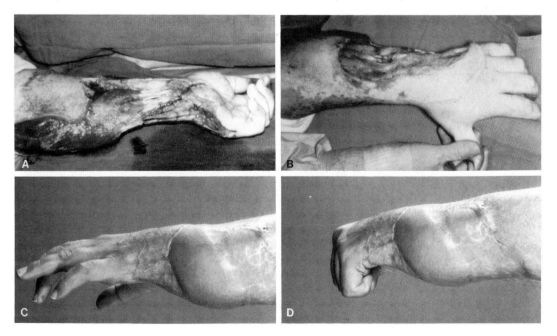

FIGURE 10. *A* and *B,* Electrical injury threatening salvage of the upper extremity. Wide debridement has been performed. *C* and *D,* Long-term follow-up after limb salvage with a free latissimus dorsi flap.

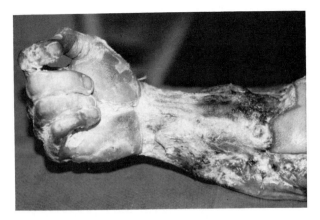

FIGURE 11. Massive destruction of the hand with no option for salvage.

dications for ablation include life-threatening sepsis, the insensate limb, and obvious unsalvageable total limb destruction (Fig. 11).

SUMMARY

Electrical injuries are devastating events that threaten the life and limbs of the victim. The extent and pattern of the injury depend on multiple factors, including voltage, current flow and path, skin resistance, and exposure time. The exact pathophysiology of tissue injury remains controversial, but the most commonly accepted mechanism of injury is the release of heat from current flowing through tissues. High-voltage injuries require aggressive techniques in both resuscitation and wound management. The initial appearance of the wound is almost always misleading, with muscle, nerve, and blood vessels sustaining more damage than the overlying skin. Victims of high-voltage injuries are subject to multiple early and late sequelae, including peripheral neuropathy, spasticity, paraplegia seizure disorders, cardiac problems, and cataracts. Survivors should have long-term medical follow-up to monitor potential problems. The use of microsurgical techniques including revascularization and free tissue transfer may offer hope of limb salvage with function in a dismal situation.

Acknowledgments

We would like to thank Drs. Warren C. Breidenbach, Joseph E. Kutz, and Henry W. Neale for the use of their cases.

REFERENCES

1. Arturson G, Hedlund A: Primary treatment of 50 patients with high tension electrical injuries. Scand J Plast Reconstr Surg 18:111, 1984.
2. Arzt CP: Changing concepts of electrical injury. Am J Surg 128:600, 1974.
3. Baxter CR: Present concepts in the management of major electrical injury. Surg Clin North Am 50:1401, 1970.
4. Bingham H: Electrical burns. Clin Plast Surg 13:75, 1986.
5. Buchanan DL, Yurel E, Spira M: Electric current arterial injury: a laboratory model. Plast Reconstr Surg 72:199, 1983.
6. Burchell HB: Electrocution: A reminder of the deadly hazard. Postgrad Med 80:21, 1986.
7. Burchell HB: Electrocution: An ever-present hazard. Postgrad Med 61:127, 1977.
8. Burke JF, Quinby WC, Bondoc C, et al: Patterns of high tension electrical injury in children and adolescents and their management. Am J Surg 133:492, 1977.
9. Burstein FD, Solomon JC, Stahl RS: Elbow joint salvage with a transverse rectus island flap: A new application. Plast Reconstr Surg 84:492, 1989.
10. Butler ED, Gant TD: Electrical injuries with special reference to the upper extremities: A review of 182 cases. Am J Surg 134:95, 1977.
11. Christensen JA, Sherman RT, Balis GA, Wicamett JD: Delayed neurologic injury secondary to high voltage current with recovery. J Trauma 20:166, 1980.
12. Daniel RK, Ballard PA, Heroux P, et al: High voltage electrical injury: Acute pathophysiology. J Hand Surg 13A:44, 1988.
13. Godina M: Early microsurgical reconstruction of complex trauma of the extremities. Plast Reconstr Surg 78:285, 1986.
14. Guinard JP, Chiolero R, Buchser E, et al: Myocardial injury after electrical burns: short and long term study. Scand J Plast Reconstr Surg 21:301, 1987.
15. Haberal MA: Electrical burns: A five-year experience. J Trauma 26:103, 1986.
16. Hammond JS, Ward CG: High voltage electrical injuries: Management and outcome of 60 cases. South Med J 81:1351, 1988.
17. Hammond JS, Ward CG: Myocardial damage and electrical injuries: Significance of early elevation of CPK-MB isoenzymes. South Med J 79:414, 1986.
18. Holliman CJ, Saffle JR, Kravitz M, Warden GD: Early surgical decompression in the management of electrical injuries. Am J Surg 144:733, 1982.
19. Hunt J, Lewis S, Parkey R, Baxter C: The use of technetium 99m stannous pyrophosphate scintigraphy to identify muscle damage in acute electric burns. J Trauma 19:409, 1979.

20. Hunt JL, Mason AD, Masterson TS, Pruitt BA: The pathophysiology of acute electric injuries. J Trauma 16:335, 1976.
21. Hunt JL, McManus WF, Haney WP: Vascular lesions in acute electric injuries. J Trauma 14:461, 1974.
22. Hunt JL, McManus WF, Haney WP: Acute electric burns. Arch Surg 115:434, 1980.
23. Jex-Blake AF: The goulstonian lectures on death by electric currents and by lightning. Br Med J 1:425, 492, 548, 601, 1913.
24. Lazarus HM, Hutto W: Electrical burns and frostbite: Patterns of vascular injury. J Trauma 22:581, 1982.
25. Lee RC, Kolodny MS: Electrical injury mechanisms: Electrical breakdown of cell membranes. Plast Reconstr Surg 80:672, 1987.
26. Lee RC, Kolodny MS: Electrical injury mechanisms: Dynamics of the thermal response. Plast Reconstr Surg 80:663, 1987.
27. Lewis GK: Electrical burns of the upper extremities. J Bone Joint Surg 40A:27, 1958.
28. Lister G: Emergency free flaps. In Green DP: Operative Hand Surgery, 2nd ed. New York, Churchill Livingstone, 1988, pp 1127–1150.
29. Luce EA, Dowden WL, Su CT, Hoopes JE: High tension electrical injury of the upper extremity. Surg Gynecol Obstet 147:38, 1978.
30. Mimoun M, Hiilgot P, Baux S: The nutrient flap: A new concept of the role of the flap and application to the salvage of the arteriosclerotic lower limb. Plast Reconstr Surg 84:458, 1989.
31. Muir IFK: The treatment of electrical burns. Br J Plast Surg 10:292, 1958.
32. Neale HW: Electrical injuries of the hand and upper extremity. In McCarthy JG: Converse's Plastic Surgery, Vol 8, 3rd ed. Philadelphia, W.B. Saunders, 1989.
33. Perotta DM, Brender J, Suarez L, et al: Occupational electrocution in Texas, 1981–85. MMWR 36:725, 1987.
34. Peterson RA: Electrical burns of the hand treatment by early excision. J Bone Joint Surg 48A:407, 1966.
35. Quinby WC, Burke JF, Trelstad RL, Caulfied J: The use of microscopy as a guide to primary excision of high tension electrical burns. J Trauma 18:423, 1978.
36. Robson MC, Murphy RC, Hegger JP: A new explanation for the progressive tissue loss in electrical injuries. Plast Reconstr Surg 73:431, 1984.
37. Rosenberg DV, Nelson, M: Rehabilitation concerns in electrical burn patients: A review of the literature. J Trauma 28:808, 1988.
38. Rouse RG, Dimick AR: The treatment of electrical injury compared to burn injury: A review of the pathophysiology and comparison of patient management protocols. J Trauma 18:43, 1978.
39. Rowlands SA: Fasciotomy: The treatment of compartment syndrome. In Green DP: Operative Hand Surgery, 2nd ed. New York, Churchill Livingstone, 1988, pp 665–708.
40. Saffle Jr, Zeluff GR, Warden GD: Intramuscular pressure in the burned arm: Measurement and response to escharotomy. Am J Surg 140:825, 1980.
41. Sances A, Larson SJ, Mykleburst JB, Cusick JF: Electrical injuries. Surg Gynecol Obstet 149:97, 1979.
42. Sances A, Mykleburst JB, Larson SJ, et al: Experimental electrical injury studies. J Trauma 21:589, 1981.
43. Salisbury RE, Dingeldein GP: Peripheral nerve complications following burn injury. Clin Orthop Res 163:92, 1982.
44. Salisbury RE, Hunt JL, Warden GD, Pruitt BA: Management of electrical burns of the upper extremity. Plast Reconstr Surg 51:648, 1973.
45. Salisbury RE, Dingeldein GP: The burned hand and upper extremity. In Green DP: Operative Hand Surgery, 2nd ed. New York, Churchill Livingstone, 1988, p 2135.
46. Silverberg B, Banis JC, Verdi GD, Acland RD: Microvascular reconstruction after electrical and deep thermal injury. J Trauma 26:128, 1986.
47. Shen T, Yonghua S, Doxing C, Naiguo W: The use of free flaps in burn patients: Experiences with 70 flaps in 65 patients. Plast Reconstr Surg 81:352, 1988.
48. Wang XW, Bartle EJ, Roberts BB: Early vascular grafting to prevent upper extremity necrosis after electric burns: Additional commentary on indications for surgery. J Burn Care Rehabil 8:391, 1987.
49. Wilkinson C, MacDonald W: High voltage electric injury. Am J Surg 136:693, 1978.
50. Zelt RG, Daniel RK, Ballard PA, et al: High voltage electric injury: Chronic wound evolution. Plast Reconstr Surg 82:1027, 1988.

Chapter 19

EMERGENCY MANAGEMENT OF THERMAL, ELECTRICAL, AND CHEMICAL BURNS

Leland R. Chick, M.D., and Graham D. Lister, M.B., Ch.B.

THERMAL BURNS

The treatment of hand burns must have begun moments after the discovery of fire. The first therapeutic maneuver is unrecorded, but it was likely the self-administration of warm, homologous saliva, a practice since discredited although still widely used by the layity. Over the years, a variety of potions and medicants have been prescribed by shamans, witch doctors, and physicians, and many of them are still in use today.

Currently the emphasis in treating burns is on immediate surgical excision of deeper wounds. This emphasis requires the primary physician to determine early which burns to refer to a surgeon. Through a combination of experience and knowledge, the physician should be able to differentiate first-, second-, and third-degree burns of the hand. Fabry proposed the first formal differentiation of burns 200 years ago on the basis of appearance. He recorded three degrees of burn: (1) redness and blistering of the skin; (2) withering of the skin without charring; (3) eschar formation and charring.[21] This classification is still useful nearly two centuries later.

First-degree burns are characterized by an inordinate amount of pain, erythema, and an edematous appearance. Second-degree burns are primarily characterized by profuse blistering and bullae filled with gelatinous material (Fig. 1). Deeper second-degree burns may not have blisters, or the blisters may not be intact, and the burns may extend down to the deeper dermis, which appears white. These burns are often difficult to differentiate from third-degree burns, which are full-thickness penetrations through the epidermis and dermis. Classically, the third-degree burn is characterized by a lack of sensation, which may be confirmed by a pinprick. This test, however, is not entirely reliable. The physician should also recognize that the depth of a burn is not a static phenomenon. Over 48–72 hours burn depth increases unless therapeutic interventions are started and sometimes in spite of this. Douglas Jackson in 1953 first described the now classical zones of coagulation, microvascular stasis, and hyperemia.[21] In this scenario the initial zone of coagulation is always lost, whereas the zones of stasis and hyperemia may potentially be salvaged by therapeutic maneuvers.

ACUTE MANAGEMENT OF THERMAL BURNS

This section describes the management of burns of the upper extremity, making the assumption that they are the only burns sustained. If large portions of the remaining body are involved, then resuscitation procedures necessarily are employed. These protocols are

259

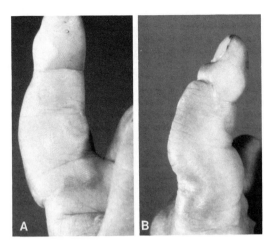

FIGURE 1. Blistering consistent with second-degree burn.

not discussed here, but health care providers must be familiar with them.[34]

Cold Water

Acute management of thermal burns of the extremities often begins with cold water, which laboratory studies have shown to have a beneficial effect on local burn metabolism. Cold water reduces the local metabolic rate by as much as 75%, absorbs the residual heat that was transferred by the accident, inhibits histamine and kinin release, and has even been shown to slow remote edema formation.[1,12] The water administered should be cold but not iced, and the patient must not be allowed to become hypothermic. Therefore, the cold water used should be limited to less than 10% of the body surface area. Most of the distal upper extremities can be treated with this amount of water. This therapy is effective when given within the first hour of the burn. After administration of cold water and relief of pain, the depth of the burn needs to be determined. Further therapy is based on this information.

Topical Therapy

First-degree burns are easily managed with topical ointments and dressings. Dressings incorporating antibacterial ointments, aloe vera gels, or silver sulfadiazine have been described. The primary choice at our medical center is a 75% aloe vera ointment, or Bacitracin. An aloe vera ointment should *not* con-

tain an alcohol vehicle and should be reapplied two to three times a day until the burn is no longer painful. The primary purpose of these ointments is to provide antisepsis and prevent desiccation of the wound. First-degree burns rapidly reepithelialize and heal within 48–72 hours. The major concern of the patient is most likely to be pain management. Removing the burn from exposure to air by covering it with moist dressings or ointments is helpful in pain management, in combination with analgesics as necessary.

Second-degree burns are also usually managed initially by topical therapy. If the burn blisters are still intact, they are left alone and usually are covered with an ointment as described above. With second-degree burns, our choice of ointments is either Silvadene or Bacitracin. Dressings are changed twice a day regardless of ointment used. Once the blisters are ruptured, the overlying blister skin is debrided and the gelatinous material is removed by gentle washing. Hand dressings are composed of a nonadherent layer such as Adaptic and wrapped loosely with a gauze wrapping such as Kerlex. In both first- and second-degree burns, motion of the hand is encouraged from the initial dressing change. With second-degree burns, hydrotherapy is often useful to cleanse the hand and to facilitate range-of-motion exercises, which are more comfortably done under water. This is usually less painful to the patient and often facilitates these exercises.

Splinting

At night the hand is often splinted in an orthoplast material with Velcro fasteners. Splinting is done with the wrist in neutral, the thumb abducted, the metacarpophalangeal joints at 60–70 degrees of flexion, and the interphalangeal joints at neutral. The splint is used only for long periods of inactivity, such as during sleep; during the day movement of the hand should be encouraged. Use of the hand in daily activities such as eating and performing toilet activities should also be encouraged. Almost by definition, superficial second-degree burns should heal within 10–14 days and should not require skin-graft coverage.

Biobrane Gloves

Another method of treating superficial second-degree burns is with Biobrane gloves.

Biobrane is an artificial membrane composed of a Silastic backing with one surface covered by bovine collagen. The collagen is held in place by very fine nylon threads attached to the Silastic. The Biobrane Company manufactures gloves of several sizes that are quite useful for large, second-degree hand burns. The glove or Biobrane patch is applied to the hand on the first day of the burn, and a light dressing is used to maintain position. After 48 hours, the dressing may be removed and the Biobrane exposed. At this time the Biobrane is usually adherent but must be protected from shear forces. Active range-of-motion exercises may begin after the dressing change. Care must be taken to remove any fluid accumulations under

the glove. After a week, neovascularization has penetrated the bovine collagen, and the collagen becomes incorporated into the wound. Reepithelialization occurs underneath the Silastic. The glove is left in place and the Silastic slowly comes off by itself in 2–3 weeks. The patient is encouraged to trim the material as it comes off. Range-of-motion exercises can be done quite well with the glove in place starting from the initial day of the burn. A major disadvantage of Biobrane gloves is cost and the necessity of keeping fluid collections from amassing under the glove material (Fig. 2).

Surgical Gloves and Silvadene

A cheaper method of managing hand burns initially, allowing early range of motion, involves the use of sterile surgical gloves and Silvadene. A glove size about a half size larger than the patient's hand is chosen. A moderate amount of Silvadene is applied to the hand, and the hand is placed in the glove and sealed with a snug, but not tight, rubber band at the wrist. Range-of-motion exercises are encouraged, and the hand may also be splinted at night, if necessary, while in the glove. Twice a day the glove is changed and the hand cleansed of old Silvadene (Fig. 3). Maceration of the hand may occur with this method, but it is usually not a serious problem.

Surgical Therapy

Deeper second- and third-degree burns are usually managed by surgical therapy. As noted before, these burns are characterized by a whitish appearance; they often have a leathery eschar and are usually insensate. Optimally they are treated by early tangential excision and skin

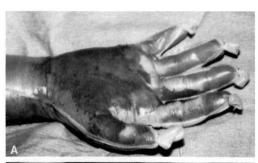
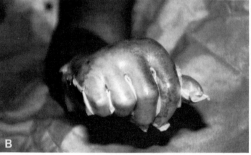

FIGURE 2. *A*, A Biobrane glove covering second-degree burns of the hand. *B*, Immediate range-of-motion exercises are possible with Biobrane gloves.

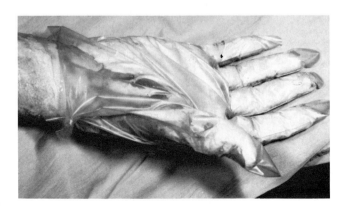

FIGURE 3. Hand treated with surgeon's glove and topical therapy. Early range of motion is encouraged.

grafting in the first 72 hours. Before surgery, they should be treated much like second-degree burns with topical therapy and splinting. For third-degree burns, Silvadene is the topical agent of choice. The use of early tangential excision and immediate grafting of these deeper burns has been associated with better functional and cosmetic results, and with less time in the hospital.[11,19,38]

Tangential excision is done with the use of a dermatome to sequentially excise the burn down to punctate bleeding (signifying viable tissue). Hemostasis must be assured, and then skin grafts are applied. When skin-grafting the hand, meshed grafts are generally not used because they allow more contraction and produce poor functional and cosmetic results (Fig. 4). When grafts extend over the digital joint surfaces, K-wire fixation of the fingers with the

metacarpophalangeal joints in flexion and the interphalangeal joints in extension is indicated for 7–10 days. After this time the K-wires are removed and range of motion is begun. The exercises should initially involve only active range of motion because passive range of motion may still shear the skin grafts in the second week. After 2 weeks, passive range-of-motion exercises may begin.

Burns of the more proximal upper extremity are treated in a similar fashion to hand burns. Deep burns of the axilla are maintained in an airplane splint with the arm abducted to nearly 90 degrees when range-of-motion exercises are not being performed. Elbows are kept extended when burns extend across the flexor surface. When small areas on the upper extremity are burned, especially where there is lax skin (such as on the dorsum of the hand or

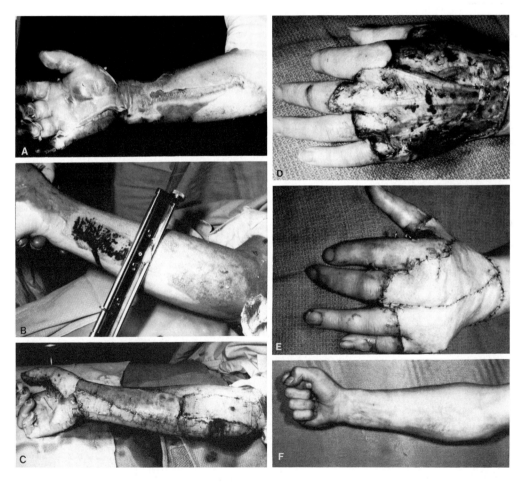

FIGURE 4. *A*, Full-thickness burn of the hand and forearm. *B*, The forearm burn is tangentially excised with the Humby knife to viable tissue. *C*, Split thickness skin grafts are applied to the forearm after tangential excision. *D*, The dorsum of the hand after burn excision. *E*, Unmeshed split-thickness grafts applied to the dorsum of the hand. *F*, The arm and hand 1 year after the burn.

the flexor surface of the forearm), excision and primary closure should be considered. This procedure leaves linear scars and decreases the risk of infection and of later contracture and cosmetic deformities. However, situations in which this method can be used are not common.

FOLLOW-UP OF THERMAL HAND BURNS

Infections

Several complications may occur after the initial therapy of upper extremity burns. Within the first 2 weeks, infection is the most common complication. The burn wound itself is usually sterile for the first 48–72 hours, but after this time, it becomes colonized. Currently the use of prophylactic antibiotics is indicated only for extreme and gross contamination of the burn wound or for exposed joint or bone. Within 48–72 hours the most likely pathogen causing infection, manifesting as a local cellulitis, is a streptococcus. These infections are easily treated with penicillin. After 5–7 days, staphylococcal infections become more commonplace. Hospitalized patients are at risk of developing infections from other pathogens, such as *Pseudomonas* and *Proteus* species. Infections of the hand should be taken seriously; hospitalization and intravenous antibiotics are usually required. Infected hands should be splinted and made immobile, and the extremity should be elevated. When significant infections occur, excision of the burn eschar should be done expediently to minimize loss of tissue. After skin graft coverage or secondary healing has occurred, infection is rarely a problem.

Boutonnière Deformity

Full-thickness burns on the dorsum of the hand may expose tendons, especially over the proximal interphalangeal joints. A common sequel of hand burns is the boutonnière deformity, which results, in this case, from nonrecognition of the exposure of the central extensor tendon and ensuing necrosis of the tendon. When tendons become exposed, they need to be covered expediently to protect them from desiccation. This can be done with local skin flaps if available, or with more distant flaps, either as free vascularized tissue transfers or

as pedicled flaps, depending on the expertise of the surgeon.[4,13,26,36]

Contractures

Contractures of the hand are perhaps the most feared long-term complication of hand burns (Fig. 5). Flexion contractures of the digits, wrist and/or elbow, and quite often of the axilla, are usually involved. Contractures are best managed by prevention, which requires early graft or flap coverage of deep second-degree and full-thickness defects, and by proper splinting and range-of-motion exercises. When the hand is burned, the most common position for it to assume, if left alone, is with the metacarpophalangeal joints in extension, the interphalangeal joints in flexion, and the thumb adducted and flexed. This is the position of the claw hand, which is difficult to correct. Contractures are caused by wounds that remain open and inactive for prolonged periods of time, allowing myofibroblasts to close the wound by contracture. Repair of these contractures requires release of the scar bands and replacement of tissue lost with either local (or distant) skin flaps or full-thickness skin grafts. Split-thickness skin grafts are not commonly used because they permit wound contraction. For burns in children, scar releases must often be repeated throughout the growing stages, because scar and skin grafts often do not grow at the same rate as normal skin. With severe digital contractures, amputation must be considered. If proximal interphalangeal contractures are long-standing, release of the checkreins (volar plate adhesions)[37] or collateral ligaments[7] may be necessary. Tenolysis of the extensor and flexor tendons is occasionally required.

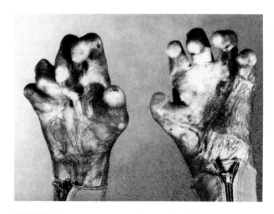

FIGURE 5. Severe contractures of both hands seen after grafting of burns.

Contractures over the flexor surface of the elbow and the axilla are usually manifested as bands. They can sometimes be released and Z-plasties performed to obtain more tissue in the area of the burn. Occasionally flaps or full-thickness skin grafts are necessary.

When contractures develop early, splinting in combination with the use of pressure garments can sometimes decrease scar hypertrophy. Pressure garments have long been recognized to decrease scar hypertrophy and should be indicated in almost all hand burns beyond the first degree. The Jobst Company (Toledo, OH) makes the largest selection. Pressure garments are designed to maintain a pressure of 24 mmHg and are custom-fitted for each patient. They are available as gloves, gauntlet sleeves, or entire upper-body garments. When prescribed, they are used for at least 6 months or until the scars become pale and do not blanche when pressed. Use may well extend beyond a year. The garment should not be removed for more than $\frac{1}{2}$ hour at a time. We have found pressure garments useful after wounds have healed by secondary intent or after grafting. They are also useful after scar releases to prevent recurrence.

Close cooperation between the treating physician and the hand therapist is necessary. The use of splinting techniques, both static and dynamic, can be helpful in managing contractures.

ELECTRICAL INJURIES OF THE UPPER EXTREMITY*

Electrical burns result from direct conversion of electrical energy into heat, which is dependent upon current (amperage), voltage, and resistance, as expressed by Ohm's law. Generally speaking, voltage is the most important variable for predicting the amount of tissue destruction in an electrical burn. The amperage is often impossible to ascertain. Electrical injuries are often broken down into low-voltage and high-voltage injuries. By arbitrary agreement, high-voltage injuries involve more than 1000 volts. The type of current, direct or alternating, is also important. Alternating current is more likely to cause immediate death from ventricular fibrillations, respiratory arrest, or asphyxia from diaphrag-

matic tetany. The local burns caused by alternating current usually result from low voltage and are often minor. Direct current is less likely to cause immediate death, but the local effects are more serious.

High-tension lines may carry up to 350,000 volts, and other lines often have well over 10,000 volts. In a series of high-tension electrical injuries to the upper extremity,[27] the voltage seen in 40 burns averaged more than 14,000 volts. Only 5 of the 40 patients suffered injuries at less than 4000 volts. The mean percentage of body surface area involved was nearly 18%. An average of four operations per hospitalization was done, and 11 patients suffered extremity amputations. An additional 7 patients lost fingers or toes. The average duration of hospital stay was nearly 38 days, demonstrating the extreme severity of high-tension electrical injuries.

High-tension electrical injuries are usually suffered when the upper extremity comes in contact with a high-tension line; the electricity exits either through the feet or through some other portion of the body that is in contact with a grounded surface. The entrance wounds are usually full-thickness wounds, typically leathery or charred. In contradistinction, the exit wounds often look "exploded"; they have a larger and more impressive appearance. There may be more than one entry site and more than one exit site.

An arc burn may be produced by current coursing external to the body, either from contact to ground or across joints. Most commonly it crosses the wrist joint, the elbow joint, and the axilla. It may also be related to a violent flexion contraction of the limb stimulated by electricity to bring the wrist, forearm, and axilla adjacent to each other. Burns sustained in the arcing may be severe; temperatures up to 4000°C have been recorded.[28] The hand may be severely charred; the wrist itself may appear to be less involved with a deep burn in the distal forearm. Other burns may also be sustained when clothing catches fire, as it often does in arc burns. Cutaneous thermal burns may further complicate the situation.

Proximal to the upper extremity, the physician should be very cautious of the cardiopulmonary effects of electrical burns and of their effects on other portions of the body. Specifically, resuscitation of these patients requires much more fluid than with thermal burns of a similar body surface area. In general, these patients require twice as much fluid for the

---

* See also Chapter 18.

same calculation of body surface area. We usually calculate the requirement to be at least 4 cc of lactated Ringer's solution per kg per percentage of cutaneous burn in the first 24 hours, and 2.5 cc per kg per percentage of cutaneous burn in the second 24 hours.[28] The patient should be monitored for cardiac arrhythmias, and the ABCs of trauma therapy should be observed from the outset. The patient may have fallen some distance when burned, and care must be taken to assess cervical spine injuries. The hospital course may be complicated by myoglobinuria and renal failure. This should be monitored by urinalysis over the first 24 hours and treated aggressively if myoglobinuria is seen.

At the site of injury, the extremity should be placed in clean dressings, which may be dampened with saline solution to prevent further desiccation. Transport to a surgical facility or burn unit is mandatory after high-tension electrical injury. Resuscitation should begin immediately as should tetanus prophylaxis. Antibiotics are generally not given unless there is severe contamination. At the burn unit or hospital, serious consideration should be given for escharotomy and fasciotomies of the upper extremity. Subfascial edema develops after high-voltage electrical burns and results in compartment syndromes. Indications for fasciotomy should include paresthesias of the distal extremity, loss of sensation, obvious circulatory problems including loss of pulse or of capillary refill, or merely concerns about muscle compartments. It is our belief that excessive tissue turgor is an indication for fasciotomy. We therefore do not routinely do intercompartmental pressures and frequently perform fasciotomy and escharotomy in these cases. These procedures can often be accomplished without anesthesia in deep burns. Local infiltration or regional nerve blocks are useful, if anesthesia is necessary.

Fasciotomies are usually done in the operating room. They are often quite bloody and may require blood transfusions despite careful hemostasis. In the upper extremity, the fasciotomy is done on the ulnar and radial aspects of all five digits, combined with release of the intrinsic muscle compartments and of the carpal tunnel. Release of Guyon's canal may be done at the same time as carpal tunnel release. Longitudinal incisions should be used in the palm and on the dorsum of the hand, and more serpentine longitudinal incisions are made over the volar and dorsal forearm compartments.

Care is taken to release all compartments. The wounds are then dressed without closure.

At our institution silver sulfadiazine is the primary chemotherapy. Over very deep, charred eschar, Sulfamylon, which penetrates deeply, may be useful to reach deeper tissues. However, care should be taken not to use Sulfamylon over more than 20% of the body surface area because metabolic acidosis may result. After the initial escharotomies, further tissue debridements are necessary. Generally the first debridement is done within the first 48 hours to remove grossly nonviable tissues. Further debridements are often necessary before definitive skin coverage can be obtained. Amputations are quite common in this group because of extensive burns of the distal extremity, specifically to tendons and nerves. We have found free tissue transfers to be useful in many acute situations to salvage distal extremities. These transfers should be considered when appropriate expertise is available.

Low-voltage injuries—that is, injuries at less than 1000 volts—often leave local burns. However, these full-thickness burns can often be excised and closed primarily. Injuries to nerves and tendons are much less common. Care should be taken not to allow contractures to occur after these injuries, and range-of-motion exercises and splinting should be done early, if they are necessary.

Outdoor workers are subject to lightning injuries. Cardiopulmonary resuscitation is the major concern after a lightning injury. Many patients are reported to have survived lightning strikes even though vital functions have been absent for prolonged periods of time. Therefore, cardiopulmonary resuscitation should be initiated on anyone found after a lightning strike, regardless of the time since injury. The management of extremity burns after lightning strikes is much the same as that for high-tension injuries. Fasciotomies are performed as necessary, and debridement and amputations are often necessary. Interestingly, many nerve deficits that are seen early resolve without sequelae after lightning strikes.[28]

CHEMICAL BURNS

Chemical burns are not particularly common as compared with thermal burns. However, more than 25,000 different chemicals used in industry can cause burns.[6] Twenty years ago the number of chemical burns requiring professional care exceeded 60,000 per year.[6] This number can only have increased since then.

Fortunately, the initial treatment for most chemical burns is massive lavage with water. Notable exceptions include burns from hydrofluoric acid, phenol, elemental sodium, and potassium, and, to some extent, white phosphorus. Management of these specific burns is described in this section. After dilution of the chemical, wound care is generally similar to that for other burns, involving topical ointments and dressings described previously, with surgical debridement and wound coverage as necessary. Successful decontamination at the accident site may prevent the need for surgical intervention.

Chemical burns are discussed below in alphabetical order.

Alkyl mercuric agents.[22]   Burns from alkyl mercuric agents characteristically present as erythema with blister formation. The blister fluid may cause deepening of the burn unless the blister is debrided and liberally irrigated with water. This phenomenon may be due to free metallic mercury within the blister fluid. Furthermore, cutaneous absorption of the mercury occurs and may be fatal at more than 5 mg of the compound per kg of body weight.

Ammonia (NH_4).[9]   Ammonia is a very common, strong alkali capable of causing severe liquefaction necrosis of tissues. Injury is dependent on concentration and duration of exposure. Respiratory sequelae are possible with prolonged exposure to fumes. Removal of contaminated garments and copious lavage are mandatory before transportation to a medical facility.

Asphalt/tar.[18]   Asphalt or tar is used extensively in roofing and road construction; it is useful only when heated to temperatures of 250–500°F. Upon contact with skin, it adheres, becomes enmeshed in hair, and is quite difficult to remove physically. Resulting burns are often deep owing to prolonged contact. Immediate cooling of the asphalt/tar and body area with cold water is required, and the substance is then best removed by a petroleum-based compound, such as Bacitracin or Neosporin ointments. Removal of the asphalt/tar is not as important as cooling the area. Further therapy depends on the depth of the burn, which is treated as a thermal burn. Prophylactic antibiotics may be considered, although wound infections were not seen in one large series.[18]

Calcium hydroxide.   See Lye.

Chromic acid ($CrO3$).[22,32]   Chromic acid is a pungent, yellow, viscid liquid used in metal cleaning. A potent oxidizer, it causes ulceration and blister formation with coagulation necrosis after skin contact. Burns often leave deep holes in the skin surrounded by peeled areas ("chromeholes"). These may be filled with pus as a result of coagulation necrosis. The lesions are often painless. Removal of contaminated clothing and copious lavage with water are indicated.

Cantharide.[22]   In the past, cantharide was used as a veterinary aphrodisiac (the "Spanish fly"). It is a potent vesicant, causing papules of 0.5–1.0 cm and a severe histamine response. Partial-thickness burns are common. Water lavage is indicated.

Cement.[31]   Burns from prolonged exposure to wet cement are not uncommon. They are most likely due to the production of calcium hydroxide during manufacture of the cement, which, together with hydrolysis of complex silicates when cement is mixed with water, produces a pH in the range of 12–14. Treatment is water lavage and topical therapy. Pike[31] suggests the use of an Unna's boot to allow early ambulation.

Creosol, creosote.[10]   Creosol and creosote are related substances used as chemical intermediaries, disinfectants, and wood preservatives. They commonly cause skin dermatitis on exposure. The depth and severity of burns are related to phenol content (see Phenol).

Dichromate salts.[22,25]   Used primarily in metal electroplating, dichromate salts are highly corrosive to skin and mucosa. Chronic exposure may result in indolent ulcerations of skin, dermatitis, and perforations of the nasal septum. If ingested, the lethal dose may be as low as 500 mg. Death from cutaneous absorption has been reported.[25] In smaller burns, generous water lavage is indicated; in larger exposures, immediate excision should be considered.[25]

Formic acid ($HCOOH$).[10,33]   Formic acid is used in tanning, in manufacture of airplane glue and cellulose formate, and in European agriculture as a hay preservative. It is a metabolite of formaldehyde and methanol when these are ingested. After cutaneous exposure, severe metabolic abnormalities and hemolytic anemia and hemoglobinuria have been reported.[33] Burned skin may take on a greenish color and blister later. Early water lavage is indicated.

Freon.[10]   Freon is a fluorocarbon widely used as a refrigerant and propellant and in the manufacture of polytetrafluoroethylene (Teflon).

Thermal decomposition may result in hydrofluoric acid, hydrochloric acid, and phosgene. Cutaneous exposure results in frostbite burns. Rapid rewarming of frozen tissues, aspirin for antiprostaglandin action, and topical therapy are indicated.

Gasoline and hydrocarbons.[16,20,34] Gasoline and hydrocarbons are fuels and solvents that are primarily skin irritants; prolonged exposure is required for burns of the skin. At least theoretically, cutaneous exposure to leaded gasoline may result in acute toxicity through absorption of tetraethyl lead.[34] After extensive exposure, serum and urinary lead levels should be monitored. Inhalation of gasoline fumes may result in pulmonary, hepatic, and renal dysfunction. At initial therapy removal of sources of contamination should be followed by prolonged (more than 1 hour) water lavage. Cutaneous burns are afterward treated with topical therapy and surgery as necessary.

Hydrofluoric acid.[2,3,8,14,23] Hydrofluoric acid is widely used in industry in production of fluorocarbons, high octane fuels, glass and metal cleaning, rust-removing compounds, and silicon chip etching. Burns are characterized by (1) an intense, deep pain that may be delayed in onset by several hours, (2) coagulative skin necrosis, (3) progressive tissue destruction eventually causing bony erosions, (4) a predilection for subungual necrosis. Death has been reported as a consequence of exposing 1% of body surface area, secondary to sudden and severe hypocalcemia.[14] Symptoms are related to the concentration of the solution and are thought to be related to fluoride binding to intracellular calcium and magnesium, causing cell death, which re-releases the fluoride ion. Symptoms may progress over several days.

Initial treatment should consist of removal of contaminated gloves or clothing, copious lavage, and most importantly, binding of the fluoride ion. This may be done initially by application of a calcium gluconate gel; alternately, we have described a calcium carbonate mixture that can be easily prepared.[3] If symptoms persist, local injection of a 10% calcium gluconate solution is required.[8] Because relief of pain is the end-point of therapy, anesthesia is contraindicated. Intra-arterial injections of calcium gluconate are occasionally useful.[23] Follow-up of these patients is mandatory. In-hospital monitoring is required for (1) ≥1% total body surface area exposure to a 50% or greater solution, (2) >5% of total body surface area exposure to any solution, and (3) inhalation of a 60% solution.

Hydrochloric acid (muriatic acid.)[10] Hydrochloric acid is used in dye and chemical synthesis, metal refining, and plumbing. Coagulative necrosis follows skin exposure, and severe scarring may result. Copious water lavage after removal of contaminated clothing is required.

Lithium.[10,25] Lithium is used in nuclear reactor coolants, alkaline storage batteries, and alloy manufacturing. It is a strong, corrosive alkali. Water lavage is indicated as an initial therapy and should be prolonged for at least 1 hour. **Elemental lithium** fragments must be removed and covered with mineral oil before irrigation; otherwise serious burns result.

Lye.[14] Lye is the general term for corrosive alkalis, including sodium hydroxide, calcium hydroxide, and potassium hydroxide, among many others. Cutaneous burns tend to result from liquefaction necrosis and may penetrate deeply (Fig. 6). Prolonged water lavage is man-

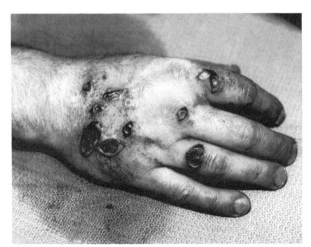

FIGURE 6. Deep, penetrating local burns due to lye splattering.

datory for at least an hour, with recommendations of up to 24 hours. Hydrotherapy tank baths may be useful.

Muriatic acid. See Hydrochloric acid.

Nitric acid.[10] Nitric acid is used in engraver's acid, electroplating, and fertilizer manufacturing. A peculiar yellow color occurs in the area of a burn. Water lavage is indicated initially.

Phenol.[10,30] Used in disinfectants, solvents, and wood preservatives, phenol causes protein denaturation resulting in a relatively painless coagulum. When absorbed through skin, larger exposures may result in arrhythmias, convulsions, and cardiovascular collapse. Patients should be monitored closely for several hours after exposure. Initially, high-flow water lavage is necessary (i.e., a shower); if a shower is not available, polyethylene glycol, glycerol, or vegetable oil may be used to remove the substance.

Phosphorus (white phosphorus).[29] Used in munitions manufacture, phosphorus is most often associated with military casualties. In the presence of air, it is rapidly oxidized in a severe exothermic reaction. The fire may be extinguished by immersion in water to remove oxygen exposure. Reexposure to air reignites the process. The phosphorus particles must be removed to prevent reignition. They are best seen and removed with the aid of a Wood's lamp. A dilute (1%) copper sulfate solution has been recommended; however, systemic absorption of the copper sulfate may result in massive hemolysis and renal failure. Major efforts should be directed toward removal of affected clothing, maintaining a wet environment, and removal of all particles of phosphorus. Mineral oil is useful for coating the burn and particles to prevent air exposure.

Potassium (elemental potassium).[5] Potassium reacts explosively in the presence of water. Water lavage is thus contraindicated. Initial therapy consists of removal of clothing and removal of particles of potassium attached to skin. Mineral oil (or any other available oil) is then applied to burn areas. In hospital, the wounds are debrided further to remove all fragments. Potassium fragments are disposed of by immersion in pure *tert*-butyl alcohol.

Potassium hydroxide. See Lye.

Potassium permanganate.[10] Used in the photographic, pharmaceutical, and chemical industries, potassium permanganate causes a coagulative necrosis with surrounding deep purple staining. Initial therapy consists of copious lavage with water.

Povidone-iodine. Prolonged exposure to pools of povidone-iodine may cause burns. Initial therapy consists of removal of contamination and water lavage.

Propane (liquid).[17] Propane may produce deep tissue injuries with massive subcutaneous and subfascial edema, as well as cutaneous burns. Fasciotomies may be required. Wounds are otherwise treated like frostbite injuries; surgical debridement may be necessary.

Sodium (elemental).[5] Sodium reacts explosively with water owing to a severe exothermic reaction. Treatment consists of removal of particles and clothing and covering burns with mineral oil (or any available oil). In the hospital, further debridement of burns is often required. Elemental sodium particles may be disposed of in pure isopropyl alcohol (<2% water).

Sodium hypochlorite. Sodium hypochlorite is used in bleaches and in medicine as Dakin's solution. See Lye.

Sodium hydroxide. Sodium hydroxide is a severe caustic used in drain cleaners. See Lye.

Sulfuric acid.[10] Sulfuric acid is used as a 90–95% solution in chemical, munitions, and fertilizer industries. Solutions of 25–30% are used in machinery and batteries; toilet bowl cleaners use a 10% solution. Skin injury is dependent on duration of exposure and concentration of solution. Injuries range from erythema and blisters to penetrating ulcers. Initial treatment consists of removal of contaminated clothing and copious water lavage.

Trichloroacetic acid.[10] Solutions of 60% trichloroacetic acid are used in hat making, printing, and rayon manufacture. More dilute concentrations are used in disinfectants and hair-wave neutralizers. Burn severity is dependent on concentration and the length of exposure. Initial treatment consists of removal of contaminated clothing and copious water lavage.

REFERENCES

1. Boykin JV, Eriksson E, Sholley MM, Pittman RN: Histamine-mediated delayed permeability response after scald burn inhibited by cimetidine or cold-water treatment. Science 209:815–817, 1980.
2. Brown TD: The treatment of hydrofluoric acid burns. J Soc Occup Med 24:80–89, 1974.
3. Chick LR, Borah GB: Treatment of hydrofluoric acid burns of the hand. Plast Reconstr Surg (in press).

4. Chow JA, Bilos J, Hui P, et al: Groin flap in reparative surgery of the hand. Plast Reconstr Surg 77:421–425, 1986.
5. Clare RA, Krenzelok EP: Chemical burns secondary to elemental metal exposure. Am J Emerg Med 6:355–357, 1988.
6. Curreri PW, Asch MJ, Pruitt BA: The treatment of chemical burns. J Trauma 10:634, 1970.
7. Curtis RM: Management of the stiff hand. In Hunter JR, Schneider LH, Mackin EJ (eds): Rehabilitation of the Hand. St Louis, C.V. Mosby, 1978, pp 209–215.
8. Dibell DG, Iverson RE, et al: Hydrofluoric acid burns of the hand. J Bone Joint Surg 52A:931–936, 1970.
9. Edelman PA: Chemical and electrical burns. In Achaver BM (ed): Management of the Burned Patient. Norwalk, CT, Appleton & Lange, 1987, pp 183–202.
10. Ellenhorn MJ, Barceloux DG: Medical Toxicology: Diagnosis and Treatment of Human Poisoning. New York, Elsevier, 1988.
11. Engrav LH, Heimback DM, Rues JL, et al: Early excision and grafting vs. nonoperative treatment of burns of indeterminate depth: A randomized prospective study. J Trauma 23:1001–1004, 1983.
12. Eriksson E, Robson M: New pathophysiological mechanism explaining post-burn edema. Burns 4:153, 1977.
13. Gilbert, DA: Overview of flaps for hand and forearm reconstruction. Clin Plast Surg 8:129–139, 1981.
14. Greco RJ, Hartford CE, Haith LR, et al: Hydrofluoric acid-induced hypocalcemia. J Trauma 28:1593–1596, 1988.
15. Gruber RP, Laub DR, Vistnes LM: Effect of hydrotherapy on the clinical course and pH of experimental cutaneous chemical burns. Plast Reconstr Surg 55:200–204, 1975.
16. Hansbrough JF, Zapata-Sirvent R, Dominic W, et al: Hydrocarbon contact injuries. J Trauma 25:250–252, 1985.
17. Hicks LM, Hunt JL, Baxter CR: Liquid propane cold injury: A clinicopathologic and experimental study. J Trauma 19:701–703, 1979.
18. Hill MB, Achaver BM, Martinez S: Tar and asphalt burns. J Burn Care Rehabil 5:271–274, 1984.
19. Hunt JL, Sato R, Baxter CR: Early tangential excision and immediate mesh autografting of deep dermal hand burns. Ann Surg 189:147–151, 1979.
20. Hunter GA: Chemical burns of the skin after contact with petrol. Br J Plast Surg 21:337–341, 1968.
21. Jackson DM: The diagnosis of the depth of burning. Br J Surg 40:588–596, 1953.
22. Jelenko, C: Chemicals that burn. J Trauma 14:65–72, 1974.
23. Kohnlein HE, Achinger R: A new method of treatment of hydrofluoric acid burns of the extremities. Chir Plast 6:297–305, 1982.
24. Laseter GF: Management of the stiff hand: A practical approach. Orthop Clin North Am 14:749–765, 1983.
25. Leonard LG: Chemical burns: Effect of prompt first aid. J Trauma 22:420–422, 1982.
26. Lister GD: Local flaps to the hand. Hand Clin 1:621–640, 1985.
27. Luce EA, Gottlieb SE: "True" high-tension electrical injuries. Ann Plast Surg 12:321–326, 1984.
28. Monafo WW, Freedman BM: Electrical and lightning injury. In Boswick J (ed): Art and Science of Burn Care. Rockville, MD, Aspen, 1987, pp 241–252.
29. Monzingo DW, Smith AA, McManus WF, et al: Chemical burns. J Trauma 28:642–647, 1988.
30. Pardoe R, Minami RT, Sato RM, Schlesinger SL: Phenol burns. Burns 3:29–41, 1977.
31. Pike J, Patterson A, Arons MS: Chemistry of cement burns: Pathogenesis and treatment. J Burn Care Rehabil 9:258–260, 1988.
32. Saydjari R, Abston S, Desai MH, Herndon DN: Chemical burns. J Burn Care Rehabil 7:404–408, 1986.
33. Sigurdsson J, Bjornsson A, Gudmundsson ST: Formic acid burn—Local and systemic effects. Burns 9:358–361, 1983.
34. Simpson LA, Cruse CW: Gasoline immersion injury. Plast Reconstr Surg 67:54–57, 1981.
35. Thornton JW: Resuscitation. In Achauer BM (ed): Management of the Burned Patient. Norwalk, CT, Appleton & Lange, 1987, pp 67–77.
36. Upton J, Rogers C, Durham-Smith G, Swartz WM: Clinical applications of free temporoparietal flaps in hand reconstruction. J Hand Surg 11A:475–483, 1986.
37. Watson HK, Light TR, Johnson TR: Checkrein resection for flexion contracture of the middle joint. J Hand Surg 4:67–71, 1979.
38. Wexler MR, Yeschua R, Neuman Z: Early treatment of burns of the dorsum of the hand by tangential excision and skin grafting. Plast Reconstr Surg 54:268–273, 1974.

Chapter 20

PERIPHERAL NERVE INJURIES AND THEIR MANAGEMENT

R. Frederick Torstrick, M.D.

While not nearly as dramatic or as common as a severely angulated fracture, vascular lesion, or extensive superficial laceration, peripheral nerve injuries of the upper extremity can ultimately be functionally devastating to the injured patient. In a survey conducted by Yale University School of Medicine, Kelsey et al. noted an estimated 21,000 peripheral nerve injuries for 1977, compared to an estimated 819,000 upper extremity disorders during the same time period.[12] Of those neurologic lesions, most were confined to the hand and digits. Even in skilled hands, the prognosis for an excellent outcome from treatment of a complete transection of a major peripheral nerve may be significantly decreased when compared to the management of similar lesions of the tendons, vessels, or bones. It is therefore incumbent upon the treating physician to be able to diagnose and institute the appropriate care of these injuries.

HISTORICAL BACKGROUND

Relatively little attention was directed toward the treatment of peripheral nerve injuries until the late 19th century. Hippocrates of Cos simply accepted the fact that a severed nerve or tendon would not spontaneously repair itself and actually did not differentiate between these two structures.[9] Salicetti, a 13th century Italian surgeon, demonstrated how to repair a nerve, while Ferrara, a fellow countryman, reported

on an experimental neurorrhaphy in 1608.[19] Paget, in 1847, reported to the Royal College of Surgeons on two methods of nerve healing and noted that if a nerve was cut, union would occur if the two nerve ends were in contact.[2]

The past 100 years has seen our most dramatic advances in the care of peripheral nerve injuries, in large part secondary to war injuries. S. Weir Mitchell first described the management of causalgia in his experience as head of a hospital for nervous diseases during the Civil War.[2,19] Similar opportunities to observe nerve injuries were experienced by Tinel during World War I, and Sir Herbert Seddon in England and Sir Sidney Sunderland in Australia during World War II.[2,19,20,26] More recently, Burkhalter and Omer have had the opportunity to evaluate experiences with peripheral nerve injuries during the Vietnam conflict.

Perhaps the greatest technical advances in the 20th century have come as an outgrowth of Carl Olaf Nylen's utilization of the microscope as an intraoperative instrument in 1921. Thereafter, we are indebted to the creation of the binocular microscope by Holmgren and Zeiss in 1923.[17] Testament to its usefulness are the advances achieved by Sunderland, Bunke, and Millesi during the past two decades.

ANATOMY

To understand the pathophysiology of nerve injury and its subsequent repair, it is beneficial to review briefly normal peripheral neuroanatomy.

Peripheral nerves are composed of several elements of either ectodermal or mesodermal origin. Nerve fibers (axons) are the distal extension of the anterior horn cells or dorsal sensory ganglia. These fibers may be either myelinated or unmyelinated. Myelinated fibers conduct impulses much more rapidly (50 meters per second) and function in balance, proprioception, vibratory feedback, and motor function. Unmyelinated fibers are slow conducting (1 meter per second) and provide feedback of visceral pain and so forth.[25] Endoneurium is the connective tissue that protects the axon, resists elongation under tension, and forms the supporting wall of the endoneural tube. A fascicle (funiculus) is several axons bundled together and surrounded by a thin layer of connective tissue composed of up to 12 layers of tightly packed cells, the perineurium. This structure is 1.3 to 100 microns thick and is essential in ionic transport of materials, acting as a diffusion barrier, as the regulator of axoplasmic flow, in the maintenance of proper endoneural pressure, and in resisting stretch. The fasciculi are separated from endoneurium and supported by areolar connective tissue that contains the major vasculature of the nerve, the epineurium. The epineurium constitutes 30 to 75% of the cross-sectional area of the peripheral nerve and is thickened at its periphery to form the epineural sheath; it functions primarily to protect the nerve against compression. Finally, the microcirculation to the peripheral nerve is both segmental and longitudinal in configuration.[6,11,15,19,26]

PATHOPHYSIOLOGY

When a nerve is completely transected, axons with their encircling Schwann cells and myelin sheath are divided, with loss of nerve conductivity within 72 hours. Subsequently, the distal portion of the nerve fiber degenerates to about 50% of its normal size,[6] with subsequent degeneration of axons and phagocytosis of the surrounding myelin. Proximally, an increase in metabolic activity and hyperactivity of the central cell body occurs between the 4th and 20th day after injury. Within 2 to 8 weeks, Schwann cells digest the myelin of the endoneural tube, followed by proximal axonal sprouting 4 to 21 days after the injury, which grows distally at a rate of 1 to 5 mm per day after a 1-month delay at the site of transection.[6,15,25] If there is no obstruction to the newly budding axons that are migrating distally, then there exists the possibility that sensory and motor fibers will direct themselves into the empty distal endoneural tubes, aided by any neurotrophic factors. One hopes that reinnervation of their respective sensory and motor nerve endings without excessive crossover will occur before irreversible motor atrophy. The goal of the hand surgeon, then, is to intervene in those instances when a nerve is not in continuity to attempt to increase the likelihood of successful distal reinnervation of end organs.

CLASSIFICATION

Peripheral nerve injuries may be subdivided into degrees of severity based upon the anatomical components that are involved.[15,19,20] Seddon (1943) described his concept of neural lesions as neurapraxia, axonotmesis, and neurotmesis. Sunderland has grouped these types of nerve lesions into five types (Table 1). Type I is equivalent to Seddon's neurapraxia. Types II and III are equivalent to Seddon's axonotmesis with and without disruption of the Schwann cell membrane, respectively. Types IV and V are equivalent to Seddon's neurotmesis with and without an intact epineurium, respectively.

TABLE 1.   Classification of Neural Lesions*

Structures Involved	Sunderland Injuries				
	I (Neurapraxia)	II (Axonotmesis)	III	IV (Neurotmesis)	V
Myelin	±	+	+	+	+
Axon		+	+	+	+
Endoneurium			+	+	+
Perineurium				+	+
Epineurium					

*Modified from Mackinnon SE, Dellon AL: Surgery of the Peripheral Nerve. New York, Thieme Medical Publishers, 1988, p 35.

Lesions of **neurapraxia** are lesions associated with a physiologic block in nerve conduction, without wallerian degeneration. Three types have been noted: ionic, vascular, and mechanical. The patient may present with a loss of motor and/or sensory function that should recover within a 6- to 8-week period without neurologic crossover.[23] Failure to do so would suggest a lesion of greater magnitude. Notable exceptions are radial nerve palsies secondary to distal humeral fractures that have been noted to have a 90% recovery rate if given 3 to 4 months to recover.[6,17]

An **axonotmesis** may be associated with axonal disruption and subsequent wallerian degeneration with (Sunderland II) or without (Sunderland III) an intact Schwann cell sheath. The epineurium and perineurium, however, are intact. Low-velocity and some high-velocity gunshot wounds are examples of such lesions, which may take up to 6 months for recovery with a functional result closely approximating that of neurapraxia.[6,17] Sunderland III lesions, on the other hand, involve disruption of the endoneural tube, and therefore crossover occurs with some resultant disorientation of sensory and motor fibers. Typical of these lesions is the crossover of sensory fibers normally supplying one digit that subsequently innervate a contiguous digit. The patient therefore experiences some altered pattern of sensation and sensory reeducation may be necessary.

A **neurotmesis** is due to a complete disruption of the peripheral nerve (Sunderland V) or all elements of the nerve with the exception of the epineurium (Sunderland IV). The clinical presentation of either of these lesions is similar, with a Sunderland IV injury being typical of neuroma in continuity as compared to a Sunderland V lesion being exemplified by a completely disrupted nerve. It is these latter two lesions to which the majority of surgical management is usually directed.[23]

TREATMENT

General Considerations

While the previously noted classification is useful for understanding the pathophysiology of the peripheral nerve, most injuries demonstrate characteristics of more than one degree of lesion. Therefore, a nerve injury may manifest elements of a neurapraxia, axonotmesis, and/or a neurotmesis. From a practical standpoint—usually if a patient presents with hypesthesia or motor weakness of acute onset due to a closed injury, a negative Tinel's test, and progressive return of sensory or motor function within 1 to 2 months—the treating physician is usually dealing with a neurapraxia. Should symptoms persist more than 3 months, one might then consider exploration and a possible neurolysis of the peripheral nerve to minimize the likelihood of progressive demyelination.[19,26]

However, when a patient presents with a sharp laceration and a positive Tinel's test, most likely the axon itself has been injured. If the two ends of the axon are reapproximated, healing will occur at a slower rate secondary to wallerian degeneration. Subsequent distal axonal remyelination averaging approximately 1 inch a month after a 1-month initial delay[6] will usually occur, with potential reinnervation of the distal sensory motor end organs.

The more proximal the lesion, the longer it will take to have a functional return, and therefore usually a poorer prognosis exists. Thus, an axonotmesis of the ulnar nerve in the proximal forearm might take at least 12 to 18 months to achieve maximal functional recovery as compared to a similar injury at the wrist in Guyon's canal. Unfortunately, this may often result in permanent atrophy of the hand intrinsics innervated by the ulnar nerve, necessitating possible consideration of tendon transfers to help restore lost function.

Finally, should a patient on initial presentation demonstrate a positive Tinel's sign, as well as motor or sensory dysfunction that fails to show signs of distal advancement after more than several months, there is a low likelihood of neural regeneration distal to that point. Wilgis[26] feels that a failure to note progressive distal advancement 3 to 4 months after the initial repair is an indication to consider exploration of the area of injury. At exploration, neurolysis, excision of an existent neuroma, and a secondary epineural repair with or without possible nerve grafting may be necessary.

Penetrating Injuries

Initial evaluation of the patient should be directed to his or her general medical status. Once the patient has been stabilized, and after life-threatening injuries have been assessed and treated, one may then focus on assessing the neurologic status of the involved upper extremity. Motor and sensory testing of the upper extremity is essential to localizing the particular area of injury.

In general, one should initially perform a sensory examination of the hand, remembering that the median nerve usually provides sensation to the volar surface of the thumb, index finger, middle finger, and radial border of the ring finger. Volarly, the ulnar side of the ring and the entire small finger are usually supplied by the ulnar nerve. Dorsally, the first web space is usually innervated by the radial nerve. Anatomic variations do occur secondary to communications between the median and ulnar nerves in the palm (Riche-Cannieu) or forearm (Martin-Gruber).[19] These anatomical variations should be kept in mind if sensory and motor testing does not correlate with the anatomical site of injury. Sensation may be tested by pinprick, two-point discrimination,* and observation for the presence of sweating. Children may be evaluated by noting the normal wrinkling of the digital pulp when placed in water, as described by O'Riain.[18] Finally, motor function may be assessed by observing digital and wrist extension for radial nerve function, flexion of the thumb, and distal interphalangeal joints of the index finger for median nerve function. Ulnar nerve function may usually be assessed by asking the patient to abduct and adduct the middle finger, as well as by noting whether the small finger is unable to be adducted (Wartenburg's sign). Froment's sign† may also be of benefit.

Once any abnormality in neurologic function is detected, the condition of the wound and the mechanism of injury should be noted. Sharp, penetrating injuries have a low likelihood of spontaneous recovery. However, they have a much better prognosis than a blunt penetrating injury with crushing disruption and contusion to a peripheral nerve. Gunshot wounds and neurologic loss secondary to displaced fractures (i.e., fracture of the distal humerus) are often due primarily to a neurapraxia or axonotmesis and have a much better prognosis according to Omer than one might initially expect. In his series, he noted full recovery in 65 to 70% of gunshot wounds,[17] although one should follow the specific injury to confirm a distal progression of a Tinel's test and motor reinnervation. Dirty wounds with vascular insufficiency, excessive scarring, granulation tissue, soft tissue loss, and gross contamination should be addressed before consideration of a neurorrhaphy.[22,23] Should there be concern about the wound condition, it is best to perform a delayed primary repair or secondary neurorrhaphy. Usually a delay of up to 2 to 3 weeks, at least in digital nerve injuries, will not significantly compromise the functional end result[6] and will allow for soft tissue inflammatory response to begin to subside.

However, assuming the wound is "clean," sharp, and has adequate vascularity and soft tissue coverage, a primary repair of the nerve should be entertained. Garrett et al. have noted differences in functional return with delays in animal studies of no more than 2 to 3 weeks.[1] Usually, a primary neurorrhaphy can be achieved if it is attempted within the first several days and if the prior criteria can be met. A delayed secondary neurorrhaphy may also be accomplished after resection of any fibrous tissue, possibly augmented by limited local nerve mobilization without damage to the intravascular blood supply. Should a nerve gap of 3 to 7 cm be noted, interfascicular nerve grafting should be strongly considered,[26] either primarily or secondarily depending upon the expertise and discretion of the surgeon.

Primary neurorrhaphy may be accomplished by epineural repair, group fascicular, or fascicular repair, again at the discretion of the attending surgeon. Epineural repair has the advantage of placement of a minimal degree of foreign material (suture) in the area of the nerve, although it does not allow as accurate a coaptation of the bundles of axons.[22] Group fascicular repairs, on the other hand, appear to be extremely attractive in those lesions of mixed motor and sensory nerves in which frequent

---

*Two-point discrimination may be performed by spreading two blunt points of a paperclip 5 to 6 mm apart on the volar pulp of the radial or ulnar aspect of each digit with the points aligned along the longitudinal axis of the finger. Normally, a patient can discern two-point spread 5 to 8 mm apart if a digital nerve is functioning normally. Complete transection of a nerve will result in an inability to detect two-point spread 20 mm or greater.

†Normally, pulp-to-pulp pinch between the thumb and index finger is achieved with the thumb interphalangeal joint maintained in extension. If, however, an ulnar nerve palsy has occurred, the patient will utilize the median innervated flexor pollicis longus to flex the interphalangeal joint of the thumb in order to obtain strong pulp-to-pulp pinch, because the ulnar innervated thumb intrinsics and adductor pollicis that normally help extend the thumb interphalangeal joint are paralyzed. This test is useful in determining loss of motor function to the thumb intrinsics innervated by the ulnar nerve.

crossover may occur and groups of fascicles can be easily identified both proximally and distally. Gaul,[5] Jabaley,[11] and Hakistan have each advocated intraoperative nerve stimulation to help to reapproximate more accurately the nerve fibers.

Should an excessive gap exist, then nerve grafting techniques should be considered. Opinions vary as to the degree of gap, but, in general, studies indicate that the results of a microscopic neurorrhaphy augmented with grafting have a better outcome than an excessively mobilized secondary neurorrhaphy under tension.

Donor sites for nerve grafts may be from multiple sites,[7] including the medial and lateral antebrachial cutaneous nerves[21] of the forearm for digital nerve lacerations, as well as the terminal branch of the posterior interosseous nerve. For group fascicular nerve grafting over a larger gap or involving more proximally based peripheral nerves, sural nerve grafts are frequently utilized.

Probably the most common nerve injuries are those to the digital nerves. In general, lacerations to the digital nerves of the thumb and the border digits (especially the radial digital nerve of the index finger and the ulnar digital nerve of the small finger) should be repaired, if possible, as they provide essential sensory feedback in one's daily activities. At about 3 to 5 mm distal to the distal interphalangeal joint, the digital nerve will begin to arborize into at least three terminal branches. Beyond this point, neurorrhaphy is technically very difficult, even with the benefit of magnification.[25]

Finally, other sensory nerves, particularly the dorsal sensory branch of the radial or ulnar nerve, also merit discussion. Although not on the "working" (volar) surface of the hand, neuromas of these two areas can be extremely debilitating. No definite sensory return can be assured to the patient, but neurorrhaphy will frequently decrease the likelihood of an excessively tender neuroma that often can be more symptomatic than the associated hypesthesia. Surprisingly, some sensory reinnervation frequently will be achieved, although it can never be guaranteed preoperatively.

Rehabilitation

Postoperatively, the hand therapist may play a key role in the sensory reeducation and functional recovery of the patient. Baseline measurements of range of motion and grip strength, as well as instruction in activities of daily living required by the patient, will aid the patient's early return to a functional status. Splints may be required to assist the patient during this recovery, such as a cock-up splint for a radial nerve palsy. Passive range-of-motion exercises should be initiated to prevent joint stiffness, followed by active assisted range-of-motion exercises when motor recovery begins to occur. Nerve stimulation of temporarily denervated muscle groups may also help to minimize atrophy and promote tendon excursion. Biofeedback and sensory and motor reeducation techniques are also important adjuncts in achieving maximal functional recovery.[4,26]

COMPLICATIONS OF PERIPHERAL NERVE INJURIES

Painful Neuromas

These lesions are extremely debilitating, often difficult to treat, and occasionally lead to development of reflex sympathetic dystrophy if unattended. Neuromas of symptomatic sensory nerves are best managed by local steroid injection, delayed neurorrhaphy, or mobilization and subsequent relocation of the neuroma into a deep, well-vascularized, soft tissue bed away from the prehensile area of the hand.[8] Care should usually be taken to leave the neuroma stump intact. However, Wood has found neuroma resection and delayed repair useful in selected cases of intractable painful neuromas of major peripheral nerves.[27] If adjacent to an amputated stump, a stump revision with more proximal bony resection may be of benefit, with an associated proximal resection or relocation of the digital neuroma into deeper soft tissue. Sensory retraining and desensitization under the supervision of a hand therapist are frequently of great benefit to these patients.[8,23]

Neuroma in Continuity

Failure of a nerve repair or injury to demonstrate a distal progression of Tinel's test below the area of injury or repair within 3 to 4 months should alert the treating physician that there is a low likelihood of distal regeneration of nerve fibers. If serial electrodiagnostic studies fail to show motor reinnervation distal to the area of injury, one should consider reexploration. This type of a procedure should be performed with the assistance of an operating microscope and, if available, an intraoperative nerve stimulator to allow the surgeon to determine the efficacy of a neurolysis as compared to a resection and secondary repair with or without nerve grafting. Occasionally, tendon transfers may also be considered either as internal splints, as advocated by Burkhalter,[3] or as the definitive procedure, if the lesion is a proximal one and there is a low likelihood of functional motor recovery.

Reflex Sympathetic Dystrophy

Although a comprehensive discussion of this disorder is beyond the scope of this chapter, briefly, reflex sympathetic dystrophy is a pathologic condition of the extremities characterized by severe pain, swelling, discoloration, and stiffness due to increased sympathetic tone caused by some noxious stimulus, usually of traumatic origin. Major causalgia, initially described by Weir Mitchell in 1864, usually involves a partial injury to one of the major peripheral nerves with associated motor and sensory components. Minor causalgia may be secondary to a neuroma of a sensory nerve, most commonly a digital nerve or the dorsal sensory branch of the radial or ulnar nerve. Treatment in either case should initially be directed at alleviation of the noxious agent, thereby breaking the pain cycle. Sympatholytic and antiinflammatory medications, regional or stellate ganglion blocks, mood-elevating drugs, and an intensive hand therapy program of gentle, nonpainful, passive range-of-motion exercises and edema control, followed by active range of motion, desensitization, and occasional splinting, are all important adjuncts in treatment of this most difficult problem.[13,14,16]

SUMMARY

Treatment of peripheral nerve injuries of the upper extremity is a challenging problem. As Jabaley has stated, the treatment of peripheral nerve injuries "may be the last frontier of hand surgery."[10] Perhaps, in the not too distant future, additional research will be able to advance even further our management of these most interesting lesions.

REFERENCES

1. Bolesta MJ, Garrett WE, Ribbeck BM, et al: Immediate and delayed neurorrhaphy in a rabbit model: A functional histological and biomechanical comparison. J Hand Surg 13A:352–357, 1988.
2. Boyes JH: On the Shoulder of Giants. Philadelphia, J. B. Lippincott, 1976, p 65.
3. Burkhalter WE: Early tendon transfer in upper extremity peripheral nerve injury. Clin Orthop Rel Res 104:68, 1974.
4. Fess EE: Rehabilitation of the patient with peripheral nerve injury. Hand Clin 2:207–215, 1986.
5. Gaul JS: Electrical fascicle identification as an adjunct to nerve repair. Hand Clin 2:709, 1986.
6. Gelberman RH: Nerve Injury and Regeneration. New Orleans, American Academy of Orthopaedic Surgeons Instructional Course, 1990.
7. Greene TL, Steichen JB: Digital nerve grafting using the dorsal sensory branch of the ulnar nerve. J Hand Surg 10B:37–40, 1985.
8. Herndon JH: Neuromas. In Green DP (ed): Operative Hand Surgery, 2nd ed. New York, Churchill Livingstone, 1988, pp 1405–1422.
9. Lloyd GER (ed): Hippocratic Writings. Harmondsworth, Middlesex, England, Penguin Books, 1978, p 228.
10. Jabaley ME: Current concepts of nerve repair. Clin Plast Surg 8:33–44, 1981.
11. Jabaley ME: Peripheral Nerve Repair. In McCarthy JG (ed): Plastic Surgery, Vol 7, 3rd ed. Philadelphia, W.B. Saunders, 1990, pp 4757–4762.
12. Kelsey JL, Patides H, Kreiger N, et al: Upper Extremity Disorders: A Survey of Their Frequency and Cost in the United States. St. Louis, C.V. Mosby, 1980, p 44.
13. Lankford LL: Reflex sympathetic dystrophy. In Omer GE, Spinner M (ed): Management of Peripheral Nerve Problems. Philadelphia, W.B. Saunders, 1980, pp 216–244.
14. Lankford LL: Reflex sympathetic dystrophy. In Green DP (ed): Operative Hand Surgery, 2nd ed. New York, Churchill Livingstone, 1988, pp 633–663.
15. MacKinnon SE, Dellon AL: Surgery of the Peripheral Nerve. New York, Thieme Medical, 1988.
16. Merritt WH: Reflex sympathetic dystrophy. In McCarthy JG (ed): Plastic Surgery, Vol 7, 3rd ed. Philadelphia, W.B. Saunders, 1990, pp 4884–4921.
17. Omer GE, Spinner M: Management of Peripheral Nerve Problems. Philadelphia, W.B. Saunders, 1980, p 362.
18. O'Riain S: New and simple test of nerve function in hand. Br Med J 3:615–616, 1973.
19. Spinner M: Injuries to the Major Branches of Peripheral Nerves of the Forearm, 2nd ed. Philadelphia, W.B. Saunders, 1978, p 2.
20. Sunderland S: Nerves and Nerve Injuries, 2nd ed. Edinburgh, Churchill Livingstone, 1978.
21. Tank MS, Lewis RC Jr, Coates PW: The lateral antebrachial cutaneous nerve as a highly suitable autograft donor for the digital nerve. J Hand Surg 8:942–945, 1983.
22. Urbaniak JR: Nerve Injury and Regeneration. New Orleans, American Academy of Orthopaedic Surgeons Instructional Course, 1990.
23. Van Beek AL: Management of nerve compression syndromes and painful neuromas. In McCarthy JG (ed):

Plastic Surgery, Vol 7, 3rd ed. Philadelphia, W.B. Saunders, 1990, pp 4817–4821.

24. Van Beek AL, Eder MA, Zook EG: Nerve regeneration—evidence for early sprout formation. J Hand Surg 7A:79–83, 1982.

25. Van Beek AL: Techniques of nerve repair and grafting including neuroma management. Dallas-Fort Worth, American Society for Surgery of the Hand, Second Annual Comprehensive Review Course in Hand Surgery, 1989.

26. Wilgis EF Shaw: Nerve repair and grafting. In Green DP (ed): Operative Hand Surgery, 2nd ed. New York, Churchill Livingstone, 1988, pp 1373–1403.

27. Wood VE, Mudge MK: Treatment of neuromas about a major amputation stump. J Hand Surg 12A:302–306, 1987.

Chapter 21

DIAGNOSIS AND MANAGEMENT OF OCCUPATIONAL DISORDERS OF THE SHOULDER

Elin Barth, M.D., and Edward W. Berg, M.D.

As in most areas of medicine, the history is by far the most important aspect of the diagnosis of a work-related shoulder disorder. Occupational injuries or chronic overuse syndromes are frequent causes of shoulder pain, but other possible etiologies include arthritis of the cervical spine, carpal tunnel syndrome, metastatic tumor, Pancoast tumor, and problems of the elbow, spine, and wrist that may give rise to pain of the shoulder.

The shoulder is a complex construction consisting of several articulations and is capable of a wide range of motion. Its extensive mobility is achieved at the cost of stability. As a consequence, the shoulder is particularly vulnerable to dislocation and also to the ravages of degenerative changes such as shoulder impingement, rotator cuff tear, and arthritis of the acromioclavicular (AC) joint.

The shoulder may be a frequent site of trauma because of its exposed position. Also, active sports participants are subject to painful shoulder problems ranging from overuse syndromes to acute rotator cuff tears. Rather than enumerate all possible causes of the painful shoulder, this chapter reviews the main elements in diagnosing and managing the shoulder problems seen most often (Table 1). It characterizes the frequently encountered causes, then reviews important steps in the history, physical examination, and radiological study. Finally, it suggests management approaches to frequent diagnoses.

SURGICAL ANATOMY AND FUNCTION

The primary purpose of the shoulder is to position the hand for use. As stated, the shoulder pays for its tremendous range of motion with relative instability. The glenohumeral joint, of course, is not only the shoulder joint but a complex of four separate articulations: the scapulohumeral, the sternoclavicular, the acromioclavicular, and the scapulothoracic joints. Any motion of the shoulder joint includes motion of the scapula and clavicle. The glenohumeral joint is enveloped by muscles from the scapula, the infraspinatus, the supraspinatus, the teres minor posteriorly, and the subscapularis anteriorly. Bursal inflammation in the scapulothoracic "joints" may refer pain to the corresponding extremity. However, abnormalities of the scapulothoracic junction rarely cause work-related problems.

Anatomy

Figure 1 is a schematic illustration of normal right shoulder anatomy.

The coracoacromial ligament extends from the acromion to the coracoid, a bony projection from the scapula. These structures directly overhang the humeral head and are in close relationship with it. An irregularity or hypertrophy of the humeral head can be obstructed during abduction by the coracoacromial arch,

TABLE 1.   Common Causes of Shoulder Pain

Local	Other
Bursitis	Thoracic outlet syndrome
Bicipital tendinitis	Naffziger's syndrome
Frozen shoulder	Cervical rib
Impingement syndrome	Carpal tunnel syndrome
	Shoulder-hand syndrome
	Pancoast tumor

the so-called impingement syndrome. The most lateral surface of the scapula gives rise to the small, shallow glenoid, which is the articulating surface for the head of the humerus. The glenoid labrum surrounds the periphery of the cavity and gives added stability. It is the labrum that is injured primarily in dislocation of the shoulder.

The long head of the biceps tendon traverses the notch between the greater and lesser tuberosities crossing the shoulder joint and lies in close approximation to the humeral head. A very small part of the surface of the humeral head articulates with the glenoid fossa. The bicipital sulcus is covered by the musculotendinous cuff, the so-called rotator cuff. The capsule is a redundant structure from the capsular border of the labrum and forms a synovial recess anteriorly. The inner aspect of this capsule is lined by synovium extending into the anterior synovial recess and along the bicipital groove. It communicates with the numerous bursae about the shoulder. The broad, flat tendons of the rotator cuff envelope the head and become incorporated into and strengthen the shoulder joint capsule. This musculotendinous cuff or rotator cuff is the primary stabilizing force of the shoulder. Acute and chronic injuries of the rotator cuff lead to pain, instability, and disability. The coracohumeral ligament from the coracoid reaches the bicipital groove and inserts into both greater and lesser

tuberosities of the humerus. It forms an integral part of the rotator cuff and helps to check external rotation. In the frozen shoulder syndrome, the subscapularis contracts and limits external rotation. The three muscles attaching to the greater tuberosity are the teres minor, the infraspinatus, and the supraspinatus. Attaching to the lesser tuberosity is the subscapularis.

Osteoarthritis of the acromioclavicular joint with osteophytes may set up an irritative subacromial tendinitis and may act as an impingement in shoulder abduction. The constant bursae are the subcoracoid and the subacromial, which may communicate with each other and occasionally with the intra-articular portion of the glenohumeral joint. In lesions of the humeral head, the rotator cuff and the overlying arch may have an inflammatory reaction of the bursae, which may give rise to shoulder pain. They also may be involved with sepsis, gouty arthritis, and rheumatoid arthritis.

The neurovascular bundle, including the axillary nerve with its branch to the teres minor, and the vessels cross anteriorly to the subscapularis, separating it from the inferior aspect of the glenoid. Anatomically this separation explains why the typical anterior inferior glenohumeral dislocation seldom involves nerve injury. The long head of the triceps attaches to the inferior aspect of the glenoid and acts as a stabilizing force. The deltoid muscle from the outer border of the acromion and the scapular spine and clavicle inserts into the deltoid tubercle of the proximal humerus. The deltoid is innervated by the axillary nerve and may be injured in glenohumeral dislocations. Because of the inferior entrance of the nerve to the deltoid, surgical approaches avoid the more distal part of the deltoid in order to avoid nerve injury.

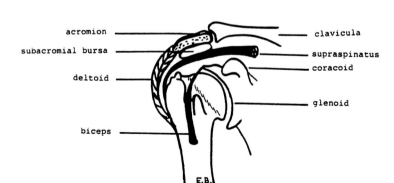

FIGURE 1. Schematic, simplified anteroposterior view of the shoulder joint with some anatomical landmarks pertinent to various causes of shoulder pain.

Function

The muscles attaching the scapula and humerus to the axial skeleton act as a unit; motion takes place simultaneously at the glenohumeral, acromioclavicular, thoracoscapular, and sternoclavicular junctions and within the biceps tendon sheath. With elevation of the arm, the scapula stabilizes and moves with a ratio to humeral motion of 1:2, meaning that with every 20 degrees of elevation of the arm, there are 10 degrees of thoracoscapular motion. Loss of motion in either articulation means loss of shoulder motion; glenohumeral fixation causes twice as much restriction as thoracoscapular fixation. Thoracoscapular motion can provide elevation of the arm to approximately 65 degrees even with a glenohumeral arthrodesis. This is the so-called shrugging motion, which can substitute for glenohumeral motion.

With paralysis of the deltoid muscle, the arm cannot be abducted beyond a few degrees. Deltoid abduction is initiated by other stabilizing muscles before the deltoid begins to come in beyond 30 degrees. The trapezius, rhomboids, levator scapulae, serratus anterior, and pectoralis minor act to stabilize the scapula. If the scapular stability is impaired by weakness of these muscles, through either inflammation or loss of innervation, elevation of the arm above the horizontal is made more difficult. If the scapula becomes fixed—as, for example, after a thoracic operation—abduction is not possible.

UNDERLYING CAUSES OF SHOULDER PAIN

Local Conditions

Most of the common causes of shoulder pain are local (see Table 1), including bursitis, bicipital tendinitis, frozen shoulder, impingement syndrome, acute and chronic rotator cuff tears, and degenerative and post-traumatic arthritis. Note that degenerative arthritic changes in the shoulder are usually post-traumatic. Primary degenerative arthritis of the glenohumeral joint is rare without preexisting injury. Another rare cause of shoulder pain is syringomyelia, which may present as a painful or nonpainful degeneration of the glenohumeral joint. The cause is in the spinal canal. Recur-

rent dislocation of the shoulder appears to predispose to degenerative arthritis of the glenohumeral joint. More common is degenerative arthritis of the AC joint, which may result from an old AC injury or may be a primary degenerative joint disease. Osteophyte production and narrowing of the subacromial space can be a part of the impingement syndrome.

Other Conditions

Several conditions originating outside of the shoulder area can cause shoulder pain (see Table 1). A quick technique that helps in differentiating shoulder pain referred from cervical disorders from intrinsic shoulder pain is to ask the patient to point to the pain (Fig. 2).

Thoracic Outlet Syndrome. This syndrome may be caused by constriction of the neurovascular bundle as it emerges from the thorax and may cause referred pain to the shoulder. It includes the scalenus-anticus syndrome also known as Naffziger syndrome. A cervical rib and other aberrant structures in the neck can also cause thoracic outlet syndrome. Occupational use may aggravate a thoracic outlet syndrome. Nonoperative management measures are physical therapy, nonsteroidal anti-inflammatory drugs (NSAIDs), and rest. One test for vascular compromise is the Adson's test: the arm is widely abducted and externally rotated while the radial pulse is palpated. When the head and neck are rotated toward the abducted, externally rotated extremity, if the pulse disappears a presumptive

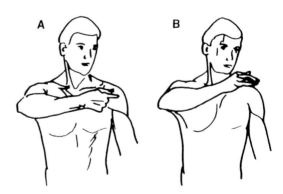

FIGURE 2. A quick test to differentiate between shoulder pain referred from cervical disorders and intrinsic shoulder pain. Patients with intrinsic shoulder pain tend to locate the pain in the area distal to the acromion process (A), whereas those with referred pain locate the pain in an area above the shoulder, roughly where a shoulder strap would lie (B).

diagnosis of impingement of the thoracic outlet vessels can be made. It can be confirmed with arteriograms. Surgical decompression may be necessary. A positive Adson's test is normal in about 20% of the population.

Carpal Tunnel Syndrome. Pain in the shoulder is the presenting complaint of 15% of patients. Carpal tunnel syndrome is compression of the median nerve under the volar transverse carpal ligament. A history of waking up at night with pain in the shoulder, arm, wrist, or hand is a likely indication of carpal tunnel syndrome. Typically patients relate shaking their arms or hands to relieve the pain. The cause is wrist flexion when the patient is sleeping. A positive Phalen's test duplicates the wrist flexion with pain and numbness into the median nerve distribution of the fingers. The presence of a Tinel's sign sometimes helps to diagnose carpal tunnel syndrome. Electromyograms and nerve conduction velocities may be helpful if the history and physical examination are not conclusive.

Shoulder-Hand Syndrome. Reflex sympathetic dystrophy may be manifested as shoulder-hand syndrome. This can occur after painful hand injuries and myocardial infarction as well as from many other causes, known and unknown. Persons who have shoulder-hand syndrome experience pain and stiffness in a shoulder and pain and swelling in the ipsilateral hand. The hand may be cool and exquisitely tender. The skin may be shiny and sweaty. Patients immobilize the shoulder joint, perhaps because of pain or feared pain, and may develop adhesive capsulitis or frozen shoulder. Shoulder-hand syndrome is a complex problem to manage. It can take weeks to months to resolve, but usually the patient does not remain totally disabled. Patience is essential in the treatment of sympathetic reflex dystrophy. In addition to a concerned, empathetic physician, these patients require closely supervised physical therapy as well as therapy with analgesics and possibly intra-articular corticosteroids. It is controversial whether shoulder manipulation under anesthesia is useful in the treatment of this entity.

Pancoast's Pulmonary Superior Sulcus Tumor. Lung cancer metastasized to the diaphragm or the apex of the lung can present as shoulder pain with concomitant Horner's syndrome. The condition is known as Pancoast tumor or syndrome. If the usual treatment for shoulder pain is not successful, an apical lordic chest x-ray to rule out metastatic tumor is indicated (Fig. 3).

DIAGNOSIS

A careful history and physical examination are the most important parts of a diagnostic workup. It is recommended that the physical examination be repeated after initiation of treatment modalities if treatment is not successful. Other diagnostic attempts, including a bone scan or magnetic resonance imaging (MRI), should be considered.

History

In the hands of the most experienced physicians and surgeons, a careful history leads to the correct diagnosis in approximately 80% of patients with a painful shoulder. Successful treatment depends on accurate diagnosis. Important information in the history includes mode of onset. Did the pain follow repeated use of the hands above the shoulders, as in a mail worker or an industrial worker who uses a textile machine with his hand over his head? Did if follow repeated motion as in a baseball pitcher who throws overhand? Regarding a recent trauma, was there an athletic injury or fall, an automobile accident, that might have aggravated the shoulder? Regarding a current disease, does the patient have a history of sys-

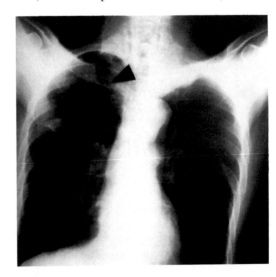

FIGURE 3. A Pancoast tumor that has partially eroded the right clavicle (*arrow*).

temic illness or coronary artery disease? Is there a history of primary tumor, rheumatoid arthritis, or past compensation award? Should malingering or secondary gain be considered?

Sudden onset of shoulder pain without any predisposing factor strongly suggests either a subacromial bursitis or a bicipital tendinitis, depending on the location of the pain.

Acute inability to abduct the shoulder may indicate a complete rotator cuff tear. Acute tears can result from indirect forces on the abducted arm often during violent sports activity, but they can also occur with minor trauma. Constant pain accompanied by an inability to abduct suggests either impingement syndrome or an incomplete rotator cuff tear.

Rupture of the long head of the biceps can also present as shoulder pain. It happens in older patients after repeated traumatic incidents or as a "wearing out" phenomenon.

In a patient with shoulder pain, a history of bronchogenic carcinoma or even of heavy smoking can lead to a diagnosis of metastatic tumor with pain referred to the shoulder joint.

The particular history of idiopathic frozen shoulder, or adhesive capsulitis, includes an incidious onset of increasing, diffuse pain. The pain subsequently resolves. The patient, typically a perimenopausal woman, has substantial loss of movement. The shoulder is tender to palpation but is not swollen or red, as it is in acute arthritis such as gout, rheumatoid arthritis, or infection.

Physical Examination

Physical examination includes (1) inspection of the shoulder; (2) palpation of the shoulder; and (3) active and passive range of motion assessment. These investigations are all critical to the diagnosis of shoulder pain.

Inspection. It is important to inspect the painful shoulder and to compare it with the opposite shoulder. Both shoulders are inspected undraped. One looks for evidence of muscle atrophy on either the anterior or posterior view. If one sees sagging of the scapula, winging of the scapula, or loss of the deltoid, supraspinatus, or infraspinatus, then significant organic pathology may be suspected. Sagging of the shoulder may indicate a chronic subluxation. This may be seen in stroke patients with muscle paralysis and subsequent development of painful shoulder; it does not

represent a true shoulder dislocation. It may also be seen in fractures of the shoulder. Sagging merely represents a relaxation of the deltoid muscle that corrects itself spontaneously when muscle strength is built up. Winging of the scapula on forward flexion may indicate impingement of the long thoracic nerve (the serratus anterior nerve). A high-riding scapula may indicate a congenital abnormality such as the Klippel-Feil syndrome. Congenital elevation of the scapula is a cosmetic rather than a pain-producing abnormality.

The shoulder joints should be examined for swelling, redness, or heat, which indicate the presence of effusion in the joint secondary to trauma, infection, or tumor.

Palpation. Patients with subacromial bursitis, bicipital tenderness, or impingement of the rotator cuff experience tenderness upon palpation. Tenderness of the AC joint may represent arthritic changes or an AC dislocation. The shoulder generally and the biceps groove and subacromial bursa specifically should be palpated.

Range of Motion Testing. Note and record active and passive range of motion in the affected shoulder compared with the opposite shoulder and also any accompanying pain. Grating in the shoulder often has no clinical significance, but it may represent destruction of the shoulder joint by conditions such as rheumatoid arthritis or osteoarthritis. As noted earlier, inability to abduct the shoulder beyond 15 degrees can represent an incomplete or complete rupture of the rotator cuff.

Demonstrate bicipital tendinitis by having the patient flex the shoulder against resistance with the elbow extended and the forearm supinated (Fig. 4). In patients with bicipital tendinitis, the pain is localized to the bicipital groove.

Impingement of the rotator cuff gives rise to the "painful arc" syndrome. The patient has pain during abduction beyond 15 degrees, but the pain disappears when abduction is continued beyond 90 degrees (Fig. 5A). Another indication of impingement is pain in the shoulder when the patient attempts to kiss the elbow: as the shoulder is abducted and the elbow internally rotated and flexed, pain is felt in the shoulder (Fig. 5B).

ROUTINE DIAGNOSTIC PROCEDURES

Diagnostic Anesthetic Injections. Injection of an anesthetic agent into the painful

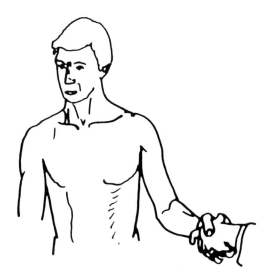

FIGURE 4.   Bicipital tendinitis symptoms can be reproduced by this test, which involves resisted supination of the forearm with the elbow flexed to 90 degrees.

area may help identify the cause of pain. With diagnostic injections, it is possible to deduce whether the pain is in the glenohumeral or the AC joint. The subacromial bursa, the long head of the biceps, and impingement syndrome may be differentiated in this manner. This diagnostic procedure should be done by an orthopedist.

Roentgenographic Studies.   At least two views taken at a 90-degree angle are required in the diagnostic workup of patients with shoulder pain (Fig. 6). Anteroposterior (AP) views of the shoulder and internal and external rotation provide insufficient information except in patients with bursitis.

A lateral view of the shoulder, preferably an axillary lateral, is obtained in all patients with shoulder pain. In the axillary lateral view, the camera is placed between the chest wall and the humerus in the axilla with the x-ray cassette opposite the glenohumeral joint. If the view is truly unobtainable (work with the x-ray technician to ascertain that this is truly the case), a transthoracic view may be substituted. In reviewing the lateral x-ray film, it is important to ensure that there is no disparity in the glenohumeral joint—that is, no dislocation or subluxation of the shoulder.

Hill-Sachs lesions can be seen on AP, internal, and external views. Hill-Sachs lesions are cartilaginous or osteocartilaginous fractures on the posterior lateral aspect of the humeral head. These lesions are a result of repeated trauma of shoulder dislocation.

A West Point view can help to demonstrate lesions of the anterior rim of the glenoid. In the West Point view, the patient is prone and the camera is angled 45 degrees to the shoulder (Fig. 7). X-ray films may reveal calcified deposits related to a subacromial bursitis. The radiographic examination may not be diagnostic in patients with soft tissue problems of the shoulder, such as rotator cuff tear. However, in these patients the roentgenographic studies can help rule out unsuspected problems—for example, fractures or lytic processes related to tumors, metastases, or other conditions.

Other Diagnostic Procedures

Special diagnostic studies used to examine the painful shoulder include arthrography (Fig.

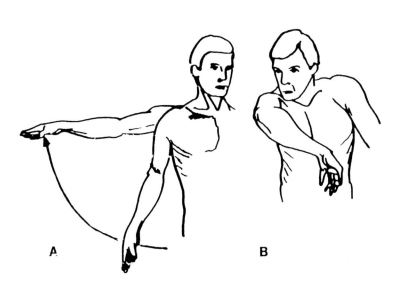

FIGURE 5.   Two tests for rotator cuff impingement. *A*, Figure demonstrates the "painful arc" syndrome: pain is felt during abduction between 15 and 90 degrees but not beyond 90 degrees. *B*, Figure shows an attempt to "kiss the elbow," which can elicit pain.

A   B

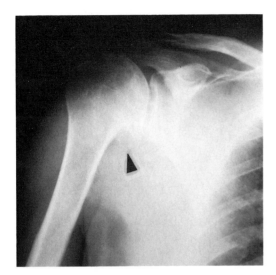

FIGURE 6. AP view of osteoarthritic shoulder. The joint space is narrowed because cartilage has been partially destroyed, and there is sclerosis of the underlying bone. Peripheral osteophyte formation is evident.

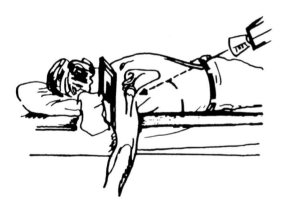

FIGURE 7. The West Point roentgenographic view in which the patient lies stomach down with a pillow underneath the shoulder to raise it. The film cassette is placed superior to the shoulder. This view best demonstrates anteroinferior lesions of the glenoid labrum.

8), computerized tomography (CT), MRI, sonography, and arthroscopy. Sonograms can demonstrate problems such as tears of the rotator cuff. Rotator cuff tears can be confirmed radiographically by arthrography with injections of dye into the glenohumeral joint.

CT scans may be particularly helpful in trauma and tumors. MRI is a useful although expensive adjunct, especially in patients with soft tissue lesions or osteonecrosis secondary to trauma, corticosteroid therapy, dysbarism, or alcohol abuse.

Finally, shoulder arthroscopy is informative in the diagnosis of rotator cuff tears (partial or

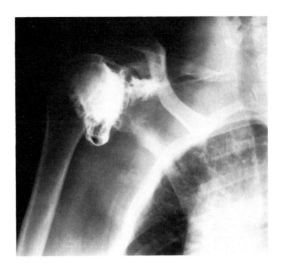

FIGURE 8. Shoulder arthrogram. This procedure is an alternative to shoulder arthroscopy in the diagnosis of rotator cuff tears.

complete) and tears of the labrum and is also being used in diagnosing instability, impingement syndrome, and degenerative joint disease.

TREATMENT

Appropriate treatment of painful shoulder is directed toward the diagnostic findings.

Subacromial Bursitis. Corticosteroid injections and physiotherapy often relieve subacromial bursitis and other shoulder problems. Physiotherapy is important to avoid a secondary problem of frozen shoulder. During physiotherapy, the therapist instructs patients in circumduction and active assistive abduction exercises. These are the Codman exercises, which were first promulgated in the 1930s and are still useful today.

Various heat modalities, active range of motion exercises, and other physical therapy modalities can be useful. The goal of therapy is to restore shoulder motion. The ultimate goal, of course, is to restore ability to position the hand for functional use in normal activities of daily living.

Surgical removal of calcium deposits in the bursae is sometimes needed to give pain relief. Injections of local anesthetic and long-acting corticosteroid agents into the deposits sometimes are helpful.

Bicipital Tendinitis. Moist heat, oral NSAIDs, and gentle, assisted range of motion exercises are the preferred treatment of bicipital tendinitis.

Impingement Syndrome. Nonoperative therapy is advised initially. Impingement of the rotator cuff may benefit from a partial resection of the acromion along with a resection of the coracoacromial ligament. This is called the Neer decompression.

Arthroscopy can be useful for both diagnostic and therapeutic purposes in patients with painful shoulder syndrome. The glenohumeral joint is a large joint and is easily amenable to arthroscopic inspection. Some shoulder arthroscopists even advocate procedures such as repair of lesions of the glenoid labrum and debridement of rotator cuff tears. This is a relatively new procedure.

Rotator Cuff Tears. Acute rotator cuff tears, particularly in young persons, may be amenable to surgical intervention. Treatment of chronic rotator cuff tears is controversial. Some authors advocate repairs in local and distant tissues (for example, grafts from fascia lata) or by using bank tissues. However, the long-term survival of these grafts is poor.

Idiopathic Frozen Shoulder (Adhesive Capsulitis). Treatment for this extremely troublesome problem demands much patience from both patient and physician. A painful frozen shoulder with no osteopenia can be gently manipulated under general anesthesia. There is an associated risk of humeral fracture or injury of the brachial plexus, and possibly dislocation. After manipulation, which is used to restore function, active and assisted range of motion exercises are important.

Degenerative and Post-traumatic Arthritis. Treatment of arthritis depends on the severity of the symptoms; last resorts may include total joint arthroplasty or a fusion (Fig. 9).

Nonlocal Conditions. Shoulder pain can be referred from a problem in the neck or from a thoracic outlet syndrome. The correct diagnosis must be obtained.

A quick check of the range of motion in the cervical spine helps to differentiate inherent shoulder pain from pain in the shoulder referred from the neck. Normal findings should rule out pain referred from the neck. As previously noted, the test shown in Figure 2 may be useful.

Shoulder pain radiating from the cervical spine is best managed with cervical immobilization, traction, and appropriate NSAIDs.

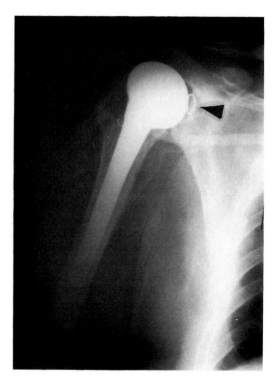

FIGURE 9. Total shoulder replacement. The glenoid component is made from a polyethylene material and is radiolucent. Its position can be assessed by means of a circular metal marker centrally in the component.

Infections, rheumatoid arthritis, and other systemic causes of shoulder pain should be managed in an appropriate manner. Aspiration of synovial fluid from the shoulder joint may be indicated. The fluid should be examined for crystals, Gram stain findings, glucose, rheumatoid factor, and total and differential white blood cell counts.

CONCLUSION

Occupational disorders of the shoulder are frequently caused by overuse. Nonoperative management with emphasis on rehabilitation usually suffices. However, one must keep in mind other important entities to exclude, including tumor, systemic disease, and causes of referred pain to the shoulder.

Acknowledgment

The authors thank the editors of *Journal of Musculoskeletal Medicine* for permission to use slightly redrawn illustrations from a previously published paper on shoulder pain by the authors.

SUGGESTED READINGS

1. Barrack R, Jacobson KE: Clinical presentation of complete tears of the rotator cuff. J Bone Joint Surg 71A:499–506, 1989.
2. Bergenudd H, Lindgaurde F, Nilsson B, et al: Shoulder pain in middle age: A case study of prevalence and relation to occupational work load and psychosocial factors. Clin Orthop 231:234–238, 1988.
3. Doody SG, Freedman L, Waterland JC: Shoulder movements during abduction in the scapular plane. Arch Phys Med Rehab 51:595–604, 1970.
4. Freedman L, Munro RR: Abduction of the arm in the scapular plane: Scapular and glenohumeral movements. A roentgenographic study. J Bone Joint Surg 48A:1503–1510, 1966.
5. Kerins CT: Evaluation and treatment of shoulder pain. Curr Concepts Trauma Care 6(2):14–18, 1983.
6. Poppen NK, Walker PS: Normal and abnormal motion of the shoulder. Surg Forum 26:519, 1975.
7. Poppen NK, Walker PS: Normal and abnormal motion of the shoulder. J Bone Joint Surg 58A:195–201, 1976.
8. Poppen NK, Walker PS: Forces at the glenohumeral joint in abduction. Clin Orthop 135:165–170, 1978.
9. Post M: Miscellaneous painful shoulder conditions. In Post M (ed): The Shoulder. Surgical and Non-surgical Management. Philadelphia, Lea & Febiger, 1988, pp. 322–363.
10. Rowe CR: Evaluation of the shoulder. In The Shoulder. New York, Churchill Livingstone, 1988.
11. Quigley TB, Freedman PA: Recurrent dislocation of the shoulder. A preliminary report of personal experience with seven Bankart and ninety-two Putti-Platt operations in ninety-nine cases over twenty-five years. Am J Surg 128:595–599, 1974.
12. Walker PS, Poppen NK: Biomechanics of the shoulder joint during abduction in the plane of the scapula [proceedings]. Bull Hosp J Dis Orthop Inst 38:107–111, 1977.

Chapter 22

DIAGNOSIS AND MANAGEMENT OF OCCUPATIONAL DISORDERS OF THE ELBOW

Ronald C. Burgess, M.D.

Injuries around the elbow are a common source of occupational disability. The elbow is the fulcrum of the arm, and large forces across it account for numerous problems that may occur at this site. Early treatment in the course of injury may forestall lost work days and prolonged disability.

ANATOMY

The elbow is composed of two separate joints, the hinge joint of the humeroulnar joint and the rotatory joint of the radiocapitellar and radioulnar joints. Both of these joints function along with the shoulder to place the hand in position to function. They can also be the prime joints used in mechanical activity. The humeroulnar joint can work as a hinge for lifting (Fig. 1). The radiocapitellar and radioulnar joints are used in rotatory activity such as using a screwdriver (Fig. 2).

The muscles associated with elbow motion are the triceps, which attaches to the olecranon and extends the elbow, and the brachialis and biceps, which attach to the ulna and radius respectively and flex the elbow. The brachioradialis attaches to the distal humerus and assists in elbow flexion.

The major flexors and extensors of the wrist and fingers have their origin near the elbow. The radial wrist extensors and the extensor dig-

itorium communis arise from the lateral epicondyle of the elbow. The wrist and finger flexors and the pronator teres have a primary attachment at the medial epicondyle.

Three major nerves cross the elbow. The ulnar nerve is posterior to the medial epicondyle; it dives through the two heads of the flexor carpi ulnaris to lie deep to this muscle. The median nerve crosses the joint anteriorly overlying the brachialis muscle. It then goes between the two bellies of the pronator teres and gives off the anterior interosseous nerve. The radial nerve lies between the brachialis and the brachioradialis proximal to the elbow. It gives off the superficial radial nerve and then dives into the supinator muscle, where it further divides into multiple muscular branches.

HISTORY AND PHYSICAL EXAMINATION

An examination of an injured worker begins with a careful history of the major complaint. It should answer the following questions: (1) Is the complaint the result of a single incident or of insidious onset? (2) Does any activity aggravate the condition? (3) What is the position of the arm and the force used during the aggravating activity? (4) Is the complaint relieved by rest? (5) Is numbness or tingling associated with the pain? (6) Is there any medical history of illness that may be associated with nerve or tendon damage?

289

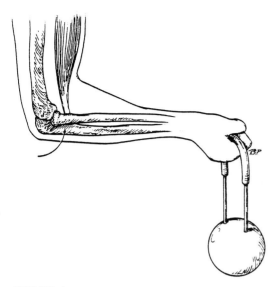

FIGURE 1. The elbow acts as a hinge joint at the humeroulnar articulation.

Using the medial and lateral epicondyles, the olecranon, and the radial head as landmarks, the examiner should localize the area of maximal tenderness. The active and passive ranges of motion should be determined for flexion, extension, pronation, and supination. Resisted muscle testing of all muscles that cross the elbow may isolate the problem to a particular muscle group. Light percussion over the major nerves helps to evaluate for hypersensitivity and possible compression neuropathy. The elbow should also be examined for areas of swelling, warmth, or redness.

X-rays of the elbow may show degenerative changes in the joint or soft-tissue calcification.

TENDINITIS

Tendinitis is the most common painful occupational disorder at the elbow. Unlike the tendinitis seen with finger and wrist complaints, tendinitis around the elbow is a true disruption and inflammation within the tendon and not tenosynovitis.[19] These injuries can be the result of a single incident, or they can be secondary to repetitive trauma, also known as "repetitive strain injury." In the latter case, minute tears within a tendon can occur in occupations that require forceful and highly repetitive tasks. These micro-tears occur in an area with poor vascularity and fill in with granulation tissue until the area becomes painful; muscular contraction of the affected muscle also causes pain. Armstrong has shown a 29-times greater risk of repetitive strain injury with occupations that require forceful and highly repetitive tasks.[2] In one study 10% of meat cutters had symptoms attributable to tendinitis at the elbow.[41] Careful attention to the position of the hand and forearm in forceful activities may help avoid tendinitis in these areas or prevent its progression.

LATERAL EPICONDYLITIS

Lateral epicondylitis, more commonly known as tennis elbow, is the most common tendinitis of the elbow.[12] The name is actually a misnomer because it is now believed that the actual area of disruption is not at the lateral epicondyle but rather in the extensor carpi radialis brevis aponeurosis just distal to the epicondyle.[11] With either a single incident or repetitive strain, a tear occurs within the tendon; it fills with granulation tissue rather than progressing to repair. This condition is most commonly seen in the fourth decade of life.[12] It may be seen concurrently with other problems, such as rotator cuff tendinitis or peripheral tendinitis.[35]

The major complaint of the patient is pain on the lateral aspect at the elbow and loss of grip strength and pain when forceably gripping an object. The major activity causing pain is

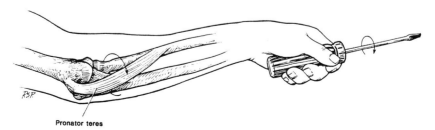

Pronator teres

FIGURE 2. The proximal radioulnar joint allows rotation of the forearm.

lifting of objects with the wrist in the pronated (palm down) position. The pain is described as burning and radiating down the arm.

On physical examination, exquisite tenderness upon palpation is present over the lateral epicondyle of the humerus. The area of greatest tenderness is 1–2 cm distal to the lateral epicondyle and anterior over the extensor carpi radialis brevis tendon. Resisted wrist extension and passive wrist flexion with the elbow in full extension both reproduce the pain. Grip strength is reduced secondary to pain. Sensory examination is within normal limits. X-rays may reveal calcification at the lateral epicondyle.[37] Both thermography and bone scan have been used in the diagnosis of questionable cases, but they are not required for most patients.

The initial treatment of a patient with acute lateral epicondylitis is rest from usual activities.[37] Ice massage is added to decrease local swelling and aid in mobilizing scar tissue. In this technique, the affected area is massaged with ice until it is numb. A small paper cup half filled with water and stored in the freezer works well as an ice cube. After the area is anesthetized by the cold, deep massage of the area is done. Nonsteroidal anti-inflammatory drugs (NSAIDs) are also of benefit in the early stages.[12,37,43]

After the acute pain is decreased, the patient is put on an exercise program to stretch and strengthen the wrist extensor muscles. This program, which is graduated, also functions as a work hardening program. The preferred program as outlined by Nirschl[36] includes:

1. Isometric exercises for wrist and finger extensors
   a. The forearm is pronated, the elbow fully extended, and the wrist and fingers maximally extended for 10 seconds 30 times a day.
   b. A tennis ball is squeezed for 15 seconds. This is done as often as possible.
2. Weight-lifting exercises
   a. The forearm is curled in flexion and extension with a 3- to 5-pound weight. The position is held for 10 seconds 20 times a day.
   b. A military press is done with a 5- to 20-pound weight. The weight and number of repetitions are increased to a goal of 40 repetitions at 20 pounds and 40 at half maximum (10 pounds).
3. Flexibility exercises for shoulder and elbow.

4. Stretching of wrist extensors until 90 degrees of palmar flexion are attained. This is done with the elbow in full extension and the forearm pronated. The stretch is held for a count of 10 seconds 15 times a day.

This program is highly successful in resolving the tendon inflammation. By strengthening and training the wrist extensors, the patient obtains greater control of the muscles. The program also increases endurance, which is important because the muscles are at greatest risk for reinjury when they are fatigued. This two-stage program resolves the pain in most cases.

Other modalities have been proposed for the treatment of lateral epicondylitis. Dimethylsulfoxide (DMSO),[38] ultrasound,[29] laser,[30] and pulsed electrical fields[9] have not been shown to have advantages over placebo treatment in controlled studies. The most common adjunctive treatment is injection of a steroid agent into the area of maximal pain.[36] This treatment has strong advocates who use it as the definitive treatment program. They claim a high rate of relief with injection alone.[5,14] Other authors believe that the local use of steroids should be reserved for patients who do not respond to other therapeutic measures and are being considered for surgery.[11] The reason for deferring local injection is that cortisone delays healing of injured tissues. Therefore, in theory, local cortisone instillation does not allow the injured tendon to recover. If steroid injections are given, they should not be repeated more than twice because a definite risk of an attrition rupture of the tendon exists upon repeated use.

The preferred method of steroid injection is to localize the area of maximal tenderness. This is most commonly 1–2 cm distal to the lateral epicondyle in the proximal aspect of the extensor carpi radialis brevis tendon. I use a one-needle, two-syringe technique of injection. The area of maximal tenderness is localized with a syringe filled with xylocaine. The area is anesthetized, the needle is left in place, and the syringe is replaced with one containing 1 cc of Celestone, which is then injected. Crystalline steroid is an irritating suspension. This two-stage technique using only one needle results in less pain than occurs with two needle injections or injection of a single combined solution.

A forearm strap that circumferentially compresses the proximal forearm has also been used for lateral epicondylitis.[37,17] Constriction of the muscles relieves the stress on the origin of the extensor muscles. This modality is of greatest use in mild cases or for a low level ache that remains after other treatments are used. It is not sufficient for the acutely painful elbow.

In approximately 5% of cases, the pain is resistant to all conservative treatment, and surgical treatment is required.[11,37,36] A variety of surgical treatments have been advocated, and good results reported for most. The most common procedure done today is excision of the granulation tissue and reapproximation of the remaining tendon.[11] Surgical treatment has been found to give excellent results in selected cases.

Lateral epicondylitis can be associated with prolonged disability. In one study of the natural history of lateral humeral epicondylitis, more than 40% of patients have prolonged minor discomfort.[5] Twenty-six percent had initial relief with treatment but recurrence of symptoms 1–5 years after initial presentation.

MEDIAL EPICONDYLITIS

Medial epicondylitis is the mirror image of lateral epicondylitis.[11] It occurs on the medial aspect of the elbow and is associated with either the pronator teres or flexor carpi radialis tendon insertions. The major activity causing pain is lifting of objects with the wrist in the supinated (palms up) position. The pain is described as burning in character and radiating down the forearm. On physical examination, exquisite tenderness is found upon palpation at the medial epicondyle. The tenderness is often worse 1–2 cm distal and slightly anterior to the medial epicondyle. Resisted pronation or resisted wrist flexion reproduces the pain. There is apparent weakness of the flexor musculature secondary to pain. The sensory examination is normal.

Treatment considerations for medial epicondylitis are the same as those for lateral epicondylitis. Ice, massage, rest, and anti-inflammatory drugs are the initial treatment. Once initial discomfort subsides, gradual muscular strengthening and stretching exercises are done to increase the muscular strength of the flexors and to gain greater control. Steroid injection and surgery are again reserved for uncommon resistant cases and are similar to procedures done with lateral epicondylitis.

RUPTURED BICEPS TENDON

Rupture of the biceps tendon at its attachment to the proximal radius can occur insidiously from osteophytes at the anterior margin of the radial tuberosity.[13,33] The osteophytes gradually erode the tendon until it spontaneously ruptures. A biceps tendon rupture can also be an acute result of lifting extremely heavy loads. The patient has a sensation of a sudden "giving away" in the arm, and the biceps bulges proximally.

On physical examination the patient is found to have exaggerated bulging of the biceps muscle on the proximal aspect of the arm. The ability to flex and supinate the arms is undisturbed because both brachialis and supinator muscles are intact.[15]

The correct treatment for this condition is surgical reinsertion of the biceps tendon into its original site.[34,6,3] If the tendon is not reattached, elbow flexion and supination will be permanently weak.[34]

BURSITIS

The elbow has multiple potential bursas.[7] The only one of clinical significance is the olecranon bursa, which lies in the posterior aspect of the elbow overlying the olecranon. This bursa is not evident on physical examination unless it is inflamed and filled with fluid. Under these conditions the bursa appears to be an enlarged ball on the posterior aspect of the elbow; it can be several centimeters in diameter. The most common cause for olecranon bursitis is post-traumatic bursitis. A direct blow to the olecranon bursa produces inflammation of the bursa, which fills with an exudate. The swelling culminates after several hours and the bursa can be markedly enlarged.

On physical examination the patient is found to have a full range of motion of the elbow. A large, fluctuant swelling with slight erythema is noted in the posterior aspect of the elbow. Despite the size of the lesion, olecranon bursitis from trauma is minimally symptomatic, except for the obvious cosmetic deformity.[21,32]

Treatment of traumatic olecranon bursitis is conservative; elbow pads prevent further damage to the bursa. Aspiration of the olecranon bursa is not indicated because the fluid rapidly reaccumulates.[32] The worker should be reassured that the olecranon will gradually assume its normal contour over a period of time. A temptation to incise the bursa to allow drainage should be resisted because the procedure may result in a secondarily infected olecranon bursa.

A second cause for olecranon bursitis is infection. Marked erythema is seen surrounding the area of the bursa, and the patient experiences tenderness in and around the inflamed bursa.[21,32,44] Pain restricts the range of motion of the elbow. Infectious bursitis may come from a penetrating injury into the bursa or occasionally without evidence of direct injury.[21,44] The bursa should be aspirated for culture and sensitivity through its edge rather than through its tip to prevent a chronic draining wound (Fig. 3). Any olecranon bursitis that is painful should be aspirated and sent for gram stain, culture and sensitivity, and examination for crystals.[21,32,44]

Treatment of a septic olecranon bursitis depends on the initial presentation. Early, mildly inflamed cases can be treated with aspiration and oral antibiotics that cover *Staphylococcus aureus* (the most commonly responsible organism).[32,44] A worker who presents with fever and marked tenderness should be admitted to a hospital for parenteral antibiotics. Repeated aspirations can remove the reaccumulating purulent fluid. Surgical drainage can be associated with chronically draining incisions, and a suction irrigation system has been proposed for use if repeat aspiration is not sufficient.[25]

A condition that can be confused with septic olecranon bursitis is gouty inflammation of the bursa.[8,32] Physical examination reveals a swollen olecranon bursa with marked erythema similar to that seen with an infected bursa. A previous history of attacks of gouty arthritis or of gout should be sought in anybody with a markedly inflamed olecranon bursa to exclude the possibility of gouty bursitis. Gouty bursitis should be considered in patients being treated for septic bursitis if cultures are negative and the response to antibiotics minimal. The correct treatment of gouty arthritis is medical treatment of the underlying condition. Incision and drainage of a gouty bursitis can lead to a chronically draining lesion and therefore should never be done.

DEGENERATIVE ARTHRITIS

Repetitive throwing can result in chronic elbow injury complicated by degenerative arthritis. This affliction is most commonly seen in athletes, especially professional baseball pitchers. It is also seen in people whose jobs require repetitive motion similar to throwing. Tullos and King have noted that in the throwing motion tension is placed on the medial side of the elbow and compression on the lateral side (radial head and capitellum).[45] This combination provides tension on the medial ligament as well as compression on the lateral aspect of the joint. Eventually the lateral joint becomes narrowed, and small osteoarthritic spurs form at the junction of cartilage and bone. The spurs may break off to form loose bodies in the joint that often settle in the olecranon fossa, where they prevent full extension of the elbow.[4]

Osteoarthritis at the elbow is usually treated by a change in work activities to reduce stress on the elbow and by NSAIDs. If loose bodies are identified they can be removed arthroscopically.[31]

NEUROLOGIC CAUSES OF ELBOW PAIN

Radial Tunnel Syndrome

The radial nerve may be the site of a compression neuropathy at or just distal to the elbow.[28,40] The radial nerve has four potential sites of compression.[39,16] The first is anterior to the radial head, where fibrous bands may compress the nerve. The second is at the juncture of the radial nerve and the radial recurrent

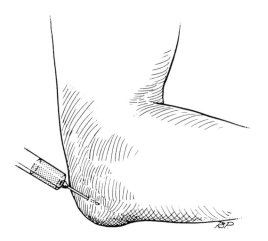

FIGURE 3. Aspiration of an inflamed olecranon bursa should be done peripherally, to prevent a chronically draining sinus.

vessels, which supply the brachioradialis and extensor carpi radialis longus. If these vessels are grouped in a fanlike pattern lying across the radial nerve; they may compress it. The third site of possible compression is the tendinous margin of the extensor carpi radialis brevis. The fourth and most common site of compression is at the arcade of Frohse, which is the fibrous proximal aspect of the superficial head of the supinator muscle. This fibrous band crosses over the deep radial nerve as it dives between the two heads of the supinator.

In distribution and manner of onset, the pain of radial tunnel syndrome is very similar to that of lateral epicondylitis. Maximal tenderness in lateral epicondylitis, however, is at the lateral epicondyle and just distal to it in the origin of the extensor carpi radialis brevis tendon.[28,40] The pain seen in radial tunnel syndrome is three to four finger breadths below the lateral epicondyle at the site of nerve compression (Fig. 4). Physical examination can also give some other clues to the location of the compression in radial tunnel syndrome. If the arm is in the fully pronated position and the patient's attempts to supinate it are resisted, re-creation of pain indicates compression at the level of the supinator muscle. If full pronation and wrist flexion reproduce the pain, especially if the pain is relieved by wrist extension, the pain can be localized to the extensor carpi radialis brevis.[16]

If radial tunnel syndrome is diagnosed, the initial treatment is rest. Stopping the muscular effort should improve the neuropathy. Electrodiagnostic studies such as electromyography and nerve conduction studies are helpful only if signs of denervation are present. The nerve conduction velocities are usually normal in radial tunnel syndrome.[28,40] If the pain of a radial tunnel syndrome is unrelieved by conservative measures, or if it returns after resumption of work, surgical decompression of the radial nerve is indicated.[16]

Cubital Tunnel Syndrome

The ulnar nerve may be entrapped as it passes along the medial aspects of the elbow.[23] The ulnar nerve passes behind the medial epicondyle in the cubital tunnel and then passes between the two heads of the flexor carpi ulnaris to lie on the anterior aspect of the flexor digitorium profundus. Compression of the nerve at this area can be caused by either osteophytes or ganglia of the elbow.[22,42] Fractures of the distal humerus can cause late symptoms of ulnar nerve compression by entrapment of the nerve in the cubital tunnel.[22] The most common site of compression is between the two heads of the flexor carpi ulnaris.[16] In 16% of normal people the ulnar nerve subluxes across the epicondyle with elbow flexion to a position where it is more vulnerable to external trauma and repetitive injury to the nerve.[10,1]

Patients with ulnar nerve symptoms have a primary complaint of pain either on the medial aspect of the elbow or the proximal aspect of the medial forearm. They will complain of paresthesias into the ring and little fingers of the hand in the distribution of the ulnar nerve. Severe cases cause weakness of the ulnar innervated muscles of the hand with loss of grip strength due to the paresis of the adductor pollicis muscle. Light percussion over the course of the ulnar nerve produces severe pain that radiates into the ring and little fingers. Vigorous percussion can cause symptoms in normal individuals and should be avoided. Recreation of symptoms when the elbow is held in full flexion for a period of 30 seconds also indicates compression of the nerve at the level of the elbow.[16,27]

Additional studies that can be obtained are elbow x-rays to look for osteoarthritic spurring or other causes of local compression. Electrodiagnostic studies such as electromyography and nerve conduction velocities are helpful in localizing the neuropathy to the level of the elbow.[18,16]

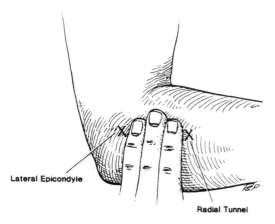

Lateral Epicondyle

Radial Tunnel

FIGURE 4. The area of maximal tenderness in radial tunnel syndrome is distal to the maximal tenderness in lateral epicondylitis.

The initial treatment of the acute onset of cubital tunnel syndrome is splinting of the elbow at 70 degrees to allow resolution of the acute inflammation.[27] The splint should be kept on for 23 of the 24 hours of the day. The supplemental use of anti-inflammatory drugs can also be of benefit. If the patient fails to respond to conservative measures, or if there is severe muscular weakness, surgical decompression of the nerve is indicated.

PRONATOR SYNDROME

Compression of the median nerve as it goes between the two heads of the pronator teres gives rise to pain in the volar aspect of the proximal forearm.[26,24] The patient may also report numbness and tingling in the distribution of the median nerve in the thumb, the index and middle fingers, and the radial half of the ring finger. The history includes increasing forearm pain and paresthesias occurring with use and relieved with rest.

One of the major difficulties with pronator syndrome is that it can be confused with the more common compression of the median nerve at the carpal tunnel. The primary diagnostic difference is that, in pronator syndrome, the maximal area of pain is localized in the proximal forearm rather than the wrist. The patient also reports that the paresthesias increase with progressive muscular use and are relieved by rest; in carpal tunnel syndrome, the symptoms are increased during rest periods.[16] Another differentiation is that in carpal tunnel syndrome, symptoms frequently occur at night; in pronator syndrome they rarely occur at night. Phalen's test may be positive in both conditions.[20]

On physical examination an area of nerve hypersensitivity is found when the proximal forearm is percussed at a level three finger breadths below the antecubital crease. The nerve at the volar aspect of the wrist may be sensitive to a minor degree. Resisted active pronation with the hand held in full supination should recreate the patient's symptoms if the nerve impingement is at the level of the two heads of the pronator. Impingement on the nerve by the fascial continuation of the biceps tendon (lacertus fibrosis) and by the fibrous edge of the sublimus muscle have also been described.[24] These conditions can be diagnosed by resisted elbow extension with the arm in a supinated position and resisted sublimus contraction.

The initial treatment of pronator syndrome is rest from muscular activity. If the compression neuropathy fails to respond to conservative care, surgical release of the nerve at the level of compression may be indicated.

REFERENCES

1. Arkin AM: Habitual luxation of the ulnar nerve. J Mt Sinai Hosp 7:208, 1940.
2. Armstrong TJ: Ergonomic considerations in hand and wrist tendinitis. J Hand Surg 12A:830, 1987.
3. Baker BE: Operative vs non-operative treatments of disruptions of the distal tendon of biceps. Orthop Rev 11(10):71, 1982.
4. Bell MS: Loose bodies in the elbow. Br J Surg 62:921, 1975.
5. Binder AL, Hazleman BL: Lateral humeral epicondylitis—A study of natural history and the effect of conservative therapy. Br J Rheumatol 22:73–76, 1983.
6. Boyd HB, Anderson MD: A method for reinsertion of the distal biceps brachii tendon. J Bone Joint Surg 43A:1041, 1961.
7. Bywaters EG: The bursae of the body. Ann Rheum Dis 24:215, 1965.
8. Caoso JJ, Yood RA: Reaction of superficial bursae in response to specific disease stimuli. Arthritis Rheum 22:1261–1264, 1979.
9. Chard MD, Hazleman BL: Pulsed electromagnetic field treatment of chronic lateral humeral epicondylitis. Am J Exp Rheum 3:330–332, 1988.
10. Childress HM: Recurrent ulnar-nerve dislocations at the elbow. J Bone Joint Surg 38A:978–984, 1956.
11. Coonrad RW: Tennis elbow. Instr Course Lect 35:94–101, 1986.
12. Coonrad RW, Hooper WR: Tennis elbow. Its course, natural history, conservative and surgical management. J Bone Joint Surg 55A:1177, 1973.
13. Davis WM, Yassine Z: An etiologic factor in the tear of the distal tendon of the biceps brachii. J Bone Joint Surg 38A:1368, 1956.
14. Day BH, Govindasamy N, Patnaik R: Corticosteroid injections in the treatment of tennis elbow. Practitioner 220:459–462, 1978.
15. Dobbie RP: Avulsion of the lower biceps brachii tendon. Analysis of fifty-one previously reported cases. Am J Surg 51:661, 1941.
16. Eversman WW: Entrapment and compression neuropathies. In Green DP (ed): Operative Hand Surgery, 2nd ed. New York, Churchill Livingstone, 1988.
17. Froimson AI: Treatment of tennis elbow with a forearm support band. J Bone Joint Surg 53A:183, 1971.
18. Gilliatt RW, Thomas PK: Changes in nerve conduction with ulnar nerve lesions at the elbow. J Neurol Neurosurg Psychiatry 23:310–320, 1960.
19. Goldie I: Epicondylitis lateralis humeri. Acta Chir Scand Suppl 339, 1964.
20. Hartz CR, Linscheid RL, Gramse RR, Daube JR: The pronator teres syndrome: Compressive neuropathy of the median nerve. J Bone Joint Surg 63A:885–890, 1981.

21. Ho G, Tice AD, Kaplan SR: Septic bursitis in the prepatellar and olecranon bursae. Ann Intern Med 89:21–27, 1978.

22. Hunt JR: Tardy or late paralysis of the ulnar nerve. A form of chronic progressive neuritis developing many years after fracture dislocation of the elbow joint. JAMA 66:11–15, 1916.

23. James GGH: Nerve lesions about the elbow. J Bone Joint Surg 38B:589, 1956.

24. Johnson RK, Spinner M, Shrewsbury MM: Median nerve entrapment syndrome in the proximal forearm. J Hand Surg 4:48–52, 1979.

25. Knight JM, Thomas JC, Mauer RC: Treatment of septic olecranon and prepatellar bursitis with percutaneous placement of a suction-irrigation system. Clin Orthop Rel Res 206:90–93, 1986.

26. Kopell HP, Thompson WAL: Pronator syndrome. N Engl J Med 259:713–715, 1958.

27. Lister G: The Hand: Diagnosis and Indications. New York, Churchill Livingstone, 1984.

28. Lister GD, Belsole RB, Kleinert HE: The radial tunnel syndrome. J Hand Surg 4:52–59, 1979.

29. Lundeberg T, Abrahamsson P, Haker E: A comparative study of continuous ultrasound, placebo ultrasound, and rest in epicondylitis. Scand J Rehab Med 20:99–101, 1988.

30. Lundeberg T, Haker E, Thomas M: Effect of laser versus placebo in tennis elbow. Scand J Rehab Med 19:135–138, 1987.

31. Morrey BF: Arthroscopy of the elbow. In Morrey BF (ed): The Elbow and Its Disorders. Philadelphia, W.B. Saunders, 1985.

32. Morrey BF: Bursitis. In Morrey BF (ed): The Elbow and Its Disorders. Philadelphia, W.B. Saunders, 1985.

33. Morrey BF: Tendon injuries about the elbow. In Morrey BF (ed): The Elbow and Its Disorders. Philadelphia, W.B. Saunders, 1985.

34. Morrey BF, Askew W, An KN, Dobyns, JH: Rupture of the distal tendon of the biceps brachii. A biomechanical study. J Bone Joint Surg 67:418–421, 1985.

35. Nirschl RP: Mesenchymal syndrome. Virginia Med U 96:659, 1969.

36. Nirshcl RP: Tennis elbow. Orthop Clin North Am 4:787–800, 1973.

37. Nirschl RP: Muscle and tendon trauma: Tennis elbow. In Morrey BF (ed): The Elbow and Its Disorders. Philadelphia, W.B. Saunders, 1985.

38. Percy EC, Carson JD: The use of DMSO in tennis elbow and rotator cuff tendonitis: A double-blind study. Med Sci Sports Exerc 13(4):215–219, 1981.

39. Riordan DC: Radial nerve paralysis. Orthop Clin North Am 5:283, 1974.

40. Roles NC, Maudsley RH: Radial tunnel syndrome. Resistant tennis elbow as a nerve entrapment. J Bone Joint Surg 54B:499–508, 1972.

41. Roto P, Kivi P: Prevalence of epicondylitis and tenosynovitis among meatcutters. Scand J Work Environ Health 10:203–205, 1984.

42. Sherren J: Remarks on chronic neuritis of the ulnar nerve due to deformity in the region of the elbow joints. Edinburgh Med J 23:500, 1908.

43. Soartoh T, Eriksson E: Randomized trial of oral naproxen or local injection of betamethasone in lateral epicondylitis of the humerus. Orthopaedics 9:191–194, 1986.

44. Thompson GR, Manshady BM, Weiss JJ: Septic bursitis. JAMA 240:2280, 1978.

45. Tullos HS, King JW: Lesions of the pitching arm in adolescents. JAMA 220:264, 1972.

Chapter 23

LIGAMENT INJURIES OF THE WRIST

Peter C. Amadio, M.D.

The wrist is the most complex joint in the human skeleton, involving the complex motions of eight carpal bones interposed between the distal radius and the metacarpals. The wrist joint has three degrees of freedom—flexion/extension, radial/ulnar deviation, and pronation/supination.[15] The center of motion is roughly within the head of the capitate; the other carpal bones rotate and translate to various degrees around the capitate as the wrist moves.[4,34,46] Injuries that interfere with the complex interplay of the carpal bones during wrist motion are common. This chapter reviews both the normal function of the wrist as a foundation for understanding wrist instability and the various types of instability encountered in clinical practice; it also summarizes general diagnosis and treatment of specific wrist ligament injuries.

NORMAL WRIST FUNCTION

The wrist is unique in the body in that it has an intercalated segment—that is, a mobile bony unit to which no tendon is attached and which thus responds only indirectly to muscle action. In the wrist, the distal carpal row of trapezium, trapezoid, capitate, and hamate are rigidly fixed to the metacarpals and to each other; this complex functions as a fixed unit to which the wrist flexors and extensors insert. This unit moves under the direct influence of muscle forces. In contrast, the proximal row of scaphoid, lunate, and triquetrum have no tendinous attachment. The proximal carpal row is, thus, an interca-

lated segment whose movements are controlled by indirect force application, modified by ligamentous constraints.[24] These constraints must be present in all three planes of movement in order to prevent collapse deformity when axial loads are applied. The proximal carpal row is not only an intercalated segment; it also contains within it another intercalated segment, the lunate (Fig. 1). Normally, the scaphoid is positioned in approximately 45 degrees of flexion and the triquetrum is slightly extended[34,24] (Fig. 2). The central axis of the lunate is typically parallel to the central axis of the radius and third metacarpal. As the wrist flexes and extends, all three bones of the proximal row flex and extend together. In radial deviation all three bones flex, as the thumb approaches the radial styloid and pushes the scaphoid into further flexion. In ulnar deviation the opposite situation occurs; the scaphoid and entire proximal row are pulled into extension. External forces tend to flex the scaphoid, whereas external forces tend to extend the triquetrum. The lunate is positioned between these opposing forces. So long as the scapholunate and triquetrolunate ligaments are intact, the proximal carpal row is in balance.

CARPAL INSTABILITY

Carpal instability is present when the wrist bones do not follow the normal, synchronous motion described above. If the abnormality is only detectable when the wrist is loaded, stressed, or moved, the instability is called **dy-**

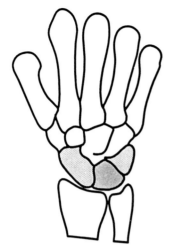

FIGURE 1. The proximal carpal row (shaded) functions as an intercalated segment within which the lunate (shaded darkest) is itself an intercalated segment. (Reproduced with permission of the Mayo Foundation.)

namic, in contrast to more obvious abnormalities evident by carpal bone malalignment even with the wrist at rest, which are called **static** instabilities[1,20,22,39] (Table 1). By convention, but also for a very logical reason, these instabilities have been described further by the position the lunate assumes (Table 2). Since the lunate is the "most intercalated" bone, it will be most sensitive to any instability. The lunate may translate dorsally,[29] palmarly,[38,41] radially (at least theoretically—it has not been reported), or ulnarly,[32] or it may angulate into flexion[24] or extension.[24] Lunate flexion insta-

TABLE 1.	Severity of Instability
	Dynamic
	Static
	Subluxation
	Dislocation

TABLE 2.	Direction of Instability
	DISI
	VISI
	Translation
	Dorsal
	Volar
	Radial
	Ulnar

DISI, dorsiflexion intercalated segment instability; VISI, volar flexion intercalated segment instability.

bility is called volar flexion intercalated segment instability or VISI; lunate extension instability is termed dorsiflexion intercalated segment instability or DISI.[24]

It must be remembered that these descriptions of lunate position describe carpal instability in the same way that the terms varus and valgus might describe instability in some other joint. They do not imply any specific etiology, which must be sought by diagnostic tests.

In addition to the classification into static and dynamic instabilities, which may be considered degrees of severity, and classification by direction of instability, wrist instabilities can

NORMAL CONJUNCT ROTATION

NORMAL SYNCHRONOUS FLEXION/EXTENSION

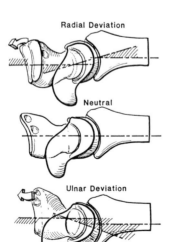

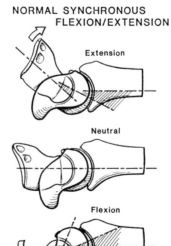

FIGURE 2. Normal conjunct rotation (see text). (Reproduced with permission of the Mayo Foundation.)

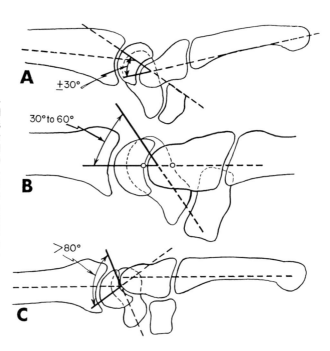

FIGURE 3. Scapholunate alignment in the lateral view. *A,* In VISI deformity the scaphoid and lunate are flexed and the scapholunate angle is low, typically less than 30 degrees. *B,* Normally the radius, lunate, and capitate are colinear and the scapholunate angle is between 30 and 60 degrees with a mean of approximately 45 degrees. *C,* In DISI deformity the lunate is extended and the scaphoid is flexed with a scapholunate angle typically greater than 80 degrees. Note also that in the VISI deformity the capitate is translated palmarly with respect to the radius, and in DISI deformity the capitate is translated dorsally with respect to the radius. (Reproduced with permission of the Mayo Foundation.)

be categorized by the site of ligament injury. Normally the scaphoid, lunate, and triquetrum move together because of the integrity of the scapholunate and triquetrolunate ligaments. If one or the other of these ligaments is disrupted, the lunate moves with the bone to which it remains associated, and the movement of the other bone is exaggerated.[24] Thus, for example, if the scapholunate ligament is disrupted, the scaphoid assumes an exaggerated flexion position over and above its normal flexion attitude of 45 degrees, and the lunate moves into extension with the triquetrum (Fig. 3). A similar situation occurs in scaphoid fracture: the distal pole falls into flexion, and the proximal pole follows the lunate into extension under the influence of the triquetrum, via the intact scapholunate and triquetrolunate ligaments.[6] Thus, a scapholunate ligament injury typically causes a DISI type of deformity. Conversely, if the triquetrolunate ligament is disrupted, the triquetrum assumes an exaggerated extended position, which typically on an anteroposterior (AP) wrist x-ray causes it to move distally on the hamate (Fig. 4). The lunate follows the scaphoid into flexion, causing a VISI type instability pattern.[33] Because these two types of instability cause a dissociation of the normally synchronous proximal carpal row they have been termed carpal instability–dissociative, or CID.[1,20,39] There are, of course, a host of capsular ligaments that also stabilize the carpal

bones (Fig. 5). If these capsular ligaments are damaged, again various collapse and translational deformities can occur. To distinguish them

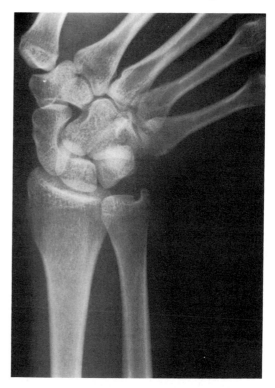

FIGURE 4. In ulnar deviation the entire proximal row extends (see also Fig. 2). This causes the triquetrum to move distally on the hamate, as shown here.

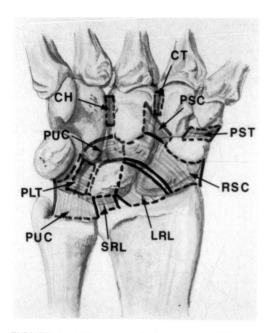

FIGURE 5. Wrist capsular ligaments form a diffuse network, especially on the volar aspect of the wrist. RSC, radioscaphocapitate ligament; LRL, long radiolunate ligament; SRL, short radiolunate ligament; PUC, palmar ulnocarpal ligament; PLT, palmar lunotriquetral ligament; CH, capitohamate ligament; PSC, palmar scaphocapitate ligament; CT, capitotrapezoidal ligament; PST, palmar scaphotrapezial ligament.

from dissociative instabilities, these capsular injuries with carpal instability have been grouped under the term carpal instability—nondissociative, or CIND.[1,20,39] In many cases CID and CIND coexist: in a perilunate dislocation, both the triquetrolunate and scapholunate ligaments are disrupted,[27] and in addition the dorsal and volar capsular ligaments are disrupted. Such instabilities can be considered carpal instability–combined, or CIC[1] (Table 3).

The complex ligamentous restraints of the wrist can be simplified to better understand nondissociative instabilities[1] (Fig. 6). Basically, the capsular ligaments are positioned dorsally and palmarly and tether the proximal row to the radius and the proximal row to the distal row. In order for the lunate to tilt into extension the proximal palmar and distal dorsal ligaments must yield (Fig. 7). Similarly, proximal

TABLE 3. Types of Instability

CID, carpal instability–dissociative
CIND, carpal instability–nondissociative
CIC, carpal instability–combined

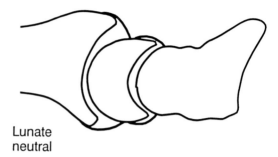

Lunate
neutral

FIGURE 6. Simplication of capsular ligaments using the lunate to represent the proximal row and the capitate the distal row. Capsular ligaments are then represented as dorsal radiolunate, dorsal lunocapitate, volar radiolunate, and volar lunocapitate. (Reproduced with permission of the Mayo Foundation.)

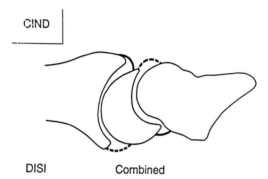

CIND

DISI   Combined

FIGURE 7. Lunate extension (DISI) deformity. (Reproduced with permission of the Mayo Foundation.)

dorsal and distal palmar incompetence create a VISI deformity (Fig. 8). Translational instabilities result from loss of the opposing restraint. For example, dorsal translation occurs after volar ligament disruption.[27,29] Carpal instability can occur with no change in lunate position if the injury is distal to the lunate.[25] The lunate may demonstrate a multidirectional instability in cases of severe multifocal capsular injury or in patients with severe generalized ligamentous laxity aggravated by injury.[9,14,21]

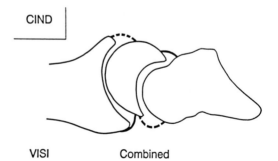

CIND

VISI   Combined

FIGURE 8. Lunate flexion (VISI) deformity. (Reproduced with permission of the Mayo Foundation.)

DIAGNOSTIC EVALUATION OF THE WRIST

The history obtained from patients with wrist ligament injuries is similar to that obtained from patients with any wrist injury. Many injuries occur as the result of a fall on the outstretched hand. Careful questioning, as well as inspection for bruising or abrasions, may help determine whether the force was directed primarily to the radial or the ulnar side of the hand. Other patients complain of a sudden pop or snap in the wrist associated with a forceful twisting action, such as turning a screwdriver against resistance. This history is typical particularly for scapholunate ligament injury.[24,42] Other patients have a history of gradually increasing wrist pain without specific injury. Symptoms suspicious for instability include sudden pain, snapping, clicking, or clunking of the wrist with movement or with forcible grip. Often the patient can demonstrate this to the examiner.

Physical examination for carpal instability is compromised by the fact that the wrist ligaments are not directly palpable. Nonetheless, a thorough circumferential examination often finds localizing signs.[2] It is best to start 180 degrees opposite to the area of the patient's maximum pain in order to avoid causing distress for as much of the physical examination as possible. A circumferential approach to the wrist ensures that all potential areas are examined.

The scaphoid tuberosity should be palpated. This may be the location of fractures or scaphotrapezial ligament injury. The anatomic snuff box is an area where the wrist capsule can be palpated; there are no ligaments in this location, but synovitis of the wrist can sometimes be felt in this region and tenderness may suggest scaphoid fracture. Tenderness over the dorsal pole of the scaphoid may be present. Often pain in this region can be exacerbated by positioning the wrist in ulnar deviation and pressing dorsally on the palmar aspect of the distal pole of the scaphoid as the wrist is brought into radial deviation. When the wrist is in ulnar deviation the scaphoid is extended. Pressing dorsally on the volar distal aspect of the scaphoid tends to displace the proximal pole of the scaphoid dorsally. As the wrist is brought into radial deviation, this tendency is exaggerated. If the scapholunate ligament is disrupted, the proximal pole of the scaphoid may actually displace dorsally with this maneuver or the maneuver may produce severe pain, reproducing the patient's symptoms. In either case this test, first described by Watson,[44] can be considered positive and suggestive of scapholunate ligament injury.

The dorsal scapholunate interval can best be palpated with the wrist flexed. Dorsal carpal ganglions in this area can be noted, as well as local tenderness. The dorsal pole of the lunate can likewise be palpated and may be tender in cases of Kienböck's disease. The triquetrolunate ligament can best be examined by positioning one hand to immobilize the lunate and the other to hold the triquetrum pisiform complex. The triquetrum and pisiform are then moved dorsally and volarly in relation to the lunate. Typically little motion should be possible.[33] If gross motion or pain is present, a triquetrolunate injury may be present.

There is an ulnar snuff box analogue to the anatomic snuff box. The ulnar snuff box is bounded by the flexor carpi ulnaris and the extensor carpi ulnaris, and within it can be palpated both the body of the triquetrum and the pisotriquetral joint. Tenderness in this area again may suggest either triangular fibrocartilage or triquetral injury. Radially directed pressure in the ulnar snuff box may reduce an ulnar translation deformity with a palpable clunk.[32] The pisiform can be grated against the triquetrum with the wrist flexed. If this is painful, pisotriquetral arthritis may be present. Intra-articular fractures can also occur at this location. On the palmar surface of the hand, the hook of the hamate can be palpated and may be tender in cases of hamate fracture. The circle is completed at the scaphotrapezial joint.

On the basis of the history and physical examination, the physician may suspect a carpal instability. Confirmation of a diagnosis depends upon the ability to demonstrate either static or dynamic carpal malalignment (Fig. 9). Routine radiographs show the lunate position at rest; if this is abnormal a static deformity exists, as shown in Figures 3 and 4. If the routine x-rays are negative, an assessment should be based on the history as to whether there is a high or low probability of ligament injury and instability. If there is a high probability of ligament injury, cineradiography can be considered as the next step. This study should be videotaped so that a thoughtful postexamination review can be performed. Cineradiography should be performed if the patient describes a click or clunk with wrist motion; the

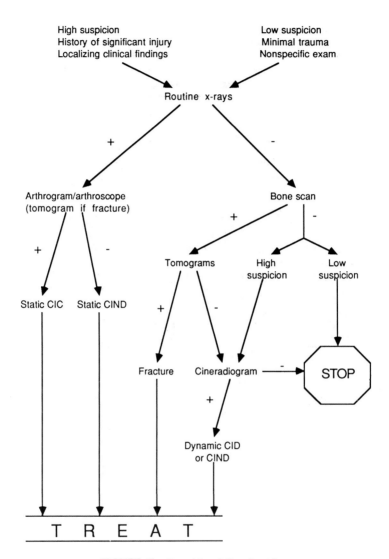

FIGURE 9. Carpal instability algorithm.

patient should be encouraged to perform the motion that causes the painful sensation while the videotaped cineradiograph is obtained in both AP and lateral projections. The examiner may also perform symptom-producing stress tests during the cineradiographic study.

An arthrogram performed at the time of cineradiography is quite useful in determining the status of the scapholunate and triquetro-lunate ligaments.[10,19] This study should also be videotaped for future view. Dye leakage from the radiocarpal to the midcarpal joint can confirm ligament injury (Fig. 10). Because some interligament injuries may function as one-way

valves, many examiners prefer to perform a separate midcarpal arthrogram as well.

Arthrography cannot determine the size of a ligament injury. A tiny pinhole perforation without clinical significance can cause dye leakage as impressively as a larger, clinically significant tear. Arthroscopy can be quite useful in determining the size of ligament injuries; it also provides an opportunity to inspect articular cartilage and to physically probe the carpal bones and ligaments to determine if an apparently intact ligament is attenuated.[45] If the probability of instability is low and routine, radiographs are negative; a bone scan may be

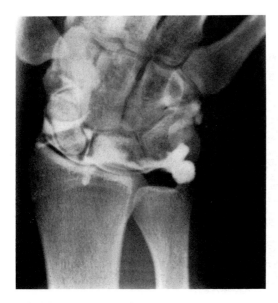

FIGURE 10. This wrist arthrogram shows dye passing through the scapholunate interval and entering the mid-carpal joint. The size of the ligament tear cannot be determined from the arthrogram.

considered as a screen. If the bone scan is also negative, the likelihood that further evaluation will yield positive data is low. If the bone scan is positive, tomography may be considered to look for fracture, and the instability workup outlined above should be continued.

With the above information the examiner can determine the severity of the injury (static or dynamic), the direction of the instability (DISI, VISI, translation), and whether the injury is dissociative, nondissociative, or both (integrity of scapholunate and triquetrolunate ligaments on arthrogram or arthroscopy).

TREATMENT OF SPECIFIC WRIST LIGAMENT INJURIES

Once a specific ligament injury has been identified and its severity is known, a treatment program can be undertaken. In general, treatment depends upon both the acuity and the severity of the injury. An acute dynamic scapholunate ligament instability often responds with simple cast protection for 6–8 weeks.[31] It can usually be safely assumed that capsular ligaments are intact; often the scapholunate injury is partial. Some surgeons prefer percutaneous Kirschner wire fixation or direct ligament repair with Kirschner wire supplementation for this injury. No clinical reports

have specifically addressed acute partial scapholunate ligament injury in detail, but the results in general are likely to be good, as a result of the fortuitous combination of early accurate diagnosis and lesser degree of injury.

An acute static scapholunate instability clearly requires reduction and stabilization. Not only is complete scapholunate ligament injury present, but capsular ligaments must at least be stretched to permit the static deformity. Thus, these injuries probably represent a carpal instability–combined. Results of direct ligament repair in such cases, with or without augmentation, are occasionally unpredictable.[11,31] Some authors favor open reduction with ligament repair, capsular augmentation, and internal fixation for this injury (Fig. 11).[3,24] In some cases, excellent dynamic and static stability is restored with near-normal strength and motion. In other cases instability has worsened after surgery. A review of published cases suggests that patients with static instability do less well than those with dynamic instability, that chronic injuries do worse than acute ones, and that the presence of any degenerative change in the joint is a relatively strong contraindication to direct ligament repair.[5,11,16,31] Because of the potential unreliability of ligament repair and reconstruction, many surgeons favor scaphotrapezial trapezoid or scaphocapitate arthrodesis.[17,42,44] This approach attempts to provide clinical stability while ignoring the site of intercarpal ligament injury. Excellent static correction can be obtained; indeed congruent reduction of the radial scaphoid articulation at the time of arthrodesis is mandatory. Incongruent reduction with arthrodesis leads to a rapidly progressive postoperative loss of joint space with pain and stiffness. Watson likens the scaphoid and scaphoid fossa to two canoes stored in a shed; if they are not nested properly, localized contact of the gunwales of one with the hull of the other will erode both.[42,44]

Although intercarpal arthrodesis can provide good static correction, it does little to restore dynamic stability, and this has raised concerns about the durability of the procedure in some quarters. The scapholunate ligament remains incomplete after scaphotrapezial trapezoid or scaphocapitate arthrodesis, and stress views postoperatively still show some gapping of the scapholunate interval, which corrects when the wrist is unloaded.[16] Many patients develop localized scaphoid radial styloid arthritis postoperatively; a styloidectomy is often advised as a routine part of scaphotrapezial trapezoid ar-

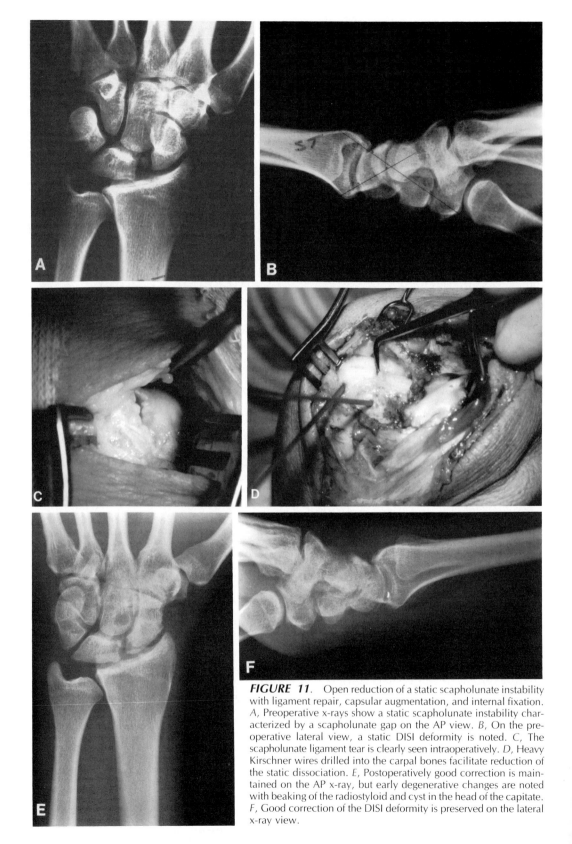

FIGURE 11. Open reduction of a static scapholunate instability with ligament repair, capsular augmentation, and internal fixation. *A*, Preoperative x-rays show a static scapholunate instability characterized by a scapholunate gap on the AP view. *B*, On the preoperative lateral view, a static DISI deformity is noted. *C*, The scapholunate ligament tear is clearly seen intraoperatively. *D*, Heavy Kirschner wires drilled into the carpal bones facilitate reduction of the static dissociation. *E*, Postoperatively good correction is maintained on the AP x-ray, but early degenerative changes are noted with beaking of the radiostyloid and cyst in the head of the capitate. *F*, Good correction of the DISI deformity is preserved on the lateral x-ray view.

throdesis.[16] Nonetheless, long-term symptomatic relief after scaphotrapezial trapezoid or scaphocapitate arthrodesis has been reported,[16] and the procedure remains a useful part of many surgeons' armamentarium. Whether ligament repair or arthrodesis is elected, 2–3 months of cast immobilization are needed after surgery, and some permanent restriction of wrist motion and strength is likely.

In chronic dynamic scapholunate instability it can be assumed that the secondary restraints within the capsule are probably intact. Because of the chronicity of the discomfort (generally defined as lasting more than 6 weeks after injury), however, the scapholunate ligament may be less likely to heal with simple immobilization, and therefore, an open repair like the one for acute static deformity is usually recommended.[24,44] Once again, some have recommended scaphotrapezial or scaphocapitate arthrodesis as an alternative.[39,44]

The treatment of chronic static scapholunate ligament injury depends upon whether or not degenerative arthritic changes are already present.[44] If they are, a salvage procedure is indicated. Typically, the arthritis begins at the radioscaphoid joint and progresses to the capitolunate articulation.[35,43] This progression is so typical that it has been given a name—scapholunate advanced collapse—and is often called acronymically the SLAC wrist.[43] Salvage treatment options include proximal row carpectomy if capitolunate degenerative changes are not present,[7] and scaphoid excision with midcarpal arthrodesis, or complete wrist arthrodesis, if capitolunate degenerative changes are present.[43] If the scaphoid is excised, the space may be filled with tendon anchovy or a silicone implant. Scaphoid excision with midcarpal arthrodesis probably functions like a proximal row carpectomy, although direct comparisons have not been made. The procedure depends upon the integrity of the radiolunate joint, which is usually preserved until very late in the progression of the SLAC wrist. If no degenerative arthritis is present, chronic static scapholunate instability can be treated as acute static instability, but the prognosis is probably worse.

Lunotriquetral instability must be differentiated from the lunotriquetral ligament perforation associated with relative prominence of the distal ulna (positive ulnar variance) (Fig. 12).[30] Essentially all cases of lunotriquetral ligament perforation associated with positive ulnar variance are symptomatic because of the ulnar carpal abutment and not because of any

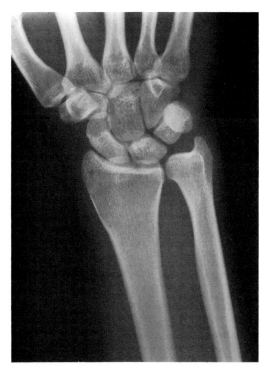

FIGURE 12. In positive ulnar variance the radial margin of the distal ulna is distal to the ulnar margin of the distal radius, as in this example. Normally the radius and ulna should be level (see Fig. 4). Relative shortening of the ulna (negative ulnar variance) is common in Kienböck's disease and is also statistically associated with scapholunate dissociation.

associated lunotriquetral instability (Fig. 13). Such cases are best treated by shortening the ulna; typically no treatment is necessary for the lunotriquetral injury itself.[30]

In patients with actual acute dynamic lunotriquetral instability, 6–8 weeks of simple cast protection with or without percutaneous Kirschner wire fixation should be sufficient to restore stability. For acute static instability, either ligament repair or lunotriquetral arthrodesis can be considered (Fig. 14).[26,33] Again, like scapholunate static instabilities, static lunotriquetral instabilities are in the CIC group, including both intercarpal and capsular ligament injury. In this case, the palmar ulnar triquetral ligaments or dorsal midcarpal ligaments are likely to be incompetent and may require repair. In some cases, repair can be accomplished by ulnar shortening; in others, by direct imbrication. Triquetral hamate arthrodesis is an option for addressing the distal aspect of this instability.[21] In the most severe cases, both triquetral lunate and triquetral hamate arthrodesis might be considered. Luno-

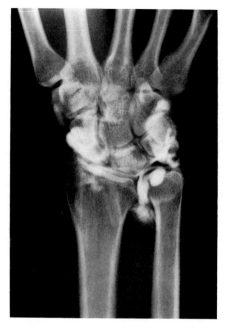

FIGURE 13. In ulnar carpal abutment syndrome the positive ulnar variance is associated with a thinner than normal triangular fibrocartilage, which may perforate, permitting the ulnar head to erode the triquetrolunate ligament. In this arthrogram leakage of dye from the radiocarpal joint into the distal radiolunar joint confirms a triangular fibrocartilage perforation. Although leakage into the midcarpal joint is evidence of a triquetrolunate perforation, both clinically and under fluoroscopy the triquetrum and proximal carpal row move normally in ulnar carpal abutment syndrome. There is no instability.

sidered, and lunotriquetral arthrodesis is a secondary option; for chronic static lunotriquetral instability, lunotriquetral arthrodesis may be most appropriate. Again, a nondissociative capsular component must be assumed; otherwise the carpal bones could not assume the abnormal static position. This component should also be addressed at the time of treatment by capsulodesis[3] or intercarpal arthrodesis.[21] In the most severe cases, a combination of triquetrolunate and triquetrohamate arthrodesis may need be considered, especially if degenerative changes are present at these joints.

Acute perilunate injuries represent the most severe form of combined dissociative and nondissociative instability (Fig. 15).[12,18,28,37] Although closed treatment can occasionally be successful if anatomic reduction is achieved and maintained, most commonly these injuries require open repair of the damaged capsular and intracapsular ligaments. Internal fixation must stabilize not only the scapholunate and lunotriquetral repairs but also the nondissociative capsular component, by pinning the reduced carpus to the radius; if this is not done, late translational instability may occur. Often both palmar and dorsal surgical approaches are needed. Acceptable, but less reliable, results from open reduction can be achieved in neglected cases up to 3 months after injury.[36]

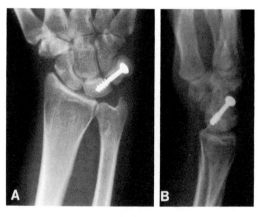

FIGURE 14. Triquetrolunate arthrodesis may be performed either with a bone screw, as shown here, or with Kirschner wires. Supplemental bone graft is also needed.

triquetral arthrodesis may be slightly more reliable than ligament repair, but nonunion of this intercarpal arthrodesis does occur.[26,33]

For chronic dynamic instability of the lunotriquetral joint, ligament repair can be con-

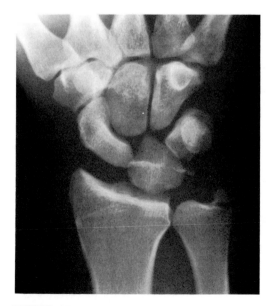

FIGURE 15. In perilunate dislocation the scapholunate and triquetrolunate ligaments, as well as the ligaments connecting the lunate to the distal carpal row, are always disrupted. The amount of disruption of the ligaments between the lunate and the radius is variable.

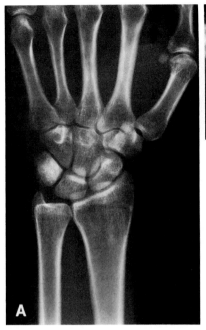

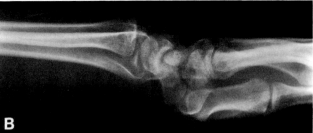

FIGURE 16. In carpal instability—nondissociative, the most common deformity is VISI. *A,* The anterior and posterior x-ray shows some foreshortening of the scaphoid, but otherwise is unremarkable. *B,* On the lateral view the marked VISI deformity can be noted.

Chronic lunate or perilunate dislocations treated beyond 3 months require some sort of salvage procedure such as proximal row carpectomy or wrist arthrodesis.[36]

Treatment of nondissociative instabilities is even less well defined than that for dissociative instabilities. Many patients with nondissociative instability have generalized ligamentous laxity as an underlying problem (Fig. 16).[14,21,25]

Such patients may have DISI, VISI, or multidirectional instabilities. Others may have had a chronic synovitis of the wrist with attenuation of the wrist capsular ligaments such as may occur, for example, in rheumatoid arthritis. In this group, translational instabilities are more common.[23,32] Translational instability can also be posttraumatic, after radiocarpal or perilunate dislocation. In the absence of degenera-

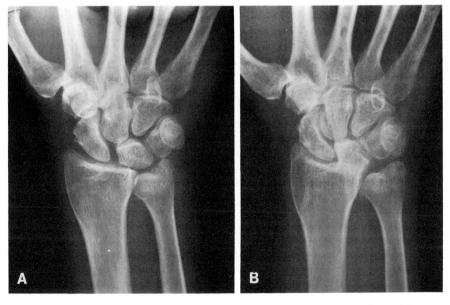

FIGURE 17. A translational instability corrected by radiolunate arthrodesis. *A,* Ulnar translation deformity is common in rheumatoid disease. *B,* The ulnar translation deformity is best corrected by radiolunate fusion.

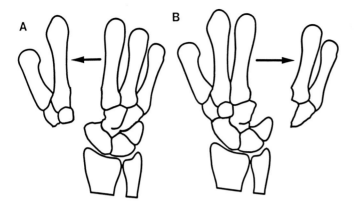

FIGURE 18. In axial carpal dislocations the disruption is within the distal carpal row. A, Axial radial disruptions involve the radial rays. B, Axial ulnar disruptions involve the ulnar rays. (Reproduced with permission of the Mayo Foundation.)

tive changes in the radioscaphoid or midcarpal joints, radiolunate arthrodesis has been reliable in correcting translational instabilities (Fig. 17).[23] Ligament reconstruction has not been successful; even when performed for acute injuries.[32] For DISI and VISI angular deformities, treatment recommendations are most unclear. It is often difficult to localize the specific ligament involved;[13] as mentioned earlier, many of these injuries are multidirectional with the lunate alternatively in DISI and VISI deformity depending upon the position in which the wrist is loaded. Various capsulodeses have been recommended; others have advised intercarpal arthrodesis. In no case have the results from published reports been sufficiently good to identify an optimal method of treatment.

One of the few types of CIND for which a well-defined and generally successful treatment program exists is the midcarpal instability that develops after malunion of a Colles fracture. In this case the dorsal angulation of the radius forces a chronic extension posture on the proximal row. A secondary flexion deformity can then develop at the midcarpal joint, with a resulting VISI appearance. The instability is usually readily corrected by osteotomy of the radius.[40]

One last type of wrist instability has recently been described. The distal carpal row bones are normally firmly adherent to each other, but they may be displaced by a strong dorsal-volar compression, flattening the carpal arch. The resulting disruption of the intercarpal ligaments of the distal row has been termed axial instability[5] (Fig. 18). Just as dissociative instabilities of the proximal row can be radial (scapholunate), ulnar (triquetrolunate), or combined radial and ulnar (perilunate), so axial dislocations can be radial, involving the first or the first and second rays; ulnar, involving the

fifth or the fourth and fifth rays; or combined radial and ulnar. Open reduction and internal fixation are mandatory for axial dislocations. These injuries are almost always secondary to violent trauma with severe crushing; permanent impairments to strength and motion are nearly universal.

CONCLUSION

Ligament injuries of the wrist present a confusing picture, both for diagnosis and for treatment. Diagnosis can be helped by a systematic approach to physical examination and diagnostic tests. The most useful diagnostic tests for characterizing wrist instability are routine radiographs, cineradiography, wrist arthrography, and wrist arthroscopy. A bone scan can be a useful screening device in doubtful cases. Both bone scans and tomograms are useful in investigating associated bony injuries. Treatment of carpal instability is difficult, particularly in cases of capsular injury with nondissociative instability, because specific localization of the site of ligament damage may be difficult or impossible. Even in intracapsular injuries to the scapholunate or triquetrolunate ligament, generally agreed-upon treatment guidelines have yet to be established. Some degree of permanent impairment is likely after any significant wrist ligament injury.

REFERENCES

1. Amadio PC: Carpal kinematics and instability. A clinical and anatomic primer. Clin Anat, in press.
2. Beckenbaugh RD: Accurate evaluation and management of the painful wrist following injury: An approach to carpal instability. Orthop Clin North Am 15:289–306, 1984.

3. Blatt G: Capsulodesis in reconstructive hand surgery. Hand Clin 3:81–102, 1987.

4. de Lange A, Kauer JMG, Huiskes R: Kinematic behavior of the human wrist joint: A roentgen-stereophotogrammetric analysis. J Orthop Res 3:56–64, 1985.

5. Eckenrode JF, Louis DS, Greene TL: Scaphoid-trapezium-trapezoid fusion in the treatment of chronic scapholunate instability. J Hand Surg 11A:497–502, 1986.

6. Fisk FR: Carpal instability and the fractured scaphoid. Ann R Coll Surg Engl 46:63–76, 1970.

7. Fitzgerald JP, Peimer CA, Smith RJ: Distraction resection arthroplasty of the wrist. J Hand Surg 14A:774–781, 1989.

8. Garcia-Elias M, Dobyns JH, Cooney WP III, Linscheid RL: Traumatic axial dislocations of the carpus. J Hand Surg 14A:446–457, 1989.

9. Garth WP Jr, Hofammann DY, Rooks MD: Volar intercalated segment instability secondary to medial carpal ligamental laxity. Clin Orthop 201:94–105, 1985.

10. Gilula LA, Hardy DC, Totty WG, Reinus WR: Fluoroscopic identification of torn intercarpal ligaments after injection of contrast material. AJR 149:761–764, 1987.

11. Glickel SZ, Millender LH: Ligamentous reconstruction for chronic intercarpal instability. J Hand Surg 9A:514–525, 1984.

12. Green DP, O'Brien ET: Open reduction of carpal dislocations: Indications and operative techniques. J Hand Surg 3:250–265, 1978.

13. Hankin FM, Amadio PC, Wojtys EM, Braunstein EM: Carpal instability with volar flexion of the proximal row associated with injury to the scaphotrapezial ligament: Report of two cases. J Hand Surg 13B:298–302, 1988.

14. Johnson RP, Carrera GF: Chronic capitolunate instability. J Bone Joint Surg 68A:1164–1176, 1986.

15. Kauer JMG: The mechanism of the carpal joint. Clin Orthop Rel Res 202:16–26, 1986.

16. Kleinman WB: Long-term study of chronic scapholunate instability treated by scapho-trapezio-trapezoid arthrodesis. J Hand Surg 14A:429–445, 1989.

17. Kleinman WB, Steichen JB, Strickland JW: Management of chronic rotary subluxation of the scaphoid by scapho-trapezio-trapezoid arthrodesis. J Hand Surg 7:125–136, 1982.

18. Kupfer KP: Dislocation of scaphoid and lunate as a unit: Case report with special reference to carpal instability and treatment. J Hand Surg 11A:130–134, 1986.

19. Levinsohn EM, Palmer AK, Coren AB, Zinberg E: Wrist arthrography: The value of the three compartment injection technique. Skeletal Radiol 16:539–544, 1987.

20. Lichtman DM, Martin RA: Introduction to the carpal instabilities. In Lichtman DM (ed): The Wrist and Its Disorders. Philadelphia, W.B. Saunders, 1988, pp 244–250.

21. Lichtman DM, Schneider AR, Swafford AR, Mack GR: Ulnar midcarpal instability—Clinical and laboratory analysis. J Hand Surg 6A:515–523, 1981.

22. Linscheid RL, Dobyns JH: The unified concept of carpal injuries. Ann Chir Main 3:35–42, 1984.

23. Linscheid RL, Dobyns JH: Radiolunate arthrodesis. J Hand Surg 10A:821–829, 1985.

24. Linscheid RL, Dobyns JH, Beabout JW, Bryan RS: Traumatic instability of the wrist: Diagnosis, classification and pathomechanics. J Bone Joint Surg 54A:1612–1632, 1972.

25. Louis DS, Hankin FM, Greene TL, et al: Central carpal instability—Capitate lunate instability pattern: Diagnosis by dynamic displacement. Orthopedics 7:1693–1696, 1984.

26. Maitin EC, Bora FW Jr, Osterman AL: Lunatotriquetral instability: A cause of chronic wrist pain. J Hand Surg 13A:309, 1988.

27. Mayfield JK, Johnson RP, Kilcoyne RK: Carpal dislocations: Pathomechanics and progressive perilunar instability. J Hand Surg 5A:226–241, 1980.

28. Minami A, Ogino T, Ohshio I, Minami M: Correlation between clinical results and carpal instabilities in patients after reduction of lunate and perilunar dislocations. J Hand Surg 11B:213–220, 1986.

29. Moneim MS, Bolger JT, Omer GE: Radiocarpal dislocation—Classification and rationale for management. Clin Orthop Rel Res 192:199–209, 1985.

30. Palmer AK: Triangular fibrocartilage lesions. J Hand Surg 14A:594–606, 1989.

31. Palmer AK, Dobyns JH, Linscheid RL: Management of post-traumatic instability of the wrist secondary to ligament rupture. J Hand Surg 3:507–532, 1978.

32. Rayhack JM, Linscheid RL, Dobyns JH, Smith JH: Posttraumatic ulnar translation of the carpus. J Hand Surg 12A:180–189, 1987.

33. Reagan DS, Linscheid RL, Dobyns JH: Lunotriquetral sprains. J Hand Surg 9A:502–514, 1984.

34. Ruby LK, Cooney WP III, An K-N, et al: Relative motion of selected carpal bones: A kinematic analysis of the normal wrist. J Hand Surg 13A:1–10, 1988.

35. Sebald JR, Dobyns JH, Linscheid RL: The natural history of collapse deformities of the wrist. Clin Orthop 104:140–148, 1974.

36. Siegert JJ, Frassica FJ, Amadio PC: Treatment of chronic perilunate dislocations. J Hand Surg 13A:206–212, 1988.

37. Stambough JL, Mandel RJ, Duda JR: Volar dislocation of the carpal scaphoid. Case report and review of the literature. Orthopedics 9:565–570, 1986.

38. Taleisnik J: Post-traumatic carpal instability. Clin Orthop Rel Res 149:72–82, 1980.

39. Taleisnik J: Current concepts review: Carpal instability. J Bone Joint Surg 70A:1262–1268, 1988.

40. Taleisnik J, Watson HK: Midcarpal instability caused by malunited fractures of the distal radius. J Hand Surg 9A:350–357, 1984.

41. Thomsen S, Falstie-Jensen S: Palmar dislocation of the radiocarpal joint. J Hand Surg 14A:627–630, 1989.

42. Watson HK, Hempton RF: Limited wrist arthrodeses. I. The triscaphoid joint. J Hand Surg 5:320–237, 1980.

43. Watson HK, Ryu J: Degenerative disorders of the carpus. Orthop Clin North Am 15:337–353, 1984.

44. Watson HK, Ryu J, Akelman E: Limited triscaphoid intercarpal arthrodesis for rotary subluxation of the scaphoid. J Bone Joint Surg 68A:345–349, 1986.

45. Whipple TL, Marotta JJ, Powell JH III: Techniques of wrist arthroscopy. Arthroscop Rel Surg 2:244–252, 1986.

46. Youm Y, McMurtry RY, Flatt AE, Gillespie TE: Kinematics of the wrist. I. An experimental study of radial-ulnar deviation and flexion-extension. J Bone Joint Surg 60A:423–431, 1978.

Chapter 24

LIGAMENT INJURIES OF THE HAND

Raymond C. Noellert, M.D., and Fred M. Hankin, M.D.

The frequency of industrial injury to the hand parallels use of the hand as an important tool. Exposure to twisting, crushing, or jamming forces is an everyday occurrence in the workplace. Because injuries of differing severity can present with a similar appearance, it becomes important for safety personnel to quickly and efficiently determine which injuries may require specialized care.

The ligaments of the hand provide impressive strength and mobility in an economy of space. Anatomically, the metacarpophalangeal (MCP) joints are similar to the interphalangeal joints of the digits. Lateral stability is provided by strong collateral ligaments, and the substantial volar (palmar plate) ligament resists extension forces. The less mobile carpometacarpal (CMC) joints of the ulnar four digits are held in place by stout interosseous ligaments reinforced by the insertions of wrist extensor and flexor tendons. Purely ligamentous injuries (sprains) occur frequently in the hand and deserve special attention because they are prone to casual treatment that might result in prolonged impairment or even permanent disability. Treatment of a significant injury to this region should be directed toward restoration of normal architecture and function. Dynamic (functional) and static (architectural) treatment goals must be incorporated in the treatment plan of any ligament injury involving the hand.

Selective positioning of the hand can help localize the area of concern on standard radiographs.[11] The difficulty of obtaining true lateral radiographic views of the overlapping metacarpals and phalanges can be managed by several methods. Multiple oblique views can help define the area of concern. Tomograms and computed tomography can also provide clarification of the overlapping structures. It is tempting to use stress radiographs to help confirm the presence of a ligament injury, but this iatrogenic manipulation can potentially convert a minor injury, treatable with simple immobilization, into a displaced intra-articular fracture requiring surgical intervention.

Immobilization, when required, should place joints in anticontracture positions. Positions of 60–90 degrees for the MCP joints and 10–20 degrees for the interphalangeal joints of the ulnar four digits maintain the maximal length of the respective collateral ligaments. The thumb should be placed in a functional attitude of opposition when immobilization is required. This provides a prehensile posture of thumb opposition. Specific patient requirements for joint position must, however, be considered if post-traumatic stiffness is expected.[2,8,13]

Interphalangeal injuries are covered in Chapter 14. Only injuries of the MCP and CMC joints are discussed in this chapter. Proper diagnosis and clinical evaluation are emphasized.

METACARPOPHALANGEAL JOINT

Thumb

Ulnar Collateral Ligament

The thumb provides a stable post about which the rest of the hand may perform activities of pinch and grasp. The ulnar collateral ligament

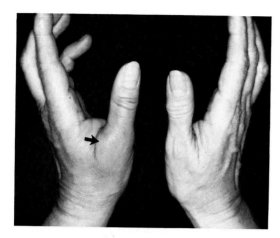

FIGURE 1. An acute injury to the UCL of the left thumb MCP joint results in localized soft tissue swelling (*arrow*) and tenderness. Stress testing demonstrates laxity, which is consistent with a tear of this ligament.

(UCL) plays a dominant role in providing this stability by resisting radial stresses across the MCP joint. The collateral ligaments have limited bone attachments and originate and insert into the original epiphyses of the proximal phalanx and metacarpal head.[6] The MCP joint UCL can be injured when the thumb is forcibly abducted or hyperextended, as, for example, when the first web space or thumb is thrust against an unyielding object, as during a fall. Straps or belts around the thumb can exert abduction forces on the thumb and disrupt the UCL. This injury has been termed "skier's thumb." "Gamekeeper's thumb" is a chronic UCL attenuation injury, historically associated with thumb MCP abduction forces used by game wardens to subdue their prey. With each of these injuries, the ligament may tear through its substance (partially or completely), or with an attached piece of bone it may be avulsed from either the proximal phalanx or the metacarpal head.[7]

The patient presents with swelling, ecchymosis, and tenderness localized predominantly to the ulnar aspect of the thumb MCP joint (Fig. 1). There is considerable weakness of pinch as well as pain. Occasionally, the end of the disrupted ligament can be palpated beneath the intact skin.

Standard radiographs should be obtained before a stress examination of the joint is done.[12] Nondisplaced fractures should not be submitted to stress, which can displace the fragment and convert a situation that is manageable by nonoperative means into one requiring surgery. Displaced fractures noted on preliminary radiographs that are associated with ligament avulsion injuries help to corroborate the clinical diagnosis (Fig. 2).

If no fracture is noted on the standard radiographs, stress examination of the thumb MCP joint can be performed. With the thumb metacarpal stabilized by one hand, the proximal phalanx is grasped by the other (Fig. 3). The MCP joint should be tested in full flexion.[12] Normally the MCP collateral ligaments are slightly lax when the joint is positioned in extension and tighten in camlike fashion over the metacarpal head as the joint is flexed. Positioning the joint in flexion serves to isolate the UCL during the stress examination.[1,12]

The examination should be consistently and carefully performed on both the injured and the uninjured thumb, and the results compared. An increase of 30–35 degrees of angulation across the stressed MCP joint is considered pathognomonic of complete ligament rupture. Lesser degrees of laxity and a distinct end point noted during the stress evaluation

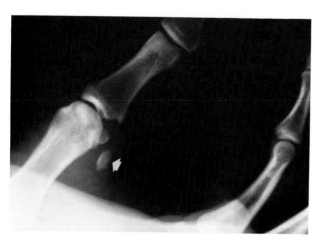

FIGURE 2. Radiograph of an acute injury to the thumb MCP joint demonstrates an avulsion of a bone fragment from the ulnar aspect of the proximal phalanx base (*arrow*). The UCL is attached to this displaced fragment.

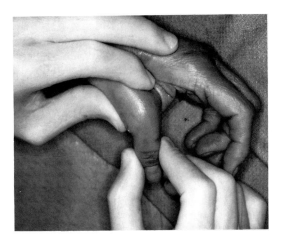

FIGURE 3. With the MCP joint flexed, radial stressing of the joint demonstrates laxity of the UCL. (Reproduced with permission.)

represent incomplete ligament injuries. The stress test may be hindered by significant pain and guarding. Diagnostic accuracy is improved with the use of local anesthesia, preferably radial and median nerve blocks at the wrist.

When doubt as to the degree of injury is present, stress radiographs may be helpful (Fig. 4). Angulation and widening of the joint space can be documented in this fashion. Only when the magnitude of injury has been ascertained may treatment proceed.

Partial ligament ruptures and nondisplaced avulsion fractures are satisfactorily treated with

immobilization in a functional position in a thumb spica splint or cast. Initially the MCP joint and the wrist should be included. After 4 weeks, a hand-based thumb splint can protect the joint for an additional 2–4 weeks (Fig. 5). The patient often can return to work with the hand-based splint. A similar device can be useful in preventing injury during high-risk activities.

Complete UCL ruptures should be splinted and referred for prompt evaluation by a hand specialist. Surgical intervention is warranted to repair a complete UCL disruption. Untreated injuries can lead to chronic instability and traumatic arthritis.

Radial Collateral Ligament

The radial collateral ligament is much less frequently damaged than its ulnar counterpart. However, its role in maintaining thumb stability is just as important, and when it is injured, guidelines for evaluation and treatment are similar to those for the UCL.[3]

A twisting injury or forced adduction is generally the mechanism of injury. Tenderness and swelling are largely confined to the radial and volar aspects of the joint. Examination and assessment of the degree of instability are performed in the same way as for injuries to the MCP joint UCL, and treatment recommendations are the same.

Hyperextension Injury (Volar Plate)

A pure hyperextension force may result in a dorsal dislocation of the MCP joint (proximal

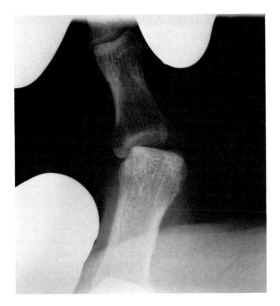

FIGURE 4. Stress radiograph demonstrates the ulnar laxity of the thumb MCP joint.

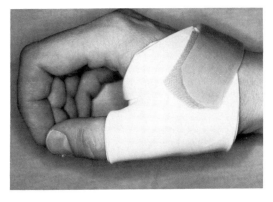

FIGURE 5. Hand-based splint made from a thermoplastic material provides effective immobilization of the thumb MCP joint.

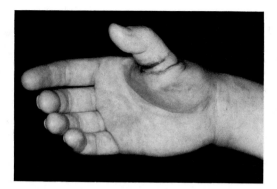

FIGURE 6. Clinical appearance of a complex dislocation of the thumb MCP joint. Mild hyperextension of the joint and a volar skin dimple are present. (Reproduced with permission.)

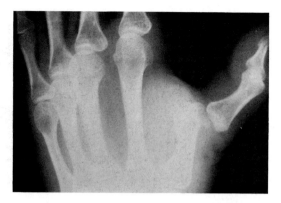

FIGURE 7. Radiograph of the complex dislocation of the thumb MCP joint demonstrates interposition of the sesamoid (volar plate) between the metacarpal and proximal phalanxes. (Reproduced with permission.)

phalanx dorsal to the metacarpal). This can occur with rupture of the volar (palmar) plate, usually the proximal attachment, without necessarily rupturing the collateral ligaments. The volar plate links the original epiphyseal portions of the joint.[6]

Clinically, the thumb is obviously deformed in a hyperextended posture at the MCP joint. Sensation and circulation should be assessed. Radiographs should be obtained before reduction attempts are made in order to discover any concomitant fractures. Local anesthesia can be provided by radial and median nerve blocks at the wrist. Reduction maneuvers should be gentle and should incorporate flexion of the proximal phalanx base across the metacarpal head. Violent longitudinal traction can potentially draw adjacent soft tissue into the joint, where it can block further reduction attempts.

After reduction of the thumb MCP joint has been accomplished and confirmed by standard radiographs, active range of motion and the stability of the collateral ligaments can be determined. If the thumb MCP joint is stable after reduction, immobilization of the joint at neutral or slight flexion in a thumb spica splint or cast for 4 weeks provides sufficient treatment. If either the radial or the ulnar collateral ligament is unstable after reduction, treatment should be directed toward that structure as outlined above.

Complex (irreducible) dislocations of the thumb MCP joint cannot be reduced by closed methods (Fig. 6). Interposition of bone, ligament, tendons, or neurovascular bundles between the joint surfaces prevents a concentric reduction of the joint (Fig. 7). Normal joint alignment is prevented by the interposition of soft tissue, which does not resolve and is sel-

dom improved by an incomplete joint reduction. Surgical consultation is required for these injuries.

Prognosis for all thumb MCP injuries is excellent if a prompt diagnosis is made and treatment guidelines are properly followed. Improperly diagnosed or treated injuries can result in impairment affecting nearly every use of the hand.

Digits

MCP Collateral Ligaments

Collateral ligament injuries of the digital joints are uncommon. Injuries may occur when the digit is twisted or when an object thrust into a digital web space forces a finger into acute radial or ulnar deviation. The degree of accompanying swelling is highly variable, and it is not unusual for the worker to delay seeking treatment. Clinical examination may reveal swelling and local tenderness. With the MCP joints extended, there is normally a wide allowance for passive radial and ulnar deviation. Stability is best tested with the MCP joint in maximum flexion in order to isolate the function of the collateral ligament. Stressing the affected ligament is invariably painful. Stress examination of adjacent and contralateral MCP joints is recommended. As with all small-joint injuries, radiographic examination is required. If small fleck of bone is avulsed, it helps to localize the injury (Fig. 8). The collateral ligaments of the MCP joints originate and insert into the original epiphyses of the articulating members.[6] Larger avulsion fractures that are

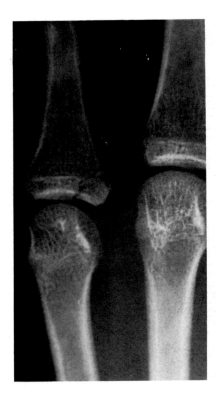

FIGURE 8. A radial deviation injury to the index finger resulted in this UCL avulsion injury to the MCP joint.

widely displaced or result in joint incongruity require surgical treatment.

Treatment of the acute MCP collateral ligament injury (less than 4 weeks) should include 3–4 weeks of immobilization with the joint held in 60–75 degrees of flexion. After this, buddy taping of the involved finger to the adjacent one should continue for several weeks until range of motion, comfort, and strength approach normal. It is not unusual for some degree of swelling and induration to persist for several months. Consideration for surgical repair is probably limited to the MCP radial collateral ligament of the index finger, which mirrors the thumb UCL in function and is essential for pinch maneuvers. Acute MCP collateral ligament injuries of the other digits do not usually require surgery. Late surgical reconstruction of the ligament can be helpful in those few cases in which pain or dysfunction persist after initial treatment.

MCP Volar Plate

Dislocation of digital MCP joints is almost invariably dorsal and represents varying de-

grees of injury to the volar plate. The border digits—index and small—are most commonly affected. The mechanism of injury is forced hyperextension, which occurs commonly during falls and with activities such as guiding lumber into a saw or planer that "kicks back" the piece into the guiding fingers.

On examination, one of two positions of the digit is noted. The first is that of exaggerated hyperextension of the involved MCP joint, which generally indicates an injury that can be easily reduced. Unlike reduction of many other musculoskeletal injuries, the maneuver for a volar plate injury should not include traction or "accentuation" of the deformity (i.e., further hyperextension). Such maneuvers may displace and interpose the volar plate into the joint, converting a reducible dislocation to a complex (irreducible) problem. Reduction maneuvers should be gentle and should incorporate flexion of the proximal phalanx base across the metacarpal head.

The second posture noted with these injuries is the so-called "bayonet" position. The digit is dorsally dislocated relative to the hand but is roughly parallel to the metacarpal. Although less dramatic in appearance, this position is commonly assumed by an irreducible dislocation that already has interposed tissue in the joint. Surgical intervention is usually required to achieve a concentric joint reduction.

After reduction of a simple dorsal dislocation, treatment is straightforward. A cast or extension block splint immobilities the joint in a position of 60–75 degrees of flexion for 3 weeks. Subsequent buddy taping to the adjacent finger in the manner described for collateral ligament injuries is recommended for several more weeks. It is unusual for these injuries to result in significant long-term impairment.

CARPOMETACARPAL JOINTS

Thumb

The thumb CMC joint differs from that of the ulnar four digits in the high degree of mobility it allows. The strongest ligamentous support is volar, connecting the base of the first metacarpal to the trapezium and the base of the second metacarpal. Injury occurs commonly from a direct blow or fall on the palm, over the thumb metacarpal. Damage may also follow hyperextension or hyperabduction of the

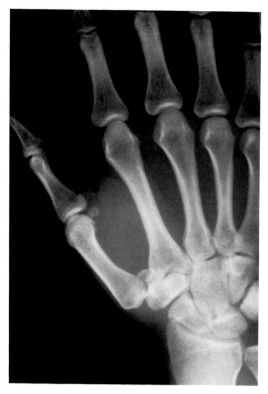

FIGURE 9. Radiograph of a fracture-dislocation of the thumb CMC joint (Bennett's fracture). Stout ligaments hold the first metacarpal fragment attached to the trapezoid and second metacarpal base while the abductor pollicis longus tendon pulls the thumb metacarpal proximally.

thumb and can occur simultaneously with injury to the MCP joint.

On examination, the degree of swelling is variable but is best seen dorsally. The patient is often unable to determine precisely the area of greatest discomfort. Tenderness may exist over a wide area, including the dorsal aspect of the CMC joint and the entire base of the thenar eminence. It may be difficult or painful to flatten the palm on a tabletop. Attempted abduction of the base of the first metacarpal is painful and may demonstrate instability. Because a wide range of laxity normally exists in this joint, comparison with the uninjured thumb is recommended.

Unless a fracture is present (Fig. 9), routine radiographs are usually normal. The CMC "stress" view can help determine the degree of instability. It consists of a single posteroanterior view of both thumbs taken while the patient firmly pushes both distal phalanges together (Fig. 10).

The overwhelming preponderance of these CMC joint ligament injuries are incomplete and easily cared for with 4–6 weeks of immobilization in a thumb spica splint or cast. Early recognition and treatment remains very important because partial, untreated injuries may develop progressive instability requiring later reconstruction (Fig. 11). Late problems related to CMC joint laxity include chronic pain, first web space contracture, and volar plate laxity (hyperextension) of the thumb MCP joint.

Digits

The digital CMC joints are inherently stable and have strong, multiplanar ligamentous support. The index and middle CMC joints are fixed and immobile.[5] Some movement (approximately 30 degrees in the anterioposterior plane) is present in the ring- and small-finger CMC joints. Together with movement of the thumb, this allows the palm to assume flattened and "cupped" positions.

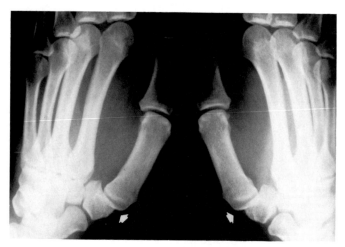

FIGURE 10. Stress radiographs demonstrate laxity (subluxation) of the thumb CMC joints (arrows).

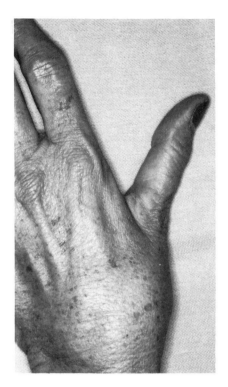

FIGURE 11. Chronic ligament laxity at the thumb CMC joint results in subluxation of the metacarpal on the trapezium. Secondary changes in the thumb include the first web space contracture and the volar plate laxity (hyperextension) of the MCP joint.

Because of strong ligamentous supports, an injury of considerable force is usually required to cause dislocation at this level.[10] An accompanying fracture[5] is frequently present (Fig. 12). However, when swelling and tenderness are present over the CMC joints and no fracture is identified, it is imperative that accurate

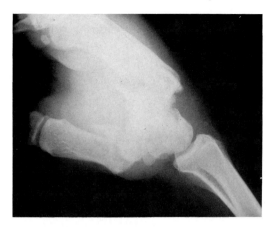

FIGURE 12. Fracture-dislocation of the CMC joints of the ulnar four digits resulted from a press injury.

radiographs be taken to exclude subluxation. Standard views are often inconclusive in this regard, and computed tomography may be required to completely assess this region (Fig. 13). Surgery is often required to reduce and stabilize the involved CMC joints.

Chronic sprains of the CMC joints can result in hypertrophy of the involved joints.[4] These CMC bosses can be associated with pain, especially during gripping maneuvers of the hand.[9] The initial injury and subsequent repetitive stress can make the joint prone to degenerative changes (Fig. 14). The patient is often able to localize symptoms to a specific joint, and manipulation of the joint by rocking the involved metacarpal against the carpus can reproduce the symptoms. Inflammation of the extensor tendons, which repetitively snap over the CMC boss, can also be a consequence of this injury. Standard radiographs may not reveal signifi-

FIGURE 13. Computed tomography of the CMC joint region can help assess the presence of fractures and subluxations in this region.

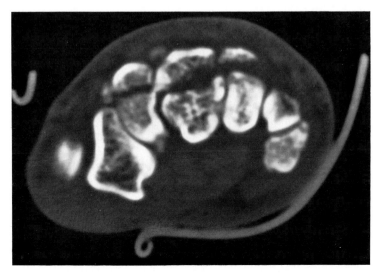

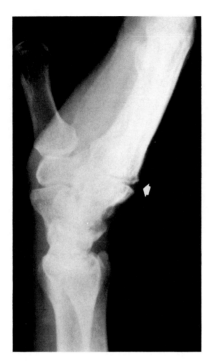

FIGURE 14. Carpometacarpal boss (*arrow*) can result from a chronic sprain of the involved joint.

subsequent referral for specialty care, great satisfaction should be derived from making the correct initial diagnosis. Effort thus spent saves many patients from unnecessary impairment.

Acknowledgment

The authors wish to express their gratitude to Ms. Helen Prussian for her expert help in the preparation of this manuscript.

cant osseous abnormalities because the boss may be predominantly cartilaginous. Radionuclide bone scans can help to confirm the specific area of involvement. Treatment includes splinting, local physiotherapy, and, infrequently, surgical removal of the boss combined with arthrodesis of the involved joint.

CONCLUSION

Ligamentous injuries to the hand are common and pose challenges to evaluation and treatment. Normal radiographs can provide a false sense of security. A careful clinical examination performed with a knowledge of the pertinent anatomy and combined with the appropriate use of local anesthesia can be rewarding. Although many problems require

REFERENCES

1. American Society for Surgery of the Hand: The Hand: Examination and Diagnosis, 2nd ed. New York, Churchill Livingstone, 1983.
2. American Society for Surgery of the Hand: The Hand: Primary Care of Common Problems. Aurora, CO, 1985.
3. Camp RA, Weatherwax RJ, Miller EB: Chronic post traumatic radial instability of the thumb metacarpophalangeal joint. J Hand Surg 5A:221–225, 1980.
4. Cuono CB, Watson HK: The carpal boss: Surgical treatment and etiological considerations. Plast Reconstr Surg 63:88–93, 1979.
5. Greene TL, Strickland JW: Carpometacarpal dislocations (excluding the thumb), In Strickland JW, Steichen JB (eds): Difficult Problems in Hand Surgery. St. Louis, C.V. Mosby, 1982, pp 189–195.
6. Hankin FM, Janda DH: Tendon and ligament attachments in relationship to growth plates in a child's hand. J Hand Surg 14B:315–318, 1989.
7. Hankin FM, Wylie RL: Gamekeeper's thumb: Injury to the ulnar collateral ligament of the metacarpophalangeal joint. Am Fam Physician 38:127–130, 1988.
8. James J: Common simple errors in the management of hand injuries. Proc R Soc Med 63:69–71, 1970.
9. Joseph RB. Linscheid RL, Dobyns JH, Bryan RS: Chronic sprains of the carpometacarpal joints. J Hand Surg 6:172–180, 1981.
10. Kleinman WB, Grantham SA: Multiple volar carpometacarpal joint dislocation. J Hand Surg 3:377–382, 1978.
11. Lane CS: Detecting occult fractures of the metacarpal head: The Brewerton view. J Hand Surg 2:131–133, 1977.
12. Louis D, Huebner JJ, Hankin FM: Rupture and displacement of the ulnar collateral ligament of the metacarpophalangeal joint of the thumb. J Bone Joint Surg 68A:1320–1326, 1986.
13. Swanson AB: Fractures involving the digits of the hand. Orthop Clin North Am 1:261–274, 1970.

Chapter 25

WORK-RELATED VASCULAR INJURIES AND DISEASES

Anthony C. Berger, M.B.B.S., FRACS, and James M. Kleinert, M.D.

Industrialization in modern society has, by and large, greatly improved the quality and length of life for the vast majority of people. The increasing complexity and sophistication of machinery used to produce goods and perform tasks previously performed by hand have rapidly increased the productivity of the modern work force. Unfortunately, modern production line techniques combined with a demand for productivity at low cost have resulted in major injuries for many workers. The frightful injuries caused by earlier machines have thankfully decreased in number due to the implementation of modern safety standards. Unfortunately, operating modern machinery for prolonged time periods can result in more subtle injuries, some of them debilitating, although obvious only to the sufferer. Occupational vascular disorders of the upper extremity are an example of a subtle cumulative injury.

Although arterial lacerations, amputations, burns, electrical injuries, and post-traumatic sympathetic dystrophy have obvious vascular components, they are not specific to an occupational setting and are not discussed here. This chapter concentrates on the less obvious vascular diseases and injuries that are typically related to occupation. It covers the various presentations and assessments of vascular disease and then examines in detail the major occupational vascular diseases.

THE PRESENTATION OF OCCUPATIONAL VASCULAR DISEASE

Modern work-related vascular disorders are subtle. The pathological changes may take years to develop, symptoms are often intermittent, and objective findings scarce. Medical skepticism may make it difficult for the patient to get help for a long time. Occasionally patients may present with clear signs such as a mass overlying a traumatic aneurysm or arteriovenous fistula, or obvious cold, pale fingers with tip necrosis. There may be vague symptoms of burning, tingling, numbness, coldness, heaviness, swelling, color changes, or inability to work. By far the most common presentation of work-related vascular disorders in the upper extremity, however, is cold intolerance or Raynaud's phenomenon.

THE ASSESSMENT OF VASCULAR PATHOLOGY

The clinical presentations of vascular pathology are wide and varied. Symptoms, including those listed above, are often highly subjective and intermittent. Careful examination for physical signs and further testing is needed to diagnose and appropriately treat these conditions.

319

A basic profile for each patient including age, handedness, and smoking history must be constructed. Symptoms should be reviewed, and any history of diabetes mellitus should be noted. Specific information about occupational exposure to vibration, trauma, and chemicals also should be sought.

The examination starts with inspection of the hands for callosities, scars, and areas of obvious necrosis or trophic changes. The color and temperature of the hands in relation to the ambient temperature also should be noted. Pulses should be palpated at the radial, ulnar, brachial, axillary, and subclavian levels, documenting the strength, vessel size, and presence of a thrill. Allen's testing should be performed to detect any occlusion of the wrist or digital vessels. Auscultation of these vessels also should be performed to detect any bruit indicating turbulent flow. Brachial pressures are then measured in each arm. A difference of more than 20 mmHg indicates significant proximal stenosis. If thoracic outlet compression is suspected, pulse measurement during Adson's test and costoclavicular and hyperabduction positioning should be performed.

A neurological examination should be performed to exclude any associated neurological pathology, such as carpal tunnel syndrome, Guyon's canal compression, cubital tunnel syndrome, or thoracic outlet compression. Motor and sensory testing and evaluation for a Tinel's sign along the distribution of the peripheral nerves are performed.

Finally, one should be aware of any pathonomic signs that may help in the diagnosis or detection of associated diseases, such as skin changes seen with some chemical exposures and liver masses in patients exposed to polyvinyl chloride (PVC). Plain radiographs of the hand may reveal carpal cysts from vibration disorders, acro-osteolysis from PVC poisoning, or vascular calcification from Buerger's disease. Radiography of the neck is indicated in patients with thoracic outlet compression to exclude a cervical rib and other outlet anomalies.

Clinical examination combined with the patient's history usually enables the physician to determine the major pathological process (e.g., vasospasm, vascular occlusion, or aneurysm formation) and to determine the etiology as vibrational, traumatic, chemical, secondary to thoracic outlet compression, or some nonoccupational cause. Further evaluation of these patients may require more specific noninvasive and invasive vascular testing.

The most useful tools in assessing patients with suspected vascular pathology are the noninvasive vascular studies. These groups of tests are relatively safe and inexpensive, and they provide both static and dynamic information about the patient's vascular system.[48] It is very important to assess not only the anatomic problem, but also its effect on the vascular dynamics of the limb. Only in this way can appropriate management be undertaken.

Our assessment of patients with suspected vascular disorders includes a combination of tests, each of which looks at a specific aspect of the patient's vasculature. Blood pressure measurements taken at brachial, forearm, and digital levels reveal any significant occlusions in the arterial tree.[42] A drop in blood pressure between two adjacent segments of more than 20 mmHg indicates a significant intervening stenosis. A digital brachial index (digital pressure divided by brachial pressure) in the range of 0.56 ± 0.27 indicates significant ischemia to the digit.[89] Pulse volume recordings are then taken for each digit to assess the compliance and state of the digital vessels—whether they are normal, stenosed, or occluded[20] (Fig. 1). A Doppler map of the wrist and hand shows areas of arterial occlusion, aneurysm formation, turbulent flow, and flow reversal (Fig. 2). Finally, the patients with suspected vasospastic disorders or Raynaud's phenomenon can be assessed with various cold stress tests.[49] To observe abnormal sensitivity to and prolonged recovery from a cold stimulus, digital temperature or pulse volume recording is measured after immersion of the hands in cold water (60°F).

Tests for thoracic outlet arterial compression involve accurate measurement of digital blood flow with shoulder and neck posturing as mentioned previously. Either digital blood pressure, pulse volume recording, or photoplethysmographic measurements are taken. These results, however, must be interpreted with care because a significant number of people with normal circulation show digital blood flow reduction with some of these postures.[36,84]

If, after the above tests are performed, the diagnosis is still uncertain, further investigations may be indicated. Intravenous radionuclide angiography is useful in assessing the vascular competency of the upper limb. It gives valuable information about vascular flow in the hand and can be used to assess accurately the

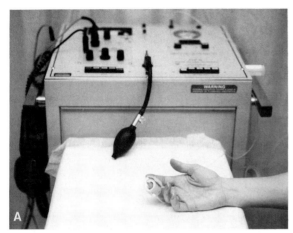

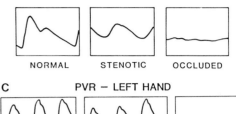

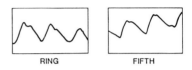

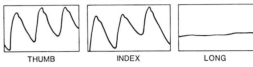

B   PVR TRACINGS

NORMAL   STENOTIC   OCCLUDED

C   PVR — LEFT HAND

THUMB   INDEX   LONG

RING   FIFTH

FIGURE 1. A, Pulse volume recording (PVR) is performed using Life Sciences Pulse Volume Recorder. B, PVR tracings from a normal digit, a partially occluded (stenotic) digit, and a completely occluded (occluded) digit. C, PVR tracing showing thrombosis of both digital arteries to the left long finger.

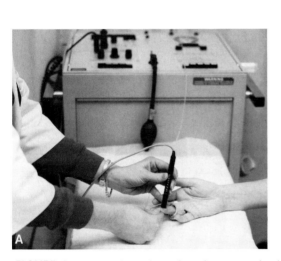

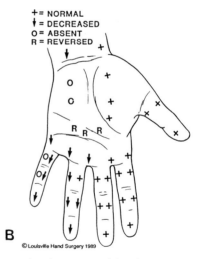

+ = NORMAL
↓ = DECREASED
O = ABSENT
R = REVERSED

© Louisville Hand Surgery 1989

FIGURE 2. A, Use of Doppler probe to locate superficial arch, common digital arteries, and digital artery. B, Doppler mapping of a symptomatic hand with ulnar artery thrombosis.

presence and degree of any subclavian or distal stenosis.[50] Arteriography occasionally may be used, especially for proximal lesions.

RAYNAUD'S PHENOMENON

The complex of symptoms and signs known as Raynaud's phenomenon has been the source of much confusion since the original description by Maurice Raynaud in 1862.[87] In his 1879 inaugural thesis for the Academy of Medicine, entitled "*De l'asphyxie locale et de la gangrene*

symetrique des extremités," he described episodes of vascular instability in the digits induced by cold and concluded that they were due to increased sensitivity of the sympathetic nervous system. Since that time the terminology, pathology, and clinical features of this most confusing syndrome have been considerably clarified.

A distinction must be made between primary Raynaud's phenomenon and secondary Raynaud's phenomenon. Both disorders are characterized by a disturbance of peripheral circulatory control induced by a number of internal and external stresses. Secondary Raynaud's phenomenon is a fluctuating vascular disturbance secondary to associated and contributory conditions and diseases such as trauma, neurogenic lesions, and autoimmune diseases. This condition has been called Raynaud's syndrome. Primary Raynaud's phenomenon or Raynaud's disease occurs in the absence of any identifiable predisposing cause (Table 1).

The typical presentation of primary Raynaud's phenomenon commences with color changes in one or more digits after a triggering event. The color changes start distally and may involve the more proximal parts of the hand in later stages. They may entail only cyanosis or pallor, but classically they are triphasic, showing pallor, cyanosis, and rubor. Pain may or may not be a prominent feature. Paresthesias, however, are common. During an attack, cutaneous sensibility may be reduced,[64] and it has been shown that manual dexterity also is reduced,[21] an important factor for patients working with dangerous machines in cold environments. Gaydos[34] has shown that a drop in fingertip temperature is responsible for this impairment. In primary Raynaud's phenomenon, episodes are bilateral, involve females five times more frequently than males, usually start before the third or fourth decade, and are triggered by cold or emotional upsets (Fig. 3). Secondary Raynaud's phenomenon does not have a high female preponderance, is more often unilateral, and has identifiable predisposing conditions or diseases.

The clinical presentation of Raynaud's phenomenon appears, at least initially, to be due to episodes of arterial and possibly venule spasm in the digital vessels. Capillary and venule dilation may or may not follow. The initial spasm produces digital pallor due to emptying of the vascular bed. Later, cyanosis is caused by slow return of sluggish blood flow that, combined with areas of stasis and possible venule reflux, produces a blotchy appearance. Finally, when the spasm ceases, a reactive hyperemia causes the rubor phase. With increased duration of the disease, intimal thickening, vessel wall hypertrophy, and occlusive lesions may supervene. In these late stages digital necrosis may develop.

Secondary Raynaud's phenomenon has a similar clinical presentation. However, it is more often intermittent and unilateral and is found in slightly older age groups with a sexually more equal or slightly male-biased distribution. Occupationally induced secondary Raynaud's phenomenon occurs most frequently in four settings:

1. Vibration syndromes
2. Occupational occlusive diseases
3. Chemical exposure
4. Thoracic outlet compression

Despite numerous investigations, the exact mechanism of the observed vasospasm is unknown. It is clear, however, that patients with primary Raynaud's phenomenon have a much lower capillary flow in warm and cool rooms than people with normal circulation. Also, body cooling significantly reduces digital blood flow in patients with Raynaud's phenomenon.

TABLE 1.   Classification of Raynaud's Phenomenon

Primary Raynaud's phenomenon	I.
Secondary Raynaud's phenomenon	II.
Post-traumatic	A.
Occupational	1.
After injury or surgery	2.
Neurogenic	B.
Thoracic outlet syndrome	1.
Carpal tunnel syndrome	2.
Vaso-occlusive disease	C.
Atherosclerosis	1.
Buerger's disease	2.
Postembolism or thrombosis	3.
Miscellaneous	D.
Scleroderma	1.
Systemic lupus erythematosus	2.
Rheumatoid arthritis	3.
Cryoglobulinemia	4.
Myxedema	5.
Ergotism	6.

ANEURYSM FORMATION

Aneurysms of the upper extremity are more often traumatic, whereas those of the lower extremity are usually atherosclerotic. Two types of aneurysm are found in the injured worker. The **false aneurysm**, due to a partial laceration of an artery or repeated blunt trauma, results in a walled off hematoma communicating with the arterial lumen. This presents as a painful, post-traumatic mass. It is pulsatile and painful and usually has an overlying scar (Fig. 4).

True aneurysms in the hand are very rare. In the occupational setting, they occur in the subclavian artery at the thoracic outlet. This type of aneurysm can present in a number of ways. Most obviously there is a painful, tender,

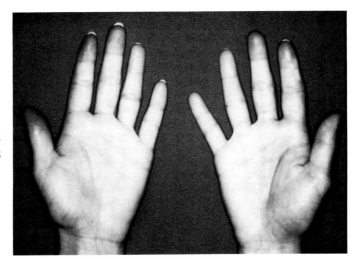

FIGURE 3. *A,* Otherwise healthy, white, 24-year-old woman with primary Raynaud's phenomenon. No underlying etiological factors are known.

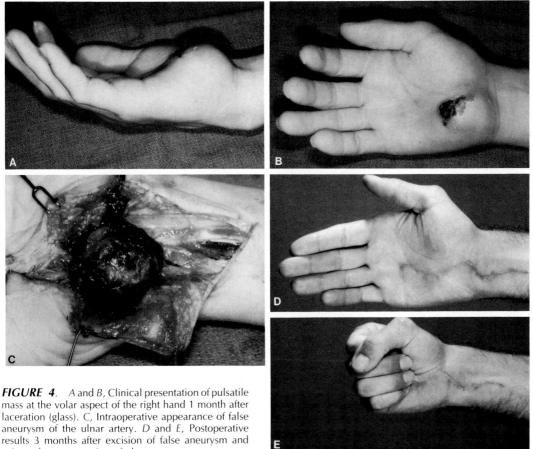

FIGURE 4. *A* and *B,* Clinical presentation of pulsatile mass at the volar aspect of the right hand 1 month after laceration (glass). *C,* Intraoperative appearance of false aneurysm of the ulnar artery. *D* and *E,* Postoperative results 3 months after excision of false aneurysm and vein graft reconstruction of ulnar artery.

pulsatile mass overlying the involved artery. The mass may be due to a localized aneurysm or, more often, a tortuous dilation of the vessel. Mural thrombus within the aneurysm may fragment, resulting in distal embolization. The emboli may present with a sudden onset of pain, pallor, cyanosis, or pulselessness.

The vascular sympathetics to the digital vessels travel in the digital nerves and in the adventitia of the major palmar and digital arteries. Aneurysmal dilation or arterial thrombosis can induce a perivascular inflammation or fibrosis that may stimulate these nerves. This sympathetic stimulation is a possible cause of Raynaud's phenomenon in patients with ulnar artery aneurysm or thrombosis.

THROMBOSIS

Spontaneous arterial thrombosis in the hand is uncommon, representing 1–5% of all peripheral vascular disease.[46] It occurs secondary to a number of disease processes, notably thromboangiitis obliterans. In the occupational setting, however, thrombosis of an artery is more often seen with repeated trauma, similar to that causing aneurysms to form. Von Rosen proposed that repeated trauma to a vessel resulting in intimal damage causes thrombosis and, if the media is damaged, an aneurysm forms.[102] A tortuous aneurysm with mural thrombus also may thrombose with time and repeated trauma. Thrombosis can occur as a result of severe Raynaud's phenomenon with vessel wall hypertrophy.

The presentations of arterial thrombosis are varied. The effect of the thrombosis is determined by the site of the lesion, the efficiency of the collateral circulation, the presence of other disease, and the rapidity of the vascular narrowing. The patient may, therefore, be asymptomatic or present with ischemic changes. More often, however, the patient has a relative ischemia that only becomes symptomatic during times of stress, such as cold exposure. This is similar to Raynaud's phenomenon secondary to aneurysm formation.

Subclavian artery stenosis secondary to thoracic outlet compression can present with relative ischemia producing arm claudication. The patient is usually asymptomatic at rest. On use of the arm, however, pain and cramping with occasional paresthesias may occur. These symptoms resolve with rest only to recur when work is recommenced.

NEUROLOGICAL SYMPTOMS

Neurological symptoms secondary to occupational vascular pathology are uncommon. They can occur, however, with aneurysm formation or thrombosis of the ulnar artery at Guyon's canal. The result may be compression neuropathy of the ulnar nerve causing motor and sensory changes. The neurological features seen with subclavian aneurysm formation are more often due to a common etiology (thoracic outlet compression) rather than secondary to any vascular disorder.

VIBRATION SYNDROMES

Modern hand-held machines used in primary and secondary industries rely heavily on tools that function by compressed-air–operated piston reciprocation, electrically driven rotary motors, or air turbines. These tools release variable amounts of vibration energy. Pneumatic tools were first used in French mines around 1840 and were slowly introduced in other industries and other countries. After the 1880s they found widespread use in many industries. Electric and gasoline motors began to be used in vibratory tools during the late 1940s.

In 1911, Loriga first reported a relationship between vibration and Raynaud's phenomenon in Italian quarrymen.[58] Subsequently, at the recommendation of Dr. J.C. Miller of Chicago, Dr. Alice Hamilton[41] investigated a number of cases of vibration-induced Raynaud's phenomenon in limestone cutters in Indiana in 1917 and 1918. As a result of this study she stated, "I discovered a very clearly defined localized anemia of certain fingers which is undoubtedly associated with the use of the air hammer and which, while it lasts, makes the fingers numb and clumsy, causing the workman more or less discomfort and sometimes hampering his work."

The recognition of vibration-induced disease has been delayed owing to difficulties with measuring vibration levels and with establishing a relationship between exposure and disease. Only in April 1985 was vibration white finger accepted by the Department of Health and Social Security of the United Kingdom as a prescribed occupational disease.

Many names have been given to this condition, including dead finger, white finger,[41] dead hand,[94] pneumatic hammer disease,[63] vibration-induced white finger,[101] traumatic vasospastic disease,[39] and Raynaud's phenomenon of occupational origin.[1] At a recent symposium on the hand and arm effects of local vibration, it was determined that the condition should be called the hand-arm vibration syndrome.[92] The list of occupations in which this condition has been reported is extensive and includes almost every occupation that involves the use of hand-held vibrating machinery.

The reported prevalence of this condition has been quite staggering, particularly in the northern latitudes of the Northern Hemisphere—that is, Scandinavia, Poland, Canada, the United States, and Japan. Alice Hamilton[41] reported an incidence of vibration white finger in Indiana stonecutters of 89.5%, Olsen and Nielsen[72] reported an incidence of 72% in Danish granite quarrymen, Futatsuka et al.[32] reported a frequency of 84% in rock drill operators and 50% in sawyers in 1984, Agate[1] reported a 66.2% incidence in tool operators, and Taylor and Pelmear[91] reported a 40–90% incidence in forestry workers. These figures are of some concern. Unfortunately, even with advances in occupational health and the development of standards, improvement has been limited. Taylor revisited the quarries that Alice Hamilton had visited more than 60 years earlier and reported a vibration white finger prevalence of 63% in limestone workers and 80% in stonecutters and carvers.[93] These percentages translate into a large number of potential sufferers among the more than 1.2 million workers exposed to hand-arm vibration in the United States.[106]

The main reasons for the lack of progress in this disease are the highly subjective and intermittent nature of the symptoms, the lack of any reproducible technique of quantifying vibration exposure, and the difficulty of setting safe standards for exposure. As a result, industry has few guidelines for safe tool manufacture and worker protection.

Most frequently, the manifestations of prolonged vibration exposure include:

1. Raynaud's phenomenon
2. Peripheral neuropathy and muscle weakness
3. Bone changes.

Many other symptoms and signs have been attributed to vibration syndrome, such as headache, insomnia, tinnitus, palmar hyperhidrosis, bradycardia, cardiac hypertrophy, deafness, and impotence. However, an association between them and vibration exposure has not been demonstrated.

Clinical Features. Workers initially report tingling and later numbness of the fingers after vibration exposure. Prolonged exposure causes the fingers to feel swollen, painful, and inflexible. After a latent period of some years, fingertip blanching occurs; it is usually precipitated by cold. The latent period between exposure and blanching is related to the frequency, amplitude, and intensity of exposure. The shorter the latent period, the more rapid the progression of the disease. The average latency is about 10 years, with a range of 1.6–27 years, depending on the exposure intensity.[76] The disease progresses proximally up the involved finger and later spreads to other digits. The level of neurological change is more proximal than the level of vascular change.[61] The effect is often asymmetric, involving more severely those fingers with greater exposure. The index, middle, and ring fingers are most often affected, the thumbs rarely.[15,16] Raynaud's phenomenon is the main component of vibration white finger. It is provoked by cold exposure, and episodes increase in frequency and severity with continued vibration exposure. With continued exposure, the episodic nature of the vascular injury is replaced by a continuous cyanotic appearance of the fingers, the reactivity of the vessels being lost as their walls thicken and lumens narrow. Less than 1% of patients, however, develop digital atrophy, necrosis, or gangrene.

With vascular deterioration, the neurological deterioration progresses. The numbness and paresthesias that occur intermittently early in the disease process may progress to the point of sleep disturbance and later reduction in grip strength, tactile sensitivity, and manipulative dexterity with permanent sensorimotor loss.[7] Compression neuropathies, particularly carpal tunnel compression, have been associated with vibration diseases. Boyle, Smith, and Burke[16] found electrical evidence of carpal tunnel syndrome in 12 of 19 patients with vibration white finger. Färkkilä found evidence of median nerve disease in 36% of lumberjacks; however, he concluded that this was not a vibration-induced neuropathy.[27] Wasserman found fewer than 2%

of patients with vibration white finger to have concomitant carpal tunnel syndrome.[105]

Soviet investigators have claimed that other features are part of the vibration syndrome. They have concluded that the major pathology is mediated by the central nervous system and have included symptoms of excess sweating, vertigo, headache, insomnia, irritability, forgetfulness, loss of concentration, and impotence as part of the stress syndrome. They regard the etiology of this vibration syndrome to be the combination of stress from vibration, cold, and noise.[61] This view is, however, not widely held.

Classification.   Two classifications are now commonly used. The usefulness of both, however, is limited in that very little objective assessment is used to stage the disease, and all grading is based on highly subjective criteria. The Taylor-Pelmear classification[91] (Table 2) groups the disease into four stages based on the condition of the digits and a subjective evaluation of the disease's effects on social activities and work. This classification has been widely adopted in the United States, the United Kingdom, and Canada. In 1986 a Stockholm workshop revised this classification to diminish the subjectivity associated with social and personal impairments. A score was added to indicate the number of digits involved; and sensory testing, cold provocation, and vibration assessments were added to improve the objectivity of the classification.[35] In Japan, the USSR, and Eastern Europe, the classification is based on the work of Andreeva-Galanina[92] (Table 3).

Measurement of Vibration.   Vibration is defined by the following parameters: frequency (cycles per second or Hz), amplitude (meters), acceleration (meters per second squared), direction of application, duration of application, and whether continuous or intermittent. The vibrations produced by a machine, however, are not pure but are composed of a spectrum of frequencies and amplitudes. Vibration is now measured with the use of three piezoelectric crystal accelerometers measuring in three perpendicular axes linked to a computer. The computer then displays the vibration "fingerprint" of the machine. The human response to vibration depends on the body's resonance, which actually amplifies any incoming vibration energy. The resonance level for the hand is 50–150 Hz and for the lower arm, 16–30 Hz. Vibration transmission tests by Reynolds and Angevine imply that vibrations of 150–200 Hz are isolated in the hand and fingers; only vibrations of less than 100 Hz are transmitted to the forearm.[80]

Futatsuka et al.[33] have concluded that the effects of vibration depend on the dominant frequency. Frequencies less than 40 Hz with amplitudes of several centimeters produce osteoarticular lesions. Frequencies between 40 and 300 Hz with amplitude of about 1 cm produce vasomotor disturbances after a long latency period. Higher frequencies and smaller amplitudes produce these changes much earlier. Pelmear et al.[75] have concluded that the limited medical evidence suggests that the most vascular damage occurs at frequencies of 30–200 Hz and around 480 Hz and that neurological damage occurs between 250 and 350 Hz (range 60–700 Hz).

Pathogenesis.   The exact mechanism of vasospasm induced by vibration is unknown. In early stages hypertrophy of the vessel media either causes the vasospasm or is secondary to it. In late phases, extensive hypertrophy of the

TABLE 2.   Taylor-Pelmear Classification for Vibration-induced Disease*

Stage	Conditions of Digits	Work and Social Interference
0	No blanching of digits.	No complaints.
0-T	Intermittent tingling.	No interference with activities.
0-N	Intermittent numbness.	
1	Blanching of one or more fingertips with or without tingling and numbness.	No interference with activities.
2	Blanching of one or more complete fingers; numbness usually confined to winter.	Slight interference with home and social activities. No interference at work.
3	Extensive blanching usually of all fingers bilaterally. Frequent episodes, summer and winter.	Definite interference at work, at home, and with social activities. Restriction of hobbies.
4	Extensive blanching of all fingers. Frequent episodes, summer and winter.	Occupation changed to avoid further vibration exposure because of severity of signs and symptoms.

* From Taylor and Pelmear, Acta Chir Scand 45(Suppl):27, 1976, with permission.[91]

TABLE 3.   Andreeva-Galanina Classification of Hand-Arm Vibration Syndrome[92]

Level I	Numbness, intermittent pain in the fingers and forearm, and light palmar sweating.
Level II	Occasional secondary Raynaud's phenomenon, increasing numbness, pain, coldness, stiffness. Decline in muscle power and grip strength. Dull headaches and increasing palmar sweating.
Level III	Frequent Raynaud's phenomenon, muscle contracture, occasional ulnar nerve palsy. Bone changes in elbow may be detected; occasional nausea and vertigo.
Level IV	Very frequent and prominent Raynaud's phenomenon. Muscle contracture, nerve paralysis, and bone changes all increase. Nervous instability and neurosis may increase.

intima and media and near closure of the lumen occur.[4] In this stage, the digits become permanently cyanotic. In yet later stages, thrombosis has been identified in some of the vessels.[45] Muscle hypertrophy in the vessel wall in the early stages may exaggerate the response to cold exposure, which markedly reduces digital blood flow. At a critical closing pressure, the vessel collapses and an attack of vibration white finger occurs. In the early stages of the disease, vessel reactivity is still present. With time, the intimal fibrosis and thickening result in loss of reactivity and a permanently low flow state.

Welsh has shown that vibrations of 120 Hz significantly reduce digital blood flow by about 70% in normal volunteers and that the reduction is greater when the amplitude is increased.[107] (Chain-saw vibrations peak at 125 Hz). Using finger pulse plethysmography, Pyykkö, Hyvärien, and Färkkilä have revealed similar vasoconstriction at frequencies of 80–125 Hz. This vasospasm is more marked in patients with vibration white finger[79] and is exacerbated by body cooling and loud noise.[78] A number of theories attempt to explain this increased vasoconstrictive response to vibration. Magos and Okos have suggested a vascular hypersensitivity due to an overactive biochemical vasoconstrictor mechanism or an accumulation of vasoactive substances that cannot be destroyed.[60] Ekenvall and Lindblad[25] give further evidence for this mechanism. They found that the vasoconstriction induced by α_1 receptors is reduced by cold and that induced by α_2 receptors is increased by cold. Subjects with higher percentages of α_2 receptors have an exaggerated response to cold, which is seen in patients with vibration white finger. The exaggerated response may be due to a vibration-induced damage to α_1 receptors. In dogs, Azuma and Ohhashi[5] have demonstrated a vibration-induced hyper-responsivity to noradrenaline that produces local vasoconstriction.

Most current research focuses on the influence of the sympathetic nervous system on vibration white finger. At present there seems to be much evidence that a sympathetic vasoconstrictive response to cold plays a dominant role in the cause of vibration white finger.[71] The importance of the sympathetic system and central reflex arcs is reinforced by Pyykkö's [78] and Matoba's[62] observations that the vasoconstrictive response to vibration is amplified by noise and body cooling. Hallbäck and Folkow have demonstrated increased vascular tone in rats with chronic vibration exposure, which appears to be mediated by the sympathetic nervous system.[40]

Some authors now believe the vasoconstrictive response is mediated by stimulation of the pacinian corpuscles. These are shown to be most sensitive to vibrations of 60–700 Hz,[66] similar to the range known to produce vibration injury most effectively. Pacinian corpuscles also are very slow to adapt, meaning that frequent vibration exposure can lead to continuous neural stimulation. With time, stimulation could lead to vasospasm and vessel medial hypertrophy via central reflex arcs.[79] The vibration threshold curve for vasoconstriction is parallel to the threshold curve for Pacinian corpuscle stimulation.

Narem[68] has investigated the effects of vibration on blood flow characteristics and sheer stress on the endothelial lining. A viscous flood, such as blood, moving over a surface produces a frictional force related to flow velocity and viscosity. The normal sheer stress in digital vessels is about 25 dynes per square centimeter. Above a critical level, endothelial damage and swelling occur; higher levels may result in endothelial cell loss. Narem has shown that vibration produced by a jack hammer or pneumatic chisel produces vessel wall sheer stresses well in excess of the levels that produce vascular damage. He believes this frictional force may be a direct cause of endothelial damage.

Une and Esaki[99] have shown an increase in noradrenalin excretion in patients with vibration white finger, indicating an increase in the activity of the sympathetic nervous system. Bovenzi,[14] however, showed no correlation between catecholamine secretion and digital blood pressure.

Other factors thought to be involved in the pathogenesis of vibration white finger are blood viscosity and immunoglobulin levels. Okada et al.[70] and Turczyński et al.[98] found significantly higher blood and plasma viscosity in patients with vibration white finger and have proposed viscosity as a useful discriminatory test. Okada found increased IGG, IGA, and IGM levels in chain-saw workers. Knutsson[47] in 1975 and Bovenzi[14] in 1988, however, found no increase in immunoglobulin levels in patients with vibration white finger.

Sivertsson and Ljung[86] have demonstrated that vibration acting on isolated vascular smooth muscle causes relaxation. They have proposed that relaxation may induce an increased sympathetic vasoconstrictive tone to restore the normal basal tone. When the vibration is removed, the resultant vascular muscle hypertrophy may lead to the condition of vibration white finger.

Despite the lack of proof for these theories, it is evident that the disease is related to the cumulative energy entering the hands. Deterioration is clearly correlated with continued exposure to vibration. A shorter latent period implies a more hazardous vibration. Vibration white finger is more common in smokers,[96] more common with the use of light-weight tools that do not dampen the vibrations as well as heavier tools,[92] more common in workers who have to grip tools firmly,[28] and more common with poorly maintained equipment.

Diagnosis. The diagnosis of vibration white finger requires the presence of Raynaud's phenomenon in a worker with chronic exposure to vibration in the absence of any other identifiable cause of vasospasm. The latent period for the vascular phase of vibration white finger often exceeds that for the neurological phase; therefore, a patient presenting for the first time with episodes of vasospasm is likely to have some neurological features already. In studying foundry workers, Behrens et al. identified a median latency for tingling of 7 months, for numbness of 9 months, and for blanching of 17 months.[9]

Objective tests for vibration white finger attempt to detect and quantify an abnormal vascular response to cold exposure. These tests can include skin temperature measurement, photoplethysmography, Doppler studies,[59] digital blood pressure measurements in response to either local digital or whole-body cooling, and radionuclide scanning.[113] Other investigations have included measurement of blood viscosity and occasionally arteriography.[92] Unfortunately, many attempts to reproduce vibration white finger with exposure to local cold, whole-body cold, noise, and vibration have failed. To date, no single objective test is available that reproduces accurately an episode of vibration white finger, even though population studies show an increased incidence of abnormal cold stress testing.[16,90] As a result, the diagnosis of vibration white finger essentially becomes a clinical one. One test that is often used is the measurement of digital systolic pressure in response to cooling of the hand, usually to 10°C. Although this cold exposure does not always induce an episode of vibration white finger, it demonstrates a dramatic drop in the digital blood pressure.[13,22,24] Other tests, however, are probably only useful in establishing a baseline for pre-employment levels before vibration exposure.[92]

Exposure Standardization. Investigators attempting to identify safe exposure limits for vibration in industry have not, as yet, been successful for three reasons. First, the diagnosis of the disease is purely clinical and based on subjective evaluations of the patient. Second, the grading system is also subjective, and no objective investigation is available to quantify the disease state accurately. Third, there is no commonly accepted standardized method of measuring vibration exposure both quantitatively and qualitatively. Variables such as total operating time, frequency and amplitude of vibration, grip strength, coupling between hand and source, and the effects of wear and aging on machinery all combine to make this calculation extremely difficult.

Current standards issued by the International Standards Organization, British Standards Institute, American National Standards Institute, and the American Conference of Governmental Industrial Hygienist Threshold Limit Values have attempted to set exposure limits for vibration. In 1986, ISO/DIS/5349 standards were adopted. This sets out procedures for the measurement of vibration exposure but does not set vibration limits as Griffin recommended.[37] Pelmear et al.[75] summarized the many attempts to set actual limits for safe vibration exposure. These exposure limits, however, use the same weighting for different types of machines. Measurements of the vibration spectra of different types of machines have shown a wide range of frequencies. Some machines produce frequencies that appear to be more damaging to the peripheral nervous system, whereas others produce frequencies more damaging to the vascular system. Also, dose–effect relationships for each of the standards do not take into account the type of machine used. At present, these guidelines may overestimate or underestimate exposure risk, depending on the type of machinery used.[15] Further work is needed to measure vibration in a standardized fashion and to calculate safe exposure limits for each type of vibrating machine on the basis of medical evidence.

Treatment. At present, no treatment exists beyond palliation of symptoms. There is evidence that patients in stage 1 and early stage 2 (Taylor-Pelmear scale) improve with time; however, there is less evidence for improvement in stage 3.[92] At least 3 years without exposure to vibration may be required before any subjective improvement can be expected.[23] Most treatments have been aimed at reducing the sympathetic input to the digital vessels through chemotherapeutic or surgical maneuvers. Drugs such as nifedipine, Ketanserin, Verapamil, and some prostaglandins may have some benefits; however, their effects have not been predictable.[5,56,81] Chemotherapeutic vasodilation is only palliative therapy, and its effectiveness requires that the patient be removed from vibration exposure. Because this therapy requires some reactivity of the vessels, it is only useful in early stages before the development of occlusive lesions and vascular fibrosis. Surgical sympathectomy, either digital or cervical, causes immediate vasodilation,[18,29] which, however, is only temporary owing to increasing sensitivity to circulating catecholamines and recurrence of symptoms in 3–6 months.[90,92] Biofeedback may offer a promising long-term therapy for these patients.[30] Biofeedback with cold stress training in some reports has produced a 92.5% reduction in symptom frequency and good long-term retention.

Because increased viscosity has been implicated in the etiology of vibration white finger, defibrinogenating therapy has been attempted.[69] It has been shown to increase digital blood flow without vasodilation and with a subsequent increase in skin temperature, an increase in digital blood pressure, and improved cold provocation tests lasting up to 1 year after therapy.

Because of the progressive nature of the disease and the lack of predictable treatments, it would be prudent to remove from exposure patients identified as being in stage 1 or early stage 2 and await the natural regression of the symptoms.

Prevention. Although some success has been seen with the introduction of vibration-isolating handles and improved work techniques and machinery, the prevalence of this disease is still quite high. Taylor and Brammer have suggested a number of preventive measures to minimize the hazard of severe vibration white finger.[90] These include: (1) implementing pre-employment screening for primary and secondary Raynaud's phenomena, (2) identifying previous vibration exposure, (3) requiring annual examinations, (4) using power tools with vibration reduction devices and maintaining them properly, (5) wearing sufficient clothing and gloves to keep warm (gloves do not dampen vibrations in the harmful range), (6) avoiding continuous vibration exposure by instituting 10-minute breaks every hour, (7) using a minimum hand grip consistent with work safety, (8) resting the tool on the work base if possible, and (9) removing the worker from vibration exposure as soon as stage 1 or stage 2 is identified.

Conclusion. Vibration white finger is a vasospastic disorder brought about by exposure to vibration. The disease appears to be progressive; neurological features present early and are followed by vasospastic disorder. The patient initially complains of episodic pallor and burning sensation in one or more digits, which progresses to involve the entire hand if vibration exposure is continued. No cure is presently available for this condition; even removing the patient from chronic vibration exposure does not guarantee resolution of the symptoms. Treatment at present is purely palliative. Prevention of the condition is the major aim.

Although the symptoms are annoying during leisure-time activities in cold weather, they appear to have minimal effect on work time and efficiency. Grounds[38] concluded that in most patients the symptoms are not bad enough to give up a job. Kylin et al.,[53] however, found some moderate disability in 45% of workers with vibration white finger; most of the job and wage reduction was due to the neurological features of the disease.

OCCUPATIONAL OCCLUSIVE DISEASES

Occupational occlusive diseases of the hand include a group of conditions with a common etiology: repetitive blunt trauma to the palm of the hand resulting in occlusive or aneurysmal disease of the digital or palmar vessels. Von Rosen[102] was first to report and treat a case of ulnar artery thrombosis due to a contusion of the hypothenar eminence. The patient was successfully treated by simple excision of the thrombosed segment and ulnar nerve decompression. Subsequently Barker and Hines strengthened the association between repetitive trauma and ulnar artery thrombosis by reporting 11 cases in 1944. The vessels most often involved are either the radial[103] or ulnar arteries, and occasionally, the palmar arch[2] or the digital vessels.[73]

The most typical and best described example of this condition is the hypothenar hammer syndrome described by Conn et al.[19] Typically the patient uses the hypothenar area of the palm as a hammer. Repetitive blunt trauma to the area causes damage to the ulnar artery as it courses over the hook of the hamate. A number of outcomes are possible. The ulnar artery may thrombose, become aneurysmal, or shower distal emboli into the digits (Fig. 5). Periarterial fibrosis around the injured vessel may induce a Raynaud's phenomenon involving the ulnar digits or may cause direct compression of the ulnar nerve in Guyon's canal. Although this is the most common form of occupational occlusive disease, the physician should be aware of other possible sites of repetitive trauma in the hand that can result in arterial injury.

Hypothenar hammer syndrome is probably underdiagnosed owing to a large number of asymptomatic causes. In an extensive review of 966 patients with Raynaud's phenomenon, Vayssairat et al. found an incidence of 1.7%.[100] Little and Ferguson in 1972 examined 127 workers with Raynaud's phenomenon in two government vehicle maintenance workshops; 79 gave a history of habitual use of the hand as a hammer, and 14% of these workers showed ulnar artery occlusions.[57] They discovered a significant relationship between duration of employment and the presence of ulnar artery occlusion. All patients were symptomatic. The

exact cause of thrombosis or aneurysm formation is unclear. Von Rosen has suggested that damage to the intima causes thrombosis, whereas damage to the media causes aneurysms to form.

Occlusive vascular disease occurs in many occupations (Table 4). A latent period of about 15 years precedes the onset of symptoms.[100] Patients may be asymptomatic or have symptoms as severe as ischemic rest pain and ulceration. Most often, however, patients present with Raynaud's phenomenon and a persistent coldness of the digits indicating arterial compromise.[88] The ulnar three digits are most affected with episodes of coldness, color changes, and pain with tenderness in the hypothenar area and an occasional palpable mass. Occasionally the patient experiences paresthesia and numbness due to associated ulnar nerve compression or fibrosis within Guyon's canal. These symptoms may occur spontaneously or may be aggravated by exposure to cold.

The ischemia seen with ulnar artery thrombosis or aneurysm formation has three causes. First, in the presence of an incomplete or inadequate arch or in an ulnar-artery–dominant hand, the collateral flow from the radial side may be insufficient for the needs of the ulnar side of the hand. In a radial-artery–dominant hand, an ulnar artery thrombosis often may be asymptomatic. Second, if the hand is radial artery dominant, ulnar artery thrombosis or aneurysm formation may induce vascular spasm secondary to excitation of the perivascular sympathetic nerves. This results in a Raynaud's phenomenon involving the ulnar three digits. Third, aneurysmal dilation of the ulnar artery can allow mural thrombus formation and subsequent distal embolization.

Diagnosis. Occupational occlusive disease should be suspected in a worker with unilateral Raynaud's phenomenon or vascular compromise when there has been definite occupational exposure to repetitive trauma to the palm. Bilateral hypothenar hammer syndrome occurs, although rarely.[108,110] In the clinical setting, a positive Allen's test indicating ulnar artery occlusion is presumptive diagnosis of a hypothenar hammer syndrome. It is important to exclude other causes of Raynaud's phenomenon, such as vibration exposure, and to exclude Buerger's disease in smokers. The diagnosis is most easily confirmed with noninvasive vascular studies[48,89] (Fig. 6). A Doppler map-

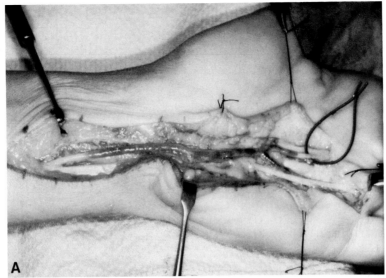

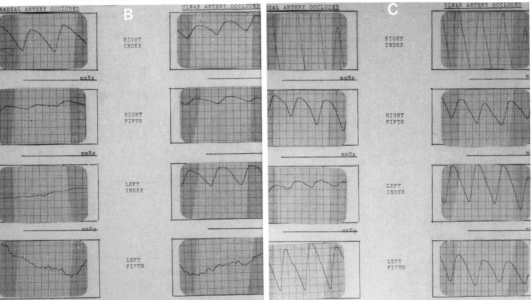

FIGURE 5. *A,* Example of ulnar artery thrombosis in 43-year-old white woman (hypothenar hammer syndrome). *B,* Preoperative noninvasive Allen's test using pulse volume recording demonstrates left ulnar artery thrombosis. Pre- and postoperative digital blood pressures show the following changes after ulnar artery reconstruction with a vein graft interposition (see table below). *C,* Postoperative pulse volume recording demonstrates patency of the ulnar artery graft.

Pre- and Postoperative Digital Blood Pressures

Digit	Blood Pressures	
	Preoperative	Postoperative
Thumb	80	95
Index	85	100
Long	40	80
Ring	45	90
Fifth	20	80

TABLE 4. Occupations Associated with Occupational Occlusive Disease of the Hand

Steamfitter
Cotton gin operator
Pneumatic drill machinist
Toolmaker
Mechanic
Farmer
Bricklayer
Metalworker
Tiler
Painter
Carpenter
Storekeeper
Stonecutters
Truck driver
Karate practitioner
Sculptor
Fruit juicer
Artificial inseminator
Butcher
Forestry worker
Cashier
Pharmacist
Obstetrician
Jackhammer operator

ping of the hand shows the extent of the ulnar occlusion and the presence of any other distal occlusions (see Fig. 2). Digital plethysmography, pulse volume recording, and blood pressure measurement show the dynamic status of the vasculature to the involved digits. We have found the correlation between noninvasive vascular examination, arteriography, and surgical findings to be 96%.[10] Noninvasive vascular examination helps predict the possible outcomes of ulnar artery reconstruction. Finally, cold stress testing with and without ulnar artery

sympathetic block demonstrates the presence of any sympathetic hyperactivity. Brachial arteriography anatomically delineates the problem but unfortunately does not provide information about digital pressures or sympathetic activity.

Treatment. Occupational occlusive disease is initially managed conservatively by cessation of smoking, protection of the hand, avoidance of cold exposure, and a trial of chemotherapeutic agents such as nifedipine to reduce the sympathetic influence.[81] Surgery is reserved for patients with thrombotic disease after failure of conservative treatment or for those with aneurysmal dilation of the ulnar artery.[43] Resection of the involved area has a number of benefits: first, it removes (by local sympathectomy) any sympathetic overactivity; second, it removes a possible source of distal embolization; third, it removes a painful or tender palmar lesion; and fourth it decompresses the ulnar nerve within Guyon's canal.

The major decision, however, involves the use of reversed vein grafts to restore vascular continuity. Unfortunately the long-term patency rate for vein grafts or arterial repairs at the wrist level is 50% and appears to be related in part to the vascular dynamics of the collateral circulation in the hand.[52] A number of noninvasive methods are used to predict which patients will benefit from reconstruction of the ulnar artery.[43] If the preoperative noninvasive vascular studies show poor digital pressures and low digital brachial indices in the ulnar three digits, then reconstruction should be at-

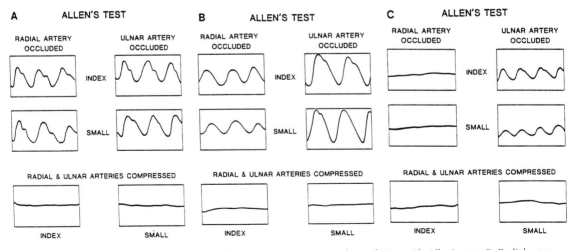

FIGURE 6. A, Pulse volume recording (PVR) tracing showing normal circulation with Allen's test. B, Radial artery dominance with increased flow to the hand via the radial artery as compared to the ulnar artery. C, Ulnar artery occlusion.

tempted. Normal pressures indicate a likely radial-artery–dominant hand and an ulnar artery reconstruction probably would thrombose. Another technique is to measure the intraoperative digital pressures after resection of the ulnar artery. If these are low or the backflow pressure is low, reconstruction is necessary.[50] If the digital pressures are high, then simple resection of the segment is indicated. In general, good results are reported in most series, irrespective of treatment methods.[100]

Prevention.   As in many occupational vascular diseases, the final disease is the result of cumulative injuries. The best prevention, therefore, is to avoid the repetitive injury. Each person must look at his work practices and avoid using the hand as a hammer. Management should provide appropriate tools for workers' use. Occupational health services should become aware of the possibility of this condition and should regularly screen with Allen's testing workers in industries where the hand is habitually used as a hammer. It is interesting to note that hypothenar hammer syndrome is still not a compensable condition in the United Kingdom.[65]

CHEMICALLY INDUCED VASCULAR PATHOLOGY

The increasing sophistication of the synthetic manufacturing industries and the use of more and more volatile agents has led to an increasing number of chemically induced diseases. Some of the chemicals implicated influence the peripheral vascular system. The most widely reported condition is the vasculopathy associated with vinyl chloride exposure. Cutaneous vasculitis is the only symptom of exposure to most chemicals, including aluminum and fluorides produced by the Soderberg aluminum electrolysis process[6,82] and silver behenic acid from photocopier fumes.[95] These chemicals do not cause significant diseases of the large vessel.

Other chemicals, however, have been reported to induce rare vascular disorders. Carbon disulfide has been thought to induce small-vessel sclerosis,[97] and arsenic has been implicated in Raynaud's phenomenon in smelter workers after long-term exposure.[54] The vasospastic tendency of patients with arsenic exposure seems to result from functional alterations in the vessels due to inhalation of arsenic

oxides. Nickel and chromium exposure also has been implicated as a cause of a vasospastic disorder of the upper extremity.[77]

Vinyl Chloride Disease.   Raynaud's phenomenon, scleroderma-like skin induration, and acro-osteolysis form a triad classically attributed to the non-neoplastic vascular lesions associated with chronic vinyl chloride exposure. Other manifestations of this exposure include noncirrhotic portal hypertension, angiosarcoma of the liver, arthralgia and arthritis, pulmonary fibrosis, thrombocytopenia, skin nodules, finger clubbing, and vasculitic purpura.

Vinyl chloride was first polymerized to polyvinyl chloride (PVC) in Germany in the 1930s. Its association with acro-osteolysis and hepatic changes, however, was not noticed until the late '60s and '70s. Wilson noted an incidence of hepatic changes of 31 per 3000 workers in the PVC industry and an involvement of the majority of patients in cleaning autoclaves.[111] The actual pathophysiology of the disease process is unclear. The disease appears to be mediated by both immunological and direct toxic mechanisms. Vinyl chloride has been shown to be directly toxic to vascular endothelium, causing hyperplasia and swelling of endothelial cells leading to ultimate fibrosis. Biopsies have revealed lymphocytic and histiocytic infiltration around the walls of the dermal arterioles. Multiple occlusive vascular lesions have been seen on arteriography of patients with vinyl chloride disease.[26] The susceptibility to clinical disease after exposure to vinyl chloride may be increased by the presence of tissue antigens human leukocyte antigen (HLA)-DR5, for the mild form of the disease, and HLA-B8 and -DR3, for the severe form.[11] Evidence of an immunological mechanism for the vascular injury is mounting. Reports suggest that vinyl chloride disease is an immune complex disorder initiated by adsorption of vinyl chloride or a metabolite onto a tissue or plasma protein.[104] Immunoelectrophoresis has shown an increase in polyclonal immunoglobulins and cryoglobulins due to an altered immunological response. There is also evidence of an altered cellular immunity in patients who develop vinyl-chloride–induced malignancies.[55]

A specific treatment for vinyl chloride disease is not available. Symptomatic therapy with vasodilators is useful for palliation of the vasospastic disorder. Removing the patient from exposure is the best way to prevent disease progression, and some of the symptoms may reverse with time.[31] Prevention obviously includes reducing exposure to vinyl chloride by providing adequate ventilation and by developing techniques for cleaning autoclaves without resorting to manual labor. Again, screening of exposed workers is very important so that those in early stages of the disease can be removed from further exposure.

THORACIC OUTLET COMPRESSION

Thoracic outlet compression is a term used to describe a large number of syndromes related to compression of various structures in the region of the thoracic outlet, specifically the brachial plexus, subclavian artery, and subclavian vein. Compression of each of these structures produces specific complexes of symptoms. The compression can occur at different levels within the thoracic outlet. It has been suggested that the development of thoracic outlet compression correlates not so much to the heaviness of the work as to difficult work postures and constant muscular tension in the shoulder girdle.[83] Difficult postures, plus possible anatomical and developmental anomalies, may increase the likelihood of developing clinically significant compression.

The prevalence of thoracic outlet compression in the general population is unknown, although one study of a normal population by Sällström and Thulesius revealed an incidence of provoked thoracic outlet compression of 9.5%.[84] In a study of 191 workers by Sällström and Schmidt, 18% had symptoms of compression of the thoracic outlet, 13% had evidence of arterial compression, and 4% had evidence of venous compression.[83] These patients showed a significant female preponderance and an incidence of compression that increased with duration of employment. The symptom complex of neurological thoracic outlet compression consists of pain, paresthesia, numbness on the ulnar side of the hand, and fatigue. It occurs initially after prolonged arm elevation, and with progression of the compression, the symptoms may occur at rest. The symptoms of arterial compression may vary from none to Raynaud's phenomenon, forearm claudication, or later ulceration.[12] Venous compression produces swelling, cyanosis, and engorgement of veins across the shoulder and the upper arm.[88] Sällström and Schmidt[83] found no relationship between neurological and vascular types of thoracic outlet compression.

Subclavian artery compression produces symptoms of forearm claudication by restricting the blood flow to the arm below what is needed for normal cell metabolism. Continued activity of the forearm musculature in the presence of relative ischemia leads to a buildup of metabolites that produces pain and cramps within the involved muscles. With time and progression of the disease, a fixed stenosis may develop at the site of compression owing to repetitive intimal trauma. This stenosis, through its hemodynamic influences, may lead to a poststenotic dilation or aneurysm formation in the subclavian artery. When this occurs, ischemia may be present at rest and may be accompanied by distal embolization from mural thrombus. Thrombosis of the subclavian artery may occur rarely.[85] Bouhoutsos et al. believe that unilateral Raynaud's phenomenon is due to reduced blood flow, most often from subclavian stenosis resulting from extraliminal factors.[12]

Three sites of compression of the neurovascular bundle may result in thoracic outlet compression: (1) (most frequently) in the costoclavicular space between the clavicle and the first rib, (2) in the triangle between the scalenus anterior, the scalenus medius and the upper border of the first rib, and (3) in the angle between the coracoid process and pectoralis minor insertions (Fig. 7). Compression of vascular structures at each of these sites can be accentuated by a number of anatomical or pathological variations. In the scalene triangle, the space can be reduced by muscular hypertrophy, by a broad fibrous or common insertion of the scalenus anterior and scalenus medius muscles, or by the presence of a cervical rib or fibrous anlage elevating the floor of this triangle. In hyperabduction syndrome, the vessel can become kinked under the insertion of the pectoralis minor to the coracoid process. This compression may be accentuated by muscular hypertrophy or by variations in the shape of the coracoid process. Costoclavicular compression, which occurs between the clavicle and first rib, is accentuated by the presence of a horizontal clavicle (possibly related to the female preponderance), drooping of shoulders, or prior clavicular fractures and malunion. All of these variations plus occupational stresses may lead to thoracic outlet arterial compression.[88]

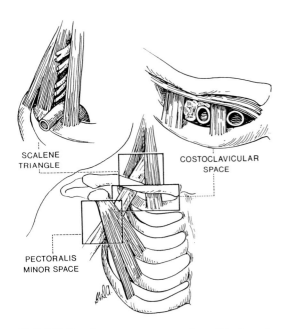

FIGURE 7. Three common areas of possible thoracic outlet compression: scalene triangle, costoclavicular space, and pectoralis minor space.

On examination, differentiation of vascular compression from the more common neurological compression should present no difficulties. At rest, arterial examination is usually normal. Occasionally the fullness of a cervical rib or the pulsation of a post-stenotic dilation of the subclavian artery may be felt and a bruit may be audible in the supra- or infraclavicular fossa if a fixed stenosis is present. Examination of the patient at rest should include palpation of all the distal pulses, Allen's testing, and blood pressure measurement of both upper limbs. Stress testing is useful for suspected vascular compression of the thoracic outlet. Using various maneuvers to compress the artery, the examiner may be able to elicit a reduction in pulse or blood pressure in the arms. The sensitivity of this test can be greatly increased by employing noninvasive vascular studies, such as measurement of digital blood pressure, pulse volume recordings, and Doppler flow patterns during these maneuvers.[3,112] A bruit in the region in the subclavian artery during these maneuvers also indicates a significant compression. The three tests used to stress the thoracic outlet are the costoclavicular maneuver, hyperabduction, and Adson's test. These abnormalities must be interpreted with care, however, because many asymptomatic patients may have an abnormal test.[36] The costoclavicular

maneuver involves adopting the exaggerated military position with the shoulders drawn backward and downward. This position may occlude the subclavian artery in the angle between the clavicle and the first rib. For the hyperabduction test the shoulders are at 0 degrees, the arms externally rotated, and then again the shoulders abducted 180 degrees. Adson's test involves inhaling and holding the breath, extending the neck, and turning the head toward the side being tested. During each of these maneuvers, the radial pulse should be examined along with osculation of the area around the clavicle to elicit a possible bruit.

Before any surgery, the state of the subclavian vessels and an accurate localization of the compression site must be documented. Although contract angiography has been the recommended standard, safer and less invasive techniques are available, particularly isotope scanning and digital subtraction angiography. These give a relatively accurate and detailed anatomic picture of the subclavian artery after a single intravenous injection. Scans taken during the appropriate stress maneuvers show the site of disease, and the static pictures show the presence of any fixed stenosis or aneurysm formation. Distal noninvasive vascular studies are also useful to exclude sites of distal embolization or the presence of more systemic vascular disease.

Treatment. Although the treatment of neurological thoracic outlet compression is conservative for the majority of patients, those with documented vascular involvement are best treated surgically. If no anatomical anomaly, aneurysm, or distal embolization is evident, then a trial of physiotherapy aimed at elevating the shoulder girdle to reduce compression is indicated. If the patient has Raynaud's phenomenon alone, then a trial of vasodilators also may be beneficial. If, however, anomalies, stenosis, aneurysm, or embolization is evident, surgical repair is indicated. Once the site of obstruction is identified, release is performed. Compression most often involves the first rib or scalenus anterior muscle, and resection of either of these is usually required. For costoclavicular compression or scalene triangle compression, a first rib resection via the axilla is performed or scalenectomy is done by the supraclavicular approach. If the compression is secondary to a prior clavicle fracture, then a clavicle osteotomy and fixation may be indicated. In hyperabduction syndrome, division of the pectoralis minor muscle is indicated. The management of the subclavian artery depends on the amount of damage already sustained. If a stenosis is present, along with releasing the compression, a vascular reconstruction or a resection with repair or grafting is needed. In some centers, transluminal angioplasty to dilate the stenotic segment is an alternative. If an aneurysm or embolization is present, then resection and grafting are needed. If the patient has evidence of Raynaud's phenomenon secondary to thoracic outlet arterial compression or distal embolization, a sympathectomy may be performed at the time of rib resection and vascular repair. The sympathectomy can usually be performed between the second and third ribs; the lower third of the stellate and the upper four thoracic sympathetic ganglia are removed. Some recovery of sympathetic tone, however, results in only temporary improvement for most patients. The addition of a vasodilator such as nifedipine may be useful in these patients.

Prevention. Prevention of this type of vascular compression is difficult because of the wide range of occupations that involve overuse of the upper extremity and the high prevalence of normal workers with evidence of posture-induced arterial impingement. In patients with suspected thoracic outlet compression, the avoidance of prolonged overhead work or awkward postures, the use of frequent rest periods, and physical therapy may avoid progression of the condition.

VENOUS OCCLUSIONS

Upper extremity venous occlusion, often called effort thrombosis, is uncommon in the workplace. The incidence of venous thrombosis in the upper extremity is approximately 1–2% of that in the lower limbs. Most patients are male, the average age is 31 years, and involvement is more common in the dominant arm. The precipitating cause seems to be unusual exertion of the arm or repetitive trauma. The patient presents with pain, swelling, cyanosis, and venous engorgement of the arm. The axilla may be tender over the subclavian or axillary vein. Hughes[44] and Campbell et al.[17] believe this condition is due in most cases to some underlying anomaly resulting in venous compression. A number of cases have been reported in laborers carrying objects, such as hay

bales and wooden planks, on their shoulders, where direct trauma to the veins may be implicated.[109] Venous compromise can also occur without thrombosis in a mechanism similar to thoracic outlet compression. Nakada reported a case of venous claudication of the upper extremity due to stenosis of a duplicated axillary vein beneath a hypertrophied pectoralis minor muscle. The symptoms resolved after a confirmation by venography and transluminal angioplasty.[67] Venous claudication is a difficult diagnosis and only becomes evident with stress testing and exercises of the upper limb.

After clinical suspicion is raised, the diagnosis is best made via impedance plethysmography[74] or venography. The initial treatment is rest and intravenous anticoagulation. There is a small but significant risk of fatal pulmonary embolus. In a review of 25 cases of upper extremity vein thrombosis, Campbell found three pulmonary emboli, two of which were fatal. Despite anticoagulation and apparent resolution of the thrombus, three out of four patients with effort thrombosis remained mildly symptomatic, and all patients with identifiable extrinsic compression of the thoracic outlet remained symptomatic. Reconstruction surgery to remove this external compression has had limited success.[17]

CONCLUSION

Occupational vascular disorders appear some time after exposure to an initiating cause. The resultant disease is the effect of cumulative trauma from vibration, repetitive blunt trauma, chemical exposure, or postural stress, occasionally in association with genetic or developmental predisposing fractures. This chronic exposure may leave a permanent vascular disorder that is refractory to all treatments. The patient may be unable to continue work at the previous level and may be at risk for digital ischemia.

Identification of people at risk requires thorough knowledge of these conditions and use of simple screening tests. When symptoms are identified, early treatment or work modification is needed. Ultimately, prevention of these diseases depends on the collection of accurate epidemiological data, the identification of easily applied objective tests, the development of standards for risk exposure, and the development of machinery and work techniques with reduced harmful forces and substances.

REFERENCES

1. Agate JN: An outbreak of cases of Raynaud's phenomenon of occupational origin. Br J Ind Med 6:144, 1949.
2. Annetts DL, Graham AR: Traumatic aneurysm of the palmar arch: Lemon squeezer's hand. Aust NZ J Surg 52:584, 1982.
3. Archie JP, Larson BO: Noninvasive vascular laboratory evaluation of subclavian artery occlusion. South Med J 71:482, 1978.
4. Ashe WF, Cook WT, Old JW: Raynaud's phenomenon of occupational origin. Arch Environ Health 5:333, 1962.
5. Azuma T, Ohhashi T: Pathophysiology of vibration-induced white finger: Etiological considerations and proposals for prevention. In Brammer AJ, Taylor W (eds): Vibration Effects on the Hand and Arm in Industry. New York, John Wiley, 1982, pp 31–38.
6. Balic J, Kansky A, Wolf A: Skin telangiectasias, heavy sweating and diffuse itching in aluminum potroom workers. Arh Hig Rada Toksikol 37:337, 1986.
7. Banister PA, Smith FV: Vibration-induced white fingers and manipulative dexterity. Br J Ind Med 29:264, 1972.
8. Barker NW, Hines EA: Arterial occlusion in the hands and fingers associated with repeated occupational trauma. Mayo Clin Proc 19:345, 1944.
9. Behrens V, Taylor W, Wasserman DE: Vibration syndrome in workers using pneumatic chipping and grinding tools. In Brammer AJ, Taylor W (eds): Vibration Effects on the Hand and Arm in Industry. New York, John Wiley, 1982, pp 147–155.
10. Berger A, Kleinert JM: Noninvasive vascular studies: A comparison with angiography and surgical findings in the upper extremity. Paper presented at the 44th Annual Meeting of the American Society for Surgery of the Hand, Seattle, September 13–16, 1989.
11. Black C, Pereira S, McWhirter A, et al: Genetic susceptibility to scleroderma-like syndrome in symptomatic and asymptomatic workers exposed to vinyl chloride. J Rheumatol 13:1059, 1986.
12. Bouhoutsos J, Morris T, Martin P: Unilateral Raynaud's phenomenon in the hand and its significance. Surgery 82(5):547, 1977.
13. Bovenzi M: Finger systolic pressure during local cooling in normal subjects aged 20 to 60 years: Reference values for the assessment of digital vasospasm in Raynaud's phenomenon of occupational origin. Int Arch Occup Environ Health 61:179, 1988.
14. Bovenzi M: Vibration white finger, digital blood pressure and some biochemical findings on workers operating vibrating tools in the engine manufacturing industry. Am J Ind Med 14:575, 1988.
15. Bovenzi M, Franzinelli A, Strambi F: Prevalence of vibration-induced white finger and assessment of vibration exposure among travertine workers in Italy. Int Arch Occup Environ Health 61:25, 1988.
16. Boyle JC, Smith NJ, Burke FD: Vibration white finger. J Hand Surg 13B:171, 1988.
17. Campbell CB, Chandler JG, Tegtmeyer CJ, Bernstein EF: Axillary, subclavian and brachiocephalic

18. Conley JE, Endeloff GLM: Sympathectomy for upper extremity vasomotor disorders. J Cardiovasc Surg 10:436, 1969.
19. Conn J, Bergan JJ, Bell JL: Hypothenar hammer syndrome: Posttraumatic digital ischemia. Surgery 68:1122, 1970.
20. Darling RC, Raines JK, Brener BJ, Austen WG: Quantitative segmental pulse volume recorder: A clinical tool. Surgery 72:873, 1972.
21. Delp HL, Newton RA: Effects of brief cold exposure on finger dexterity and sensibility in subjects with Raynaud's phenomenon. Phys Ther 66:503, 1986.
22. Ekenvall L: Clinical assessment of suspected damage from hand-held vibrating tools. Scand J Work Environ Health 13:271, 1987.
23. Ekenvall L, Carlsson A: Vibration white finger: A follow-up study. Br J Ind Med 44:476, 1987.
24. Ekenvall L, Lindblad LE: Digital blood pressure after local cooling as a diagnostic tool in traumatic vasospastic disease. Br J Ind Med 39:388, 1982.
25. Ekenvall L, Lindblad LE: Is vibration white finger a primary sympathetic nerve injury. Br J Ind Med 43:702, 1986.
26. Falappa P, Magnavita N, Bergamaschi A, Colavita N: Angiographic study of digital arteries in workers exposed to vinyl chloride. Br J Ind Med 39:169, 1982.
27. Färkkilä M: Vibration induced injury. Br J Ind Med 43:361, 1986.
28. Färkkilä MA, Pyykkö I, Starck JP, Korhonen OS: Hand grip force and muscle fatigue in the etiology of vibration syndrome. In Brammer AJ, Taylor W (eds): Vibration Effects on the Hand and Arm in Industry. New York, John Wiley, 1982, pp 45–50.
29. Flatt A: Digital artery sympathectomy. J Hand Surg 5:550, 1980.
30. Freedman RR, Ianni P, Wenig P: Behavioral treatment of Raynaud's disease. J Consult Clin Psychol 51:539, 1983.
31. Freudiger H, Bounameaux H, Garcia J: Acroosteolysis and Raynaud's phenomenon after vinyl chloride exposure. Vasa 17:216, 1988.
32. Futatsuka M, Sakurai T, Aruzumi M: Preliminary evaluation of dose-effect relationship for vibration induced white finger in Japan. Int Arch Occup Environ Health 54:201, 1984.
33. Futatsuka M, Yasutake N, Sakurai T, Matsumoto T: Comparative study of vibration disease among operators of vibrating tools by factor analysis. Br J Ind Med 42:260, 1985.
34. Gaydos HF: Effects on complex manual performance of cooling the body while maintaining the hands at normal temperatures. J Appl Physiol 12:373, 1958.
35. Gemne G, Pyykkö I, Taylor W, Pelmear PL: The Stockholm workshop scale for the classifications of cold-induced Raynaud's phenomenon in the hand-arm vibration syndrome (revision of the Taylor-Pelmear scale). Scand J Work Environ Health 13:275, 1987.
36. Gergoudis R, Barnes RW: Thoracic outlet arterial compression. Prevalence in normal persons. Angiology 31:538, 1980.
37. Griffin MJ: Hand-arm vibration standards and dose-effect relationships. In Brammer AJ, Taylor W (eds): Vibration Effects on the Hand and Arm in Industry. New York, John Wiley, 1982, pp 259–268.
38. Grounds MD: Raynaud's phenomenon in users of chain saws. Med J Aust 22:270, 1964.

vein obstruction. Surgery 82:816, 1977.

39. Gurdjian ES, Walker LW: Traumatic vasospastic disease of the hand (white fingers). JAMA 129:668, 1945.

40. Hallbäck M, Folkow B: Cardiovascular responses to acute mental "stress" in spontaneously hypertensive rats. Acta Physiol Scand 90:684, 1974.

41. Hamilton A: A study of spastic anemia in the hands of stonecutters. Bulletin, US Bureau of Labor Statistics 236 (Industrial Accidents and Hygiene Series, No 19) 53, 1918.

42. Hirai M: Arterial insufficiency of the hand evaluated by digital blood pressure and arteriographic findings. Circulation 58:902, 1978.

43. Ho PK, Weiland, AJ, McClinton MA, Wilgis EFS: Aneurysms of the upper extremity. J Hand Surg 12A:39, 1987.

44. Hughes ESR: Venous obstruction in the upper extremity (Paget-Schrotter's syndrome): A review of 320 cases. Int Abstr Surg 88:89, 1949.

45. James PB, Galloway RW: Arteriography of the hand in men exposed to vibration. In Taylor W, Pelmear PL (eds): Vibration white finger in industry. London, Academic Press, 1975, pp 31–41.

46. Jarrett F, Hirsch SA: Current diagnosis and management of upper extremity ischemia. Surg Ann 15:207, 1983.

47. Knutsson A: Immunoglobulins in workers with traumatic vasospastic disease. J Occup Med 17:706, 1975.

48. Koman LA: Current status of noninvasive techniques in the diagnosis of upper extremity disorders. A.A.O.S.: Instructional course lectures. St. Louis, C.V. Mosby, 1983.

49. Koman LA, Nunley JA, Goldner JL, et al: Isolated cold stress testing in the assessment of symptoms in the upper extremity: Preliminary communication. J Hand Surg 9A:305, 1984.

50. Koman LA, Nunley JA, Wilkinson RH, et al: Dynamic radionuclide imaging as a means of evaluating vascular perfusion of the upper extremity: A preliminary report. J Hand Surg 8:424, 1983.

51. Koman LA, Urbaniak JR: Ulnar artery insufficiency: A guide to treatment. J Hand Surg 6:16, 1981.

52. Kutz JE, Hay EA, Kleinert HE: The fate of small vessel repair. J Bone Joint Surg 51A:792, 1969.

53. Kylin B, Lidström I-M, Liljenberg B, et al: Hälso-Och Miljöundersökning Blend Skogsarbetare. Al-Rapport 5:44, 1968.

54. Lagerkvist B, Linderholm H, Nordberg GF: Vasospastic tendency and Raynaud's phenomenon in smelter workers exposed to arsenic. Environ Res 39:465, 1986.

55. Langauer-Lewowicka H, Dudziak Z, Byczkowska Z, Marks J: Cryoglobulinemia in Raynaud's phenomenon due to vinyl chloride. Int Arch Occup Environ Health 36:197, 1976.

56. Larsen V, Fabricius J, Nielsen G, Hansen K: Ketanserin in the treatment of traumatic vasospastic disease. Br Med J 293:650, 1986.

57. Little JM, Ferguson DA: The incidence of the hypothenar hammer syndrome. Arch Surg 105:684, 1972.

58. Loriga G: Il lavoro con i Martelli Pneumatici, Boll. Inspett. Lavoro 2:35, 1911.

59. Mackiewicz Z, Jawien A: Experience with Doppler investigations in vibration syndrome. Int Angiol 7:305, 1988.

60. Magos L, Okos G: Cold dilatation and Raynaud's phenomenon. Arch Environ Health 7:402, 1963.

61. Marshall J, Poole EG, Raynaud WA: Raynaud's phenomenon due to vibrating tools. Lancet 1:1151, 1954.

62. Matoba T, Chiba M, Toshima T: Cardiovascular features of the vibration syndrome: An adaptive response. In Brammer AJ, Taylor W (eds): Vibration Effects of the Hand and Arm in Industry. New York, John Wiley, 1982, pp 25–30.

63. Mills JH: Pneumatic hammer disease in unusual locations. Northwest Med 41:282, 1942.

64. Morton R, Provins KA: Finger numbness after acute local exposure to cold. J Appl Physiol 15:149, 1960.

65. Mosquera D, Goldman M: An unusual variant of the hypothenar hammer syndrome. Br J Ind Med 45:568, 1988.

66. Mountcastle VB, La Motte RH, Carli G: Detection thresholds for stimuli in humans and monkeys: Comparison with threshold events in mechanoreceptive afferent nerve fibers innervating the monkey hand. J Neurophysiol 35:122, 1972.

67. Nakada T, Knight RT, Mani RL: Intermittent venous claudication of the upper extremity: The pectoralis minor syndrome. Ann Neurol 11:443, 1982.

68. Narem RM: Vibration-induced arterial shear stress. Arch Environ Health 26:105, 1973.

69. Nasu Y: Defibrinogenating therapy for peripheral circulatory disturbance in patients with vibration syndrome. Scand J Work Environ Health 12:272, 1986.

70. Okada A, Ariizumi M, Fujinaga H: Diagnosis of the vibration syndrome by blood viscosity. In Brammer AJ, Taylor W (eds): Vibration Effects on the Hand and Arm in Industry. New York, John Wiley, 1982, pp 67–70.

71. Olsen N, Fjeldborg P, Brøchner-Mortensen J: Sympathetic and local vasoconstrictor response to cold in vibration induced white finger. Br J Ind Med 42:272, 1985.

72. Olsen N, Nielsen SL, Voss P: Cold response of digital arteries in chain saw operators. Br J Ind Med 39:82, 1982.

73. O'Sullivan DJ, Brady MJ: Bull man's hand—an unusual occupational lesion. J Irish Med Assoc 67:102, 1974.

74. Patwardhan NA, Anderson FA, Cutler BS, Wheeler HB: Noninvasive detection of axillary and subclavian venous thrombosis by impedance plethysmography. J Cardiovasc Surg 24:250, 1983.

75. Pelmear PL, Leong D, Taylor W, et al: Measurement of vibration of hand-held tools: Weighted or unweighted? J Occup Med 31:902, 1989.

76. Pelmear PL, Taylor W, Pearson CG: Raynaud's phenomenon in grinders. In Taylor W, Pelmear PL (eds): Vibration White Finger in Industry. New York, Academic Press, 1975, pp 21–30.

77. Perbellini L, DeGrandis D: Neuro-arteriopatia verosimilmente correlata ad esposizione a nichel e cromo. Med Lavoro 4:318, 1979.

78. Pyykkö I, Hyvärinen J: Vibration induced changes of sympathetic vasomotor tone. Acta Chir Scand 465:23, 1976.

79. Pyykkö I, Hyvärinen J, Färkkilä M: Studies on the etiological mechanism of the vasospastic component of the vibration syndrome. In Brammer AJ, Taylor W (eds): Vibration effects on the hand and arm in industry. New York, John Wiley, 1982, pp 13–25.

80. Reynolds DD, Angevine EN: Hand-arm vibration. Part II. Vibration transmission characteristics of the hand and arm. J Sound Vibrat 51:237, 1977.

81. Rodeheffer R, Rommer JA, Wigley F, Smith CR: Controlled double-blind trial of nifedipine in the

treatment of Raynaud's phenomenon. N Engl J Med 308:880, 1983.

82. Rossignol M, Thériault G: Skin telangiectases and ischemic disorders in primary aluminum production workers. Br J Ind Med 45:198, 1988.

83. Sällström J, Schmidt H: Cervicobrachial disorders in certain occupations, with special reference to compression in the thoracic outlet. Am J Ind Med 6:45, 1984.

84. Sällström J, Thulesius O: Noninvasive investigation of vascular compression in patients with thoracic outlet syndrome. Clin Physiol 2:117, 1982.

85. Schein CJ, Haimovici H, Young H: Arterial thrombosis associated with cervical ribs: Surgical considerations: Report of a case and review of the literature. Surgery 40:428, 1956.

86. Sivertsson R, Ljung B: Vibration-induced changes in vascular tone. Acta Chir Surg 465:20, 1976.

87. Spittell JA: Raynaud's phenomenon and allied vasospastic disorders. In Jurgens JL, Spittell JA, Fairbairn JF (eds): Peripheral Vascular Disease. Philadelphia, W.B. Saunders, 1980, pp 554–583.

88. Spittell JA: Some uncommon types of occlusive peripheral vascular disease. Curr Probl Cardiol 8(8):6, 1983.

89. Sumner DS: Noninvasive assessment of upper extremity ischemia. In Bergan JJ, Yao JST (eds): Evaluation and Treatment of Upper and Lower Extremity Circulatory Disorders. Orlando, FL, Grune & Stratton, 1984, pp 75–95.

90. Taylor W, Brammer AJ: Vibration effects on the hand and arm in industry: An introduction and review. In Brammer AJ, Taylor W (eds): Vibration Effects on the Hand and Arm in Industry. New York, John Wiley, 1982, pp 1–12.

91. Taylor W, Pelmear PL: Raynaud's phenomenon of occupational origin. An epidemiological survey. Acta Chir Scand 465 (suppl):27, 1976.

92. Taylor W, Wasserman DE: Occupational vibration. In Zenz C (ed): Occupational Medicine: Principles and Practical Applications, 2nd ed. Chicago, Year Book, 1988, pp 324–333.

93. Taylor W, Wasserman DE, Behrens V, et al: Effect of the air hammer on the hands of stonecutters. The limestone quarries of Bedford, Indiana, revisited. Br J Ind Med 41:289, 1984.

94. Telford ED, McCann MB, MacCormack DH: "Dead hand" in users of vibrating tools. Lancet 2:359, 1945.

95. Tencati JR, Novey HS: Hypersensitivity angiitis caused by fumes from heat-activated photocopy paper. Ann Intern Med 98:320, 1983.

96. Thériault G, De Guire L, Gingras S, Laroche G: Raynaud's phenomenon in forestry workers in Quebec. Can Med Assoc J 126:1404, 1982.

97. Tolonen M: Vascular effects of carbon disulfide. A review. Scand J Work Environ Health 1:63, 1975.

98. Turczyński B, Kumaszka F, Sroczyński J: Serum viscosity in workers exposed to mechanical vibration and noise. Pol Tyg Lek 33:187, 1978.

99. Une H, Esaki H: Urinary excretion of adrenaline and noradrenaline in lumberjacks with vibration syndrome. Br J Ind Med 45:570, 1988.

100. Vayssairat M, Debure C, Cormier J-M, et al: Hypothenar hammer syndrome: Seventeen cases with long term follow-up. J Vasc Surg 5:838, 1987.

101. Vibration Syndrome. Interim report by the Industrial Injuries Advisory Council. London, DMND, 1970, p 4430.

102. Von Rosen S: Ein Fall von Thrombose in der Arteria Ulnaris nach Einwirkung von stumpfer Gewalt. Acta Chir Scand 73:500, 1934.

103. Wandtke JC, Spitzer RM, Olsson HE, Welch R: Traumatic thenar ischemia. Am J Roentgenol 127:569, 1976.

104. Ward AM, Udnoon S, Watkins J, et al: Immunologic mechanisms in the pathogenesis of vinyl chloride disease. Br Med J 1:936, 1976.

105. Wasserman DE: Raynaud's phenomenon as it relates to hand tool vibration in the workplace. Am Ind Hyg Assoc J 46:10, 1985.

106. Wasserman DE, Badger DW, Doyle TE, et al: Industrial vibration—An overview. J Am Soc Saf Eng 19, 1974.

107. Welsh CL: The effect of vibration on digital blood flow. Br J Surg 67:708, 1980.

108. Wernick R, Smith DL: Bilateral hypothenar syndrome: An unusual and preventable cause of digital ischemia. Am J Emerg Med 7:302, 1989.

109. Williams AJ, Freemont AJ, Barnett DB: Subclavian vein thrombosis due to external compression. Lancet 637, 1980.

110. Williams W, Johnson A, Wilson D: Hypothenar hammer syndrome presenting as bilateral Raynaud's phenomenon. Arthritis Rheum 30:234, 1987.

111. Wilson RH, McCormick WE, Tatum CF, Creech JL: Occupational acroosteolysis. JAMA 201:83, 1967.

112. Yao ST, Gourmos C, Papathanasiou K, Irvine WT: A method for assessing ischemia of the hand and fingers. Surg Gynecol Obstet 135:373, 1972.

113. Žák J, Rýznar V: Radionuclide angiography of the hand in occupational vasoneurosis. Acta Univ Palacki Olomuc Fac Med 117:219, 1987.

Chapter 26

MANAGEMENT OF CARPAL TUNNEL SYNDROME

Robert M. Szabo, M.D., and Michael Madison, Ph.D.

Carpal tunnel syndrome (CTS) is the commonest peripheral compression neuropathy. If left untreated, it may progress to a substantial and irreversible hand disability. However, if CTS is recognized early and treated appropriately, excellent results may be expected in most cases.

CLINICAL PRESENTATION

Classically CTS presents with a typical sequence of symptoms. The patient first complains of numbness and tingling in the hand in the distribution of the median nerve—that is, the thumb, the index finger, and the middle and radial half of the ring finger. Sometimes symptoms are recognized in only one finger, and frequently patients experience numbness in the entire hand. Pain usually follows and is aggravated by persistent exertion. The hallmark for diagnosis is night pain that awakens the patient and is relieved by hanging, shaking, massaging, or exercising the hand. Patients often claim that their hands feel swollen. With persistent compression, symptoms arising from the motor branch of the median nerve become evident. Coordinated movements of the thumb and index finger become weak, stiff, and clumsy. Simple tasks such as buttoning clothes, sewing, and winding a watch become awkward.[40,53,71,72,81,82,87]

Although symptoms are often bilateral, the dominant hand usually is affected first and more severely. Repetitious acts that load and flex the wrist aggravate symptoms. Driving a car, sweeping a floor, or repetitively cutting meat on an assembly line heightens awareness of the problem. Symptoms can radiate along the forearm to the elbow or even the shoulder. A complete history of work as well as recreational activity is necessary in addition to a medical history seeking out information about related systemic disease.

OCCURRENCE

CTS is the most commonly encountered of the peripheral compression neuropathies; occurrence in the general population has been estimated at 1%, and occasional symptoms occur in as many as 10% of adults.[62] Nathan et al.[61] measured sensory latency of the median nerve in a random sample of 471 industrial workers and found age-adjusted abnormal increases in 26%, most of them asymptomatic. While such a high incidence raises doubts about the definition of "normal," it also documents the significant occurrence of median nerve impairment in the general population.

Historically, CTS has been considered a condition of middle age or later; in a series of 1,215 patients with CTS seen at the Mayo Clinic, the mean age was 54 years, and 83% were more than 40 years old.[94] In Phalen's series of 439 patients, 82% were over 40 years of age.[71] However, in recent years we have seen an increasing number of young persons with CTS, most of them involved in repetitive manual labor. It may be that in the older series only the more severe cases were seen, and that early cases in young people are now more frequently recognized because of increased sensitivity of diagnostic tests and the widespread familiarity with CTS in the general population.[60,61] Several cases of CTS have been reported in children and adolescents,[22] and congenital cases have been described as well.[51]

Women outnumber men patients by about two to one in most of the larger clinical series; 69% of 1,215 cases were women in the Mayo Clinic series,[94] and 67% of 439 cases were women in Phalen's series.[71] In part this reflects the preponderance of women in the older population. Also, there is some evidence that women have smaller wrists but not correspondingly narrower tendons and are more susceptible to CTS for purely biomechanical reasons.[4]

Combining the results of several large clinical series reveals that CTS was bilateral in 56% of patients.[7,71,88,94] Bendler et al.[7] measured sensory and motor conduction of the median nerve bilaterally in 440 cases and found that 38% of people with only unilateral symptoms had bilateral abnormalities of nerve conduction. The high incidence of bilaterality indicates the importance of systemic disorders in the pathogenesis of CTS.[37,38]

PATHOGENESIS

The pathogenesis of CTS must be considered on three levels—the local anatomy at the carpal tunnel, underlying systemic or physiological disorders, and the patterns of use of the wrist that precipitate an episode of CTS (Table 1). Factors may be acting at each of these levels, and the examining physician must consider all three in piecing together the diagnosis.

Anatomy

The carpal tunnel is a relatively inelastic structure bounded by the concave arch of the carpal bones and by the transverse carpal ligament. Through it pass nine tendons (four flexor digitorum superficialis tendons, four flexor digitorum profundus tendons, the tendon of the flexor pollicis longus) and the median nerve. Viewed longitudinally, the carpal tunnel is nar-

rowest about 2–2.5 cm distal to its proximal margin, widening proximally and distally to this constriction.[77] The narrowest portion corresponds to the region of greatest microscopic changes in nerves, vessels, and synovium in cases of CTS.[3] As the wrist or fingers are flexed or extended, the tendons and median nerve in the carpal canal must be able to slide relative to the canal and to one another. An abnormal crowding of these structures may injure the median nerve by compression, as well as by traction, when its freedom to slide is compromised.

Compression of the median nerve in the carpal tunnel results from an imbalance in the size of the tunnel and the volume of its contents; a variety of conditions that either decrease the area of the tunnel[48,52,57,90] (e.g., traumatic deformity) or increase its contents[5,12,53,68] (e.g., flexor tenosynovitis) may result in increased pressure on the median nerve[91] (Table 1).

Physiological Disorders

In addition to its anatomic basis, CTS is also frequently associated with an underlying systemic or physiological disorder.[37,38] Indeed, CTS often is a symptom of another disorder, management of which may be important in treating the CTS. The term "idiopathic carpal tunnel syndrome" simply indicates that the diagnostician has not yet identified the pathologic process.

For convenience, we have grouped the commonest physiological correlates of CTS into three categories: neuropathic conditions, inflammatory conditions, and alterations of fluid balance (Table 1).

Occurrence of CTS in a patient with a generalized peripheral neuropathy or a more proximal lesion of the median nerve has been termed the "double crush syndrome."[69] In these cases, compromised function of the median nerve proximally lowers the threshold for symptomatic compression at the wrist, so that pressures that would be readily tolerated in a normal nerve become symptomatic of CTS in an affected nerve. Diabetic neuropathies may act in such a fashion. Phalen found that 14.5% of patients in his CTS series had associated diabetes and another 10% had a family history of diabetes.[72]

Inflammatory conditions may incite CTS by causing hypertrophy of the tendon sheath. Ya-

TABLE 1. Factors in the Pathogenesis of Carpal Tunnel Syndrome

I. Anatomy
   A. Decreased size of carpal tunnel
      1. Bony abnormalities of the carpal bones
      2. Thickened transverse carpal ligament
      3. Acromegaly
   B. Increased contents of canal
      1. Neuroma
      2. Lipoma
      3. Myeloma
      4. Abnormal muscle bellies
      5. Persistent median artery (thrombosed or patent)
      6. Hypertrophic synovium
      7. Distal radius fracture callus
      8. Posttraumatic osteophytes
      9. Hematoma (hemophilia, anticoagulation therapy)
II. Physiology
   A. Neuropathic conditions
      1. Diabetes
      2. Alcoholism
      3. Proximal lesion of median nerve (double crush syndrome)
   B. Inflammatory conditions
      1. Tenosynovitis
      2. Rheumatoid arthritis
      3. Infection
      4. Gout
   C. Alterations of fluid balance
      1. Pregnancy
      2. Eclampsia
      3. Myxedema
      4. Long-term hemodialysis
      5. Horizontal position and muscle relaxation (sleep)
      6. Raynaud's disease
      7. Obesity
III. Position and use of the wrist
   A. Repetitive flexion/extension (manual labor)
   B. Repetitive forceful squeezing and release of a tool, or repetitive forceful torsion of a tool
   C. Finger motion with the wrist extended
      1. Typing
      2. Playing many musical instruments
   D. Weight-bearing with the wrist extended
      1. Paraplegia
      2. Long-distance bicycling
   E. Immobilization with the wrist flexed, ulnarly deviated
      1. Casting after Colles fracture
      2. Awkward sleep position

maguchi et al.[94] found a frequent correlation of CTS with either a nonspecific tenosynovitis or an associated rheumatic condition. Lipscomb reported that more than half of his CTS patients had tenosynovitis.[53] Phalen observed thickening of the flexor synovialis in 203 of 212 operated hands.[72] Infection, either acute or chronic and low-grade, or even gout may trigger an inflammatory reaction of the tenosynovium, leading to CTS.[64] Rheumatoid arthritis commonly causes flexor tenosynovitis, as can scleroderma and dermatomyositis, which may result in CTS.[14,39,74]

Patency of the neural vessels depends on maintaining a pressure gradient between the blood and the surrounding extravascular tissues. Conditions that elevate the pressure of extravascular fluids may thereby decrease the transmural pressure gradient below the threshold for vessel collapse, leading to impaired nerve function.[24,27,54,84] Edema caused by pregnancy, is one such condition.[8,32,46,63,67,73,78,89] The converse is a condition in which blood pressure is lowered, thereby decreasing transmural pressure of the vessels. Perhaps the commonest fluid imbalance causing an episode of CTS occurs in sleep, when horizontal position, decreased heart rate, and muscle relaxation combine to elevate extravascular fluid pressure and decrease blood pressure simultaneously. This, combined with an awkward wrist position, may underlie the nearly universal worsening of CTS symptoms at night.

Patterns of Hand Activity

Abnormal anatomy or physiological disorders may not in themselves produce symptoms of CTS but, rather, may create a predisposition for symptomatic episodes that are triggered by certain kinds of activity. As early as 1947, direct measurements demonstrated that both flexion and extension of the wrist elevate pressure of extravascular fluid in the carpal tunnel.[10] Repetitive motions involving wrist flexion/extension and ulnar deviation, particularly when combined with application of force to a tool, may elicit symptoms of CTS. Because such activity is often inherent in performing a job, CTS has come to be known as an occupational disease.

Whether a repetitive motion can be said to "cause" CTS is an important issue; liability for workers' compensation settlements may hinge on this point. We agree with Phalen that "an occupation may aggravate, but seldom produces, a carpal tunnel syndrome." Support for this belief derives from the observation that CTS is frequently bilateral or occurs unilaterally in the nondominant hand, even if the occupation stresses only the dominant hand. In a study of 471 industrial workers in Oregon, Nathan et al.[60] found no correlation between occurrence of CTS and either type of occupational hand activity or length of employment. Nonetheless, certain occupations, such as meat packing, have a very high incidence of CTS, and occupation cannot at this point be ruled out as a primary cause.[56] In a presumed case of occupational CTS, the physician should be persistent in seeking the underlying pathologic process, treatment of which may be the key to managing the CTS. At the same time, the patient's right to workers' compensation should not be jeopardized by refusal to admit the possibility of a primary occupational cause. The field of ergonomics is developing rapidly, and ergonomic analysis of the patient's workstation may provide evidence of the role of job-related motions in the development of the CTS.

CLASSIFICATION

CTS may be acute or chronic, and the chronic condition may be subdivided into early, intermediate, and advanced.[29] Acute CTS is relatively uncommon; it usually results from trauma and is heralded by rapid and intense development of symptoms.[6,30,52,57] Casting of Colles fractures with the wrist in flexion and ulnar deviation is the commonest cause. Fractures or dislocations of the carpals or metacarpals have also precipitated acute CTS,[90] as have bleeding in hemophiliacs or patients on anticoagulation therapy, villonodular synovitis,[15] and thrombosis of a persistent median artery.[75] Acute CTS, which is analogous to an acute compartment syndrome, requires careful monitoring; if it does not resolve within a few hours, urgent surgical release should be considered.

Acute CTS must be distinguished from an acute episode of carpal tunnel symptoms resulting from overuse of the hand in an unaccustomed activity. Such an episode may be seen in the "weekend warrior" who paints his house, pulls weeds in the garden for 8 hours, or undertakes a marathon session of fly fishing. The sudden and prolonged use of the untrained extremity may cause acute symptoms of CTS that usually resolve with rest.

Early chronic CTS has findings of intermittent pain and paresthesias in the distribution of the median nerve in the hand, typically at night or after a specific activity. Sensory latencies are more likely to be prolonged than are motor latencies. Morphological changes of the nerve are absent. The underlying pathophysiology at this stage is considered to be transient epineural ischemia and impaired axonal transport, which are readily reversible.[83] These patients frequently respond well to conservative treatment of splinting and steroid injections or to modification of a precipitating activity.

In chronic CTS, paresthesias and numbness are constant. Sensory threshold testing values are elevated, and distal motor latencies are increased. The associated pathologic process involves persistent impairment of intraneural microcirculation, as well as epineural and intrafascicular edema. Conservative measures are unlikely to produce lasting improvement in these patients, and division of the transverse carpal ligament is usually the most effective therapy.[21]

Advanced chronic CTS has findings of permanent loss of sensory and motor function, as well as thenar muscle atrophy. Sensory and electrodiagnostic tests are abnormal. Long-standing endoneurial edema may have caused fibrosis of the nerves, as well as partial de-myelination and axonal degeneration.[80] Conservative treatment is ineffective. Most patients achieve partial to nearly complete resolution of symptoms after surgical release of the carpal tunnel, but some experience no relief from surgery.[40]

PHYSICAL FINDINGS AND DIAGNOSTIC WORKUP

Diagnosis of CTS comprises two parts: verification of a compressive disorder of the median nerve at the wrist, and elucidation of the underlying cause. Confirmation of the neuropathy is based on a careful history, on the patient's symptoms, on electrophysiological tests, and on sensory and provocative tests. The symptoms, as already mentioned, affect the distribution of the median nerve in the hand. Sensory symptoms typically develop before any motor involvement. Sensory symptoms may present initially in only one finger, later spreading to the rest of the distribution of the median nerve.

Although the wrist is the most frequent site of compression of the median nerve, more proximal lesions must be considered. These may be associated with a cervical rib, degenerative disc disease in the cervical spine, aberrant scalenus muscle, fracture of the clavicle, compression at the ligament of Struthers, and various fascial bands and muscle insertions through which the median nerve passes.[33] A careful history and physical examination usually distinguish among these. It is not uncommon for a proximal lesion of the median nerve to coexist with a compressive lesion at the wrist. In these cases, operative release of the flexor retinaculum at the wrist may fail to alleviate the CTS symptoms completely.

Routinely anteroposterior (AP) and lateral radiographs are obtained to look for malunited fractures or calcifications or other wrist disorders. If any abnormality is seen, an additional carpal tunnel view is obtained.

Recently, computed tomography (CT) of the wrist has been used in diagnosis of CTS.[17,41,45] On the CT scan a thickened flexor tendon or flattening or distortion of the median nerve itself can be recognized. On a routine basis, we have not found CT or magnetic resonance imaging (MRI) to be useful or necessary in the management of CTS.

When impairment of the median nerve is verified, an associated condition is considered. The patient may be worked up for possible diabetes, rheumatoid condition, hypothyroidism, coagulopathy, gout, or peripheral neuropathy. A careful history may identify particular activities that exacerbate the symptoms; modification of these activities would be an early part of conservative treatment.

Tests Of Sensibility

Tests of sensibility are of two types: innervation density tests and threshold tests.[27,86] Innervation density tests measure the innervation in multiple overlapping peripheral receptor fields and are highly dependent on cortical integration. They may remain normal even with moderately advanced nerve dysfunction. The Weber static or moving two-point discrimination test is the best known of the innervation density tests. Whereas two-point discrimination is often of little value in diagnosis of early or moderate CTS, it may confirm the other obvious symptoms in advanced and chronic cases. Two-point discrimination greater than 6 mm is considered abnormal in the hand (Fig. 1).

Threshold tests of sensibility evaluate a single nerve fiber innervating a receptor or group of receptor cells.[42–44] Such tests are considerably more sensitive than innervation density tests in detecting slight, early impairment of peripheral nerve function.[28,86] Perhaps easiest to use of the threshold tests is the Von Frey pressure test using the Semmes-Weinstein monofilaments, a series of nylon filaments of different diameters. The monofilament is applied perpendicularly to the palmar side of the digit, and pressure is increased until the filament begins to bow. Thicker filaments require greater pressure to bend, and each filament is marked with a number representing the logarithm of 10 times the force (in milligrams) required to bow the monofilament. The test is considered positive when the patient (with eyes closed) can identify which finger has been touched. It is performed on each digit of both hands so that comparisons can be made between the median and ulnar nerves. A value of 2.83 or less is considered normal (Fig. 2).

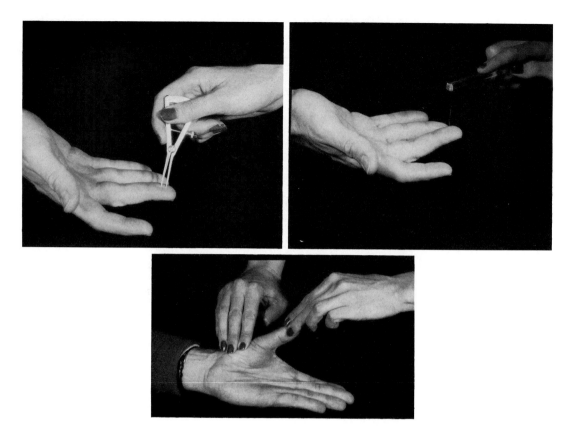

FIGURE 1 (top left). The Weber two-point discrimination test is done with blunt eye calipers or a paper clip. Pressure is applied in the longitudinal axis of the digit until the finger blanches. The distance perceived between the two points is then measured. Normal two-point discrimination is less than 6 mm. (Reproduced with permission from Szabo, RM: Carpal tunnel syndrome. In Szabo RM (ed): Nerve Compression Syndromes: Diagnosis and Treatment. Thorofare, NJ, Slack, 1989.)

FIGURE 2 (top right). Von Frey pressure test is done with Semmes-Weinstein monofilaments. The monofilament is applied perpendicularly to the palmar digital surface, and pressure is increased until the monofilament begins to bend. The response is considered positive when the patient, with eyes closed, can localize verbally which digit received pressure. (Reproduced with permission from Szabo, RM: Carpal tunnel syndrome. In Szabo RM (ed): Nerve Compression Syndromes: Diagnosis and Treatment. Thorofare, NJ, Slack, 1989.)

FIGURE 3 (bottom). The manual test of the abductor pollicis brevis. The thumb is placed in full palmar abduction, and the patient is asked to maintain this position. The examiner palpates the abductor pollicis brevis with one hand and applies downward pressure with the other hand. The strength of the muscle is then graded. (Reproduced with permission from Szabo, RM: Carpal tunnel syndrome. In Szabo RM (ed): Nerve Compression Syndromes: Diagnosis and Treatment. Thorofare, NJ, Slack, 1989.)

Koris et al.[50] have noted that this test may be more sensitive when the wrist is held in passive flexion for 1 minute before testing—i.e., when it is combined with Phalen's test.

Another useful threshold test in evaluating median nerve function employs a variable amplitude vibrometer operated at a fixed frequency of 120 hertz.[85] The vibrating head is held until the patient reports feeling vibration. The threshold is the voltage required to deliver a perceived stimulus. As with the Semmes-Weinstein monofilaments, comparisons are made between median and ulnar nerves of both hands.

In a comparative study of sensibility tests in 23 hands with carpal tunnel syndrome, Szabo et al.[86] found vibratory testing abnormal in 87% and Semmes-Weinstein monofilament tests abnormal in 83%, whereas two-point discrimination was abnormal in only 22%.

Motor Testing

The motor branch of the median nerve of the wrist comprises 6% of its total fibers. On inspection of the hand, the examiner should note the presence or absence of thenar atrophy. The strength of the abductor pollicis brevis is tested by placing the dorsum of the patient's hand on a table with the thumb pointing up toward the ceiling (palmar abduction). The examiner instructs the patient to resist his attempts to displace the thumb into the palm. The strength of the muscle is then graded (Fig. 3). One can test the opponens pollicis brevis by instructing the patient to resist attempts by the examiner to supinate the thumb while the thumb is maintained in palmar abduction. Any weakness perceived generally indicates significant muscle wasting and advanced disease.

Provocative Tests

Tinel's test is performed by lightly percussing the skin along the course of the median nerve from proximal end to distal end; the patient's report of a tingling sensation indicates the site of the compressive lesion. Phalen found a positive Tinel's sign in about 70% of patients diagnosed as having CTS.[72]

Phalen's test is performed by having the patient place his elbow on a table, hold his forearm in a vertical position, and actively but not forcibly place the wrist into flexion. If numbness or tingling in the distribution of the median nerve in the hand occurs within 60 seconds, the test is considered positive.

The tourniquet test involves inflating a tourniquet about the upper arm to above the patient's systolic pressure. If the patient reports paresthesia or numbness in the radial three and one-half digits within 60 seconds, the test is considered positive.

Paley and McMurtry[70] have described the "median nerve compression test." The examiner directly compresses with his thumb the patient's median nerve at the wrist. If the symptoms of CTS are elicited within 2 minutes, the test is considered positive.

Gellman et al.[31] compared provocative tests in both patients with electrodiagnostically proven CTS and control subjects. Phalen's test was most sensitive (71%), whereas Tinel's sign was most specific (94%). The tourniquet test was considered of no value.

Electrophysiological Tests

In applying electrophysiological and sensory tests, the patient's history must be kept in mind.

If symptoms are intermittent and appear only toward the end of an 8-hour shift at work, then testing early in the morning after a night's sleep may produce negative findings; it would be better to test the patient immediately after work at a time when the symptoms have been provoked. Similarly, if a typist or musician has symptoms only after an hour or two of activity, the likelihood of obtaining a positive test is increased by having the patient practice for an hour immediately before testing. Alternatively, a simple stress test just before electrodiagnostic measurements may increase the likelihood of an abnormal reading. Marin noted that placing the wrist in flexion for 5 minutes before testing elicited abnormal latencies in CTS patients who otherwise tested normal; this maneuver did not cause abnormal latencies in non-CTS controls.[55] With the aid of a work simulation machine, Braun developed a technique of provocative stress testing and concluded that it is useful and reliable in diagnosing very early chronic CTS, which he calls "dynamic carpal tunnel syndrome."[11]

In order to say that a measurement of nerve conduction is abnormal, we must have a concept of "normal" to compare it with. Four methods of comparison have been used.

1. Nerve conduction velocities can be compared with published population norms to see if the tested nerve falls outside the range of normal. Several caveats are in order here. First, electrophysiological testing is highly operator-dependent; the exact equipment used, type of electrodes, their placement, the testing environment, and the sequence of testing procedures all influence outcome, so that comparison to norms published by others may be unsound. Second, Nathan et al.[61] measured nerve conduction velocity of the median nerve in a large sample of normal people and found significant slowing with age, so that standards must be adjusted for age.[61] Finally, Wilson-MacDonald et al.[93] showed a diurnal variation of 6% or more in nerve conduction velocity of CTS hands, so that the timing of the tests must be standardized. Keeping these reservations in mind, distal motor latencies of more than 4.5 msec and sensory latencies of more than 3.5 msec may be considered abnormal.

2. Nerve conduction velocities of the median nerve may be compared with those of another nerve of the same patient; most commonly the ipsilateral ulnar nerve or contralateral median nerve has been used. Differences of

more than 1 msec for motor conduction or more than 0.5 msec for sensory conduction are considered abnormal.[9,49,92] Silver et al.[79] noted that 41% of hands with CTS also had abnormal electrodiagnostic results for the ipsilateral ulnar nerve. Bendler et al.[7] showed that CTS was bilateral in 61% of 440 patients. Of those who presented with unilateral symptoms, 38% had bilateral electromyographical abnormalities. The high incidence of generalized peripheral neuropathy in CTS patients makes a negative side-to-side or median-to-ulnar nerve comparison uninterpretable.

3. Different sectors of the median nerve may be compared with the "inching" technique of Kimura[47] or the antidromic versus orthodromic palmar technique of Escobar and Goka.[20] These techniques permit a particular segment with slower velocity (e.g., at the wrist) to be located. However, CTS does not always present with a discrete, site-specific reduction of nerve conduction velocity, and double crush syndromes may obscure the interpretation.

4. A specific test of the median nerve may be compared with the same test repeated on a different occasion. Although this practice may not permit differentiation between abnormal and normal, it allows the examiner to monitor progression of the disease or recovery after treatment.

We recommend measurement of median nerve conduction velocity on all CTS patients, chiefly for use in the fourth type of comparison. This establishes a baseline from which either progression of the disease or recovery after treatment can be monitored; it often is the only objective evidence of the effect of treatment.

CONSERVATIVE TREATMENT

The goal of conservative treatment is a functional patient. The symptoms of CTS are not necessarily eradicated, but they are ameliorated enough that the patient is able to accomplish his goals without undue discomfort.

The nature of conservative treatment depends on the etiology of the condition. If an underlying metabolic disorder, such as rheumatoid arthritis or diabetes, is contributing to the symptoms of CTS, then medical control of the disease is a first line of action.

If symptoms are provoked by a particular activity, modification of the activity should be tried. This may include eliminating the activity, decreasing its duration, or interrupting it with periodic breaks. A sympathetic employer may provide a rotation of work assignments to decrease exposure to overuse. In work-related cases, an ergonomic analysis of the workstation may lead to modifications of the job that diminish aggravating wrist and hand motions. Tools, especially those requiring the use of force while the wrist is flexed, may be redesigned with angled handles and appropriate grip surfaces to provide symptomatic relief. Even musical instruments may be modified, for instance by key extensions on woodwinds, to shift the placement of the hand away from a provocative position.[58,59]

In a workers' compensation case with equivocal objective findings, CTS may have a strong psychogenic component. An alienated worker in a hostile or boring work environment may have a very low threshold for perceiving disability, and he may be best treated by gentle guidance to a change in occupation.

Typically, conservative treatment in patients with mild symptoms of CTS begins with a trial of splinting the wrist in a neutral position and providing oral anti-inflammatory medications to reduce synovitis.

In the 1970s Ellis and co-workers[19] proposed that CTS may frequently be a sign of a subclinical pyroxidine (vitamin B$_6$) deficiency and that pyroxidine therapy would reverse the condition. Byers et al.[13] found that altered pyroxidine metabolic activity was associated with a generalized peripheral neuropathy that may lower the threshold for CTS; they did not comment on the possible value of pyroxidine therapy. It remains unclear whether an occasional patient with pyroxidine deficiency neuropathy (most likely in association with alcoholism) would benefit from pyroxidine therapy. As a specific therapy for CTS, vitamin B$_6$ should be considered unproven and unlikely to have widespread application.[2]*

Injection of steroids into the carpal tunnel provides relief in up to 80% of patients, but the relief is temporary.[25,34] A clinical study by Gelberman et al.[25] noted that only 22% of pa-

---

* Editor's note: Current investigations by Donald Ditmars, MD, of the Henry Ford Hospital, Philip C. Richardson, MD, of the Clayton Foundation, University of Texas at Austin, and the editor of this volume appear to indicate a place for vitamin B$_6$ in treating CTS. The use of combined vitamins B$_6$ and B$_2$ for the treatment of CTS is under study. —MLK

tients were still free of symptoms 12 months after the injection. Steroid injections were most effective in those with the mildest symptoms. Repeated injections are not recommended because the likelihood of a prolonged symptom-free interval diminishes with each injection.

The injection into the carpal tunnel is made with a 22-gauge needle 1 cm proximal to the distal wrist flexion crease between the palmaris longus and flexor carpi radialis tendons.* The needle is angled 45 degrees distally and dorsally, advanced until it touches the floor of the carpal tunnel, and then withdrawn 0.5 cm. Eight milligrams of dexamethasone acetate in 2 ml of 1% lidocaine is then injected into the carpal tunnel. A temporary block of the median nerve from the anesthetic confirms placement of the needle. Splinting the wrist in a neutral position for 3 weeks after the steroid injection seems to improve results.

Perhaps the chief value of splinting and injection of steroids is diagnostic. Short-term effectiveness of these modalities tends to confirm the diagnosis of carpal tunnel syndrome and also prognosticates a good outcome from surgical carpal tunnel release.[36] Failure of steroids and splinting to provide short-term improvement does not, however, prognosticate a poor outcome from surgery.

SURGICAL MANAGEMENT

Because surgical release of the carpal tunnel is an extremely effective, low-risk procedure, conservative regimes are of little value in cases in which CTS is clearly defined by history, physical findings, sensibility tests, and electrodiagnostic tests.[18] Indeed, when sensibility or motor disturbances are documented in addition to pain, the nerve should be considered to be in jeopardy, and surgical intervention is indicated. Conservative treatment may be recommended when the diagnosis is equivocal, or the symptoms extremely mild.[35]

Operative Technique

The carpal tunnel is approached through a curved, longitudinal incision paralleling the thenar crease and crossing the wrist crease obliquely in an ulnar direction at a point in line with the long axis of the ring finger (Fig. 4). The transverse incision should be abandoned because it does not provide adequate exposure, is associated with a high rate of incomplete division of the transverse carpal ligament, and increases the risk of injury to the motor branch of the median nerve. The transverse carpal ligament is divided on the ulnar side of the median nerve in order to avoid injury to the palmer cutaneous branch and the recurrent motor branch of the median nerve (Fig. 5). The antebrachial fascia is divided for 3 cm proximal to the distal wrist flexion crease. The contents and floor of the carpal tunnel are inspected for pathologic conditions. Tenosynovectomy is performed only when the synovium is extremely proliferative, as it sometimes is in a patient with rheumatoid arthritis.

Whether or not to perform internal neurolysis is often debated.[23,76] Proponents cite atrophy of the thenar muscles, loss of two-point discrimination, or both as indications for neurolysis. Those opposed to neurolysis claim that dissection of the epineurium results in increased scarring and strips the nerve of its blood supply, causing further damage.

We studied our own patients and found that while judicious internal neurolysis did no further harm to the median nerve, neither did it improve the results when compared with sec-

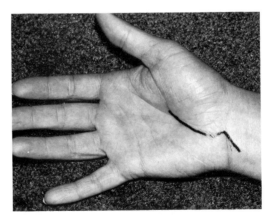

FIGURE 4. Surgery on the carpal tunnel is approached through a curved, longitudinal incision paralleling the thenar crease and crossing the wrist crease obliquely in an ulnar direction at a point in line with the long axis of the ring finger. (Reproduced with permission from Szabo, RM: Carpal tunnel syndrome. In Szabo RM (ed): Nerve Compression Syndromes: Diagnosis and Treatment. Thorofare, NJ, Slack, 1989.)

---

* Editor's note: The editor recommends injection to the ulnar side of the palmaris longus. —MLK

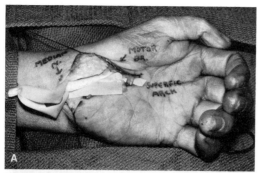

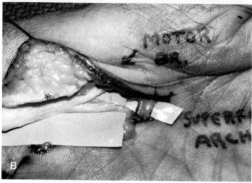

FIGURE 5. *A*, Release of the transverse carpal ligament and the anatomy of the median nerve as it courses through the carpal canal. *B*, Note the radial edge of the thick transverse carpal ligament (*). Also note the radial position of the motor branch of the median nerve and the proximity of the superficial arch at the distal edge of the transverse carpal ligament. (Reproduced with permission from Szabo, RM: Carpal tunnel syndrome. In Szabo RM (ed): Nerve Compression Syndromes: Diagnosis and Treatment. Thorofare, NJ, Slack, 1989.)

tioning of the transverse carpal ligament alone.[26,76]

Many patients with CTS also have symptoms of ulnar nerve compression at the wrist. Most patients can be treated with carpal tunnel release alone, and it is rarely necessary to explore and release Guyon's canal.[79]

Postoperative Course

Many patients have persistent pain in the palm after carpal tunnel release. The pain is not associated with neuroma, is poorly described in the literature, and is not well understood. Referred to as "pillar pain," it may represent a periostitis caused by altered mechanics after carpal tunnel release. On the other hand, it may be a form of sensitive scar with skin, palmar fascia, and transverse carpal ligament all healing in one layer. The pain eventually

goes away, but it may take 6 months to 1 year to completely resolve.

Persistent palmar pain and early recurrent symptoms in the workers' compensation patient have become an increasing unsolved problem for patient, physician, and industry. Standard carpal tunnel release without job modification and prolonged time off full duty often leads to failure. Endoscopic carpal tunnel release is being investigated as a new method of treatment. If the transverse carpal ligament can be safely and effectively released without creating a big incision and scar across the palm, the morbidity of surgery in the working patient might be considerably less. We now know that it is technically possible to perform this surgery,[1,16,65,66] and we await definitive study of its efficacy.

REFERENCES

1. Agee J: Personal communication.
2. Amadio PC: Pyridoxine as an adjunct in the treatment of carpal tunnel syndrome. J Hand Surg 10A:237, 1985.
3. Armstrong TJ, Castelli WA, et al: Some histological changes in carpal tunnel contents and their biomechanical implications. J Occup Med 26(3):197, 1984.
4. Armstrong TJ, Chaffin DB: Some biomechanical aspects of the carpal tunnel. J Biomech 12:567, 1979.
5. Backhouse KM, Churchill-Davidson D: Anomalous palmaris longus muscle producing carpal tunnel-like compression. Hand 7:22, 1975.
6. Bauman TD, Gelberman RH, Mubarak SJ, et al: The acute carpal tunnel syndrome. Clin Orthop 156:151, 1981.
7. Bendler EM, Greenspun B, Yu J, et al: The bilaterality of carpal tunnel syndrome. Arch Phys Med Rehabil 58:362, 1977.
8. Benz RL, Siegfried JW, Teehan BP: Carpal tunnel syndrome in dialysis patients: Comparison between continuous ambulatory peritoneal dialysis and hemodialysis populations. Am J Kidney Dis 11(6):473, 1988.
9. Borg K, Lindblom U: Diagnostic value of quantitative sensory testing (QST) in carpal tunnel syndrome. Acta Neurol Scand 78:537, 1988.
10. Brain WR, Wright AK, Wilkinson M: Spontaneous compression of both median nerves in the carpal tunnel. Lancet 1:277–282, 1947.
11. Braun RM, Davidson K, Doehr S: Provocative testing in the diagnosis of dynamic carpal tunnel syndrome. J Hand Surg 14A:195–197, 1989.
12. Butler B, Bigley EC: Aberrant index (first) lumbrical tendinous origin associated with carpal tunnel syndrome. J Bone Joint Surg 53A:160, 1971.
13. Byers CM, Delisa JA, Frankel DL, Kraft GH: Pyridoxine metabolism in carpal tunnel syndrome with and without peripheral neuropathy. Arch Phys Med Rehabil 65:712–716, 1984.
14. Chamberlain A, Corbett M: Carpal tunnel syndrome in early rheumatoid arthritis. Ann Rheum Dis 29:149, 1970.
15. Chidgey LK, Szabo RM, Wiese DA: Acute carpal tun-

nel syndrome caused by pigmented villonodular synovitis of the wrist. Clin Orthop Rel Res 228:254, 1988.

16. Chow JCY: Endoscopic release of the carpal ligament: A new technique for carpal tunnel syndrome. Arthroscopy 5:19–24, 1989.

17. Cone RO, Szabo R, Resnick D, et al: Computed tomography of the normal soft tissues of the wrist. Invest Radiol 18:546, 1983.

18. Cseuz KA, Thomas JE, Lambert EH, et al: Long-term results of operation for carpal tunnel syndrome. Mayo Clin Proc 41:232–241, 1966.

19. Ellis JM, Folkers K, Levy M, et al: Response of vitamin B-6 deficiency and the carpal tunnel syndrome to pyridoxine. Proc Natl Acad Sci 79:7494, 1982.

20. Escobar PL, Goka RS: Carpal tunnel syndrome: Palmar sensory latencies to third digit and wrist. Orthop Rev 14(10):49, 1985.

21. Eversmann WW, Ritsick JA: Intraoperative changes in motor nerve conduction latency in carpal tunnel syndrome. J Hand Surg 3:77, 1978.

22. Feingold MH, Hidvegi E, Horowitz SJ: Bilateral carpal tunnel syndrome in an adolescent. Ann J Dis Child 134:394–396, 1980.

23. Fissette J, Onkelinx A: Treatment of carpal tunnel syndrome: Comparative study with and without epineurolysis. Hand 11:206–210, 1979.

24. Fullerton PM: The effect of ischaemia on nerve conduction in the carpal tunnel syndrome. J Neurol Neurosurg Psychiatry 26:385, 1963.

25. Gelberman RH, Aronson D, Weisman MH: Carpal tunnel syndrome—Results of a prospective trial of steroid injection and splinting. J Bone Joint Surg 62A:1181, 1980.

26. Gelberman RH, Pfeffer GB, Galbraith RT, et al: Results of treatment of severe carpal tunnel syndrome without internal neurolysis of the median nerve. J Bone Joint Surg 69A:896–902, 1987.

27. Gelberman RH, Szabo RM, Hargens AR: Pressure effects on human peripheral nerve function. In Hargens A (ed): Tissue Nutrition and Viability. New York, Springer Verlag, 1986, pp 161–183.

28. Gelberman RH, Szabo RM, Williamson RV, et al: Sensibility testing in peripheral-nerve compression syndromes. J Bone Joint Surg 65A:632, 1983.

29. Gelberman RH, Rydevik BL, Pess GM, et al: Carpal tunnel syndrome: A scientific basis for clinical care. Orthop Clin North Am 19:115, 1988.

30. Gelberman RH, Szabo RM, Mortensen WW: Carpal tunnel pressures and wrist position in patients with Colles' fractures. J Trauma 24:747, 1984.

31. Gellman H, Gelberman RH, et al: Carpal tunnel syndrome: An evaluation of the provocative diagnostic tests. J Bone Joint Surg 68A:735, 1986.

32. Gilbert MS, Robinson A, Baez A, et al: Carpal tunnel syndrome in patients who are receiving long-term renal hemodialysis. J Bone Joint Surg 70A:1145, 1988.

33. Goldner JL: Median nerve compression lesions—Anatomical and clinical analysis. Bull Hosp J Dis Orthop Inst 44:199, 1984.

34. Goodman HV, Foster JB: Effect of local corticosteroid injection on median nerve conduction in carpal tunnel syndrome. Ann Phys Med 6:287–294, 1962.

35. Goodwill CJ: The carpal tunnel syndrome: Long-term follow-up showing relation of latency measurements to response to treatment. Ann Phys Med 8:13, 1965.

36. Green DP: Diagnostic and therapeutic value of carpal tunnel injection. J Hand Surg 9:850, 1984.

37. Grokoest AW, Dermastim FE: Systemic disease and the carpal tunnel syndrome. JAMA 155:635, 1954.

38. Grossman LA, Kaplan JH, Ownby FD, et al: Carpal tunnel syndrome—Initial manifestation of systemic disease. JAMA 176:259, 1961.

39. Herbison GJ, Teng C: Carpal tunnel syndrome in rheumatoid arthritis. Am J Phys Med 52:68, 1973.

40. Inglis AE, Straub LR, Williams CS: Median nerve neuropathy at the wrist. Clin Orthop Rel Res 83:48–54, 1972.

41. Jetzer TC, Webb AG: The use of computer assisted tomography in the analysis of carpal tunnel syndrome in VDT users and assemblers. Abstract for Cumulative Trauma Symposium, 1986.

42. Johansson RS, Landstrom U, Lundstrom R: Sensitivity to edges of mechanoreceptive afferent units innervating the glabrous skin of the human hand. Brain Res 244:27–32, 1982.

43. Johansson RS, Vallbo AB: Detection of tactile stimuli: Thresholds of afferent units related to psychophysical thresholds in the human hand. J Physiol 297:405–422, 1979.

44. Johansson RS, Vallbo AB, Westling G: Thresholds of mechanosensitive afferents in the human hand as measured with von Frey hairs. Brain Res 184:343–351, 1980.

45. John V, Nau HE, Nahser HC, et al: CT of carpal tunnel syndrome. AJNR 4:770–772, 1983.

46. Kellgren JH, Ball J, Turron GK: The articular and other limb changes in acromegaly—A clinical and pathological study of 25 cases. Am J Med 21:405, 1952.

47. Kimura J: Carpal tunnel syndrome: Localization of conduction abnormalities within the distal segment of median nerve. Brain 102:619–635, 1979.

48. Kinley DL, Evarts CM: Carpal tunnel syndrome due to a small displaced fragment of bone. Cleve Clin Q 35:215, 1968.

49. Kopell HP, Goodgold J: Clinical and electrodiagnostic features of carpal tunnel syndrome. Arch Phys Med Rehabil 49:371, 1968.

50. Koris M, Gelberman RH, Duncan K, et al: Carpal tunnel syndrome: Evaluation of a quantitative provocational diagnostic test. Clin Orthop 251:157–161, 1990.

51. Leslie BM, Ruby LK: Congenital carpal tunnel syndrome. Orthopedics 8:1165, 1985.

52. Lewis MH: Median nerve decompression after Colles's fracture. J Bone Joint Surg 60B:195, 1978.

53. Lipscomb PR: Tenosynovitis of the hand and the wrist: Carpal tunnel syndrome, de Quervain's disease, trigger digit. Clin Orthop 13:164–181, 1959.

54. Lundborg G, Myers R, Powell H: Nerve compression injury and increased endoneural fluid pressure: a "miniature compartment syndrome." J Neurol Neurosurg Psychiatry 46:119–1124, 1983.

55. Marin EL, Vernick S, Friedmann LW: Carpal tunnel syndrome: Median nerve stress test. Arch Phys Med Rehabil 64:206, 1983.

56. Masear VR, Hayes JM, Hyde AG: An industrial cause of carpal tunnel syndrome. J Hand Surg 11A:222, 1986.

57. McClain EJ, Wissinger HA: The acute carpal tunnel syndrome: Nine case reports. J Trauma 16:75, 1976.

58. Moore AE, Wells RP: Response of biomechanic correlates of cumulative trauma disorders in the carpal tunnel and extrinsic flexor musculature to stimulated working conditions. Abstract #256 submitted to 12th International Congress of Biomechanics, UCLA, 1989.

59. Moore AE, Wells RP, Ranney D: A system to predict internal factors related to the development of cumu-

lative trauma disorders of the carpal tunnel and extrinsic flexor musculature. Abstract #257 submitted to 12th International Congress of biomechanics, UCLA, 1989.

60. Nathan PA, Meadows KD, Doyle LS: Occupation as a risk factor for impaired sensory conduction of the median nerve at the carpal tunnel. J Hand Surg 13B:167, 1988.

61. Nathan PA, Meadows KD, Doyle LS: Relationship of age and sex to sensory conduction of the median nerve at the carpal tunnel and association of slowed conduction with symptoms. Muscle Nerve 11:1149, 1988.

62. Occupational Injuries and Illnesses in the United States by Industry. Bureau of Labor Statistics Bulletin 2130. Washington, D.C., Government Printing Office, 1982.

63. O'Duffy JD, Randall RN, MacCarty CS: Median neuropathy (carpal tunnel syndrome) in acromegaly. Ann Intern Med 78:379, 1973.

64. Ogilvie C, Kay NRM: Fulminating carpal tunnel syndrome due to gout. J Hand Surg 13B:43, 1988.

65. Okutsu I, Ninomiya S, Takatori Y, Ugawa Y: Endoscopic management of carpal tunnel syndrome. Arthroscopy 5:11–18, 1989.

66. Okutsu I, Setsuo N, Hamanaka I, et al: Measurement of pressure in the carpal canal before and after endoscopic management of carpal tunnel syndrome. J Bone Joint Surg 71A:679–683, 1989.

67. Ordeberg EO, Salgeback S, Ordeberg G: Carpal tunnel syndrome in pregnancy. Acta Obstet Gynecol Scand 66:233–235, 1987.

68. Oster LH, Blair WF, Steyers CM: Large lipomas in the deep palmar space. J Hand Surg 14A:700, 1989.

69. Osterman AL: The double crush syndrome. Orthop Clin North Am 19:147–155, 1988.

70. Paley D, McMurtry RY: Median nerve compression test in carpal tunnel syndrome diagnosis reproduces signs and symptoms in affected wrist. Orthop Rev 14:41, 1985.

71. Phalen GS: The carpal tunnel syndrome: Seventeen years experience in diagnosis and treatment of 654 hands. J Bone Joint Surg 48A:211, 1966.

72. Phalen GS: The carpal tunnel syndrome: Clinical evaluation of 598 hands. Clin Orthop Rel Res 83:29, 1972.

73. Purnell DC, Daly DD, Lipscomb PR: Carpal tunnel syndrome associated with myxedema. Arch Int Med 108:751–756, 1961.

74. Quinones CA, Perry HO, Rushton JG: Carpal tunnel syndrome in dermatomyositis and scleroderma. Arch Dermatol 94:20, 1977.

75. Rayan GM: Persistent median artery and compression neuropathy. Orthop Rev 15:89, 1986.

76. Rhoades CE, Gelberman RH, Szabo RM, Botte M: The results of carpal tunnel release with and without internal neurolysis of the median nerve for severe carpal tunnel syndrome. Orthop Trans 10:206, 1986.

77. Robbins H: Anatomical study of the median nerve in the carpal tunnel and etiologies of the carpal tunnel syndrome. J Bone Joint Surg 45A:953, 1963.

78. Schwarz A, Keller F, Seyfert S, et al: Carpal tunnel syndrome: A major complication in long-term hemodialysis patients. Clin Nephrol 22:133, 1984.

79. Silver MA, Gelberman RH, Gellman H, et al: Carpal tunnel syndrome: Associated abnormalities in ulnar nerve function and the effect of carpal tunnel release on these abnormalities. J Hand Surg 10A:710, 1985.

80. Sunderland S: The nerve lesion in the carpal tunnel syndrome. J Neurol Neurosurg Psychiatry 39:615, 1976.

81. Szabo RM: Carpal tunnel syndrome. In Szabo RM (ed): Nerve Compression Syndromes—Diagnosis and Treatment. Thorofare, NJ, Slack, 1989.

82. Szabo RM, Gelberman RH: Peripheral nerve compression—Etiology, critical pressure threshold and clinical assessment. Orthopedics 7:1461, 1984.

83. Szabo RM, Gelberman RH: The pathophysiology of nerve entrapment syndromes. J Hand Surg 12A:880, 1987.

84. Szabo RM, Gelberman RH, Williamson RV, et al: Effects of increased systemic blood pressure on the tissue fluid pressure threshold of peripheral nerve. J Orthop Res 1:172, 1983.

85. Szabo RM, Gelberman RH, Williamson RV, et al: Vibratory sensory testing in acute peripheral nerve compression. J Hand Surg 9A:104, 1984.

86. Szabo RM, Gelberman RH, Dimick MP: Sensibility testing in patients with carpal tunnel syndrome. J Bone Joint Surg 66A:60, 1984.

87. Tanzer RC: The carpal tunnel syndrome—A clinical and anatomical study. J Bone Joint Surg 41A:626, 1959.

88. Thomas JE, Lambert EH, Cseuz KA: Electrodiagnostic aspects of the carpal tunnel syndrome. Arch Neurol 16:635–641, 1967.

89. Voit AJ, Mueller JC, Farlinger DE, Johnson RU: Carpal tunnel syndrome in pregnancy. Can Med Assoc J 128:277–281, 1983.

90. Weiland AJ, Lister GD, Villarreal-Rios A: Volar fracture dislocations of the second and third carpometacarpal joints associated with acute carpal tunnel syndrome. J Trauma 16:672, 1976.

91. Werner C, Elmquist D, Ohlin P: Pressure and nerve lesion in the carpal tunnel. Acta Orthop Scand 54:312, 1983.

92. White JC, Hansen SR, Johnson RK: A comparison of EMG procedures in the carpal tunnel syndrome with clinical EMG correlations. Muscle Nerve 11:1177–1182, 1988.

93. Wilson-Macdonald J, Caughey MA: Diurnal variation in nerve conduction, hand volume, and grip strength in the carpal tunnel syndrome. Br Med J 289:1042, 1984.

94. Yamaguchi DM, Lipscomb PR, Soule EH: Carpal tunnel syndrome. Minn Med 48:22–33, 1965.

Chapter 27

CUMULATIVE TRAUMA DISORDERS AND COMPRESSION NEUROPATHIES OF THE UPPER EXTREMITIES

Linda H. Mosely, M.D., F.A.C.S., Roberta M. Kalafut, D.O., Paula D. Levinson, P.T., and Sue A. Mokris, O.T.R.

The return from your work must be the satisfaction which that work brings you and the world's need of the work.

W.E.B. du Bois—1958
in an address commemorating his 90th birthday.

Cumulative trauma disorders (CTD) and nerve compression syndromes, which are occupationally related, have an enormous socioeconomic impact on the injured worker. Some industries, i.e., poultry plant operations, have almost epidemic numbers of CTD and nerve compression problems.[1] This chapter discusses CTD with a specific focus on cervicobrachial disorders, compression neuropathies, and ergonomics pertinent to these conditions.

Cumulative trauma disorders are defined as "disorders of the nerves, muscles, tendons, and bones that are caused, precipitated, or aggravated by repeated exertions or movements of the body."[7] Injuries of the upper extremity are classified as acute or chronic. *Acute injuries* usually occur suddenly during a single event or accident. *Chronic injuries* such as CTDs develop over a long period of time and usually from repeated physical stresses.[7]

Ergonomics is the study of work and the workplace. The word is derived from the Greek words *ergos* (work) and *nomos* (natural law). The science of ergonomics had its beginning in World War II, when researchers began studying soldiers in order to improve the efficiency of the fighting forces.[10]

Ergonomics is an interdisciplinary approach composed of engineering, physiology, psychology, and philosophy. It revolves around a simple idea: Adapt the manmade world to man, rather than man to the manmade world. Ergonomics blends human characteristics with the living and working environment.[9]

Our discussion of pertinent ergonomics at the end of each section of this chapter highlights preventive measures and solutions for work-related CTDs and compression neuropathies.

From a historical perspective, in antiquity the Romans knew how to protect their reclining guests at receptions and banquets by having them place their elbows on special cushions called cubitales,[11] perhaps reducing cubital tunnel syndrome as a complication of Roman bacchanalia. Occupational disorders were not mentioned in the medical literature until the Middle Ages. It was left to the father of occupational medicine, Bernardo Ramazzini,[12] in the 18th century to describe work-related disorders in his book, *De Morbis Artificum Diatriba* ("Disease of Workers"). Ramazzini noted two causes for occupational problems:

> The first and most potent is the harmful character of the materials that they handle for these emit noxious vapors and very fine particles inimical to human beings and induce particular diseases; the second cause I ascribe to certain violent and unnatural postures of the body, by reason of which the natural structure of the vital machine is so impaired that serious diseases gradually develop therefrom.[12]

The Industrial Revolution that followed the Civil War in the United States profoundly affected the individual worker. Population shifted from rural areas to cities, and with the growth of factories, assembly lines came into vogue. Skilled craftsmen were replaced by machines run by workers performing repetitive, monotonous tasks.[4] Garraty, in *The American Nation*,[5] noted that when the Civil War began, the country's industrial output, while important and increasing, did not approach that of major European powers. By the end of the 19th century, America had become a giant among world manufacturers; its production dwarfed that of Great Britain and Germany. Conditions for workers, however, were frequently poor and sometimes deplorable. In *The Jungle*, published in 1906, novelist Upton Sinclair depicted the squalid working conditions in a Chicago slaughterhouse.[13] This novel, which could easily steer the reader to vegetarianism, marked Sinclair's conversion to socialism, and it also prompted the progressivist President Theodore Roosevelt to send inspectors to Chicago to evaluate the meat-packing plants. The resulting report was so shocking that Roosevelt orchestrated Congress's passage of not only a meat inspection bill, but also the Pure Food and Drug Act.[6]

To begin our study of the modern worker's propensity to develop CTD, it is instructive to consider a task such as **woodcutting**. Figure 1 (also reproduced in the frontmatter of this book) is a painting of a woodcutter at work, by the French artist Jean Francois Millet.[8] Because of its repetitive nature, manual woodcutting is a potential mechanism of CTD. Modernization

of saws has not completely eliminated the problem.

Work is an important part of daily life, but job stress and the repetitive nature of many tasks in modern industry are leading to CTDs, not to mention job frustration. Fortunately, today many companies are increasingly motivated to make the workplace a safe and pleasant environment, with a view toward prophylaxis of job-related ailments, among which CTD and compression neuropathies are prominently featured.[14]

This chapter concentrates on two main categories of CTD, (1) **cervicobrachial disorders** and (2) **nerve compression syndromes**, as outlined below:

   I. Cervicobrachial Disorders
      A. Myofascial pain disorders
      B. Cervical spondylosis
      C. Thoracic outlet syndrome
  II. Nerve Compression Syndromes
      A. Brachial plexus neuropathy-occupational entrapment
      B. Peripheral nerve compression syndromes
         1. Median nerve syndromes
            a. Pronator syndrome
            b. Anterior interosseous nerve syndrome
            c. Carpal tunnel syndrome
            d. Median nerve branch entrapments
         2. Ulnar nerve entrapment
            a. Cubital tunnel syndrome
            b. Ulnar nerve compression in the forearm
            c. Guyon's canal compression syndrome
         3. Radial nerve syndromes
            a. Radial nerve entrapment at the brachium
            b. Radial tunnel syndrome
            c. Posterior interosseous nerve syndrome
            d. Wartenberg's syndrome
         4. Multiple crush syndrome

CERVICOBRACHIAL OCCUPATIONAL DISEASES

In the years between 1960 and 1980, an epidemic of occupational cervicobrachial disorders was reported in Japan.[27,30,32] The initial reports of cervicobrachial problems were noted among punch card perforators in 1958, but subsequently the disorder was found to affect **typists, telephone operators, office keyboard operators**, and **process workers**. It was also seen

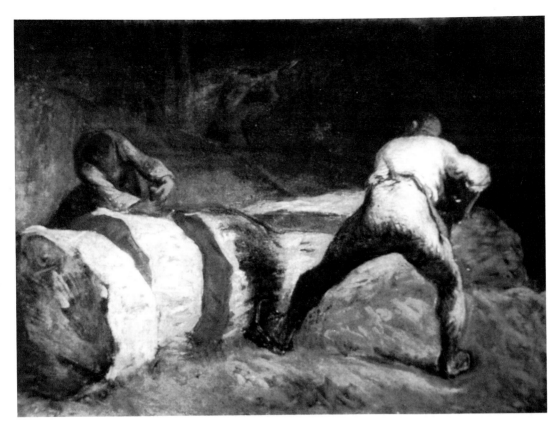

FIGURE 1. "Woodsawyers," by Jean Francois Millet (1850). Woodcutting is a repetitive task that can precipitate CTD and compression neuropathies. In the 1850s a simple saw was exclusively used to cut wood. Even today, power saws do not eliminate occupational disorders. (Reproduced with permission from the Victoria and Albert Museum, London.)

in **calculator** and **cash-register operators**, and in **packing-machine** and **assembly-line workers**. According to McDermott,[28] the problem became so widespread that in 1964 the Japanese Ministry of Labor set ergonomic guidelines for **keyboard operators**, limiting their workday to 5 hours and ordering 10-minute rest breaks each hour. Cervicobrachial disorders have been discussed frequently in the Scandinavian[23] and British literature,[16] and American industrial managers are beginning to heed the socioeconomic importance of avoiding neck strain in their workers.[14]

In a study of various staff members at the University of Hong Kong, back and neck problems were found to be more prevalent in the 31–40 age category and to have an increased incidence in the female sex.[19]

Myofascial Pain Syndrome

Cervicobrachial pain of mainly soft tissue or muscle origin has been termed myofascial pain syndrome (MFPS). A variety of terms have been used to describe MFPS, including tension neck syndrome, fibrositis, myalgia, and fibromyalgia. Travell and Simons[36] have defined a trigger point as a "hyperirritable spot, usually within a taut band of skeletal muscle or fascia, that is painful on compression and can give rise to characteristic referred pain, tenderness, and autonomic phenomena." Simons[34] has listed eight characteristics that identify a trigger point:

1. A history that identifies an activity or movement that has overloaded a muscle.
2. A characteristic pain pattern of muscles causing pain.
3. A restricted range of motion as a result of involved muscles.
4. Palpation of a tender trigger point causes the patient to "jump" or "wince" in pain.
5. A palpable taut band harboring the trigger point is found in the muscle.
6. A visible local twitch response (cutaneous reflex phenomenon) is elicited by application of compression or digital pressure to the trigger point.

7. Reproduction of pain upon palpation of the trigger point.

8. Semiobjective muscle testing reveals weakness or "give way" sensation secondary to pain.

Trigger points often refer pain to a well-defined, distant region. The referred pain from trigger points is described as "dull and aching, often deep, with intensity varying from low-grade discomfort to severe."[35] The pain can be elicited and reproduced by deep digital pressure of the trigger point. The painful areas of referred pain do not follow a peripheral nerve distribution or dermatome.[34]

Laboratory or diagnostic testing is unrewarding in MFPS. Sedimentation rate and muscle enzymes are usually normal. If a systemic illness (i.e., rheumatoid arthritis) is a perpetuating cause, laboratory testing may help identify the illness and aid in the resolution. Thermograms use the "cutaneous reflex phenomena characteristic of myofascial trigger points"[35] to measure skin temperature changes and thus help to document the trigger points, which often show up on a thermogram as "hot spots."

Myofascial pain syndrome can be perpetuated by a variety of etiologies. It often arises in disc disease, spondylosis, peripheral nerve entrapments, and—the most frequent cause—trauma. Chronic overloading of the muscle due to chronic posturing has been a mechanical cause of MFPS. **Computer operators, cashiers, slaughterhouse workers**, and **assembly-line workers**[33] have increased incidences of MFPS owing to the need for persistent shoulder elevation to complete the task. The worker frequently reports pain in the neck, upper shoulder, and mid-thoracic region. Palpation of the cervical paraspinals, upper trapezius, and rhomboids reveals well-defined trigger points.[34] Cilley has called attention to a condition he dubbed "intern's neck" or "house officer's headache"; it is probably a nuchal myofascial disorder that is more common in **interns** and **junior house officers** who carry heavy paraphernalia (training manuals, diagnostic equipment, and dressings) in their pockets. Apparently the condition is usually self-limited and tends to resolve as the medical trainee advances in rank and concomitantly lightens the loads carried in the white coat.[20]

In the worker with recurrent MFPS, an ergonomic evaluation is a must. The chair used must have adequate height so that the heels rest comfortably on the floor. Adequate room

should be allowed for the backs of the knees to clear the seat. The chair should have a backrest that is contoured to the normal lumbar lordosis. When prolonged arm abduction is required, as it is for **keyboard operators**, elbow support should be provided.[35] Finally, the overall body position and its relationship to the task must be evaluated.

Treatment. The cornerstone of treatment for myofascial pain syndrome is a well-defined stretching program of the muscles involved (Fig. 2).

A referral to a physiatrist and a psychologist for a comprehensive treatment plan is appropriate. The patient undergoes physical therapy consisting of the traditional modalities, the use of vapocoolant spray—"spray and stretch"—followed by a home stretching program. Simons[35] describes spray and stretch as the "quickest and least painful way to resolve a single-muscle trigger point" (Fig. 3A).

Injections of a local anesthetic such as Lidocaine into the trigger points followed by regular stretching have been beneficial in eliminating trigger points. In the worker who reports recurrent or persistent myofascial pain, other perpetuating causes must be sought. Perpetuating causes of MFPS include mechanical stresses, nutritional inadequacies, metabolic and endocrine dysfunctions, and chronic infection. Anxiety and tension in the worker may result in a state of constant muscle contraction with overloads and stresses. In these cases, in addition to physical therapy, a program of stress management, biofeedback, and a home stretching program may be beneficial (Fig. 3B).

Ergonomics. In sedentary jobs such as **data entry**, work stations must be adjustable to fit the worker. The screen work should be done with the neck in a neutral position. Telephone head sets should be used to eliminate cradling of the receiver between the ear and shoulder. Carrying heavy items with shoulder straps should be avoided if possible, or the strap should be removed at frequent intervals.[22]

Cervical Spondylosis

Cervical spondylosis (CS) may also play a role in perpetuating cervicobrachial pain in the aging worker. Often, patients with pain referred to the neck and arm have radiologic evidence of CS. Since CS is frequently silent clinically, the diagnosis is purely radiologic. Typical radiologic findings in CS (Fig. 4) are[24]:

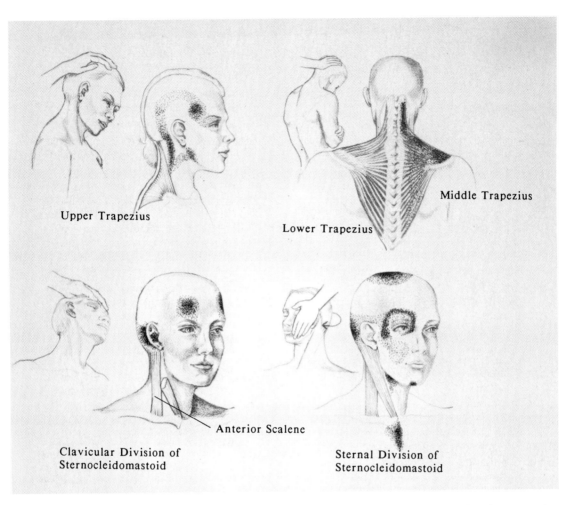

FIGURE 2. Trigger points for myofascial pain disorders of the neck and shoulder regions. Darkened areas are the actual trigger points, lighter areas are the zones of referred pain. Stretching exercises are diagrammed.

1. Intervertebral disc space narrowing
2. Anterior and posterior osteophyte formation at the vertebral body margin
3. Sclerosis of the bone beneath the vertebral endplate
4. Osteophyte formation adjacent to the neurocentral lip
5. Osteoarthritic changes in apophyseal joints with osteophyte formation
6. Narrowing of the sagittal diameter of the spinal canal

Weed[37] and Elias[21] have found an increased incidence of CS in the "second half of life" and universality of the condition after the age of 70. Hagberg and Wegman[23] found increased incidences of CS in workers exposed to high cervical loads. Occupational groups at risk appear to be **meat carriers, dentists, miners,** and **heavy workers** including **dock workers** and **iron founders**. Cervical spondylosis has also been

noted in rural Jamaica in those who carry heavy loads on their heads.[18] Understanding the pathogenesis in CS or chronic cervical disc degeneration may help to explain its increased incidence in some occupations. In a British study comparing the incidence of spondylosis in a group of coal miners and a control group matched for age, the onset of spondylosis was advanced by 10 years in the coal miners.[31] As the disc begins to degenerate owing to biochemical and biophysical alterations, the vertebral segment becomes mechanically unstable.[26] If the worker continues to place increasing loads on the disc (e.g., **meat packers**), the disc further degenerates, and disc space narrowing and osteophyte formation are seen. As the nerve root exits the canal, it may be susceptible to compression and hence a radicular picture emerges. Thus spondylosis may present with a clinical picture similar to acute cervical disc

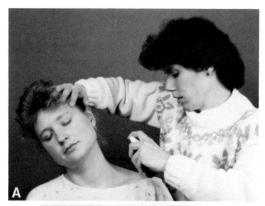

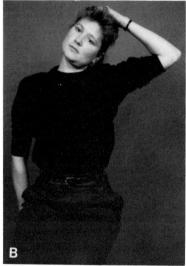

FIGURE 3. *A*, Treatment of myofascial pain disorders illustrating spray and stretch technique for the head and neck. *B*, Self-stretching exercises for nuchal myofascial pain syndrome.

herniation with nerve root impingement. Magnetic resonance imaging (MRI) has been useful in distinguishing between spondylosis and disc herniation.

Clinically, in CS, cervicobrachial pain has a more insidious onset. If lateral osteophytes are significant enough to cause nerve root compression, radicular symptoms may be present. Single or multiple nerve roots may be involved along with motor and sensory roots. Sensory symptoms of pain, paresthesias, hypesthesias, and hyperesthesias, typically predominate.[17]

On examination, pain is exacerbated by movements of the cervical spine. One must check thoroughly for spinal cord compression—i.e., positive Babinski and Hoffman's signs—as well as alteration of vibratory and position sense (posterior column involvement).

Treatment. Treatment is intimately tied in with ergonomics and prevention. Stress loads on the neck and shoulder areas of workers need to be reduced. Lighter-weight hats in mining occupations might be helpful. **Dentists** need to design their work situations to minimize stress on their neck and shoulder regions. Cervicobrachial pain produced from CS may respond to conservative treatment such as the use of a neck collar, heat, and traction.[25] Indications for surgical intervention are[25]:

1. Acute progressive signs of cord disease
2. Radicular deficit that does not resolve with conservative management
3. Intractable pain
4. Significant vertebral artery compression

The goal of conservative cervical treatment is to reduce the tightness of affected cervical muscles by removing stressors that can cause tightness. This can be accomplished by education about causative factors, in conjunction with therapeutic exercises and physical agents such as heat/ice, ultrasound, electrical stimulation, and massage. Job-site analysis as well

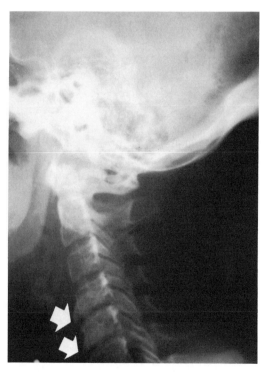

FIGURE 4. Radiographic example of cervical spondylosis. Note anterior and posterior osteophytes of the C4–6 vertebral bodies, with narrowing of the disc space and sclerosis (arrows).

as screening of home activities, hobbies, and posture are imperative.

Ergonomics. Ergonomics in myofascial nuchal pain disorders should be goal directed to design the work station to minimize conditions that cause shoulder and neck repetitive contractions. Adjustments of chair height in sitting workers or designing work tasks to avoid marked nuchal flexion or extension postures are advantageous in controlling the development of myofascial pain syndrome.[15,22,29]

Thoracic Outlet Syndrome

Thoracic outlet syndrome (TOS) is simplistically defined as a conglomerate of signs and symptoms related to a compression of the brachial plexus or the subclavian vessels at various points from the base of the neck to the axilla. The structures most at risk are the subclavian artery and vein and the lower trunk of the brachial plexus. Compression can occur in the interscalene area, between the clavicle and the first rib, and further distally, beneath the conjoined tendons of the coracoid process.[47] The thoracic outlet anatomically is defined as the triangular aperture bordered anteriorly by the scalenus anterior muscle, posteriorly by the scalenus medius muscle, and below by the first rib.[61] TOS is actually an "umbrella term" that encompasses a variety of clinical cervical rib syndromes, costoclavicular syndrome, hyperabduction syndrome, pectoralis minor syndrome, and effort vein syndrome.[55] TOS has elicited controversy because of the multiplicity of anatomic factors that can frequently cause nonspecific signs and symptoms. Adding to the confusion are the imprecise diagnostic tools available for evaluating this condition. Mackinnon and Dellon[50] believe that TOS represents primarily a brachial plexus compression of multiple crush-type lesions and that multiple sites of entrapment in a given region contribute to symptoms. They believe that a summation effect in TOS from multiple compression lesions may give symptomatic dysfunction. Roeder et al. believe that TOS is probably more common than is generally appreciated but that many people are asymptomatic even when physical findings are positive.[55]

William Harvey first described a patient with signs and symptoms compatible with TOS in *De Motu Cordis* in 1627.[45] In 1821 Sir A. Cooper[42] described a patient with a compression of the subclavian artery that resulted in vascular ischemic symptoms and signs, with "gangrenous spots" on the patient's hands. Coote[43] apparently performed the first decompression operative procedure in 1861. Thomas Murphy[51] in 1910 removed a normal first rib to relieve a patient's neurovascular symptoms. Stopford and Telford[60] and Brickner,[40] in the second and third decades of this century favored first-rib resection, and Roos[56,57] has subsequently supported first-rib resection. Roos has called attention to the fact that the first or uppermost rib forms one limb of a vise that compresses the neurovascular supraclavicular structures. The second limb of that vise can be a variety of anatomic structures. Roos[56,57] favored a transaxillary resection of the first rib, and Clagett[41] a posterior thoracoplasty approach as a decompressive procedure. Scalenotomy was first described by Adson and Coffey in 1927,[39] but the procedure fell into disfavor in the 1940s as the sole decompressive operation for TOS. It was not until 1956 that Peet et al.[53] pulled together the multiple syndromes used to describe the brachial plexus and neurovascular entrapments under one category, "thoracic outlet syndrome." Clinicians are still struggling with diagnostic and treatment modalities for TOS. For clarity in this potentially confusing condition, the clinician can refer to Sallstrom and Schmidt's[33] criteria for neurovascular compression in the thoracic outlet:

A. Symptoms and signs of brachial plexus compression—thoracic outlet
   1. *Mild compression—brachial plexus at the thoracic outlet*: Positional paresthesias and numbness on prolonged arm elevation.
   2. *Moderate compression—brachial plexus in the thoracic outlet*: Positional paresthesias and numbness together with specific muscle weakness and dysfunction.
   3. *Pronounced compression—Brachial plexus in the thoracic outlet*: Constant paresthesias, numbness, and pain in combination with muscle weakness and dysfunction of the hands.
B. Symptoms and signs of arterial compression at the thoracic outlet. Ischemic pallor of the hand and coolness and pain in the arm.
C. Symptoms and signs of venous compression at the thoracic outlet. Swelling, cyanosis, and engorgement of the superficial veins across the shoulder.

Stewart has categorized TOS into three categories[59]:

A. Neurological TOS: an uncommon focal compressive lesion producing isolated neurological symptoms.

B. Vascular TOS: a rare, isolated compressive lesion of the subclavian artery.

C. Syndrome of pain and sensory symptoms in the arm without muscle wasting or vascular symptoms: the most common TOS. We prefer Mackinnon and Dellon's[50] description of this group, which can demonstrate either neurological or vascular signs and symptoms or a combination of both. They believe it to be a "multiple crush" type of lesion of the brachial plexus (usually the lower trunk), but there may be a vascular component due to a compressive lesion of the subclavian artery.

Neurological Thoracic Outlet Syndrome

Stewart[59] describes this first category of TOS (Fig. 5A) as more common in women. It frequently presents with paresthesias along the inner aspect of the arm and may later be associated with weakness and wasting in the abductor pollicis brevis muscle and, later still, in the intrinsic musculature of the hand (thenar wasting). Radiographically there may be an elongated transverse process of C7 associated with a rudimentary cervical rib. There is a fibrous band with this lesion and the C8–T1 ventral rami of the lower trunk of the brachial plexus are stretched and angulated over this band.

Electromyography. Abnormalities are seen in muscles supplied by the lower trunk of the brachial plexus. Electromyography (EMG) of the paraspinal muscles is useful to distinguish a lesion of the spinal roots from one involving the lower trunk.

According to Wilbourn,[62] true neurogenic TOS has a distinctive electrodiagnostic picture. Changes in amplitudes of the ulnar sensory and median motor responses are the best aids in diagnosis. Reduction in amplitudes reflects "chronic axon loss occurring along the lower trunk of the brachial plexus,"[62] the area most involved with TOS. F waves are sometimes slowed and are of little help in localizing the lesion.

Treatment. Neurological TOS is a treatable surgical lesion. The operative procedure involves division of the fibrous band through a supraclavicular approach. Long-term follow-up shows that even if the wasting and weakness do not significantly improve, at least they will not worsen.[59]

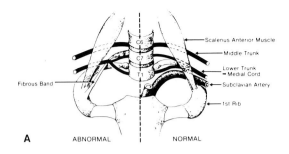

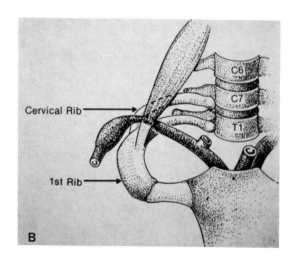

FIGURE 5. *A,* Drawing showing the normal anatomical relationships of the first rib, lower trunk, and medial cord of the brachial plexus, subclavian artery, and scalenus anterior muscle at the thoracic outlet. On the other side is depicted a small, pointed cervical rib and the fibrous band that arises from the tip of the rib to attach to the first rib. The lower trunk of the brachial plexus is angulated over this band. This abnormality can result in the neurological thoracic outlet syndrome. *B,* Drawing of the thoracic outlet showing the presence of a well-developed cervical rib. The subclavian artery is angulated over this rib and wedged between it and the scalenus anterior muscle, causing stenosis and poststenotic dilatation. This is the abnormality that produces the rare vascular thoracic outlet syndrome. (From Stewart JD: Focal Peripheral Neuropathies. New York, Elsevier, 1987, pp 110 and 111, with permission.)

Vascular Thoracic Outlet Syndrome

Intermittent blanching of the fingers or the entire hand, sometimes associated with more severe ischemia of the digits such as gangrene; is vascular TOS (Fig. 5B). It results from a cervical rib producing stenosis and poststenotic dilation of the subclavian artery. The condition can lead to thrombi and embolization of the distal vessels of the hands and digits. A bruit may be present in the supraclavicular and axillary areas. Angiography confirms the diagnosis.

Treatment. Prompt treatment is indicated. Resection of the cervical rib, exploration of the subclavian artery, and resection of thrombi are done as indicated. Embolectomy of the occluded vessels may be necessary.[59]

Syndrome of Pain and Sensory Symptoms in the Arm without Vascular Involvement[59]

The third category of TOS patients is a "grab bag" of the remaining problems that are not "pure neurogenic TOS" or "pure vascular TOS." Stewart admits that this category of TOS patients may represent a mild or early form of neurological or vascular TOS.[59] These patients present with less clearly defined symptoms of pain and numbness. The symptoms are made worse by carrying heavy objects or by holding the arms in certain positions—for example, as in drying one's hair.[50]

Evaluation of Thoracic Outlet Syndrome

Mackinnon and Dellon[50] have devised the following protocol for evaluation of TOS patients.

Clinical historical data:

A. Aching pain, discomfort, or heaviness in the neck, shoulder, and upper arm region is followed by discomfort or numbness and tingling along the inner aspect of the arm.

B. Abnormal sensations may be felt in the neck or axilla, accompanied by neck tightness and posterior cervical and occipital headaches.

C. Sleeping in the prone position with the arms outstretched around pillows may produce nocturnal symptoms, but not usually the paresthesias seen with carpal tunnel syndrome.

(Raskin et al.[54] have found headache as a presenting symptom in 26 of 30 patients with TOS. They found a high frequency of neck pain.)

Physical examination findings of TOS:

A. Positive Tinel's sign is found over the brachial plexus beneath the scalene muscle.[52]

B. The hyperabduction test is performed by having the patient sit with the arms held at a 90-degree angle from the chest and the elbows flexed 90 degrees with the shoulders slightly braced. The patient opens and clenches the fingers for 3 minutes. With a positive test, the arms drop.[58]

C. Positive pressure, when applied over the brachial plexus posterior to the anterior scalene muscle, and when held 10–60 seconds, will *re-*

produce the patient's symptoms which *may* include numbness in the hand.

D. Elevation of arms directly above the head produces profound fatigue and discomfort in the affected upper extremity.

E. Increased vibratory threshold occurs. After provocative maneuvers, the patient perceives a vibratory stimulus only when vibration stimulation is increased.

Other Provocative Tests for TOS:

A. Adson's maneuver[38] for diagnosis of TOS in scalenus anterior syndrome: The examiner takes the patient's pulse and instructs the patient to hold a deep breath, extend the neck fully, and turn the chin to the affected side. In a positive test, the pulse is diminished on the tested side. Because the test produces 35–50% false positive results, it is nearly valueless.[50]

B. Costoclavicular maneuver[44,49]: The shoulders are drawn downward and backward by the examiner. The patient takes a deep breath and, as the costoclavicular space is compressed, the radial pulse is obliterated and symptoms may be reproduced.

C. Wright's hyperabduction test:[63] The patient is asked to place the arm above the head with the elbow flexed; symptoms are reproduced. The radial pulse may disappear, or a bruit may be heard.

TOS Incidence and Predisposing Factors. Women are more affected with TOS—female-male ratio is 5:1—and it usually occurs in the 20–40 year age category.[47] Predisposing conditions include underlying congenital fibrous muscular bands near the brachial plexus[47] and congenital rib. Leffert[47] points out that cervical ribs occur in 1% of the population and should not hasten a diagnosis of TOS; they are frequently incidental findings. Clavicular abnormalities, both congenital and post-traumatic, may be contributory factors.[47] The configuration of the female chest cage, along with the postural descent of the shoulder girdle and, in some cases, pendulous large breasts[46] may be contributory elements in TOS. Mackinnon and Dellon have found TOS commonly in long-necked women with drooping shoulders.[50]

Occupations in which Thoracic Outlet Syndrome Has Been Described. Assembly-line workers, painters, and plasterers who frequently work with arms outstretched are at a risk for TOS.[50] The syndrome has been described in the Scandinavian literature as an occasional finding among slaughterhouse workers.[23] It occurs more frequently in musicians[48] and has also been described in cash register operators and heavy workers.[23] Feldman et al. find welders and hikers who carry heavy loads at increased risk for TOS.[22] They also found TOS in a **crane operator** in whom repetitive abduction-adduction movements of the shoulder and arms resulted in hypertrophy of the subclavius muscle and pectoral muscles. They described TOS symptoms in a **bookkeeper** who abducted her right arm, extending it backward to reach a calculator repetitively during her workday.

Work-up for Thoracic Outlet Syndrome.[50]

1. Cervical radiographs and CT scan with contrast media.

2. Diagnostic nerve blocks to rule out other nerve lesions.

3. Work-up for shoulder bursitis.

4. Work-up to rule out specific peripheral nerve lesions.

5. Electrodiagnostic tests to rule out radiculopathy in peripheral nerve entrapment.

Treatment for Thoracic Outlet Syndrome.[50]

1. Once the diagnosis is established, conservative treatment is instituted for at least 6–12 months. Treatment is initially directed to strengthening the shoulder girdle muscles and injection of trigger points.

2. Resting of the involved structure.

3. **If surgery is required, the surgical procedure of choice is** decompression of the brachial plexus through a supraclavicular approach, with release of constricting compression points.[50] Anterior scalenotomy is done, including removal of any specific bony structures encroaching on the plexus. It is not always necessary to remove the first rib. This is a controversial subject.

NERVE COMPRESSION SYNDROMES: BRACHIAL PLEXUS NEUROPATHY

The brachial plexus is a network of nerves arising from the fifth through the eighth cervical and first thoracic nerve roots and is most commonly injured by stretch or avulsion injuries related to automobile or motorcycle accidents (Fig. 6).[64,78] However, occupational trauma can occur from stretch or direct compression. As the brachial plexus evolves—forming from medial to lateral as roots, trunks, divisions, and cords—there are potential anatomic compression sites, including the scalene muscles, clavicle, and first rib. The roots lie between the anterior and middle scalene muscle. C5, C6, C7 roots exit above their numbered vertebrae and the C8–T1 root junctures.

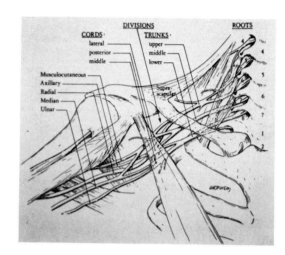

FIGURE 6. The anatomy of the brachial plexus relating the roots, trunks, divisions, and cords to the scalene muscles and clavicle. (From Mackinnon SE, Dellon AL: Surgery of the Peripheral Nerve. New York, Thieme Medical, 1988, with permission.)

The presence of Horner's syndrome suggests root avulsion at the origin of the plexus. Cervical sympathetic fibers C8 and T1 controlling oculopupillary action accompany the trigeminal nerve to the orbit. The ciliary nerve supplies Muller's muscle, and ptosis is caused by disruption of the nerve supply to Muller's muscle.[64,75] Thus Horner's syndrome is (1) miosis, (2) relative enophthalmus, (3) ptosis, and (4) anhidrosis.

There are two clinically important nerve branches from the nerve roots closer to the origin of the plexus. The first is the long thoracic nerve comprised of cervical roots of C5, C6, and C7. The long thoracic nerve innervates the serratus anterior, an important shoulder stabilizer, and injury to this nerve can produced a winged scapula (Fig. 7).

The second important nerve branch coming off the root is the dorsal scapular nerve, a branch of the fifth and sixth cervical roots, which innervates the levator scapulae and the rhomboid muscles. If the rhomboid and serratus anterior are not functioning, it suggests a root avulsion with no proximal nerve usable for reconstruction.[76]

Formation of Trunks.[75,76] Trunks lie in the lower part of the cervical triangle:

Upper trunk: C5, C6

Middle trunk: C7

Lower trunk: C8, T1

Another important nerve is the suprascapular nerve arising from the upper trunk of

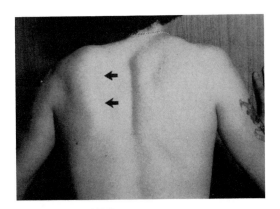

FIGURE 7. Example of a long thoracic nerve palsy resulting in winging of the left scapula due to weakness in the serratus anterior muscle. (From Mackinnon SE, Dellon AL: Surgery of the Peripheral Nerve. New York, Thieme Medical, 1988, with permission.)

the plexus originating from the 4th, 5th, and 6th cervical roots. The nerve courses deep to the trapezius through the bony suprascapular notch to supply the supraspinatus and infraspinatus muscles, the shoulder abductor, and the external rotator, respectively (Fig. 8A).

The nerve is susceptible to entrapment by either traction or compression at the suprascapular notch, as it is relatively fixed at this site by the superior transverse scapular ligament. **Backpackers**[22,67] or other types of workers that carry loads with straps about the shoulder may experience weakness about the shoulder girdle and difficulty abducting the arm. Typically there are no sensory symptoms in a suprascapular nerve palsy. Motor nerve conduction studies are helpful in demonstrating a slowing through the notch. Electromyographic examinations of the supraspinatus and infraspinatus muscles often display characteristic denervation (Fig. 8B).[74]

The lateral pectoral nerve (C5, C6) is a branch of the lateral cord and innervates the clavicular head of the pectoralis major muscle. Thus, if weakness of the clavicular head of the pectoralis major is present, it implies injury to the lateral cord.[76]

The medial pectoral nerve arises from the medial cord and, along with branches from the lateral pectoral nerve, innervates the sternocostal head of the pectoralis major. Careful examination of the pectoralis major muscle will be critical in localizing the injury at the cord level.

Level of the Division of the Brachial Plexus-clavicular Level.[75,76] The three trunks divide into anterior and posterior divisions at the level

of the clavicle. The cords are formed below the clavicle and have been termed the "infraclavicular plexus."

Formation of the Cords.

Lateral cord: The anterior divisions of the upper and middle trunks form the lateral cord (C5, C6, C7).

Posterior cord: The three posterior divisions unite to form the posterior cord (C5, C6, C7, C8, T1).

Medial cord: The anterior divisions of the lower trunk continue as the medial cord.

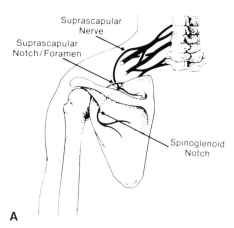

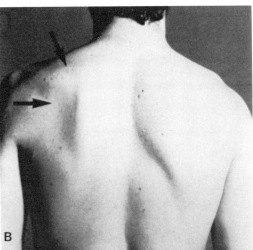

FIGURE 8. A, Posterior view of the left shoulder showing the origin and course of the left suprascapular nerve. (Reproduced from Stewart JD: Focal Peripheral Neuropathies. New York, Elsevier, 1987, p 110, with permission.) B, Injury to the suprascapular nerve (C5, C6) with wasting of the left supraspinatus and infraspinatus muscles (arrows). Note, prominence of spine of the scapula on affected side compared with the normal side. (From Mackinnon SE, Dellon AL: Surgery of the Peripheral Nerve. New York, Thieme Medical, 1988, with permission.)

Axillary Area—Transition of Cords to Nerves. The three cords are named to correspond to their position with respect to the axillary artery and are located just below the pectoralis minor muscle. Most of the branches of the brachial plexus originate from the cords.

Median Nerve. Formed by contribution from the medial and lateral cords. The medial cord contributes the innervation of the intrinsic hand muscles. The lateral cord contributes the sensory component to the median nerve.

Ulnar Nerve. Formed by a continuation of the medial cord after the cord gives a terminal branch to the medial head of the median nerve.

Radial Nerve. Radial nerve is a direct continuation of the posterior cord.

Axillary Nerve. This is the terminal branch of the posterior cord and it travels through the quadrilateral space (boundaries of quadrilateral space: above, by the subscapularis, teres minor, and capsule of shoulder joint; below, by the teres major, surgical neck of the humerus laterally, and the long head of the triceps medially).[80] The axillary nerve innervates the deltoid muscle.[81] It supplies a sensory innervation over the lateral deltoid region in a nondermatomal distribution.

Musculocutaneous Nerve—Lateral Cutaneous Nerve of the Forearm. The musculocutaneous nerve is a mixed motor and peripheral sensory nerve originating from roots of C5, C6, and C7 and the anterior division of the brachial plexus. At the level of the axilla, the nerve innervates the coracobrachialis (a flexor and adductor of the arm). It then travels deep and through the coracobrachialis, supplying the brachialis and biceps muscles (flexors of the arm). It becomes superficial after piercing the deep fascia of the biceps brachii muscle at the level of the elbow. From there on it travels obliquely as the lateral cutaneous nerve of the forearm, providing sensation to the lateral aspect of the forearm as the name implies (Fig. 9).

Brachial Plexus Occupational Injuries

Long Thoracic Nerve. This nerve can be injured by carrying heavy loads and individuals in occupations such as **furniture moving**[71] are at risk. **Backpackers** hauling heavy weights on their upper back and shoulders put the long thoracic nerve on stretch or set the stage for this nerve's entrapment.[72] Excess use of the shoulder has been implicated in damage to the

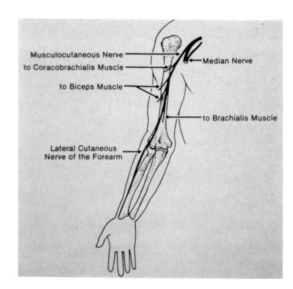

FIGURE 9. Anterior view of the right upper chest and shoulder showing the origins and course of the musculocutaneous nerve. (Modified from Haymaker W, Woodhall B: Peripheral Nerve Injuries: Principles of Diagnosis. Philadelphia, W.B. Saunders, 1953, with permission.)

long thoracic nerve, including activities such as **chopping wood**,[81] and when using the arm to control various machines.[66,79] Paresis of the long thoracic nerve causes a winged scapula (see Fig. 7).

Suprascapular Nerve. Injury to this nerve can occur from obvious acute shoulder trauma or from chronic pressure or inflammation in the shoulder region. It has been described by Feldman[22] in a **letter carrier** whose symptoms could be reproduced by pulling his right arm across the body, but not by raising his arm vertically. It was surmised that chronic pressure from the letter bag strap on his shoulders caused the patient's suprascapular nerve symptoms. It has been described in **students** carrying heavy school bags and in **cargo loaders**.[22,77] The most common complaint for suprascapular nerve entrapment is pain at the lateral and posterior aspects of the shoulder. An example of supraspinatus-infraspinatus muscle wasting in a suprascapular palsy is shown in Figure 8B.

Injury to Upper Trunk of the Brachial Plexus. This brachial plexus compression of the upper trunk was described in 17 **soldiers** in the U.S. Army who carried a "rucksack" in the Republic of Vietnam.[70] The rucksack was lightweight and had an aluminum frame and heavy webbed shoulder straps. The soldiers carried at least 40 lb of weight, and those who developed symptoms displayed muscle wasting similar to those with Erb's palsy. The muscles involved were supplied by the upper trunk of the brachial plexus, i.e., the biceps, deltoid, supraspinatus, and infraspinatus muscles (Fig. 10).

Musculocutaneous Nerve. This is a peripheral nerve, but it is included with lesions of the brachial plexus because it is more likely to be entrapped as part of the multifocal brachial plexus paralysis than as an isolated neuropathy.[81] Reported cases of isolated musculocutaneous nerve entrapment in the literature are usually the result of strenuous resistive exercise (Fig. 11).[69,73]

The primary site of entrapment in the arm is where the nerve travels through the coracobrachialis, thus sparing this muscle, an important point to remember in the differential diagnosis. Strengthening resistive exercise with the elbow flexed can lead to coracobrachialis muscle hypertrophy. It has been hypothesized that with the increase in muscle bulk or through a strong contraction, pressure ischemia-in-duced neuropraxia or, more serious, Wallerian degeneration can occur.[69] Cervical radiculopathy of the roots of C5 and C6 should be considered in the differential diagnosis. However, most helpful in establishing the diagnosis is electrophysiologic testing. In a musculocutaneous nerve root entrapment, there is no abnormal involvement of the cervical paraspinal muscles on EMG. Nerve conduction studies show a slowing of motor conduction velocity when compared to the "normal side."[74]

Lateral Cutaneous Nerve. Another common site of entrapment is in the sensory distribution of the nerve. As the musculocutaneous nerve travels on, it pierces the deep fascia of the biceps brachii at the elbow and continues on in an oblique fashion as the lateral cutaneous nerve of the forearm (see Fig. 9). The nerve is somewhat fixed as it pierces this fascia, hence rendering the nerve susceptible to compression injuries as seen in workers doing frequent elbow extension with the arm pronated.[65]

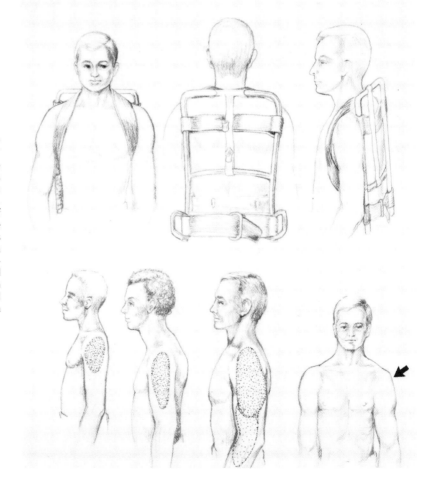

FIGURE 10. Top, View of the military "rucksack" without its load. Note the wide anterior shoulder straps conducive to compression injury to the brachial plexus. Bottom left, Distribution of sensory loss from moderate to severe in brachial plexus compression injury from a rucksack. Bottom right, Arrow indicates deltoid and shoulder girdle atrophy seen in longstanding brachial plexus compression from a rucksack.

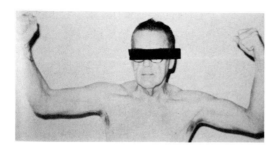

FIGURE 11. Example of a right bicipital atrophy from musculocutaneous nerve injury and persistent forearm dysesthesias (hatched areas). (Reproduced from Braddom RL, Wolfe C: Musculocutaneous nerve injury after heavy exercise. Arch Phys Med Rehabil 59:290–293, 1978, with permission.)

The patient frequently complains of pain over the lateral epicondylar region, which is often misdiagnosed as lateral epicondylitis. In addition, these patients have decreased sensation over the lateral aspect of the forearm. Electro-diagnostic studies can be of benefit in helping the clinician in evaluating this entrapment.

NERVE ANATOMY, PHYSIOLOGY, AND PATHOMECHANISMS FOR THE DEVELOPMENT OF NERVE COMPRESSION DISORDERS

In this section, the anatomy of peripheral nerve is discussed. The focus is on the mechanism of compression neuropathies and the underlying occupational contributory factors, which include repetitive trauma and stressful postural changes in the upper extremities.

Hippocrates (460–377 B.C.) gave us the first description of nerves.[104] Sir Charles Bell[104] (1774–1843) first attributed motor function to the ventral roots, and Magendie[104] (1783–1855) localized sensory function to the dorsal roots of the spinal cord. Remak[98] (1815–1865) recognized myelinated and unmyelinated (fiber of Remak) nerve fibers. Theodore Schwann discovered the cell as the building block of all living tissues. Ranvier (1835–1922) showed segmental interruption in the myelin sheath (nodes of Ranvier). Claude Bernard[104] (1813–1873) was the foremost physiologist of the 19th century, whose research on curare blockage of the neuromuscular transmitters set the stage for later work on synaptic and neurotransmitters. Silas Weir Mitchell (1892–1914) described clinical sequelae following peripheral nerve lesions in his classic text, *Injuries of Nerves*, based on examination of Civil War casualties.[104]

In the "modern era," as problems with nerve compression became more recognized and documented, researchers worked to find answers to the mechanisms of neural compression. Peripheral nerves are longitudinal structures composed of nerve fibers, connective tissue, lymphatics, blood vessels, and ectodermally derived specialized supportive cells.[104] To construct the peripheral nerve (Fig. 12), we start with the nerve cell body, the *neuron*, which is the functional unit of the nervous system. The neuron has much in common with other cells, in that it contains a nucleus, a cytoplasm, mitochondria, and a Golgi apparatus.[89] The *nerve axon* is an extension of the nerve cell cytoplasm, has neurotransmitting function, and is extremely long in length relative to the nerve body cell.[94,101]

The axonal neurotransmitting function is facilitated by neurotransmitter molecules and metabolic by-products that are carried retrograde to the nerve cell body. When a peripheral nerve is damaged at some point along its course, the clinical significance is that the transport system impairment contributes to nerve dysfunction.[101]

In this discussion, a nerve fiber is equivalent to axon and satellite cells.[104] The nerve fibers within peripheral nerves are either myelinated or unmyelinated. *Myelin sheath* is composed of lipoproteins and phospholipids and provides an insulatory membrane with a low electrical capacity for the axonal membrane, the axolemma.[104] The myelin sheath is formed from compacted layers of Schwann cell plasma membrane. There are small gaps called the nodes of Ranvier, which are important in the propagation of action potentials[101,104] in the neurotransmission process. The proportion of unmyelinated to myelinated fibers in a peripheral nerve trunk varies with the nerve function, but in most peripheral nerves, 75% are unmyelinated.[101] Within a nerve trunk, individual nerve fibers, whether myelinated or unmyelinated, are invested by a collagenous connective tissue, the *endoneurium*. Nerve fibers and their related endoneurial tubes are grouped in bundles called fascicles, with each fascicular bundle enveloped by another connective tissue layer, the *perineurium*.[101] The connective tissue outer sheath is called the *epineurium*. The epineurium may occupy up to 50% of the cross-sectional diameter of the nerve. This outer layer epineurium is contiguous with the *mesoneu-*

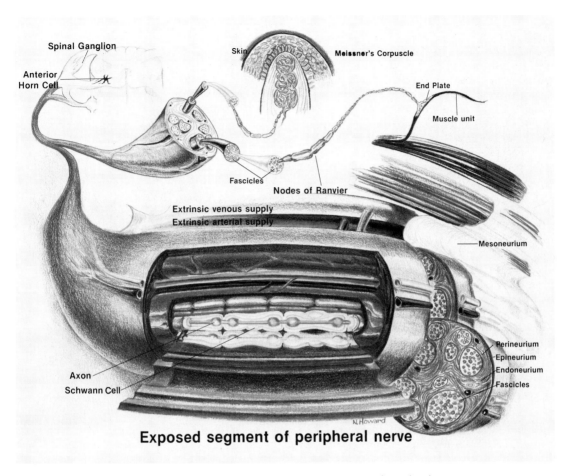

Exposed segment of peripheral nerve

FIGURE 12. Anatomy and cross-sectional appearance of peripheral nerve.

rium,[94] which is a suspending expansible mesentery containing the blood vessels, segmentally arranged. It is this same mesentery that allows the nerve to shorten and lengthen when adjacent joints go through range of motions. The expansible properties of the mesoneurium are lost when the nerve develops scarring related to repetitive trauma, and this process ultimately leads to focal neural entrapment.[101]

The blood supply to the nerves is extrinsic as well as intrinsic. There are large vessels found in the epineurium and perineurium, but only a capillary network exists in the endoneurial environment. Focusing on the blood supply, the endoneurial blood vessels, like those of cerebral vessels, are linked by tight junctions and constitute a blood-nerve barrier. It is this blood-nerve barrier that is permeable to sugars and may be important in diabetic neuropathies.[94] Additionally, the multi-lamellated perineurium has unique permeability properties. The internal milieu of the nerve fascicles is thus jointly controlled by the vascular endothelium and the perineurium. Trauma can cause the endothelial barrier to become "leaky," and when both endoneurial and intrafascicular edema increase, a compartment-like syndrome can develop. Thus, nerve compression can occur from within (inside out), as well as from outside in, as in external compressive forces.[94] Damage to these structures by ischemia, such as one can get with repetitive trauma, causes alteration in the endoneurial environment, which in turn interferes with nerve function.[94,101]

Stewart has nicely summarized and reviewed the pathomechanisms of nerve injuries. Nerves can be injured from *lacerations, external pressure, stretching*, or a combination of these damaging forces. Our discussion is on focal peripheral neuropathies. *Pressure* and *stretching* can be definite etiologic factors in CTD of nerves.[101]

External pressure may be applied abruptly, as when a nerve is crushed between a hard object and underlying bone. If the pressure is continued over time, one can get a problem such as the "Saturday night palsy"[101] from a pressure on the radial nerve. Underlying anatomic structures can also be a contributing factor causing nerve compression (i.e., fiber bands, scar tissue, abnormal muscles), or it can occur when a nerve passes through fibro-osseous spaces, such as the carpal tunnel. Resultant chronic compression syndromes are called *entrapment neuropathies*.[101] External pressure may also be applied repetitively over time and cubital tunnel syndrome can develop from habitual elbow leaning, as an example. Repeated manual injury resulting from external forces, such as holding a tool in a certain manner, or uncomfortable posturing of the body for long periods of time may cause chronic syndromes of nerve dysfunction. Nerve impingement can occur within a ligamentous bony tunnel. Other ischemic injury may occur by squeezing of the nerve between muscle edges during repetitive motion.[22] These are some of the mechanisms for nerve injury.

We now focus on the acute and chronic entrapment neuropathies. The discussion begins with acute nerve injuries. According to Stewart,[101] in acute compression myelinated nerves respond in three ways, depending on the severity and duration of the compression force:

1. Rapid reversible physiological block
2. Focal demyelination
3. Wallerian degeneration.

Acute Nerve Compression

Rapid Reversible Physiological Block. In acute nerve compression, when the neural response is a rapidly reversible physiological block, the patient has a familiar experience of the limb "falling asleep." The mechanism by which acute compression affects the peripheral nerve is not well understood, but both mechanical and ischemic factors have been implicated as the primary etiologies for nerve compression.[90–93,97,102] It is clear, however, that exceeding capillary perfusion pressure embarrasses the neural microcirculation.[102]

In both acute and chronic entrapment neuropathies, sensation is generally affected earlier than motor function and manifestations of motor involvement, i.e., weakness and muscle wasting are usually late findings.[83,88,103]

Use of Vibration Testing to Determine Decrease in Nerve Function Due to Acute Compression. It has been determined in numerous clinical and neurophysiologic studies that there is an important correlation between nerve compression and the large group-A fibers.[84,88] Light touch and vibration sensation are mediated through these group-A fibers, and the use of vibration testing has been shown to be a noninvasive technique to determine whether acute pressure is causing nerve dysfunction. Human volunteers have had wick catheters[95] placed in the carpal tunnel, and when pressures of 50 mmHg were produced in the carpal tunnel by a special external compressive device, changes in cutaneous vibratory thresholds occurred. Changes in perception of a 256 cps vibratory stimulus is one of the earliest signs of nerve compression.[102]

Sensory testing was performed to document a decrease in nerve function.[102] Static and moving 2-point discrimination remained normal until all nerve conduction ceased.[84] Then there was an abrupt cessation of all 2-point discrimination at pressures of approximately 50 mmHg.

Focal Myelin Degeneration. Focal demyelination produces weakness, sensory loss, and an electrophysiologically demonstrable conduction block that may last for days or even months. It is usually a mild compression of the peripheral nerve that results in focal demyelination at the site of compression. However, depending upon the amount of proximal axonal damage, conduction through the damaged area may be decreased and even severely compromised. Complete recovery may take anywhere from 3–10 weeks until remyelination has been achieved.[101]

Wallerian Degeneration. As acute nerve compression persists, or increases in severity, the peripheral nerve begins to lose its excitability to conduct, and a condition known as axonotmesis and Wallerian degeneration ensues. According to Mackinnon and Dellon,[94] Wallerian degeneration changes occur only in the myelinated fibers in the distal nerve segment beyond a zone of compression. In Wallerian degeneration, the myelin deteriorates and Schwann cells proliferate. Schwann cells then phagocytize the myelin debris. As a consequence, Wallerian degeneration begins to take place after nerve transection, and in severe entrapments all end-organs supplied by the nerve begin to exhibit the typical signs of denervation. Electromyographic testing will show marked fibrillations and positive waves. The degree of recovery can vary, depending on the extent of injury and the number of axons surviving.[101]

Chronic Nerve Compression

A number of researchers have delineated the pathophysiology of chronic compression neuropathies, including Lundborg,[92,93] Fowler,[87] and Mackinnon.[94] The diagrammatic schema (Fig. 13, abstracted from Eversmann)[85] shows an example of how repetitive flexion or prolonged wrist flexion in the carpal tunnel region sets in motion circulatory dysfunction that creates anoxic nerve segments and endoneurial edema, with resultant scarring and nerve compression.

Figure 13 shows that when the wrist is held in prolonged flexion, there is obstruction to venous return, resulting in slowed circulation in the epineurial, perineurial, and intrafascicular nerve complex. Anoxia of the nerve leads to dilatation of the small vessels and capillaries within the nerve segment, increasing the edema, which aggravates the effect of the original compression. The edema over a period of time sets the stage for fibroblastic proliferation and subsequent scarring that further restricts circulation and nutrient exchange.[85] With ischemic changes, connective tissue layers, and perineurial and epineurial thickening occur. Central fascicles are initially spared, but with progression of the ischemia and compression, either in degree or duration, diffuse fiber changes are noted (Fig. 14).[100]

Sir Herbert Seddon[99] classified acute nerve injuries in an attempt to correlate nerve injury with recovery and introduced the terms *neuropraxia, axonotmesis,* and *neurotmesis:*

Neuropraxia refers to nerve dysfunction lasting approximately one week to six months

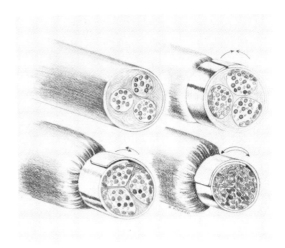

FIGURE 14. Schematic drawing of progressive peripheral nerve compression. Note the fibroblastic proliferation restricting circulation and the progressive thickening of the perineurium and epineurium. Diffuse fiber changes are also present.

after sudden blunt injury. The nerve dysfunction probably results from focal demyelination, hemorrhage, and changes in the vasa nervorum and the blood nerve barrier. The nerve dysfunction is seldom complete, and the condition is considered a conduction block, i.e., Saturday night palsy.

Axonotmesis is a physical interruption of the axons with an intact epineurium. These result from *crush* or *compression* injuries and recovery is variable. Upper arm injuries usually recover at a rate of 8 mm/day and more distal recovery at a slower rate, of approximately 1.5 mm/day.[94,101]

Neurotmesis is a nerve transection.

Pathology of Neural Entrapment. Normal peripheral nerves have a spiral series of transverse bands that are seen microscopically and are called the *bands of Fontana.*[86,94] These bands in the peripheral nerve are related to the nerve's undulating course and tend to disappear when the nerve is subjected to tension and stretching. The bands of Fontana usually return after appropriate neurolysis of the entrapped nerve. Also, Renaut bodies can be observed microscopically at neural entrapment sites in some nerves (Fig. 15).

Mackinnon and Dellon observed that these Renaut bodies do not represent normal components of a peripheral nerve but probably do represent a pathological response to traction or stretching. It is interesting that these authors have *not* seen these Renaut bodies in nerves

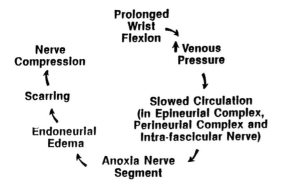

FIGURE 13. Pathophysiology of nerve compression as a result of persistent wrist flexion (with resultant carpal tunnel syndrome). (Adapted from Green DP (ed): Operative Hand Surgery, 2nd ed. New York, Churchill Livingstone, 1988, p 1424.)

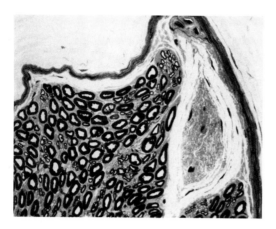

FIGURE 15. Transverse section of a Renaut body. This structure in the subperineurial space demonstrates an occasional cell nucleus in an amorphous connective tissue background. Toluidine blue ×500. (Reproduced from Mackinnon SE, Dellon AL, Hudson AR, Hunter DA: Chronic human nerve compression: A histological assessment. Neuropathol Appl Neurobiol 12:547–565, 1986, with permission.)

subjected to *direct compression without the association of repetitive motion and traction.*[94]

Figure 16 diagrammatically shows the common median and ulnar focal neuropathy sites.

MEDIAN NERVE COMPRESSION

The median nerve is a blending of roots of C5 through C8 as well as fibers from the first thoracic nerve. It is a union of the lateral and medial cords, and after it emerges from the axilla, it travels along the medial aspect of the arm in close proximity to the brachial artery. Upon reaching the elbow, the median nerve lies medial to the biceps tendon and the brachial artery.[125] The mnemonic MAT is helpful in recalling these anatomic arrangements, respectively, to the median nerve, brachial artery, and biceps tendons from medial to lateral in the proximal forearm,[125] just proximal to the lacertus fibrosis.[122]

The median nerve enters the forearm from the medial side of the cubital fossa by passing under the lacertus fibrosis and between the superficial and deep heads of the pronator teres. Although the relationship to this muscle and its superficial and deep heads is variable, the median nerve gives off branches supplying that muscle. The median nerve then goes on and pierces another muscle, the flexor digitorum superficialis. It then passes under the tendi-

nous arch connecting the humeroulnar and radial heads of the flexor digitorum superficialis, and courses distally in the forearm between the flexor digitorum superficialis and profundus muscles.[125] At this point the nerve divides, and one branch becomes the anterior interosseous nerve (AIN), which is predominantly a motor nerve coming off the radial side of the parent median nerve about 5–8 cm from the lateral epicondyle of the humerus.[122] The AIN supplies the flexor pollicis longus of the thumb and the flexor digitorum profundus of the index and middle digits, and the pronator quadratus. It terminates to supply sensory fibers to the wrist joint. The sensory component of the AIN may be a source of wrist pain.[107] The median nerve continues into the forearm. At a variable distance above the wrist the median nerve gives off a sensory branch supplying sensation to the skin of the thenar eminence. The main trunk of the median nerve continues on under the transverse carpal ligament and through the carpal tunnel, where it divides once again. Motor branches go on to innervate the thenar eminence and the first two lumbricales. Sensory branches usually supply the volar aspect of the thumb, index, middle and radial aspect of the ring fingers.[125]

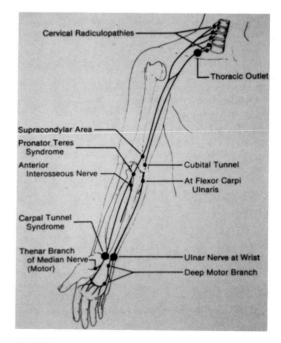

FIGURE 16. Common areas of local pathology for neural pathways traveling in median and ulnar nerves. (Reproduced from Chaplin E, Kasdan ML, et al: Occupational neurology and the Hand. Hand Clin North Am 2:517, 1986, with permission.)

Sites of Median Nerve Compression (Pronator Syndrome)

The four principal sites of median nerve compression in the proximal forearm (pronator syndrome)[85] are:

1. Distal one-third of the humerus, beneath the supracondylar process and the ligament of Struthers

2. Lacertus fibrosis (bicipitus brachii)

3. Pronator teres between the superficial and deep heads (by hypertrophy of the pronator or by aponeurotic fascial compression of the superficial surface of the deep head of the pronator)

4. Arch of the flexor digitorum superficialis (Fig. 17). Other less common anatomic entrapment sites include Gantzer's muscle.[115]

Pronator Teres Syndrome

The pronator teres syndrome (PTS) is the most proximal median nerve lesion in the

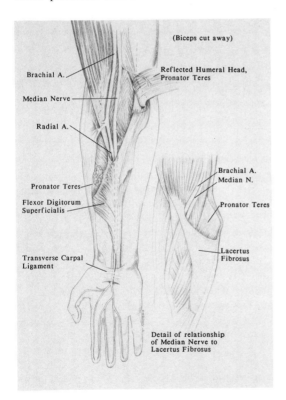

forearm and was described for the first time by Seyffarth in 1951.[121]

Symptoms. The only early subjective symptom may be aching in the proximal forearm. Other symptoms include easy fatigability and paresthesias and numbness of the thumb, index, and middle fingers.[121] Nocturnal paresthesias, such as one encounters frequently in CTS, are uncommon in pronator teres syndrome.[115]

Signs. A sign of PTS is tenderness over the proximal pronator tunnel aggravated by pronation of the forearm (Fig. 18).

Provocative Tests for Median Nerve Entrapment in the Forearm (Fig. 18).[119]

A. Symptoms reproduced with resisted pronation with a clenched fist suggest entrapment beneath the pronator teres.

B. Resisted middle finger sublimis testing suggests entrapment at the sublimis arch if these resisted movements create pain or aching in the proximal forearm. There may be a positive Tinel over the pronator tunnel.

C. Symptoms reproduced with forearm flexion and supination suggest entrapment beneath the lacertus fibrosis.

Occupational Causes for Pronator Teres Syndrome. PTS is more common in women according to Hartz's series, in which 29 out of 39 cases were female.[109] Repetitive pronation-supination activities associated with exertional grasping seem to be underlying factors. The syndrome is seen with increased frequency in those who hang clothes, and Nigst notes that it has been seen in those who cradle babies on the forearm, which presumably causes compression of the forearm structures.[118] It has been dubbed "honeymoon paralysis" from continued low grade pressure of the partner's head on the proximal forearm (Fig. 19).[106]

PTS is seen in the following occupations: **fork lift operators, carpenters, hospital dietary personnel, unrestrained weight lifters,** and **tennis players.**[112] Other authors have found PTS in **housewives**,[108,112] **nurses**,[108] **farmers**,[108] **dentists**,[105] **cutters**,[22] **writers**,[22] **musicians**,[22] **electricians**,[108] in an avid **wood worker**,[116] in a **stock clerk**,[114] and in **assembly line workers** where pronation-supination motions are constantly repeated,[115] particularly if associated with forced finger flexion as in manipulating levers.[22]

Mackinnon and Dellon[115] view PTS as an early phase of median nerve compression in the proximal forearm, with aching pain as the predominant sign. In later phases, when the

Labels on figure:
(Biceps cut away)
Reflected Humeral Head, Pronator Teres
Brachial A.
Median Nerve
Radial A.
Pronator Teres
Flexor Digitorum Superficialis
Transverse Carpal Ligament
Brachial A.
Median N.
Pronator Teres
Lacertus Fibrosus
Detail of relationship of Median Nerve to Lacertus Fibrosus

FIGURE 17. Anatomy of the median nerve in the proximal forearm with particular focus on the relationships of the median nerve to the pronator teres and flexor digitorum superficialis. Inset depicts the relationship of the median nerve to the lacertus fibrosis.

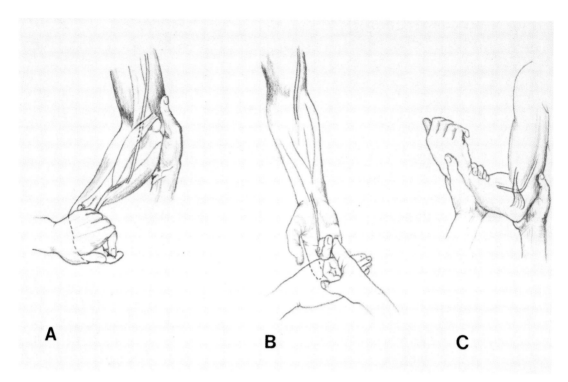

FIGURE 18. Physical examination techniques that provide a provocative test for median nerve entrapment in the forearm. *A*, Pain in the proximal forearm increased by resistance to pronation of the forearm and flexion of the wrist is a positive sign of median nerve compression at the level of the pronator teres. *B*, Pain in the proximal forearm reproduced by resistance to flexion of the flexor superficialis of the long finger is a positive sign for compression of the median nerve at the flexor digitorum superficialis arch. *C*, Pain in the proximal forearm increased by resistance to forearm supination and elbow flexion is a positive sign for compression of the median nerve at the lacertus fibrosis. (Modified from Spinner M: Injuries to the Major Branches of Peripheral Nerves of the Forearm, 2nd ed. Philadelphia, W.B. Saunders, 1978, with permission.)

condition worsens, the anterior interosseous nerve (AIN) becomes compressed and the motor palsy characteristic of the AIN may develop. The PTS is distinguished from anterior interosseous nerve syndrome in that in PTS there is a normal pinch mechanism indicating sparing of the flexor pollicis longus (FPL) and the flexor digitorium profundus (FDP) in the index finger.[122,123] PTS is also considered by these same authors to be a multiple crush lesion, because multiple sites of entrapment of the median nerve can occur (pronator heads, superficialis, crossing vessels, and Gantzer's muscle).[115] Hartz also notes that PTS can coexist with or be preceded by carpal tunnel syndrome (7 out of 39 patients were considered to have double-crush lesions). PTS is *usually distinguished from the carpal tunnel syndrome* by the fact that the *findings are related to the forearm and not to the wrist or thenar area*, and the positive Tinel is over the pronator region and not over the wrist, although there are

exceptions. Carpal tunnel syndrome does not involve the palmar cutaneous branch.

Electrodiagnostic Studies. A normal electrophysiologic test does not rule out PTS.[110,125] When the test is positive, there is a characteristic denervation pattern in median nerve-innervated muscles distal to the pronator teres. Motor nerve conduction velocity of the median nerve is slowed in the forearm, with normal distal latencies and sensory amplitudes.[74]

Treatment for Pronator Teres Syndrome. When the test is positive spontaneous pronator syndrome, conservative treatment is usually recommended as the initial treatment. This usually involves splinting and anti-inflammatory agents. If no improvement in 8 weeks, operative decompression of the median nerve may be indicated.[118]

Ergonomics and Pronator Teres Syndrome. PTS is associated with occupations that require pronation-supination and external-internal rotation and abduction of the forearm,

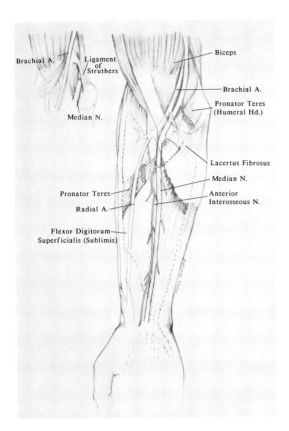

FIGURE 19. Anatomy of the median nerve in the proximal forearm with detail of the anterior interosseous nerve.

often aggravated by forceful finger flexion. Tools should be used that can be grasped with the forearm in the neutral position. Scheduled short breaks should be added to the work shift to decrease continuous time spent on an activity. Rotating work stations to change job tasks will also decrease repetitive trauma.[22]

Anterior Interosseous Nerve Syndrome

Historical Perspective. In reviewing the historical background on anterior interosseous nerve (AIN) syndrome, Spinner notes that Tinel in 1918 described two cases under the heading of "dissociated paralysis of the median nerve."[122]

In 1948 Parsonage and Turner[120] reviewed 136 cases of brachial neuritis and reported six patients who had paralysis of the flexor pollicis longus and the flexor digitorum profundus of the index finger. Kiloh and Nevin[113] in 1952 described two cases of isolated anterior interosseous nerve palsies.

Description of AIN Compression Syndromes. AIN compression is an entrapment neuropathy of a motor branch of the median nerve that results in paresis or paralysis of the innervated muscle-tendon units: the flexor pollicis longus (FPL), the flexor digitorum profundus (FDP) of the index finger and sometimes the middle finger, and the pronator quadratus. Entrapment along the AIN results from fascial bands or muscle hypertrophy of the pronator teres and/or the flexor digitorum superficialis. Chronic forearm pronation and elbow flexion can lead to the complete AIN syndrome. The patient presents with complaints of pain in the proximal forearm that develops insidiously over several hours. The pain is followed by weakness of the muscles innervated by the AIN. According to Spinner,[123] this is manifested in the "pinch attitude" of the thumb and index finger. Normally when a patient is asked to make the "O" sign with his thumb and index finger, the interphalangeal joint of the thumb and index finger flex and the pads of these fingers touch one another. With an AIN palsy, there is loss of flexion in the interphalangeal joints of the thumb and index finger, with resultant extension at these joints (Fig. 20). Deterioration of writing ability has been described as a predominant, presenting symptom of patients with AIN.[124]

These muscles (FPL, FDP index) are abnormally weak, and the "O" is easily broken

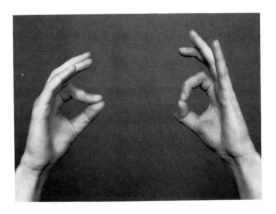

FIGURE 20. Diagnosis of an anterior interosseous nerve palsy. *Right*, Normally when a patient is asked to make the "O" sign with his thumb and index finger, the interphalangeal joint of the thumb and index finger flex, and the pads of these fingers touch one another. *Left*, With an anterior interosseous nerve palsy, there is loss of flexion in the interphalangeal joints of the thumb and index finger, with resultant extension of these joints. (From Mackinnon SE, Dellon AL: Surgery of the Peripheral Nerve. New York, Thieme Medical, 1988, adapted with permission.)

with minimal resistance by the examiner. In normal subjects, the examiner is unable to break this "O" with his or her finger looped through the patients. Testing for pronator quadratus weakness is done by eliminating the strong pronator teres by elbow flexion. Weakness of the pronator quadratus then can be determined by resisting forced pronation.

Complete Anterior Interosseous Nerve Palsy.   This palsy is manifested by an inability to flex the thumb at the interphalangeal joint, the index finger at the distal interphalangeal joint, and at times the middle finger at the interphalangeal joint. Howard[112] has delineated three principal etiologic factors contributing to the entrapment of the AIN: (1) edema, (2) traction, and (3) entrapment due to compression bands.

Edema.   Edema within the entrapment area of the AIN is thought to be the most common cause of this entrapment neuropathy in those who overused their flexor pronator muscles.[112] This includes people in occupations such as **assembly-line workers**, (who require consistent repetitive forearm pronation-supination), **typists, bank tellers**, and **furniture movers**; and avocations including **unrestrained weight lifting** and **tennis playing**. Approximately 50% of AIN patients with edema will clear with conservative treatment consisting of rest and sometimes immobilization.

Traction.   Traction of the AIN from a displaced supracondylar fracture. Fracture reduction and observation over time usually shows a return of function.

Entrapment Due to Compression Bands. This is the least common etiologic factor in AIN.

Occupational case reports of complete anterior interosseous nerve palsy also include: **newspaper carrier**,[123] **plumber**,[123] **assembly line worker**,[112] **typist**,[112] and **Coast Guardsman**.[117]

Incomplete Anterior Interosseous Nerve Syndrome.   AIN palsy can also present as an isolated paralysis of the FPL or the FDP of the index finger. Most commonly the isolated lesion of the AIN involves the inability to flex the interphalangeal joint of the thumb (Fig. 21).[111] This is due to injury or compression of the nerve near the site of origin as it innervates the FPL near where the flexor digitorum superficialis crosses it. Spinner cites examples of incomplete AIN neuropathies in **bank tellers** and a **bass player**.[123] Hill et al.[111] reported 33 patients with incomplete AIN paralysis involv-

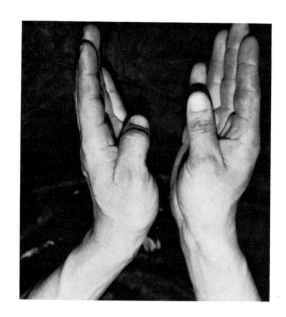

FIGURE 21.   Demonstration of an incomplete anterior interosseous nerve palsy in a 26-year-old male construction foreman with an isolated flexor pollicis longus weakness of the right thumb.

ing isolated lesions of either the FPL or the thumb or FDP of the index fingers, collected over a 15-year period. In Hill's series, the following jobs were associated with incomplete AIN paralysis: **Mechanics, bank tellers, press operator, dental technician, electrical worker**, and **housewife**. Two cases were caused by lifting heavy furniture (**piano mover**).

Hill recommended in the differential diagnosis ruling out tendon rupture, stenosing or adhesion tenosynovitis, and peripheral neuropathy. A baseline EMG and nerve conduction velocity should be performed and repeated in 12 weeks[111] if clinical improvement has not occurred. Consideration should be given to exploration and external neurolysis of the AIN, if no improvement, clinically or electrophysiologically, has occurred in 12 weeks.

Ergonomics and Anterior Interosseous Nerve Syndrome.   Since compression can be the cause of AIN syndrome, objects should not be carried on the forearm and carts should be used to transport items when possible.

Carpal Tunnel Syndrome— Median Nerve Compression at the Wrist

History.   Compression of the median nerve at the wrist has been known by many names: acroparesthesia, median compressive neuropathy, median neuritis, tardy median palsy, and carpal tunnel syndrome (CTS).[130,134] CTS is the most common compressive neuropathy in the upper extremity.[85] The increasing incidence of CTS is considered to be primarily due to the increased use of the hand in vocational as well as avocational settings that require repetitive wrist and finger motion.[134,143]

In 1833, Ormerond presented an excellent clinical description of CTS, including night pain, digital dysesthesias, and onset with manual work.[153] He did not have a clear concept of the etiology.[130]

Some authors have attributed the original description of CTS to Sir James Paget, who noted the clinical stigmata of the syndrome in 1863.[146] Pathological changes of the median nerve were described by Marie et Foix in 1913.[137] J. R. Learmonth performed the first carpal tunnel release by sectioning of the transverse carpal ligament in 1930.[147] Moersch coined the name of the syndrome in 1938, and Cannon and Love described the first series of patients with median nerve compression in 1946.[135] Beginning in 1950, in a series of articles, Phalen repeatedly directed the attention of the American and international communities to CTS.[85,150–152]

Anatomy of the Median Nerve—Wrist Level. The median nerve gives off the palmar cutaneous branch to the thenar area prior to entering the hand at the carpal tunnel level (Fig. 22). The median nerve is accompanied by nine flexor tendons in the carpal tunnel, which has the following boundaries:[85]

    Floor: Volar radiocarpal ligament and the volar ligamentous extensions between the carpal bones.
    Roof: Transverse carpal ligament (thick fibrous band that arches over the concave surface of the carpal bones).
    Lateral (radial) wall: Tuberosity of the scaphoid and the tubercle of the trapezium.
    Median (ulnar) wall: The pisiform and the hook of the hamate.

Thus the boundaries of the carpal tunnel are either bony or ligamentous and unyielding.[142] The median nerve itself ordinarily lies superficial, directly beneath the transverse carpal ligament.[130] Once through the tunnel, the nerve divides into motor and sensory branches. The motor branches supply function to the thenar muscles: abductor pollicis brevis, opponens pollicis, and the short head of the flexor pollicis brevis, as well as the first and second lum-

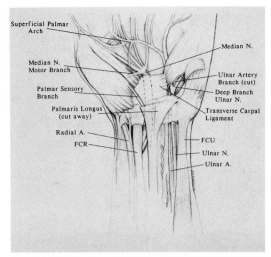

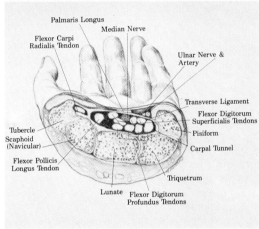

FIGURE 22. *A,* Anatomy of the median nerve at the wrist level including the carpal tunnel area. *B,* Cross-sectional anatomy of the median nerve in the carpal tunnel region.

bricales. The sensory branches usually innervate the volar surface of the thumb, index, middle, and radial half of the ring fingers.

Robbins explained that the median nerve's susceptibility to compromise by wrist flexion was due to[154]:

1. The nerve becoming superficial just proximal to the wrist and therefore not easily being displaced during acute flexion.

2. The transverse carpal ligament's sharp proximal border impinging on the nerve when the wrist is flexed.

3. The anterior part of the lunate bone rotating so much during wrist flexion, that the bone projects volarward, thereby decreasing the volume of the carpal canal.

The signs and symptoms of CTS are caused by the median nerve being pushed against the unyielding roof of the carpal tunnel. Flexor synovitis is the most common etiology for the CTS. CTS affects women in a 3:1 ratio over men, at age 30 to 50 years.

Diagnosis—Signs and Symptoms. Compression of a nerve at any location along its course impedes conduction of the nerve impulse distally beyond that point.[22,139] Lack of motor power in muscles with incomplete nerve supply is expressed as weakness and decreased ability to perform usual functions, such as grasping, holding, or lifting. Disturbances in perception of sensation, such as numbness, ringing, or "pins and needles" sensation occur in areas of skin over the extremities to which the nerve supply has been interrupted.[22,139] There are slight tingling and numbness in the tip of the middle finger,[149] and frequently the whole finger is numb. Involvement of radial aspect of the tip of the ring finger and the tips of the index and thumb is also present.[149]

Classically, CTS presents with paresthesias in its sensory distribution, initially waking the patient at night in order to shake the hand out. Chronic compression of the nerve with subsequent venous congestion has been proposed as a casual factor. Arminio[126] describes that perineurium of the median nerve as "unyielding with increasing intrafunicular pressure," thus compromising the nerve.

A feeling of coldness and sweating in the hand is present. Attention has been drawn to the association of CTS and vasospasm (Raynaud's phenomenon), since Phalen stated that such disturbances could be expected because the median nerve carries the greater part of sympathetic innervation to the hand.[149]

A nonspecific burning feeling, pain, and swelling of the hand radiate into the forearm further proximally. Pain characteristically occurs at night. The individual counters this by shaking, rubbing, or allowing the hand to hang out of bed. Pain can recur in the course of daily work.[149]

As compression persists, symptoms may become more constant in nature. Weakness of the median innervated hand muscles may become evident. The patient may begin to complain of forearm pain as well.

The patient experiences loss of dexterity and weakness of the hand, and can either no longer pick up fine objects or tends to let them fall. This is due to the distal innervation of the abductor pollicis, abductor brevis, opponens pollicis, and flexor pollicis. In longstanding cases, thenar atrophy can occur.[149] The clinician should

exclude a co-existing cubital tunnel syndrome as a cause of dropping objects and clumsiness in the hand. These are usually early signs in cubital tunnel syndrome, whereas they represent late manifestations in carpal tunnel syndrome.

There is a loss of protective sensation and rarely the development of ulcers in longstanding cases.[149]

Provocative Testing for CTS. Physical findings including paresthesias on percussion of the median nerve (Tinel's sign). Phalen's test is positive in 70% of cases (Fig. 23A).[142] This test involves acute flexion of the wrist (70 degrees) for 30–60 seconds. The test may be modified by adding the forced flexion of the index finger (Fig. 23B). The reverse Phalen's test with the wrist held in a dorsiflexed position can reproduce CTS symptoms as well (Fig. 23C). Allen's test[94] (Fig. 23D) may be used as a provocative test to rule out ulnar artery occlusion and to reproduce carpal tunnel symptoms.

Sensory Testing for CTS. Vibratory sense is one of the earliest sensory parameters affected in CTS. Testing with a 256 Hz tuning fork applied to the finger pulp has been described as a sensitive means of detecting early nerve dysfunction[94] (Fig. 24A).

Cutaneous pressure threshold can be quantitated through the use of Semmes-Weinstein monofilament testing (Fig. 24B). Further testing can be used to quantitate cutaneous sensibility changes with CTS, including the static and moving 2-point discrimination tests. In the more severely involved cases, the static 2-point is affected[94] (Fig. 24C).

Motor Testing for CTS. Thenar wasting may be seen in late cases, giving the hand a Simian appearance. Apart from the first and second lumbricales, only two hand muscles receive exclusive median nerve innervation, the abductor pollicis brevis and opponens pollicis. Intrinsic muscle function can be assessed by the opponens pollicis and abductor pollicis brevis tests. The testing of the APB muscle is shown in Figure 25.

The etiology of CTS is extensive. One must keep in mind that although a work-related causal relationship appears evident, metabolic or other factors can not be overlooked (Table 1).

Occupational Causes of Carpal Tunnel Syndrome. The most common cited etiology is related to jobs in which repetitive wrist flexion and extension is used with the fingers flexed.[156] Although CTS can be caused or associated with a host of conditions, it is flexor synovitis that

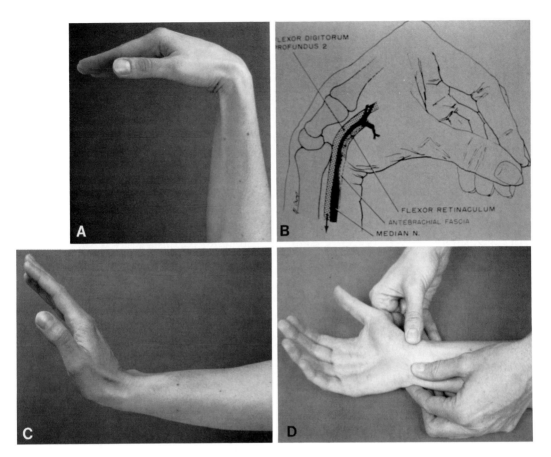

FIGURE 23. *A*, Phalen's test: the test is positive for median nerve entrapment at the wrist if the patient develops paresthesias and numbness in the median nerve distribution while maintaining the wrist in acute flexion (70 degrees) for 30–60 seconds. *B*, Compression of median nerve between tensed tendon of flexor digitorum profundus and underlying flexor retinaculum during wrist flexion. (From Smith EM, et al: Carpal tunnel syndrome: contribution of flexor tendons. Arch Phys Med Rehabil 58:385, 1977, with permission.) *C*, Reverse Phalen's test: wrist dorsiflexion for 30–60 seconds reproduces symptoms in the median nerve distribution. *D*, Allen's test: both the radial and ulnar artery are occluded at the wrist level and the patient is asked to open and close the hand. Paresthesias may be stimulated if there is compression of the median nerve in the carpal tunnel.

is the most common etiologic factor, because flexor synovitis is stimulated by repetitive wrist motions.

CTS has been described in multiple occupations, some of which include: **assembly line workers,**[22,139] **butchers,**[138] **meat processors,**[131] **poultry workers,**[127,129] **farmers,**[22] **mechanics,**[22] **garment workers,**[22,132,139] **dentists,**[22] **surgeons, occupational and physical therapists, carpenters,**[155] **musicians,**[22] **janitors,**[22,139] **gardeners,**[22] **painters,**[22] and occupations in which hand-held vibrating instruments are used.[135,157] This is just a partial list of occupations with an increased prevalence of CTS. It appears that CTS knows no socioeconomic bounds. What these occupations do have in common are: (1) positional stress, (2) mechanical stress, and (3) repetitive stress. These factors are common to

all the aforementioned occupations with risk for development of CTS.[128]

Gelberman et al.[140] measured intracarpal canal pressures using a wick catheter in 15 patients with CTS and in 12 controls. In CTS patients, there was a near threefold increase from abnormal baseline pressures when the wrist was flexed and extended. Baseline pressures in these subjects were 32 mmHg compared to 2.5 mmHg in normals. This increase in pressure combined with an ungiving perineurium of the median nerve can lead to both mechanical and vascular compromise.

Gordon et al.[141] studied the ratio of the anteroposterior wrist diameter divided by the mediolateral diameter in 80 automobile factory workers over a 3-year period. Seventy-four percent of those workers with ratios greater

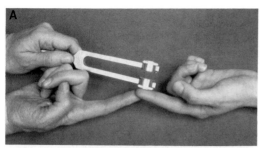

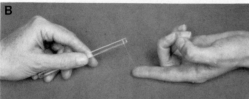

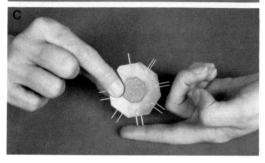

FIGURE 24. A, Sensory testing for median nerve deficits related to the carpal tunnel syndrome. The 256 cps tuning fork is used to assess qualitative vibratory perception. Note the "wrong end" of the tuning fork is used, because the amplitude at this end of the tuning fork is greater than that at the single prong end of the tuning fork. At both ends, the vibration is 256 cps, but the amplitude varies greatly from one end of the tuning fork to the other. The goal is to use a stimulus intensity sufficiently high enough that if the patient does not perceive the stimulus, it is due to a nerve problem, not just a subthreshold stimulus. B, Semmes-Weinstein monofilaments can be used to quantitate the cutaneous pressure threshold of the slowly adapting fiber receptor system. C, The Disk-Criminator is used to evaluate static two-point discrimination. In this instance, the pulp of the index finger is being tested (autonomous zone of the median nerve). (From Mackinnon SE, Dellon AL: Surgery of the Peripheral Nerve. New York, Thieme Medical, 1988, adapted with permission.)

than 0.70 developed symptoms of CTS and indeed had abnormal electrodiagnostic tests to confirm the diagnosis.

Carpal canal stenosis has been proposed by Bleecker and associates[131] as a cause for median nerve entrapment. Carpal canal size was evaluated by CT scan in symptomatic electricians and controls. The cross-sectional area was markedly diminished in these individuals compared with controls.

Smith et al.[156] felt that during wrist flexion, not only is the median nerve compressed against the transverse carpal ligament, but also it is subject to compression by the taut flexor tendons. Tension of the flexor tendons can be further increased and thus compromise the nerve to an even greater extent by flexing the fingers with the wrist flexed (see Fig. 23B).

This type of chronic posturing, as seen in **assembly workers**, leads to repetitive damage, intrafascicular fibrosis and focal demyelination. Phalen's test can, therefore, be modified to include this principle and increase sensitivity. While the wrist is acutely flexed, ask the patient to pinch his thumb against his index and middle fingers. If symptoms are reproduced, it is a positive test.

Ditmars et al.[136] noted that during flexion of the metacarpophalangeal joints, the lumbricales can actually retract into the tunnel. This would also be a mechanism for nerve compression, possibly explaining occurrence of symptoms while pinching items for any length of time.

Finally, vibration through its production and dissipation of heat, especially in sensitive nervous tissues, causes vascular congestion and subsequent nerve entrapment. This appears to be a form of CTD as well. It is frequently seen in **jackhammer** or **power tool users**.[136]

Electrodiagnostic studies are the most valuable tool in diagnosing CTS. Nerve conduc-

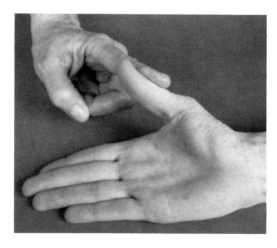

FIGURE 25. Assessment of median nerve intrinsic muscle function is best tested by having the patient abduct the thumb at 90 degrees from the palm of the hand. The examiner then asks the patient to keep the thumb in this position and resist this movement. (From Mackinnon SE, Dellon AL: Surgery of the Peripheral Nerve. New York, Thieme Medical, 1988, adapted with permission.)

TABLE 1. Conditions Predisposing to Carpal Tunnel Syndrome*

I. Inflammation
   a. Flexor tenosynovitis
   b. Rheumatoid tenosynovitis
   c. Acute calcific tendonitis
   d. Suppurative tendonitis
   e. Osteoarthritis
   f. Polymyalgia rheumatica
II. Trauma
   a. Wrist fractures
      1. Colles
      2. Carpal with dislocation
      3. Distal radial epiphysis
      4. Distal radius and ulna
   b. Volkmann's ischemic contracture
III. Neoplasias and other masses
   a. Benign or malignant tumors
   b. Aberrant muscles
      1. Flexor digitorum sublimis
      2. Lumbricales
   c. Tuberculous granuloma
IV. Deposition of biosynthetic product
   a. Primary and secondary amyloidosis
   b. Mucopolysaccharidosis
   c. Gout and pseudogout
V. Abnormal vasculature
   a. Thrombosis of aberrant median artery
   b. Permanent shunt for renal dialysis
VI. Other system conditions
   a. Diabetes mellitus
   b. Pregnancy
   c. Myxedema
   d. Acromegaly

* From Shuman S, Osterman L, Bora FW: Compression neuropathies. Sem Neurol 7:76–87, 1987, with permission.

tion studies help confirm the diagnosis by demonstrating a slowing in electrical conduction of the nerve through the tunnel. Slowing of the sensory nerve action potential is most frequently seen, although slowing of the motor conduction by itself can also be noted. Also studied are the latency and amplitudes, by comparison of the ulnar and radial nerves.[133,141,158] Needle exam of the abductor pollicis brevis in severe cases can demonstrate denervation, a sign of severe chronic compression.

Treatment of Carpal Tunnel Syndrome

Treatment of CTS can be broken down into two categories, conservative and surgical.

Conservative Treatment of CTS. Conservative treatment approaches include volar splinting with the wrist in approximately 20 degrees of extension to control wrist motion. If the splint cannot be worn on the job, then it should be utilized during non-working hours and during sleep. In conjunction with splinting, rehabilitation techniques to reduce pain and edema may be helpful.[144] A job analysis can be beneficial in minimizing repetitive trauma to the wrist and recurrence of a person's symptoms by means of work station and tool redesign, or by simply changing the position in which a task is performed.

Medications utilized to control the symptoms of CTS include anti-inflammatory agents, steroids, diuretics, and vitamin B6.[118] Cortisone injections at the wrist in the carpal canal are used for pain relief,[142] but cortisone injections are not universally accepted because of the possibility of nerve damage. Reduction of highly repetitive movements of the wrist and fingers is one of the mainstays of conservative treatment.

Surgical Treatment of CTS. In cases with severe symptoms and signs, such as atrophy of the thenar eminence, with increasing symptoms, and in longstanding situations where conservative measures are ineffective, or at best, give only transient improvement, surgery may be necessary.[22] Techniques for surgical carpal tunnel releases vary among surgeons. Attempts should be made to avoid injury to the median nerve with its palmar cutaneous and motor branches while releasing the distal end of the carpal tunnel, which is the site of most compressions.[145] Most procedures are done on an outpatient basis in an ambulatory surgical setting.[148]

Ergonomics and Carpal Tunnel Syndrome. Because of the alarming increase in CTS, the discipline of ergonomics is playing a larger role in the workplace. For example, redesigning the height of containers an employee must reach into on the assembly line can reduce wrist flexion. A word processor job can be modified to be more energy efficient by padding the edge of the table where the keyboard sits and decreasing mechanical stress (pressure) on the wrist. Redesigning the handle on a pair of pliers can minimize repetitive stresses.[15,22,29,127]

In the long run, job site analysis, ergonomics, and education as to the cause of cumulative trauma disorders associated with repetitive stress will be more cost effective than the loss of manpower at work and insurance claims paid to manage CTS. Preventive measures are critical (Fig. 26).

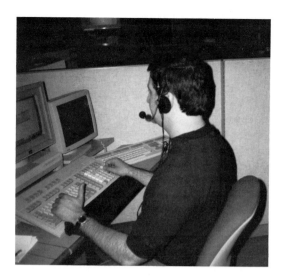

FIGURE 26. Ergonomics at the Bell Atlantic Plant in Washington, D.C. Note the forearm and wrist support for prevention of carpal tunnel syndrome. (Permission granted by S.A. Kosiak, Director Safety, Bell Atlantic.)

Occupational Injuries to Median Nerve Branches in the Palm and Digits

Occupational and avocational injuries to median nerve branches in the palm and digits are now discussed.

Opponens Branch Injury of the Median Nerve. Feldman described an entrapment injury of the motor branch of the median nerve that comes from pressing tools into the palm, pounding safety levers, and operating a stamping machine.[22] Signs and symptoms include weakness in precision grip, atrophy of the thenar muscles, and tenderness over the nerve at the edge of the transverse ligament. Occupations where opponens nerve entrapment are seen include **painters, carpenters, stable hands** (using horsebrush), **timekeepers**, and **receipt processors.**[22]

In relation to ergonomics, designing tools to avoid pressure on the thenar area is one important way to reduce the incidence of this condition.

Median Palmar Digital Neuropathy. Cases have been reported in **bowlers** and **seamstresses.**[171,175] Nerve conduction studies reveal a decrease in sensory amplitudes of the digital median nerve.[169]

Thumb Neural Entrapments. Digital nerve neuropathy has been described in a **cherry pitter** (cherry pitter's thumb)[178]; it has been reported as an occupational hazard in **flutist**[161] (first common digital nerve neuropathy), and

in **jewelers**, as a digital nerve thumb compression problem. It has been reported as an occasional problem in **surgeons** related to wearing tight gloves, and in **bowlers**. Prevention of the digital nerve entrapment is directed at reducing the repetitive pressure on the digital nerve. In the case of the cherry pitter, wearing special neoprene gloves solved the problem. Avoiding tight surgical gloves is a solution to the occupational hazard that surgeons potentially face.

ULNAR NERVE COMPRESSION SYNDROMES

Anatomy. The ulnar nerve is formed by the C8 and T1 nerve roots with a small contribution from C7. It arises as the continuation and terminal branch of the medial cord of the brachial plexus after the medial cord contributes to the median nerve. In the proximal axilla it lies medial to the axillary and then to the brachial artery down to the middle third of the humerus, and then courses posteriorly at the midpoint in the upper arm. The nerve then pierces the medial intermuscular septum that separates the flexor and extensor muscle groups. It then inclines somewhat posteriorly to lie close to the humerus and medial head of the triceps muscle to the groove between the olecranon and the medial epicondyle of the humerus.[177]

The cubital tunnel begins at the so-called ulnar groove just behind the medial epicondyle of the humerus (Fig. 27). In the cubital tunnel the ulnar nerve is covered by multiple fascial layers of the flexor carpi ulnaris and can be readily palpated coursing behind and beneath the medial epicondyle of the partially flexed elbow. The cubital tunnel is roofed first by the aponeurotic arch and then the belly of the flexor carpi ulnaris. The floor is formed by the medial ligaments of the elbow and the flexor digitorum profundus muscle. There are three principle anatomic parts in the cubital tunnel[85]:

1. The entrance of the canal just posterior to the medial epicondyle.

2. The fascial aponeurosis joining the two heads of the flexor carpi ulnaris.

3. The muscle bellies of the flexor carpi ulnaris.

The nerve courses through the rest of the forearm between the flexor digitorum profundus and flexor carpi ulnaris muscles.[177] When the nerve is in a particularly shallow groove or

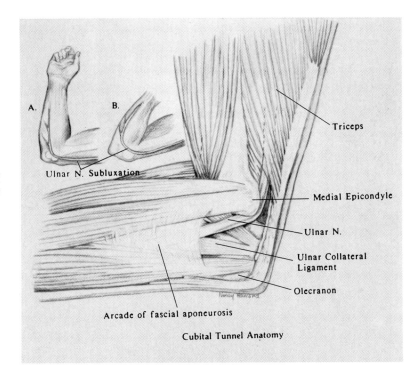

FIGURE 27. Anatomy of the ulnar nerve in relation to the cubital tunnel.

is hypermobile, it is at increased risk for injury.[174]

Cubital Tunnel Syndrome

Brief Historical Perspective. From a historical review of cubital tunnel syndrome, a hypermobile ulnar nerve was described by Blattman in 1851[159] and Panas in 1878[173] described a post-traumatic ulnar nerve neuritis following elbow trauma in three patients, with the onset of symptoms delayed in one case up to 12½ years. In 1894, Oppenheim[172] drew attention to protracted elbow flexion, which may be the cause of ulnar nerve damage. It was not until 1958 that Feindel and Stratford[163] actually put the label cubital tunnel syndrome on the constellation of symptoms and signs of ulnar nerve compression at the elbow.

Elbow Posture in Relation to Cubital Tunnel Syndrome. Elbow leaners always flex the elbow to a degree and this narrows the cubital tunnel and increases the pressure on the ulnar nerve in the cubital tunnel. Elbow flexion also stretches the ulnar nerve as much as 3 cm.[174] The following list of professions that are at increased risk for cubital tunnel is divided according to elbow postures that are mainly associated with these occupations:

Protracted Elbow Flexion. In the past **telephone operators** were afflicted with cubital tunnel syndrome, and it was the left elbow, which was the side holding the earphone, that was most affected. The head-piece telephone receiver is now used instead of the hand held earphone.[174] The problem is also seen in occupations such as **watchmakers,**[174] **engravers,**[171] **jewelers,**[171] **goldsmiths, glass blowers, brass polishers,**[171] and **diamond makers** (ring).[176] It is also seen in **dress makers, cab drivers, people working with microscopes,** and **musicians.**[174] It has been reported as a transient ulnar neuritis in a **judge** who had a prolonged trial.[174]

Protracted Elbow Extension. Occupations at risk are those that require prolonged extension such as **carpentry (sawing), shovelling, digging, drilling work with pneumatic drills or hammers, work with powered handsaw or hand-held grinding machine, pushing heavy carts,** and many others. It is noted in **crystal cutters** who push the piece of crystal glass against the grinding wheel using steady pressure. Even though the elbows are flexed, there is apparently a steady pressure in extension.[174] **Wheelchair-bound patients** are also at risk for cubital tunnel syndrome.[174]

The ulnar nerve is protected against pressure, as it is situated between two bony prominences, i.e., the olecranon and medial epicondyle.[174] When leaning on the elbow, the pressure may be exerted on only one of the two bony prominences that form the groove for the ulnar nerve at the elbow. When both bony processes, the olecranon and the medial epicondyle, lie simultaneously on a hard surface, pressure may be exerted on the ulnar nerve.[174]

Entrapment of the ulnar nerve in this tunnel is second only to carpal tunnel syndrome in frequency.[179] The volume and shape of the canal is dynamic in relation to arm position. The nerve appears to be at normal resting length with the elbow held at 135 degrees (−45 degrees full extension).[164] During flexion and pronation the nerve becomes compressed in this tunnel.[155]

Symptoms of Cubital Tunnel Syndrome. These include pain over the medial aspect of the elbow and forearm, with dysesthesias of the ring and small fingers. The symptoms are frequently aggravated by elbow flexion. Activities that require a lot of elbow flexion, i.e., using a hair dryer, driving a car, or holding a phone for long periods of time, can bring on the symptoms.[170] There are also complaints of clumsiness and loss of fine manipulation. **Musicians** afflicted with cubital tunnel syndrome (**violinists** and others)[170] have difficulty manipulating their musical instruments. In time, grip strength can be impaired. The clinician should ask questions about potential systemic problems associated with cubital tunnel syndrome, such as diabetes mellitus, alcoholism, thyroid disorders.[170]

Signs of Cubital Tunnel Syndrome. On physical exam, sensation is diminished in the little finger and half of the ring finger (Fig. 28). There are abnormal perceptions of sensations

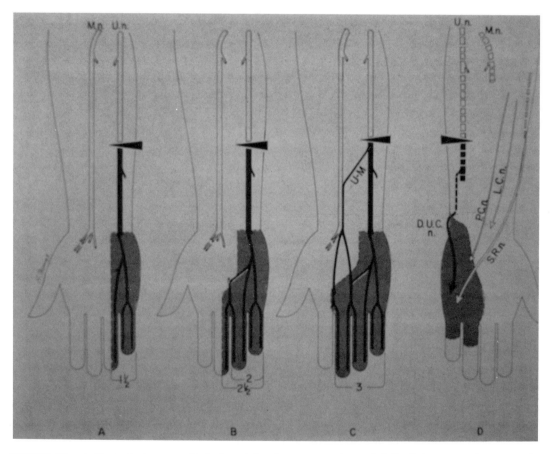

FIGURE 28. *A*, The typical sensory distribution of the ulnar nerve to the medial 1½ digits. *B*, Distribution can be increased to the adjacent digits by neural communication in the palm and *C* in the forearm. The superficial radial nerve can supply the dorsoulnar aspect of the hand, which is usually innervated by the dorsal ulnar cutaneous nerve. *D*, The posterior cutaneous nerve of the forearm (PCn) and the lateral cutaneous nerve of the forearm (LCn) can also supply some of the dorsoulnar aspect of the hand. (From Omer G, Spinner M: Peripheral Nerve Testing and Suture Techniques. American Academy of Orthopedic Surgeons Instructional Course Lectures, Vol. 24. St. Louis, C.V. Mosby, 1975, pp 122–143, with permission.)

over the dorsal ulnar aspect of the hand. Note that the dorsal ulnar branch of the ulnar nerve divides approximately 5–8 cm proximal to pisiform.[170] There is a Tinel's sign at the elbow post-condylar groove (between the medial epicondyle and the olecranon). This sign may appear more proximal to the medial epicondyle if the nerve is subluxing (see Fig. 27). A provocative test to evoke symptoms of cubital tunnel syndrome is depicted in Figure 29.

With severe ulnar nerve compression at the elbow, there is lack of flexor digitorum profundus to the little finger and, in late cases, there may be clawing of the ring and little fingers (Fig. 30).[122] Manual muscle testing may show evidence of weakness in the ulnar innervated hand muscles: the interossei, flexor pollicis brevis, flexor digitorum profundus of ring and little fingers, adductor pollicis, lumbricales four and five, and the hypothenar muscles. This is demonstrated by resisted finger abduction. Occasionally, weakness in pinch strength is seen secondary to weakness of flexor pollicis brevis, adductor pollicis brevis, and the first dorsal interossei. It is easily tested by asking the patient to hold a piece of paper between the thumb and forefinger. Weakness is manifested by the lack of effort the examiner needs in pulling the paper loose from the patient, otherwise known as Froment's sign.

Electrodiagnostic Tests for Cubital Tunnel Syndrome. Electrophysiologic evaluation can be helpful in demonstrating an ulnar compression at the elbow. In cubital tunnel syndrome, distal wrist latencies for motor and sensory nerve testing are normal. Nerve testing is then performed at the elbow, over the distal end of the tunnel, and then 10 cm proximal to this point.[164] Eisen and associates felt a 10 m/sec difference in above elbow velocity compared with the below segment, along with the slight delay in conduction at the wrist, is indicative of an ulnar lesion at the elbow.[162]

Differential Diagnosis. Differential diagnosis of CTS should include the following:

1. Thoracic outlet syndrome—tenderness over the brachial plexus, positive Roos test.

2. Brachial plexus neuropathy—involving the lower trunk.

Treatment for Cubital Tunnel Syndrome.[170]

1. *Nonoperative*
   a. Splinting techniques
   b. Medications (NSAIDs)
2. *Operative*
   a. Simple decompression

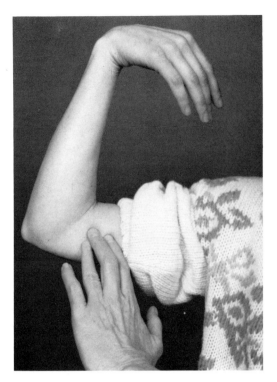

FIGURE 29. Provocative test for cubital tunnel syndrome; symptoms of ulnar nerve compression in the cubital tunnel can be provoked by elbow flexion and pressure applied over the ulnar nerve just proximal to the cubital tunnel. (From Mackinnon SE, Dellon AL: Surgery of the Peripheral Nerve. New York, Thieme Medical, 1988, adapted with permission.)

   b. Medial epicondylectomy
   c. Anterior subcutaneous nerve transposition
   d. Intramuscular transposition
   e. Submuscular transposition

Ergonomics and Cubital Tunnel Syndrome. Preventing sustained external forces on the elbows can prove beneficial in reducing the occurrence of cubital tunnel syndrome. This can be accomplished by wearing elbow pads, using padded table tops, and educating workers as to the hazards of leaning on their elbows during work. Varying the degrees of flexion and extension of the elbow at work will also minimize stress on the cubital tunnel, as opposed to holding it in a sustained position.[22]

Compression of the Ulnar Nerve in the Forearm (Between the Areas of the Cubital Tunnel and Guyon's Canal of the Wrist)

Ulnar Nerve Anatomy—Forearm. The ulnar nerve runs a straight-line course through

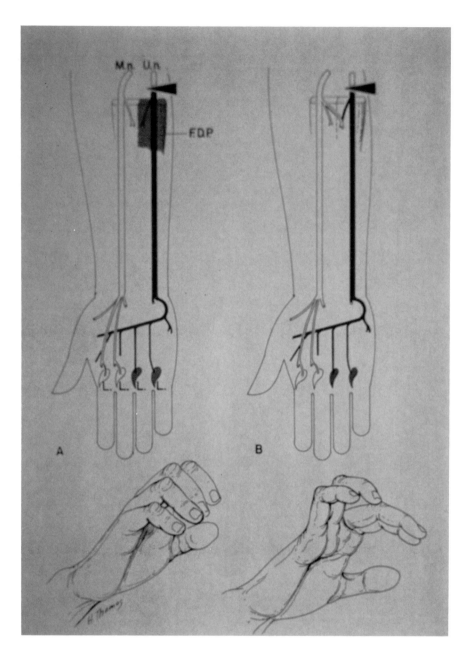

FIGURE 30.   A, A complete high ulnar nerve lesion is usually observed without digital claw deformity. B, However, complete high ulnar nerve lesions produce a clawed hand when the intact median nerve supplies the flexor digitorum profundus to the ring finger and little finger. (From Omer G, Spinner M: Peripheral Nerve Testing and Suture Techniques. American Academy of Orthopedic Surgeons Instructional Course Lectures, Vol. 24. St. Louis, C.V. Mosby, 1975, pp 122–143, with permission.)

the forearm from the level of the medial epicondyle of the distal humerus to the pisiform-hamate groove in the carpus.[122] This nerve travels between the flexor carpi ulnaris and flexor digitorum profundus and provides motor innervation to the FCU and the FDP, to the ring and little fingers. Occupational compres-

sion of the ulnar nerve in the forearm between the areas of the cubital tunnel and the Guyon's canal is not frequently reported in the literature. In fact, we could locate only one occupationally related case report of a Pakistani **rope maker** who developed ulnar nerve compression symptoms and signs related to chronic repetitive trauma to the ulnar nerve in the forearm from rope twining and unrelieved pressure on the forearm. He presented with a claw hand.[160]

Ulnar Nerve Anatomy—Distal Forearm. In the forearm, proximal to the wrist, the ulnar nerve gives off two sensory branches, neither of which travels through Guyon's canal. First, the *palmar cutaneous branch* courses down the volar aspect of the forearm to *supply the hypothenar eminence.* Second is the *dorsal cutaneous branch,* which comes off about 9 cm proximal to the pisiform to supply the dorsal surface of the ring finger and ulnar half of the little finger. Entrapment of these nerves in the forearm region has been reported after the use of handcuffs.[165] The main ulnar nerve trunk then continues to the base of the palm and enters Guyon's canal. With ulnar wrist entrapments, sensation in the palmar cutaneous and dorsal cutaneous nerve distribution is preserved. In cubital tunnel syndrome, anesthesia or hypesthesia will be noted in the sensory distribution pattern of these two nerves.

Guyon's Canal Compression Syndrome

Felix Guyon[184] in 1861, following his graduation from medical school, published a description of the canal at the base of the palm, thus the birth of the eponym Guyon's canal. Guyon's canal, which contains the ulnar nerve and artery, is superficial and medial to the neighboring carpal tunnel and is roofed by a thinner ligament.[191] There are no tendons in Guyon's canal or tendon sheaths that might cause symptoms through tendinitis and swelling.[191] Tenosynovitis is the most common cause for carpal tunnel syndrome. In ulnar nerve wrist neuropathies, space-occupying lesions such as lipoma and ganglia are more frequent causative agents.[191] Blunt trauma, repetitively applied, is the common pathway for work-related injuries to the ulnar nerve in the wrist and hand.[191]

The Guyon's canal contains the ulnar artery. The carpal tunnel contains no major blood vessel. Hypothenar hammer syndrome[180] occurs when damage to the ulnar artery causes ischemic symptoms and thus a secondary compression of the ulnar nerve.

Anatomy of the Ulnar Nerve—Guyon's Canal (Fig. 31). The ulnar nerve bifurcates into the superficial and deep branches in the pisohamate region. The superficial branch, which is predominantly sensory, first supplies sensation

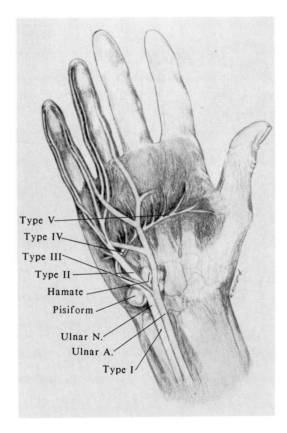

FIGURE 31. Anatomy of Guyon's canal showing the five potential areas of entrapment. (Modified from Wu J, et al: Ulnar neuropathy at the wrist: case report and review of literature. Arch Phys Med Rehabil 66:787, 1985, with permission.)

to the distal border of the palm. It then divides into two palmar digital nerves that innervate the skin of the palmar surfaces of the fifth and half of the fourth digit. The deep motor branch, in company with the artery, takes an abrupt turn about the hook of the hamate to enter the narrow interval between the origins of the abductor digiti quinti and flexor digiti minimi brevis muscles.[191] The first branches that arise from this motor branch after emergence from Guyon's canal are to the muscles of the hypothenar eminence. In the palm the ulnar nerve gives off branches to the interossei and the third and fourth lumbricales.[177] It terminates in the thenar eminence by supplying the adductor pollicis, the first dorsal interosseous, and usually half the flexor pollicis brevis.[177]

Wu and associates[194] analyzed and reclassified the ulnar nerve entrapments at the wrist into five categories, depending upon location. Most of the ulnar nerve entrapments here are due to trauma or occupations that require palm

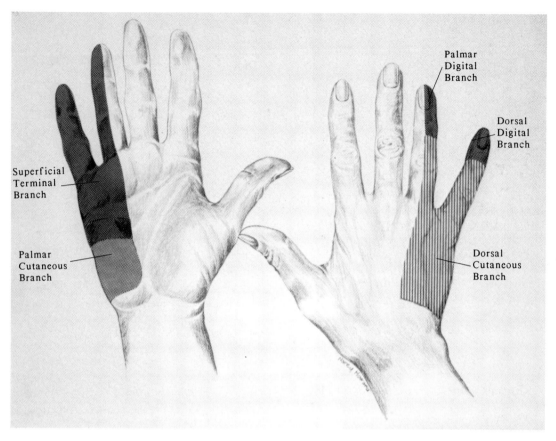

FIGURE 32.   Sensory pattern for ulnar nerve lesions.

pressure. Depending on the location of the lesion, the patient may experience only motor or sensory symptoms, or a combination of the two. There may be wasting of the intrinsic muscles on inspection. Nerve conduction studies complemented with a thorough electromyographic examination of the ulnar innervated hand muscles should help to establish the site of the lesion.

Classification of Ulnar Neuropathies at the Wrist

Type I (Mixed Motor and Sensory).   This lesion is proximal to the bifurcation, occurring usually at the proximal end of Guyon's canal. Characteristic symptoms include motor impairment in the ulnar intrinsic muscles and sensory impairment in the little finger and the ulnar side of the ring finger.[194]

Signs.   Sensory deficits in the ulnar half of ring and in the little finger (Fig. 32). Clawing of the digits may be present (see Fig. 30).

Figure 33 demonstrates muscle testing of the first dorsal interosseous muscle.

Electrodiagnostic Tests.   A prolonged distal latency may be seen when the motor nerve is stimulated at the wrist and recorded either from the hypothenar or the first dorsal interosseous. Sensory distal latency is prolonged and denervation seen in all ulnar innervated muscles.[194]

Type II (Pure Sensory).   This lesion involves the superficial branch of the ulnar nerve at the wrist, distal to the branch to the palmaris brevis muscle.

Symptoms.   Symptoms include sensory impairment to the ulnar innervated digits which include the ulnar half of the ring and little finger.[194]

Signs.   There are no motor deficits in ulnar innervated hand muscles.

Electrodiagnostic Test.   Electrophysiologic abnormalities are limited to sensory function.

Type III (Pure Motor).   This lesion of the deep branch of the ulnar nerve is distal to the superficial branch, but proximal to the branch going to the hypothenar.[194]

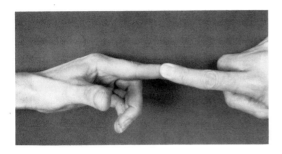

FIGURE 33. Ulnar nerve intrinsic muscle function can be tested by assessing the function of the first dorsal interosseous muscle by having the patient demonstrate a lateral key pinch and noting contraction in this muscle, or, as is shown, resisting abduction of the index finger and noting the contraction of the first dorsal interosseous muscle. (From Mackinnon SE, Dellon AL: Surgery of the Peripheral Nerve. New York, Thieme Medical, 1988, adapted with permission.)

Symptoms. No sensory complaints. Motor weakness is present.

Signs. Clawing of the hand usually results because of intrinsic impairment. Hypothenar, interossei, and adductor pollicis muscles are impaired.

Electrodiagnostic Test. Motor conduction studies are abnormal.

Type III Ulnar Nerve. Neuropathy occurs because of pathology near the pisiform.

Type IV (Pure Motor Ulnar Neuropathy with Sparing of the Hypothenar). This lesion occurs on the deep branch of the ulnar nerve distal to the origin of the superficial branch and distal to the branch going to the hypothenar. Anatomically the lesion occurs usually close to the hook of the hamate.

Symptoms. Sensation is normal.

Signs. The patient will have weakness of all muscles supplied by the ulnar nerve except the hypothenar.

Electrodiagnostic Test. There is normal sensory and motor conduction to the hypothenar, but motor conduction to the first dorsal interosseous muscle is abnormal, and there are denervation patterns in the adductor pollicis.

Type IV Ulnar Nerve. Entrapment occurs with disease near the hook of the hamate.

Type V (Distal Motor). This lesion occurs just proximal to the branches going to the first dorsal interosseous and the adductor pollicis muscles.

Symptoms. Sensation is normal and the patient has motor deficit with weakness of the involved muscles.

Electrodiagnostic Studies. Sensory conduction is normal but there is abnormal motor conduction recorded from the first dorsal interosseous. There are denervation patterns in the adductor pollicis and the first dorsal interosseous on EMG.

Type I, III, and IV ulnar nerve entrapments are the more common with the Type V the less common.

Occupational Causes of Distal Ulnar Neuropathies. Gessler in 1880[181] described a peculiar form of muscle atrophy in **gold polishers** but did not recognize the lesion as an ulnar neuropathy. Hunt [187] documented occupational trauma involving the deep motor branch in 1908. In surveying the literature on distal ulnar neuropathies, one is struck by the variety of classifications of this compression lesion. **Cyclists**[185,189] (amateur and professional), **carpenters,**[22] **builders, farmers, pizza cutters,**[188] **jewelers, brass polishers,**[171] **cobblers,**[186] **machine operators, meat cutters** and **meat packers,**[192] **dressmakers,**[193] **factory workers,**[193] **metal workers,**[191] and **amateur weight lifters**[194] have all been reported.

Mechanisms of Trauma for Distal Ulnar Neuropathy. The problem occurs where the nerve passes into the hand through a shallow opening between the pisiform and the hook of the hamate. Damage to the palmar nerve can occur when repetitive forces are applied to the base of the hypothenar eminence, which can occur when striking the palm of the hand or hitting a palm activated button on certain machinery.[22]

Mechanics and **carpenters** using tools, such as pliers, planes, staplers, and pneumatic drills are at risk for this neuropathy. **Gardeners** using shears,[190] **bootmakers** using a knife,[186] and **electronic assembly workers** using needle nose pliers are also at risk.[183]

Occupational entrapment of the deep motor branch of the ulnar nerve has been reported: Most of the occupational traumas to the distal ulnar nerve seemed to fall into Wu's category III, but no statistical analysis was made of the data.

Management of Distal Ulnar Neuropathies. If occupational causes for the neuropathy can be identified and subsequently avoided, many patients recover spontaneously.[191] Surgical exploration should be considered if:

1. No clear cause for the neuropathy can be identified and the lesion is either severe or worsening.

2. If an occupational cause has been found,

but in spite of avoiding further nerve trauma the condition is worsening.

3. A swelling is palpable or visible radiographically.[191]

RADIAL NERVE COMPRESSION NEUROPATHIES

The radial nerve is most commonly injured by fractures and blasts,[204,205] and less commonly afflicted by cumulative trauma. However, there are some occupational CTDs that can affect the radial nerve. It has been postulated that the virtuoso composer and pianist Robert Schumann, who was plagued by mental illness, suffered from partial posterior interosseous nerve palsy that caused weakness and apparently extensor lag in the index and middle fingers.[199] Schumann led a tortured life and died in a mental institution in 1856 where he had been hospitalized since 1854 following a suicide attempt.

We will discuss four important radial nerve compression syndromes:

1. Radial nerve at the brachium (high radial nerve palsy wrist-drop syndrome)
2. Radial tunnel syndrome
3. Posterior interosseous nerve syndrome
4. Wartenberg's syndrome (sensory nerve entrapment of the radial nerve).

Anatomy of the Radial Nerve.   The radial nerve is the continuation of the posterior division of the brachial plexus (Fig. 34). It has fibers from roots of C5 through the T1 nerve root.[122] In the axilla it is located laterally, and soon thereafter it travels obliquely. It gives off muscular branches to the triceps and anconeus. It then curves around the proximal humerus in close proximity to the spiral groove supplying the brachioradialis and extensor carpi radialis brevis and longus. This close association with the bony humerus makes it susceptible to direct compression. The most common cited example is "Saturday night palsy."[101] The nerve travels anterior 10 cm above the elbow.[122] At the level of the elbow, usually the radial nerve divides into two branches: the superficial radial sensory nerve and the posterior interosseous nerve, a pure motor branch (Fig. 35).

The superficial radial nerve branch lies beneath the brachioradialis muscle and tendon and travels under the brachioradialis musculotendinous unit. It exists at the distal third of the forearm, at which point it goes dorsally and

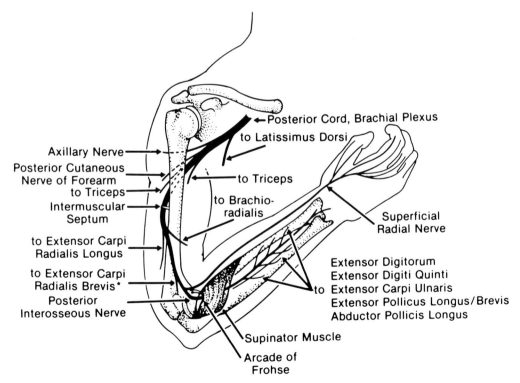

FIGURE 34.   Lateral view of the right arm, showing the course, clinically relevant anatomical relations, and major branches of the radial nerve. (Modified from Lotem M, et al: J Bone Joint Surg 53B:505, with permission.)

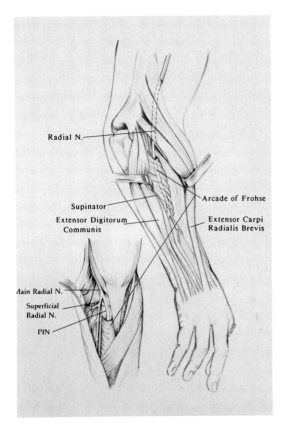

FIGURE 35. Radial nerve course in the distal arm and proximal forearm. Note the arcade of Frohse (supinator canal). (Adapted from Green DP: Operative Hand Surgery, 2nd ed. New York, Churchill Livingstone, 1988, with permission.)

superficially to supply sensation on the dorsal radial aspect of the hand.[202]

The deep motor branch of the radial nerve, the posterior interosseous nerve, passes into the radial tunnel. Entrapment of the radial nerve in the radial tunnel can produce the radial tunnel syndrome.[203] Its symptoms closely mimic those of lateral humeral epicondylitis (tennis elbow). The radial tunnel begins just after the takeoff of the motor branches to the brachioradialis and extensor carpi radialis longus and brevis. At the entrance of the tunnel,[202] the radial nerve is bordered medially by the brachialis muscle and the biceps tendon, laterally by the origin of the brachioradialis muscle, and posteriorly by the lateral humeral epicondyle. As the radial nerve progresses distally, it becomes crossed by the extensor carpi radialis brevis, which can compress the nerve against the bony capitellum.[202] It is important at the onset to note the proximity of the radial tunnel and the more distal supinator canal with the

arcade of Frohse,[196] which in fact overlap in some cases but have different symptoms and signs.[196,202]

Occupational Causes of Radial Nerve Palsy. The radial nerve can suffer damage due to external pressure at the upper arm as it winds around the posterior aspect of the humerus. Wrist drop occurs related to weakness of the extensor muscles of the forearm, because of which the paralyzed extensors of the wrist and fingers are unable to position the joints for leverage. This renders inadequate the flexion and pinching performed by the median and ulnar innervated muscles (Fig. 36).[22] Wrist drop may occur in those whose work position results in pressure of the radial nerve against the underlying bone.[22]

Occupations Associated with Radial Nerve Entrapment at the Brachium (High Radial Nerve Palsy). **Porters** who carry heavy parcels that press on the inner aspect of the upper arms and **military recruits** who shoot rifles with the sling tightly fastened around the upper arm are at risk.[195] Any kind of tourniquet may produce a high radial nerve palsy. Testing for wrist strength and extensor tendon function is important (Fig. 37). There is also a sensory deficit in the radial sensory nerve distribution. The wrist and digital posture in Figure 37 should be compared with Figure 38, which shows a posterior interosseous nerve palsy in which wrist extension is preserved because the extensor carpi radialis is not denervated.

The radial nerve passes between the heads of the supinator muscle and innervates that muscle. In 1908 the German anatomist, Frohse,[196] with Frankel described the area

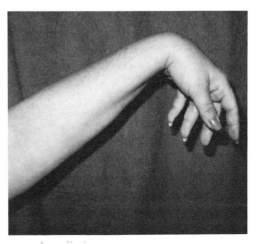

FIGURE 36. Example of a complete high radial nerve palsy. Note the wrist drop and digital extensor lag.

where the two heads of the supinator muscle arose from the lateral and medial edges of the lateral humeral epicondyle. Spinner found a fibrous arch in 30% of his dissections, which he termed the arcade of Frohse.[122,206]

The radial nerve exits from the distal border of the supinator muscle and gives off multiple branches that supply the following muscles:

1. More superficial layer of muscles
   a. Extensor digitorum communis
   b. Extensor digiti quinti
   c. Extensor carpi ulnaris
2. Deeper muscles
   a. Abductor pollicis longus
   b. Extensor pollicis longus
   c. Extensor pollicis brevis
   d. Extensor indicis proprius.[122]

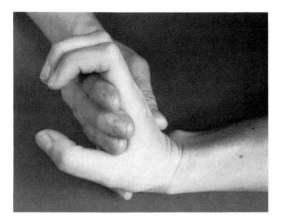

FIGURE 37. Testing for wrist strength and extensor tendon function is important in diagnosing radial nerve disorders. (From Mackinnon SE, Dellon AL: Surgery of the Peripheral Nerve. New York, Thieme Medical, 1988, adapted with permission.)

Radial Tunnel Syndrome

Radial tunnel syndrome is best described as having pain without palsy. The pain is usually dull and aching over the extensor supinator area in the proximal forearm, and it can radiate into the distal forearm and hand. The pain is usually initiated and intensified by repetitive movements incorporating forearm pronation, often with wrist flexion, presumably because pain is caused by wrist dorsiflexion of strong power grasp.[201] The radial tunnel syndrome is more frequently encountered than the paralysis of the posterior interosseous nerve syndrome.[112]

Tests for Radial Tunnel Syndrome. *Resisted middle finger extension* causes more pain to be referred to an area beneath the mobile muscle mass than does resisted extension of the little or ring finger.[201,202] This is based on the mechanism of symptom induction by compression of the nerve by the extensor carpi radialis brevis origin. The extensor carpi radialis brevis inserts at the base of the third (middle) metacarpal (Fig. 39).

Resisted supination creates a pain referred to the mobile muscle extensor mass. Palpation of the radial nerve in this region causes pain (Fig. 40).[202] The lateral humeral epicondyle is tender with tennis elbow.

Occupations and Avocations Associated with Radial Tunnel Syndrome. Carpenters, builders,[22,203] **housewives,**[203] **maintenance builders,**[203] **plant operator** using a pneumatic drill,[203] **secretary,**[203] **assembly line workers,**[112] **weight lifters**, and occasionally **tennis players** have been reported.[112]

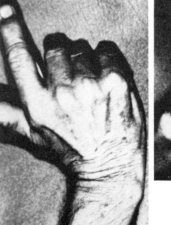

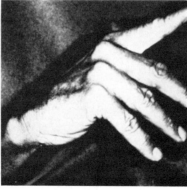

FIGURE 38. Example of complete posterior interosseous nerve palsy. Note that radial wrist extension is maintained because of an intact extensor carpi radialis. (From Compression neuropathies in the anterior forearm. Hand Clin 2:743, 1986, with permission.)

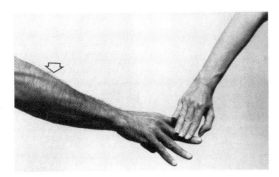

FIGURE 39. Diagnosis of radial tunnel syndrome. Resisted middle finger extension causes more pain to be referred to an area beneath the mobile muscle wad (arrow) than does resisted extension of the little or ring finger. Mechanism of symptom induction is compression of the nerve by extensor carpi radialis brevis, which inserts at the base of the third ("middle") metacarpal. (From Mackinnon SE, Dellon AL: Surgery of the Peripheral Nerve. New York, Thieme Medical, 1988, with permission.)

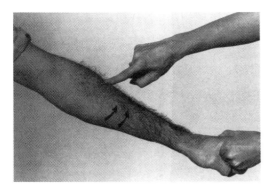

FIGURE 40. Diagnosis of the radial tunnel syndrome. Resisted supination creates pain referred to the mobile muscle wad (arrows). Palpation of radial nerve in this region causes pain. (The lateral humeral epicondyle is where resisted wrist and finger extension produce pain with lateral humeral epicondylitis—tennis elbow.) (From Mackinnon SE, Dellon AL: Surgery of the Peripheral Nerve. New York, Thieme Medical, 1988, with permission.)

Differential Diagnosis. The differential diagnosis includes lateral epicondylitis of the elbow.[203] Tests including resisted middle finger extension and resisted supination should be performed, as discussed above. Injections with Xylocaine may be utilized to localize the lesion.

Treatment. The treatment is surgical with release of constricting points in the radial tunnel, if splinting and rest do not relieve symptoms.

Posterior Interosseous Nerve Syndrome (PINS)

While the radial tunnel syndrome is associated with aching pain without palsy, the posterior interosseous nerve syndrome (PINS) starts as pain, followed by progressive weakness and motor loss. Cases of compression on the dorsal aspect of the forearm have been reported in **bricklayers**.[200] In performing their trade, they lay bricks on the forearm while handling cement with the other arm. Most cases of entrapment of the posterior interosseous nerve occur as the result of forceful supination, dorsiflexion, or radial deviation of the wrist. This has been reported in **musicians** such as **oboists** and **orchestra conductors**.[171] Mandel in fact noted that PINS was first described in an orchestral conductor[112,197] in 1905, whose baton movements of repetitive pronation-supination were thought to be causative factors. Other occupations include **violinist, dairymen, barmen**, and **roofers**.[112]

There is loss of digital extension at the MCP joints and a loss of thumb abduction. The extension at the IP joints is preserved because of intrinsic innervation. There is no wrist drop because the extensor carpi radialis is intact, but wrist extension drifts into radial deviation owing to the paralysis of the extensor carpi ulnaris muscle (see Fig. 38). This can be distinguished from radial nerve lesions above the bifurcation, in which wrist drop and sensory symptoms predominate (compare Figs. 36 and 38).

Tendon ruptures (seen in rheumatoid arthritis) need to be differentiated from posterior interosseous nerve syndrome. This can be done by utilizing the tenodesis effect, so that when the wrist is flexed normally, the fingers become extended, and when the wrist is extended, the fingers become flexed. The tenodesis effect is maintained in PINS, but it is lost in the event of tendon rupture. Electromyography is also helpful in diagnosing the location of the lesion.[202]

Ergonomics. Instruct workers not to carry items on their forearm or allow straps from heavy bags to place sustained pressure in this area. Workers can also be instructed in alternate hand positions with varying degrees of supination, extension and radial deviation of the wrist, which appears to be the location in which most cases are reported.[15,22,29,198]

Wartenberg's Syndrome (Radial Sensory Nerve Entrapment)

Radial sensory neuropathy in the distal radial forearm was first described in 1932 by Robert Wartenberg,[209] a German neurologist. He reported on a series of five patients who had complaints of area of pain or numbness over the dorso-radial hand associated with palpable tenderness of the radial sensory nerve.

Radial Sensory Nerve (RSN). The RSN lies beneath the brachioradialis muscle in the forearm and is superficial to the radial artery (Fig. 35). This nerve exists from the distal border of the brachioradialis, emerging between the tendons of the brachioradialis and the extensor carpi radialis longus, at about the juncture of the distal third and middle third of the forearm.[202] The nerve can exit as far distally as the midportion of the forearm to a few centimeters proximal to the radial styloid.

Its superficial position coupled with its proximity to the radial styloid make it more likely to receive compressive forces from external bands, such as wrist watches and handcuffs.[22] Dellon and Mackinnon described radial sensory entrapment in the forearm, documenting 58 RSN entrapments in 51 patients.[207] Workmens' compensation was involved in 58 of these patients, and the problem was found to be work-related in 13%. Of the 51 patients, 35 were women and 16 were men. The patients usually gave a history of a crushing contusion. Persistent pain over the dorsal radial surface of the distal third of the forearm radiating to the dorsum of the hand, thumb, and index and middle fingers is the most common symptom.[85]

Some patients have as their initial complaint discomfort with writing, pinching, or gripping. There may be complaints of numbness and burning over the dorso-radial wrist as well.[207]

On examination, there is sensitivity to percussion over the radial nerve within a few centimeters of the radial styloid along the dorsal edge of the brachioradialis muscle.[202] The percussion sensitivity radiates to the area of pain and is often associated with numbness. Finkelstein's test is frequently positive.[202,208] This test is performed by having the thumb held under the fingers and passively moving the wrist in an ulnar position. Finkelstein's test is frequently positive both in entrapment of the RSN and in de Quervain's disease (stenosing tenosynovitis). To differentiate between the two, there is usually tenderness without numbness over the first dorsal extensor compartment in de Quervain's disease, but not in RSN entrapment.

The provocative test for entrapment of the RSN is illustrated in Figure 41A. The patient puts the forearm in hyperpronation, with the wrist held in position. Within 1 minute, symp-

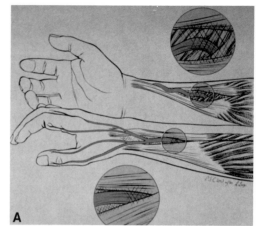

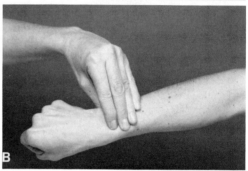

FIGURE 41. A, Diagrammatic illustration of mechanism of radial sensory nerve entrapment. With the forearm supinated, the superficial branch of the radial nerve lies beneath the fascia but without compression between the tendons of the brachioradialis and the extensor carpi radialis longus. When the forearm pronates, the extensor carpi radialis longus tendon pulls proximally, crossing beneath the brachioradialis tendon and creating a scissoring or pinching of the superficial branch of the radial nerve. B, In addition, symptoms can be provoked by pressure over the radial sensory nerve (just dorsal to the musculotendinous junction of the brachioradialis muscle) and forearm pronation with wrist ulnar flexion. (From Mackinnon SE, Dellon AL: Surgery of the Peripheral Nerve. New York, Thieme Medical, 1988, adapted with permission.)

toms of dorsal radial burning paresthesias reflect a positive test. Additionally, pressure over the intersection area of the two tendons of the brachioradialis and extensor carpi radialis longus will augment the symptoms, as will wrist flexion (Fig. 41B). Electrodiagnostic nerve conduction studies of the superficial radial sensory nerve can aid in the diagnosis of an entrapment neuropathy.[74]

There is frequently a history of trauma, such as a fall on the arm, a twisting motion of the forearm or, a history of a direct stroke or trauma to the dorsoradial wrist. There are certain occupations that can be causative factors in this neural entrapment: **assembly line workers**, using pneumatic tools, and **carpentry workers** both utilize repetitive supination-pronation movements in their work. The problem of an RSN irritation is augmented when the wrist is ulnar flexed. **Chefs, bookkeepers**, and **dishwashers** are at risk for radial nerve entrapment. People wearing bracelets, or tight watchbands are also prone to get symptoms.[202]

Treatment and Ergonomics.   Initially treatment is conservative, with splinting to include the thumb, wrist, and forearm, and restricted activities. In some instances, anti-inflammatory medications and vitamin B6 are helpful.[207] Surgical treatment is indicated if the patient is unresponsive to conservative treatment modalities, and operative intervention involves decompression of the RSN.

Avoid tight wristbands such as safety restraints. Workstation modification to allow performance of job tasks with the wrist in the neutral position and less time spent on repetitive tasks can decrease the incidence of RSN entrapment.[15,22,198] Cords of tools being used should not be wrapped around the wrist.

MULTIPLE CRUSH SYNDROMES

Multiple crush syndrome[211] is a symptom complex due to compression of a peripheral nerve at more than one site of entrapment. Upton and McComas, in 1973,[213] described multiple compression neuropathies based on their clinical observations that 70% of their patients had either carpal tunnel or ulnar neuropathy associated with evidence of cervicothoracic root lesions. These authors noted that there was an increased incidence of diabetes mellitus in carpal tunnel syndrome. They hypothesized that serial constraints on axoplasmic flow, each insufficient in itself to cause symptoms, could together summate to cause symptomatic neural dysfunction.[213] Upton and McComas coined the term *double crush syndrome*. Massey et al.[212] in 1981 described 19 patients who had carpal tunnel syndrome and cervical radiculopathy, most commonly at C6 and C7, and additionally described patients with coexisting carpal tunnel and brachial plexus neuropathy.

It is important to differentiate between multiple crush syndromes and multiple peripheral nerve entrapments. According to Mackinnon and Dellon,[211] multiple crush syndromes can be categorized as follows:

1. Multiple anatomic regions along a peripheral nerve—e.g., carpal tunnel syndrome associated with a pronator syndrome, or a cervical radiculopathy associated with a carpal tunnel syndrome.
2. Multiple anatomic structures across a peripheral nerve within an anatomic area—e.g., thoracic outlet syndrome with multiple entrapment areas.
3. Superimposed on a neuropathy—e.g., the patient begins with a Guyon's canal compression and develops a cubital tunnel syndrome.
4. Combinations of the above.

The patient with carpal tunnel syndrome and cubital tunnel syndrome *does not* have a multiple crush syndrome but has multiple peripheral nerve entrapments. Releasing a distal area of entrapment may not relieve the symptoms occurring at a proximal entrapment site.

There have been hypotheses by multiple authors as to the mechanism by which proximal nerve lesions "set the stage" for distal nerve lesions. Simplistically stated: A proximal axon lesion can render the distal nerve more vulnerable to pressure by impairing distal energy metabolism, and by proximal interruption of lymphatic or venous drainage. This renders the distal nerve more vulnerable to edema at either a proximal or distal site. Lundborg hypothesized that there is an interaction between the central cell body, the axon, and the distal innervation territory, and that each affects each other through trophic influences. With a distal compression lesion, retrograde axonal transport might be compromised. This would then cause a sick nerve cell body, which would not be able to manage the antegrade axonal transport. The lack of proper transport material required to keep axonal membranes properly functioning would be jeopardized.[210] One needs to distinguish a multiple crush type of entrapment from patients having multiple separate nerve entrapments.[211]

Multiple crush syndrome after trauma, especially work-related or motor vehicle trauma associated with litigation is difficult to manage. Frequently the patient has lived with pain and is not infrequently considered a "malingerer." Frequently, a team including the services of a hand surgeon, orthopedic surgeon, neurosurgeon, psychiatrist, and physiatrist is needed to manage the patient.

TABLE 2. Summary of Nerve Entrapments of the Upper Extremity

Nerve	Site of Entrapment	Symptoms	Physical Signs and Special Tests	Factors	Occupations
Median Nerve A. Pronator Teres Syndrome	Distal ⅓ of the humerus, beneath the supracondylar process and the ligament of Struthers Lacertus Fibrosus Between the superficial and deep heads of the pronator teres muscle Arch of flexor digitorum superficialis	Aching in the proximal forearm Easy fatigability of the forearm Paresthesia and numbness of thumb, index and long fingers Nocturnal paresthesias are uncommon	Tenderness of the pronator tunnel Pain with: —resisted pronation —resisted pronation with clenched fist —resisted forearm flexion and supination —resisted middle finger sublimis Positive Tinel's sign over pronator tunnel	Repetitive exertional grasping work with pronation and supination	Housewives, nurses, farmers, dentists, cutters, writters, musicians, wood workers, assembly line workers
B. Anterior Interosseous Nerve (AIN) Complete AIN syndrome	Proximal forearm	Pain in forearm Referred pain to the elbow	Inability to flex the thumb at IP joint and index finger at the DIP joint and variably the middle finger at the DIP joint ("O" sign) Weakened pronation	Repetitive action causing hypertrophy of forearm muscles and compression	Newspaper carriers, plumbers, typists, assembly line workers
Incomplete AIN syndrome	Proximal forearm	Pain in forearm Referred pain to the elbow	Inability to flex the thumb at the IP joint or index finger at the DIP joint	Repetitive action causing hypertrophy of the forearm muscles and compression	Bank tellers, bass players, mechanics, press operators
C. Carpal Tunnel Syndrome	Wrist	Paresthesia at night in the thumb, index, long and radial ½ of the ring fingers Pain radiating into forearm	Positive Phalen's sign Positive Tinel's sign Abnormal 2-point discrimination along the median nerve distribution in the hand. Abnormal response to vibrometer Thenar muscle atrophy Sensation of coldness and sweating.	Repetitive wrist flexion with finger flexion	Meat packers, butchers, poultry workers, workers using vibrating tools, chain saw operators, assembly line workers, garment workers, musicians
D. Palmar Digital Neuropathy	Deep transverse metacarpal ligament	Pain and numbness in the involved digit	Sensory deficit in the involved digit Positive Tinel's sign	Repetitive extension forcing the digital nerve against the deep transverse metacarpal ligament (i.e., fingers held in extension while clapping)	Cheerleaders, seamstresses, bowlers

	Site of Lesion	Complaints	Signs	Cause	Occupations
E. Opponens Branch Entrapment	Median nerve at the distal edge of the transverse palmar ligament	Tenderness over the palm area near the thumb Complaints of weak pinch and grip Numbness over the palm area near the thumb	Atrophy of the opponens muscle Weakness in pinch and grip strengths Tenderness over the nerve at the edge of the transverse ligament	Pounding or pressure into the palm against the thenar area	Painters, carpenters, stable hands, time keepers, receipt processors
F. Thumb Digital Nerve Entrapments	IP joint of the thumb and the region distal to the IP joint	Pain and numbness in the distal portion of the thumb	Varying degrees of pain and numbness in the thumb distal to the entrapment site Positive Tinel's sign	Repetitive trauma to the digital nerves of the thumb	Cherry pitter, jeweler, bowler
Ulnar					
A. Cubital Tunnel Syndrome	Elbow Entrance of the canal, just posterior to the medial epicondyle Fascial aponeurosis joining the two heads of the flexor carpi ulnaris Muscle bellies of flexor carpi ulnaris	Dysesthesia of the small finger and ulnar ½ of the ring finger	Pain over the medial aspect of the elbow and forearm Atrophy of the hypothenar and interossei Positive Tinel's sign at the cubital tunnel Positive Froment's sign Clawing of the ring and small fingers	Flexion and pronation Habitual leaning on flexed elbows Protracted elbow extension	Protracted elbow flexors: Telephone operators, watchmakers, jewelers, glass blowers, musicians, dressmakers, cab drivers Protracted elbow extensors: carpenters, people who shovel or grind, crystal cutters, people who use hand-powered or pneumatic drills
B. Guyon's Canal Type I	Proximal to the bifurcation of the ulnar nerve into the superficial and deep branches at the wrist	Numbness and tingling in the involved digits Complaints of difficulty with the use of the ring and small fingers	Motor impairment in the ulnar intrinsics Sensory deficits in the small finger and ulnar ½ of the ring finger Clawing of the digits may be present	Palm held in hyperextension or repetitive forces applied to the base of the hypothenar eminence over a long period of time	Housewives, ropemakers, mechanics
Type II	Superficial branch of the ulnar nerve at the wrist, but distal to the branch to the palmaris brevis	Pain in the involved digits Numbness and tingling in the involved digits No complaint of strength loss	Sensory impairment only to the ulnar innervated digits (small finger and ulnar ½ of the ring finger)	Palm held in hyperextension or repetitive forces applied to the base of the hypothenar eminence over a long period of time	Steel workers
Type III	The lesion of the deep branch of the ulnar nerve is just distal to the superficial branch, but proximal to the branch going to the hypothenar	Fatigability of the small fingers with loss of grip Spasms in the hypothenar muscles No complaints of numbness or tingling	Clawing of the hand Hypothenar, interossei and adductor pollicis weakness	Palm held in hyperextension or repetitive forces applied to the base of the hypothenar eminence over a long period of time	Professional and amateur cyclists, carpenters, metal workers, farmers, workers using pneumatic tools

TABLE 2. *Continued*

Nerve	Site of Entrapment	Symptoms	Physical Signs and Special Tests	Factors	Occupations
Type IV	Deep branch of the ulnar nerve distal to the origin of the superficial branch and distal to the branch going to the hypothenar, near the hook of the hamate.	Complaints of hand weakness Complaints of pain and spasms No complaints of numbness or tingling	Weakness of all ulnar nerve innervated muscles in the hand, except the hypothenar muscles	Palm held in hyperextension or repetitive forces applied to the base of the hypothenar eminence over a long period of time	Metal workers
Type V	Proximal to the branches going to the first dorsal interossei and the adductor pollicis muscles	Weakness in the thumb and index finger lateral pinch No complaints of numbness and tingling	Thenar atrophy Atrophy of the adductor pollicis and 1st dorsal interossei	Palm held in hyperextension or repetitive forces applied to the base of the hypothenar eminence over a period of time	Amateur weight lifter
Radial Nerve A. Radial Nerve Entrapment—Brachium (High Radial Nerve Palsy)	Upper arm at the posterior aspect of the humerus	Inability to extend the fingers and wrist Numbness to the dorsal aspect of the wrist and hand	Wrist drop Paralyzed extensors of the wrist and fingers render inadequate flexion and pinch Sensory deficit in the radial sensory nerve distribution	Compression of the radial nerve against the unyielding humerus	Parcel carriers, military recruits ("rifle sling palsy")
B. Posterior Interosseous Nerve (PINS)	Dorsal aspect of the forearm, just distal to the elbow.	Tingling Inability to extend the fingers and the thumb Pain with complaint of progressive weakness and motor loss	Lack of MCP joint extension of the fingers Lack of IP joint extension of the thumb	Repetitive forceful supination and extension or radial deviation of the wrist	Bricklayers, oboists, orchestra conductors
C. Radial Tunnel or Supinator Syndrome	At the elbow, where the radial nerve is bordered medially by the brachialis muscle and the biceps tendon, laterally by the origin of the brachioradialis and posteriorly by the lateral humeral epicondyle	Dull aching pain over the extensor supinator area in the proximal forearm that can radiate into the distal forearm and hand No palsy	Increased pain with resisted long finger extension compared to the ring and small fingers Increased pain with resisted supination	Repetitive resisted supination and middle finger extension	Carpenters, assembly line workers, builders
D. Wartenberg Syndrome	Distal radial forearm	Pain over the dorsal radial surface of the distal ⅓ of the forearm radiating to the dorsum of the hand, thumb, index and middle fingers. Discomfort in writing, pinching and gripping.	Sensitivity to percussion and numbness over the radial nerve, near the radial styloid Positive Finkelstein's test Hyperpronation test	Twisting motion of the forearm Strike or trauma to the dorsoradial wrist Tight wrist wear	Carpenters, assembly line workers, dishwashers, bookkeepers

CONCLUSION

We have reviewed cumulative trauma disorders and ergonomics from a historical perspective and have focused on cervicobrachial disorders and focal peripheral neuropathies (see Table 2). As jobs become more specialized and job tasks more streamlined, repetitive trauma to the worker becomes a significant concern. It is important to recognize the signs and symptoms of compressive neuropathies associated with CTD in order to minimize their occurrence. Prevention and early intervention to correct either the ergonomic problem at work or to initiate early conservative treatment are the key to minimizing serious disorder and dysfunction in the upper extremity. The control of CTD and compression neuropathies will have significant socioeconomic benefits to both the employer and the worker.

Acknowledgment

Special thanks for assistance in the preparation of this chapter to: Nancy Howard, Medical Illustrator; Diana Penning; Ruth Colson; Leslie Gilliam and Beth Rockwell, National Hospital, Arlington, VA; Esther Plotkin, Physical Medicine Department, Alexandria Hospital, VA; Kip Seymour, Media Services, Fairfax Hospital, VA (Photography); Fairfax Hospital Library Staff: Betty Brown, Alice Sheridan, Lois Culler, Phyllis Naworal, Sue Polucci, Pia Fish, Danny Overcash. Special thanks to Dr. Lee Dellon for review of this manuscript.

REFERENCES

Definition of Terms and Brief Historical Perspective

1. Armstrong T, Foulke J, Joseph B, Goldstein S: Analysis of cumulative trauma disorders in a poultry processing plant. Am Ind Hyg Assoc J 43:103–116, 1982.
2. Bartlett J: Bartlett's Familiar Quotations, 15th ed. Edited by Emily Morrison Beck, et al. Boston, Little, Brown, 1980, p 725.
3. Blair S, Bear-Lehman J: Editorial comment: Prevention of upper extremity occupational disorders. J Hand Surg 12A:821–822, 1987.
4. Garraty JA: The American Nation: A History of the United States, 6th ed. San Francisco, Harper & Row, 1987, pp 539–541.
5. Garraty JA: The American Nation: A History of the United States, 5th ed. San Francisco, Harper & Row, 1983, p 443.
6. Garraty JA: The American Nation: A History of the United States, 5th ed. San Francisco, Harper & Row, 1983, p 579.
7. Joseph BS: Ergonomic considerations and job design in upper extremity disorders. In Kasdan ML (ed): Occupational Hand Injuries. Occup Med State Art Rev 4:547–557, 1989.
8. Law: Section on Work in Art Source Book. Compiled from Bridgeman Art Library. Secaucus, NJ, Chartwell Books Inc, Publishers, 1987, p 79.
9. Leamon TB: The introduction of ergonomics: A problem of industrial practice. Appl Ergon 11:161–164, 1980.
10. Naughton TD: Making the workplace work. In Medical and Health Annual. Chicago, Encyclopedia Britannica, 1989, p 360.
11. Pechan J, Kredba J: Cubital Tunnel Syndrome. I. General Aspects. Acta University Carolin Medica, 1981, pp 5–6.
12. Ramazzini B: De Morbis Artificum (Diseases of Workers) Wri Chica. Chicago, University of Chicago, 1940, p 15.
13. Sinclair U: The Jungle. New York, New American Classic (Signet Classic), 1980.
14. Swoboda F: Work site changes let meatpackers stand tall. Washington, DC, Washington Post, December 30, 1989, pp A1, A8.

Cervicobrachial Disorders: Myofascial Pain and Cervical Spondylosis

15. Armstrong TJ, Fine LJ, Goldstein SA, et al: Ergonomics consideration in hand-wrist tendinitis. J Hand Surg 12A:830–837, 1987.
16. Bjelle A, Hagberg M, Michaelson G: Work-related shoulder-neck complaints in industry: A pilot study. Br J Rheumatol 26:365–369, 1987.
17. Bland J (ed): Disorders of the Cervical Spine: Diagnosis and Medical Management. Philadelphia, W.B. Saunders, 1987.
18. Bremner JM, Lawrence JS, Mial WE: Degenerative joint disease in a Jamaican rural population. Ann Rheum Dis 27:326–332, 1968.
19. Chan KK, Ling LC: Back and neck problems in a teaching institution. J Royal Soc Health 108:182–184, 1988.
20. Cilley RE: There are many ways to kill a resident: Try house officer's headache or intern's neck (letter). JAMA 254:1905–1906, 1985.
21. Elias F: Roentgen findings in the asymptomatic cervical spine. NY State J Med 58:320, 1958.
22. Feldman RG, Goldman R, Keyserling W: Peripheral nerve entrapment syndrome and ergonomics factors. Am J Ind Med 4:661–681, 1983.
23. Hagberg M, Wegman DH: Prevalence rates and odds ratios of shoulder-neck diseases in different "occupational" groups. Br J Ind Med 44:602–610, 1987.
24. Jeffreys E: Disorders of the Cervical Spine. London, Butterworth, 1980.
25. Leek JC, Gershwin ME, Fowler WM: Principles of Physical Medicine and Rehabilitation in Musculoskeletal Disease. Orlando, Harcourt Brace Jovanovich, 1986.
26. Macnab I: Cervical spondylosis. Clin Orthop 109:69–77, 1975.
27. Maeda K, Horiguchi S, Hosokawa M: History of the studies of occupational cervicobrachial disorders in

Japan and remaining problems. J Hum Ergol (Tokyo) 11:17–29, 1982.

28. McDermott FT: Repetition strain injury and review of current understanding. Med J Aust 144:196–200, 1986.

29. Meagher SW: Tool design for prevention of hand-wrist injuries. J Hand Surg 12A:855–857, 1987.

30. Nakaseko M, Tokunaga R, Hosokawa M: History of occupational cervicobrachial disorders in Japan. J Hum Ergol (Tokyo) 11:7–16, 1982.

31. Newell DJ: Prevalence, aetiology and treatment of pain in the neck and arm. Transactions of the Society of Occupational Medicine 17:104–106, 1967.

32. Ohara H, Aoyama H, Itani T: Health hazard among cash register operators and the effects of improved working conditions. J Hum Ergol (Tokyo) 5:31–40, 1976.

33. Sallstrom J, Schmidt H: Cervicobrachial disorders in certain occupations with special reference to compression in the thoracic outlet. Am J Ind Med 6:45–52, 1984.

34. Simons DG: Myofascial pain syndrome due to trigger points: principles, diagnosis, and perpetuating factors. Manual Med, 1985.

35. Simons DG: Myofascial Pain Syndrome Due to Trigger Points. IRMA Monograph, Series Number 1, November 1987.

36. Travell JG, Simons DG: Myofascial Pain and Dysfunction: The Trigger Point Manual. Baltimore, Williams & Wilkins, 1983.

37. Weed LL: Your Health and How to Manage It. Essex Junction, VT, Essex Publishing, 1975.

Cervicobrachial Disorders: Thoracic Outlet Syndrome

38. Adson AW: Surgical treatment for symptoms produced by cervical ribs and the scalenus anterior muscle. Surg Gynecol Obstet 85:687–696, 1947.

39. Adson AW, Coffey JR: Cervical rib: A method of anterior approach for relief of symptoms by division of the scalenus anticus. Ann Surg 85:839, 1927.

40. Brickner WM: Brachial plexus pressure by the normal first rib. Ann Surg 85:858, 1927.

41. Clagett OT: Presidential address: Research and prosearch. J Thorac Cardiovasc Surg 44:153, 1962.

42. Cooper A: On exostosis. In Cooper and Travers: Surgical Essays, 3rd ed. London, 1821, p 128.

43. Coote H: Exostosis of the left transverse process of the seventh cervical vertebra surrounded by blood vessels and nerves: Successful removal. Lancet i:360, 1861.

44. Eversmann WW Jr: Entrapment and compression neuropathies. In Green DP (ed): Operative Hand Surgery, 2nd ed. New York, Churchill Livingstone, 1988, pp 1461–1463.

45. Harvey W: Exercitatio Anatomica de Motu Cordis et Sanguinis in Animalibus (1627). Translated by C.D. Leake. Springfield, IL, Charles C Thomas, 1970, 5 ed, p 36.

46. Kaye BL: Neurologic changes with excessively large breasts. South Med J 65:177, 1972.

47. Leffert RD: Thoracic outlet syndrome. In Omer GE, Spinner M (eds): Management of Peripheral Nerve Problems. Philadelphia, W.B. Saunders, 1980, pp 592–599.

48. Lockwood AH: Medical problems in musicians. N Engl J Med 320:1989.

49. Lord JW Jr, Rosati LM: Thoracic outlet syndrome. In Ciba Clinical Symposia, Vol 23, No. 2, 1971.

50. Mackinnon SE, Dellon AL: Multiple crush syndrome. In Surgery of the Peripheral Nerve. New York, Thieme Medical, 1988, pp 360–368.

51. Murphy T: Brachial neuritis caused by pressure of first rib. Aust Med J 15:582, 1910.

52. Oschner S, Gage M, DeBakey M: Scalenus anticus (Naffziger's syndrome) Am J Surg 28:669–695, 1935.

53. Peet RM, Hendricksen JD, Guderson IP, Martin GM: Thoracic outlet syndrome. Evaluation of a therapeutic exercise program. Proc Mayo Clin 31:281, 1956.

54. Raskin NH, Howard MW, Ehrenfeld WK: Headaches as the leading symptom of the thoracic outlet syndrome. Headache 25:208–210, 1985.

55. Roeder DK, et al: First rib resection in the treatment of thoracic outlet syndrome (transaxillary and posterior thoracoplasty approaches). Ann Surg 178:49–52, 1973.

56. Roos DB: Transaxillary approach for first rib resection to relieve thoracic outlet syndrome. Ann Surg 163:354, 1966.

57. Roos DB: Experience with first rib resection for thoracic outlet syndrome. Ann Surg 173:429, 1971.

58. Roos DB, Owens JC: Thoracic outlet syndrome. Arch Surg 93:71–74, 1966.

59. Stewart JDB: Brachial plexus-thoracic outlet syndromes. In Focal Peripheral Neuropathies. New York, Elsevier Publishers, 1987, pp 109–115.

60. Stopford JSB, Telford ED: Compression of lower trunk of the brachial plexus by a first dorsal rib. Br J Surg 7:168, 1919.

61. Travell JG, Simons DG: Myofascial Pain and Dysfunction: The Trigger Point Manual. Baltimore, Williams & Wilkins, 1983, p 4.

62. Wilbourne AJ: True Neurogenic Thoracic Outlet Syndrome. Rochester, MN, Assoc of Electromyography and Electrodiagnostics, 1982.

63. Wright IS: The neurovascular syndrome produced by hyperabduction of the arms. Am Heart J 29:1, 1945.

Brachial Plexus Neuropathy

64. Barnes R: Traction injuries of the brachial plexus in adults. J Bone Joint Surg 31B:10–16, 1949.

65. Bassett F, Nunley J: Compression of the musculocutaneous nerve at the elbow. J Bone Joint Surg 64A:1050–1052, 1982.

66. Bateman JE: Nerve injuries above the shoulder in sports. J Bone Joint Surg 49A:785–792, 1967.

67. Bom F: A case of "pack palsy" from the Korean War. Acta Psychiatr Neurol Scand 28:1–4, 1953.

68. Bonney G: Prognosis in traction lesions of the brachial plexus. J Bone Joint Surg 41B:4–35, 1959.

69. Braddom RL, Wolfe C: Musculocutaneous nerve injury after heavy exercise. Arch Phys Med Rehabil 59:290–293, 1978.

70. Daube JR: Rucksack paralysis. JAMA 208:2447–2452, 1969.

71. Haymaker W, Woodhall B: Peripheral Nerve Injuries: Principles of Diagnosis, 2nd ed. Philadelphia, W.B. Saunders, 1967.

72. Ilfeld FW, Holder HG: Winged scapula: Case occurring in a soldier from knapsack. JAMA 120:448–449, 1942.

73. Kim SM, Goodrich A: Isolated proximal musculocutaneous nerve palsy: Case report. Arch Phys Med Rehabil 65:735–736, 1984.

74. Kimura J: Electrodiagnosis in Disease of Nerve and Muscle: Principles and Practice. Philadelphia, F.A. Davis, 1983.

75. Leffert RD: Brachial plexus injuries. New York, Churchill Livingstone, 1985, pp 1–38.

76. Mackinnon SE, Dellon AL: Brachial plexus injuries. In Surgery of the Peripheral Nerve. New York, Thieme Medical, 1988, pp 423–434.

77. Martinez AC, Ramirez A: Occupational accessory and suprascapular nerve palsy. A clinical and electrophysiological study. Electromyogr Clin Neurophysiol 28:347–352, 1988.

78. Millesi H: Trauma involving the brachial plexus. In Omer GE, Spinner M (eds): Management of Peripheral Nerve Problems. Philadelphia, W.B. Saunders, 1980, pp 548–568.

79. Petrera JE, Trojaborg W: Conduction studies of the long thoracic nerve in serratus anterior palsy of different etiology and neurology. 34:1033–1037, 1984.

80. Snell RS: Clinical Anatomy for Medical Students. Boston, Little, Brown, 1973, p 319.

81. Stewart JD: The nerves arising from the brachial plexus. In Focal Peripheral Neuropathies. New York, Elsevier, 1987, pp 119–132.

81a. Francel T, Dellon AL, Campbell J: Quadrilateral space syndrome. Plast Reconstr Surg (Submitted March 1990).

Nerve Compression Disorders: Nerve Anatomy, Physiology, and Pathomechanisms

82. Aguayo A, et al: Experimental progressive compressive neuropathy in the rabbit. Arch Neurol 24:358–364, 1971.

83. Dellon AL: Clinical use of vibratory stimuli to evaluate peripheral nerve injury and compression neuropathy. Plast Reconstr Surg 65:466–476, 1980.

84. Dellon AL: The moving two-point discrimination test—Clinical evaluation of the quickly adapting fiber/receptor system. J Hand Surg 3:474–481, 1978.

85. Eversmann WW: Entrapment and compression neuropathies. In Green DP Jr (ed): Operative Hand Surgery, 2nd ed. New York, Churchill Livingstone, 1988, pp 1423–1425 (Mechanism of nerve compression); pp 1425–1478 (Compression neuropathies).

86. Fontana F: Taite sur le venin de la vipere sur la poisons. Americains Vol 2. Florence, 1798.

87. Fowler RJ, Danta G, Gilliat RW: Recovery of nerve conduction after a pneumatic tourniquet: Observations on the hind-limb of the baboon. J Neurol Neurosurg Psychiatry 35:638, 1972.

88. Gelberman RH, Szabo RM, Williamson RV, Dimick MP: Sensibility testing in peripheral nerve compression syndromes. An Experimental Study in Humans. J Bone Joint Surg 65A:632–638, 1983.

89. Kleinert HE, Griffin JM: Technique of nerve anastomosis. Orthop Clin North Am 4:907–908, 1973.

90. Lundborg G: Structure and function of the intraneural microvessels as related to trauma, edema formation and nerve function. J Bone Joint Surg 57A:938, 1975.

91. Lundborg G: Ischemic nerve injury: experimental studies on intraneural microvascular pathophysiology and nerve function in a limb subjected to temporary circulatory arrest. Scand J Plast Reconstr Surg 6 (suppl):1, 1970.

92. Lundborg G, Rydevik B: Effects of ischemia on the permeability of the perineurium to protein tracers in rabbit tibial nerve. Acta Neurol Scand 49:287, 1973.

93. Lundborg G, Rydevik B: Effects of stretching the tibial nerve of the rabbit. A preliminary study of the intraneural circulation and the barrier function of the perineurium. J Bone Joint Surg 55B:390, 1973.

94. Mackinnon SE, Dellon L: Surgery of the Peripheral Nerve. New York, Thieme Medical, 1988, pp 1–87.

95. Mubarak SJ, Owen CA, Hargens AR, et al: Acute compartment syndromes—Diagnosis and treatment with the aid of the Wick catheter. J Bone Joint Surg 60A:1091–1095, 1978.

96. Ochoa J: Ultrathin longitudinal sections of single myelinated fibers for electron microscopy. J Neurol Sci 17:103–106, 1972.

97. Ochoa JT, Fowler TJ, Gilliatt RW: Anatomical changes in peripheral nerves compressed by a pneumatic tourniquet. J Anat 113:433–455, 1972.

98. Remak R: Observationes Anatomicae et Microscopicae de Systemutis Nervosi Structura. Berlin, Reimer, 1838.

99. Seddon H: Three types of nerve injury. Brain 66:237–288, 1943.

100. Spinner M: Injuries to the Major Branches of Peripheral Nerves of the Forearm, 2nd ed. Philadelphia, W.B. Saunders, 1978, p 27.

101. Stewart JD: Ch 1. The structure of the peripheral nervous system; Ch. 2, Pathology processes producing focal peripheral neuropathies. In Focal Peripheral Neuropathies. New York, Elsevier, 1987, pp 4–7, 8–22.

102. Szabo RM, Gelberman RH: The pathophysiology of nerve entrapment syndromes. J Hand Surg 2A:1987.

103. Szabo RM, Gelberman RH, Dimick MP: Sensibility testing in patients with carpal tunnel syndrome. J Bone Joint Surg 66A:60–64, 1984.

104. Terzis JK: Structure and function of the peripheral nerve. In Daniel RK, Terzis JK (eds): Reconstructive Microsurgery. Boston, Little, Brown, 1977.

Median Nerve—Forearm Level

105. Adelman S, Elsner K: Arm pain in a dentist-pronator syndrome. JADA 105:61–62, 1982.

106. Danielsson LG: Iatrogenic pronator syndrome. Scand J Plast Reconstr Surg 14:201–203, 1980.

107. Dellon AL, et al: Terminal branch of anterior interosseous nerve as a source of wrist pain. J Hand Surg 9B:316–322, 1984.

108. Gessini L, Jandolo B, Pietrangeli A: The pronator teres syndrome (clinical and electrophysiological features in six surgically verified cases). J Neurosurg Sci 1:1–5, 1987.

109. Hartz CR, Linschied RL, Gramse RR, Daube JR: The pronator teres syndrome in the proximal forearm. J Hand Surg 4:48–51, 1979.

110. Hartz CR, et al: The pronator teres syndrome:

Compression neuropathy of the median nerve. J Bone Joint Surg 63A:885–888, 1981.

111. Hill NA, et al: The incomplete anterior interosseous nerve syndrome. J Hand Surg 10A:4–16, 1985.

112. Howard FM: Compression neuropathies in the anterior forearm. Hand Clin North Am 2:743, 1986.

113. Kiloh LG, Nevin S: Isolated neuritis of the anterior interosseous nerve. Br Med J i:850–851, 1952.

114. King RJ, Dunkerton M: The pronator syndrome. Royal Coll Surg (Edin) 27:142–145, 1982.

115. Mackinnon SE, Dellon AL: Median nerve entrapment in the proximal forearm and brachium. In Surgery of the Peripheral Nerve. New York, Thieme Publishers, 1988, pp 171–196.

116. Morris HH, Peters BH: Pronator syndrome: Clinical and electrophysiological features in seven cases. J Neurol Neurosurg Psychiatry 39:461–464, 1976.

117. Nelson RM, Currier DP: Anterior interosseous syndrome—a case report. Phys Ther 60(2):1980.

118. Nigst H, Dick W: Syndromes of compression of the median nerve in the proximal forearm (pronator teres syndrome: anterior interosseous nerve syndrome). Arch Orthop Traumat Surg 93:307–312, 1979.

119. Omer GE, Spinner M: Management of Peripheral Nerve Problems. Philadelphia, W.B. Saunders, 1980, p 579.

120. Parsonage MJ, Turner JW: A neuralgia amyotrophy shoulder girdle syndrome. Lancet i:972, 1948.

121. Seyffarth H: Primary myoses in the musculi pronator teres as a cause of lesion of the nervi medianus (the pronator syndrome). Acta Psychiatr Scand 74(suppl):1, 1951.

122. Spinner M: Injuries to the Major Branches of Peripheral Nerves of the Forearm, 2nd ed. Philadelphia, W.B. Saunders, 1978, pp 80–195 (Radial nerve), 230–266 (Ulnar nerve), 160–226 (Median nerve).

123. Spinner M: The anterior interosseous-nerve syndrome. J Bone Joint Surg 52A:84–94, 1970.

124. Stern, MB: The anterior interosseous nerve syndrome (the Kiloh-Nevin syndrome). Report and follow-up study of three cases. Clin Orthop Rel Res 167:223–227, 1964.

125. Stewart J: The median nerve. In Focal Peripheral Neuropathies. New York, Elsevier, 1987, pp 134–162.

Median Nerve—Wrist Level

126. Arminio JA: Etiology of carpal tunnel syndrome. Del Med J 58:189–192, 1986.

127. Armstrong TJ: Ergonomics & cumulative trauma disorders. Hand Clin 2:553–564, 1986.

128. Armstrong TJ: An Ergonomics Guide to Carpal Tunnel Syndrome. Carpal Tunnel Syndrome Selected References. U.S. Dept of Health and Human Service Public Health Service Centers for Disease Control. NIOSH, March, 1989.

129. Armstrong TJ, Radwin RG, Hansen DJ: Repetitive trauma disorders: Job evaluation and design. Hum Factors 28:325–334, 1986.

130. Bergfield TG, Aulicino PL, Depuy TE: The carpal tunnel syndrome. Orthop Rev 7(5):1983.

131. Bleecker ML, et al: Carpal tunnel syndrome: Role of carpal canal size. Neurology 35:1599–1604, 1985.

132. Bleecker ML: Medical surveillance for carpal tunnel syndrome in workers. J Hand Surg 12A:845–848, 1987.

133. Braun RM, et al: Provocative testing in the diagnosis of dynamic carpal tunnel syndrome. J Hand Surg 14A:195–197, 1989.

134. Brown FE, Tanzer RC: Entrapment neuropathies of the upper extremity. In Flynn JE: Hand Surgery, 3rd ed. Baltimore, Williams & Wilkins, 1982, pp 460–471.

135. Cannon BW, Love JB: Tardy median palsy, Median Neuritis, and Median Thenar Neuritis Amenable to Surgery. Surgery 20:210, 1946.

136. Ditmars DM, Houin HP: Carpal tunnel syndrome. Hand Clin 2:525–532, 1986.

137. Foix et Marie: Atrophie isole de l'eminence thenar d'origine nevritique. Role due ligament annulaire anterieur de carpe dans a pathogenie de la lesion. Rev Neurol 26:647, 1913.

138. Falck B, Aarnio P: Left-sided carpal tunnel syndrome in butchers. Scand J Work Environ Health 9:291–297, 1983.

139. Feldman RG, Travers PH, Chirico-Post J, Keyserling WM: Risk assessment in electronic assembly workers: carpal tunnel syndrome. J Hand Surg 12A:849–855, 1987.

140. Gelberman RH, et al: The carpal tunnel syndrome: A study of carpal canal pressures. J Bone Joint Surg 63A:380–383, 1981.

141. Gordon C, et al: Electrodiagnostic characteristics of acute carpal tunnel syndrome. Arch Phys Med Rehabil 68:545–548, 1987.

142. Heckler FR, Jabaley ME: Evolving concepts of median nerve decompression in the carpal tunnel. Hand Clin 2:723–736, 1986.

143. Hochberg IH, Leffert RD, Heller MD, Merriman L: Hand difficulties among musicians. JAMA 249:1869–1872, 1983.

144. Hunter JM, Schneider LH, Mackin EJ, Callahan AD: Rehabilitation of the Hand: Surgery and Therapy, 3rd ed. St. Louis, C.V. Mosby, 1990, pp 640–646.

145. Lanz U: Anatomic variations of the median nerve in the carpal tunnel. J Hand Surg 2:44–53, 1977.

146. Leach RE, Odon JA: Systemic causes of the carpal tunnel syndrome. Postgrad Med 44:127–131, 1968.

147. Learmonth JR: The principles of decompression in the treatment of certain diseases of the peripheral nerves. Surg Clin North Am 13:905–913, 1933.

148. Lichtman DM, Floro RL, Mack GR: Carpal tunnel release under local anesthesia: Evaluation of the outpatient procedure. J Hand Surg 4:544–546, 1979.

149. Nigst H: Nerve compression syndromes in the upper limb. Hand Surg 1:5–17, 1988.

150. Phalen GS: Spontaneous compression of the median nerve at the wrist. JAMA 145:1128, 1951.

151. Phalen GS: The carpal tunnel syndrome: Clinical evaluation of 598 hands. Clin Orthop 83:29–40, 1972.

152. Phalen GS, Kendrick J: Compression neuropathy of median nerve in carpal tunnel. JAMA 164:524, 1957.

153. Rang M: Anthology of Orthopedics. New York, Churchill Livingstone, 1966, pp 70–72.

154. Robbins H: Anatomical study of median nerve in carpal canal and etiologies of carpal tunnel syndrome. J Bone Joint Surg 45:953–966, 1963.

155. Shuman S, Osterman L, Bora FW: Compression neuropathies. Seminars in Neurology 7:76–87, 1987.

156. Smith EW: Carpal tunnel syndrome: Contribution of the flexor tendons. Arch Phys Med Rehabil 58:Sept. 1977.

157. Wieslander G, Norblack D, Glothe CJ, Jublin L: Carpal tunnel syndrome (CTS) and exposure to vi-

bration, repetitive wrist movements, and heavy manual work: A case-referent study. Br J Ind Med 46(1):43–47, 1989.

158. Wongsam PE, et al: Carpal tunnel syndrome: Use of palmar stimulation of sensory fibers. Arch Phys Med Rehabil 64:16–19, 1983.

Median Nerve Branch

159. Blattman A: Habitual luxation of the ulnar nerve. Deutsche Klini 1851:435 (quoted by Lazaro III 1977).

160. Chen CR: Clawhand in a ropemaker—an occupational overuse. NZ Med J 10:617, 1988.

161. Cunaman KB: Flutist's neuropathy. N Engl J Med 305:961, 1981.

162. Eisen AL: Early diagnosis of ulnar nerve palsy: An electrophysiologic study. Neurology (Minneap) 24:256–262, 1974.

163. Feindel W, Stratford J: Cubital tunnel compression in tardy ulnar palsy. Can Med Assoc J 78:351–353, 1958.

164. Harding C, Halar E: Motor and sensory ulnar nerve conduction velocities: Effect on elbow position. Arch Phys Med Rehabil 64:227–232, 1983.

165. Hoffman, et al: Paired study of the dorsal cutaneous ulnar and superficial radial sensory nerves. Arch Phys Med Rehabil 69:591–594, 1988.

166. Kincaid JC: The electrodiagnosis of ulnar neuropathy at the elbow. Muscle Nerve 11:1005–1015, 1988.

167. Kisner W: Thumb neuroma: A hazard of ten pin bowling. Br J Plast Surg 29:225–226, 1976.

168. Hausmarova-Petrusewiczova I, Emeryk B, Markiewicz L, et al: Electrophysiological investigation about the mechanism of the damage of the ulnar nerve in glassworkers (in Polish). Neurology Neurochir 22:(4):509–515, 1972.

169. Lum PB, Kanakamedala R: Conduction of the palmar cutaneous branch of the median nerve. Arch Phys Med Rehabil 67:805–806, 1986.

170. Mackinnon SE, Dellon AL: Surgery of the Peripheral Nerve. New York, Thieme Publishers, 1988, pp 217–274.

171. Mandel S: Neurologic syndromes from repetitive trauma at work. Postgrad Med 82:87–92, 1987.

172. Oppenheim H: Lehrbuch der Nervenkrankheiten. Berlin, Karger, 1984.

173. Panas P: Sur une cause per connve de paralysie du nerf cubital. Arch Gen Med 142:5–22, 1978.

174. Pechan J, Kredba J: Cubital tunnel syndrome. II, Clinical Aspects. Acta Univa Carol (Med) (Pradha) 27(5–6):263–321, 1981.

175. Shields RW, Jacobs IB: Median palmar digital neuropathy in a cheerleader. Arch Phys Med Rehabil 67:824–826, 1986.

176. Spaans F, Vinken PJ, Bruyn W: Occupational nerve lesions. In Handbook of Clinical Neurology, Vol 7. New York, Elsevier, 1970, pp 326–343.

177. Stewart J: Focal Peripheral Neuropathies. New York, Elsevier, 1987, pp 163–179.

178. Viegas SF, Torres FG: Cherry pitter's thumb. Case report and review of the literature. Orthop Rev 18(3):March, 1989.

179. Wadsworth TG: The external compression syndrome of the ulnar nerve at the cubital tunnel. Clin Orthop 124:189–204, 1977.

Ulnar Nerve—Wrist Level

180. Conn J Jr, Bergan EJ, Bell JL: Hand ischemia: Hypothenar hammer syndrome. Proc Inst Med (Chicago) 28:83, 1970.

181. Gessler H: Eine eigenartige forum von progressive muskelatrophie bei goldpoliererinnen. Med Correspond des Wurtt. Arzh Landesvereins. 66:281–284, 1880.

182. Grantham SA: Ulnar compression in the loge de Guyon. JAMA 197:229–230, 1966.

183. Greenberg L, Chaffin D: Workers and Their Tools. Midland, MI, Pendell Press, 1976.

184. Guyon F: Notes sur une disposition anatomique propre a la face anterieure de la region due poignet et non encore descrite par le decteur. Bull Soc Anat Paris 6:184–186, 1861.

185. Hankey GJ, Gubbay SS: Compressive mononeuropathy of the deep palmar branch of the ulnar nerve in cyclists. J Neurol Neurosurg Psychiatry 51:1588–1590, 1988.

186. Harris W: Occupational pressure neuritis of the deep palmar branch of the ulnar nerve. Br Med Surg 1:98, 1929.

187. Hunt JR: The neural atrophy of the muscles of the hand without sensory disturbances. A further study of compression neuritis of the thenar branch of the median nerve and the deep palmar branch of the ulnar nerve. Rev Neurol Psychiatry 12:137, 1914.

188. Jones HR: Pizza cutter's palsy. N Engl J Med 319:450, 1988.

189. Noth J, Dietz V, et al: Cyclist's palsy. J Neurol Sci 47:111–116, 1980.

190. Russell WR, Whitty CWM: Traumatic neuritis of the deep palmar branch at the ulnar nerve. Lancet i:828–829, 1947.

191. Shea JD, McCalin GJ: Ulnar nerve compression syndromes at and below the wrist. J Bone Joint Surg 51A:1095–1103, 1969.

192. Streib EW, Sun SF: Distal ulnar neuropathy in meat packers. An occupational disease. J Occup Med 26:842–843, 1984.

193. Uriburu IJF, Francisco J, Morchio MD, Marin SC: Compression syndrome of the deep motor branch of the ulnar nerve (piso-hamata hiatus syndrome). J Bone Joint Surg 58:145–147, 1976.

194. Wu JS, Morris JD, Hogan GR: Ulnar neuropathy at the wrist: Case report and review of literature. Arch Phys Med Rehabil 66:785–788, 1985.

Radial Nerve: Radial Tunnel and Posterior Interosseous Syndrome

195. Burke EL: Rifle sling palsy in Marine Corps recruits. US Armed Forces Med J 8:1189–1194, 1957.

196. Frohse F, Frankel M: Die Muskeln de Menschlichen Armes. Bardelebens Handbuch der Anatomie de menschilchen Jena. Fisher, 1908.

197. Guillain G: Courtellemont l'action du muscle court supinateur dans la paralysie du nerf radial. Presse Med 1:50–52, 1905.

198. Hales T, Hobes D, Fine L, et al: NIOSH, Health Hazard Evaluation Report, April, 1984.

199. Henson RA, Urich H: Schumann's hand injury. Br Med J i:900–903, 1978.

200. Kaplan PE: Posterior interosseous neuropathies: Natural history. Arch Phys Med Rehabil 65:399–400, 1984.
201. Lister GD: The Hand: Diagnosis and Indications. Edinburgh, Churchill Livingstone, 1977.
202. Mackinnon SE, Dellon AL: Surgery of the Peripheral Nerve. New York, Thieme Publishers, 1988, Ch. 10, pp 275–288; Ch. 11, pp 289–303.
203. Roles NV, Maudsley RH: Radial tunnel syndrome: Resistant tennis elbow as a nerve entrapment. J Bone Joint Surg 54B:499–508, 1972.
204. Seddon H: Surgical disorders of the peripheral nerve. Baltimore, Williams & Wilkins, 1972.
205. Seddon H: Nerve lesions complicating certain closed injuries. JAMA 135:691–694, 1947.
206. Spinner M: The arcade of Frohse and its relationship to the posterior interosseous nerve paralysis. J Bone Joint Surg 50B:809–812, 1968.

Radial Nerve (Wartenberg's Syndrome)

207. Dellon AL, Mackinnon SE: Radial sensory nerve entrapment in the forearm. J Hand Surg 11A:199–205, 1986.
208. Finklestein H: Stenosing tendovaginitis at the radial styloid process. J Bone Joint Surg 12A:509–539, 1930.
209. Wartenburg R: Cheiralgia paresthetica (isolierte neuritis des ramus superficialis nerve radialis). Z Ges Neurol Psychiatr 141:145–155, 1932.

Multiple Crush

210. Lundborg G: The theory of the double crush syndrome. Correspondence Newsletter No. 9, Am Soc Surg Hand, Oct 24, 1985.
211. Mackinnon SE, Dellon AL: Multiple crush syndrome. In Surgery of the Peripheral Nerve. New York, Thieme Medical Publishers, 1988, pp 347–354.
212. Massey EW, Riley TL, Pleet AB: Co-existent carpal tunnel syndrome and cervical radiculopathy (double crush syndrome). South Med J 74:957–959, 1981.
213. Upton ARM, McComas AS: The double crush nerve entrapment and syndrome. Lancet ii:359, 1983.

Chapter 28

TENDINITIS OF THE UPPER EXTREMITY

*Janet R. Chipman, M.D., Morton L. Kasdan, M.D., F.A.C.S.,
and Daniel G. Camacho, M.D., F.A.C.S.*

The emphasis of this chapter is on the basics rather than the details of each form of tendinitis affecting the upper extremity. The focal point is the differential diagnosis of tendinitis.

TERMINOLOGY

As a clinical condition, tendinitis has many names. Tendovaginitis, peritendinitis, intersection syndrome, de Quervain's disease, trigger finger, lateral epicondylitis, and tenosynovitis are some of them. Adjectival qualifiers such as crepitating, stenosing, and nonspecific are added to these terms to expand the list yet further. Many authors use "tenosynovitis" and "tendinitis" interchangeably. To further confuse matters, the association of tendinitis with repetitive motion has led to the terms musculotendinous overuse syndrome, cumulative trauma disorder, and repetitive strain injury.[3,7] Part of the reason for the multiplicity of terms revolves around the basic controversy over pathology. While it seems implicit that tendinitis is inflammation of a tendon, some argue that the actual inflammation begins in the tenosynovium and involves the tendon only secondarily, if at all.[46] "Tendinitis," according to this theory, is an inaccurate term that should be replaced by "tenosynovitis." For the sake of partial clarification at this point, "tendinitis" in the upper extremity covers a spectrum of conditions. Depending upon its location, tendinitis may start with inflammation of the tendon itself or of the tenosynovium with secondary involvement of the tendon. Stenosis of the synovial compartment eventually occurs if the inflammation continues, especially in areas where the tendon sheath is restricted.

De Quervain's disease is inflammation of the tenosynovium of the first dorsal compartment of the wrist. It is also known as stenosing tenosynovitis of the abductor pollicis longus and the extensor pollicis brevis at the radial styloid. Stenosing tenosynovitis of the flexor tendon sheath is commonly called trigger finger. Peritendinitis crepitans usually means inflammation of the tenosynovium at the wrist of the second dorsal compartment, which is also known as intersection syndrome. Lateral epicondylitis is the condition known as tennis elbow, and medial epicondylitis is golf elbow. Nonspecific tenosynovitis includes the tendinitides in which no specific cause (bacterial, tuberculous, rheumatoid, or other) has been identified; it thus is usually a mechanical tenosynovitis.

In this chapter, the term "tenosynovitis" is used for inflammations of a specific musculotendinous unit in which a tendon sheath exists. The term "tendinitis" is used for the general category of musculotendinous conditions.

ANATOMY

Tendons are comprised of parallel collagen fibrils known as fibers, which are grouped into bundles called fascicles. The fascicles are surrounded by the connective tissue endotenon (endotendineum). Groups of fascicles form the tendon proper and are surrounded by the connective tissue epitenon (epitendineum), which is adherent to the tendon.[71] Although the tendon is a relatively avascular structure, having 18% of the vascularity of skin and 62% that of bone, it is not totally avascular, as was once thought.[78] The vascular supply to the midportion of the tendon runs through the mesotenon (mesotendineum) to the epitenon and then into the tendon itself. The mesotenon is connective tissue that extends perpendicularly from the undersurface of the tendon, much as the mesentery extends from the intestine.[70] In the digits, special condensations of the mesotenon are known as the vincula.

Tendons are dynamic anatomic structures that require protection from friction and attrition of areas in contact with bony prominences or located within fibrous canals. Paratendinous structures, such as bursae and tendon sheaths, serve this protective function.

A tendon sheath is much like a bursa. It wraps itself around a tendon like a long sleeve until its edges abut in a longitudinal slit along the tendon.[33] The mesotenon emerges from this slit in the sheathed regions of the tendon. The layer of the tendon sheath closest to the tendon is known as the visceral layer, and the outer layer is known as the parietal layer (much as in the pericardium). The tendon sheath is lined by synovium, which produces synovial fluid, a lubricant that permits the tendon to glide.[17,75]

The extensor tendons in the forearm and hand are relatively unrestricted except at the wrist, where there are no tendon sheaths and gliding is facilitated by another structure, the paratenon.[70] The paratenon is a semitransparent, loose, areolar connective tissue that almost completely surrounds the tendons. It is composed of multiple layers of thin, laminated sheets of connective tissue that can move back and forth, in a telescoping fashion, as the tendon moves. The innermost layer virtually moves with the tendon and each subsequent layer moves successively less; the outermost lamination remains relatively static. The tendon thus glides smoothly without friction from surrounding structures, such as skin.[70]

EPIDEMIOLOGY

Tendinitis occurs in people who subject their musculotendinous structures to an acute un-accustomed use or a chronic repetitive motion that exceeds the tolerance of the tendons or their sheaths.[22,26] Examples include (1) well-trained athletes who abruptly increase their workout intensity, (2) manual task employees who change jobs or increase their work speed, (3) musicians who increase their practice time or change their playing techniques, and (4) relatively sedentary people who become "weekend warriors." Tendinitis may also result from direct trauma or from diseases such as diabetes or rheumatoid arthritis, which increase the likelihood of flexor tenosynovitis.[48]

Tendinitis is not uncommon. It has been reported the most common cause of shoulder pain in athletes,[44] the most frequent sports-related cause of persistent wrist discomfort requiring medical attention,[80] the most frequently diagnosed upper extremity disorder in musicians,[43] and a major occupational health problem.[4] Tendinitis is generally more common in females,[54,69] perhaps because the female's tendons are "stiffer" than those of the male, as a biomechanical study has shown.[29]

In the past, tendinitis was often thought to be more common in the middle and later years, presumably owing to a decrease in tendon vascularity that predisposed the tendon to greater injury following microtrauma.[8] However, more recent studies have called into question the association of tendinitis with older age groups.[4]

ETIOLOGY

The contention that occupational factors lead to tendinitis and the resultant workmen's compensation claims have led to friction in employer-employee relations. Many studies have attempted to determine the relation of occupational environment to tendinitis. The risk factors most commonly cited and studied are repetitiveness of task, forcefulness of exertion, awkward positioning, mechanical stress, vibration, low ambient temperature, and the use of gloves.[6,72] One study showed that the risk of tendinitis of the hand and wrist is 29 times greater with highly repetitive, highly forceful jobs than with less repetitive, low-force jobs.[4] Indirectly, vibration is implicated in tendinitis because it induces short-term anesthesia in the hand and a resultant increase in exertion required to perform the task.[5] Likewise, gloves are implicated owing to a 20–30% decrease in hand strength with their use and a resultant increase in exertion.[4,69,72]

GENERAL DIAGNOSIS

The presenting complaint of most patients with tendinitis is pain, which may be well localized or diffuse.[26] There is often a localized tender swelling.[73]

Events surrounding the onset of symptoms should be determined as well as any aggravating activities, either recreational or occupational. Crepitus, snapping/catching of fingers, and weakness of involved muscles should be investigated.[26] Systemic disorders should always be considered a possible cause.

Muscle testing is an extremely useful method of diagnosing tendinitis or tenosynovitis and of localizing the particular tendon involved. This testing usually consists of contracting the involved musculotendinous unit against resistance or of stretching the involved unit. Usually the test should be performed bilaterally so that comparisons can be made.[26,48] Radiographs are useful primarily to rule out other conditions. Magnetic resonance imaging (MRI) is becoming more widely employed (see Chapter 5).

Systemic Disorders

A multitude of inflammatory diseases may include tenosynovitis/tendinitis among their manifestations. Accurate determination of cause is extremely important to effectiveness of treatment because tendinitis/tenosynovitis due to systemic disease may be treated differently than mechanical tendinitides. Some entities that must be considered before tenosynovitis is treated as an overuse injury include rheumatoid arthritis, diabetes mellitus, lupus, gout, collagen vascular diseases, seronegative spondyloarthropathies, mixed connective tissue disease, and indolent infections.[11,58,59,62,63,68,71]

In rheumatoid arthritis, the synovium of the tendon sheaths as well as the synovial joints may be inflamed. Rheumatoid tenosynovitis of the upper extremity is particularly prevalent on the dorsum of the hand and in the fingers.[62] The extensor carpi ulnaris tendon is often involved.[61] The swelling in rheumatoid tenosynovitis may be painless.[42,61] Tenosynovitis may be the first and only symptom of rheumatoid arthritis, or it may exist with other rheumatoid symptoms such as ulnar drift.[42,62] The most common radiographic finding is a lobulated soft-tissue swelling. In the case of extensor carpi ulnaris tenosynovitis, radiographs may show surface resorption of the outer aspect of the distal ulna beneath the inflamed tendon sheath.[62]

Less common than rheumatic tenosynovitis is tendon sheath involvement as part of the seronegative spondyloarthropathies (ankylosing spondylitis, psoriasis, and Reiter's syndrome). The considerable associated soft-tissue swelling may result in a "sausage-shaped" digit.[62]

Indolent infection with tuberculosis, atypical *Mycobacterium* species, fungi (sporotrichosis, disseminated coccidioidomycosis), protozoa (acquired toxoplasmosis), or bacteria such as *Neisseria* species may also cause tenosynovitis. Tuberculosis most commonly affects the radial and ulnar bursae of the hand and the flexor tendons of the fingers; other tendon sheaths in the upper extremity are only rarely involved.[60] In tuberculous tenosynovitis, a soft-tissue swelling, often doughy in consistency, is associated with little pain.[42] Osteoporosis and soft-tissue swelling may be shown by radiographs.[60] It occurs most often in males and in people 20–50 years of age.[38]

The most common atypical *Mycobacterium* tenosynovitis is *M. marinum* infection, which usually results from some exposure to fish—either a bite or contaminated water. There is often a history of a puncture wound 2–3 months before symptoms appear.[76] Because of the association with fish, the condition is sometimes called "fish fancier's digit."

GENERAL TREATMENT OF TENDINITIS

The goals of treatment of nonspecific tenosynovitis are first to address the acute inflammatory condition (and thus to reduce the swelling and tenderness) and to prevent any further generation of fibrous adhesions or scarring due to chronic inflammation. Aggravating activities must be avoided. Part of the initial treatment must center around education of the patient. If possible, any inciting occupational or recreational activities should be restructured. Once the acute condition is controlled, exercises for stretching and strengthening are begun to prevent recurrences. The patient is instructed to warm up adequately before work. A change in technique or equipment may be necessary. In addition to education, some of the recommended modalities of treatment are rest, splinting, ice, heat, alternating ice with heat, ultrasound, stretching and strengthening exercises, transcutaneous electronic nerve stimulation, nonsteroidal anti-inflammatory drugs (NSAIDs), and corticosteroid injections.

Rest is the cornerstone of treatment for acute tendinitis. However, rest is a relative state, the degree needed depending upon the severity of the acute inflammation.[45,51] Immobilization should be limited in order to avoid stiffness. Because it is important to maintain range of motion, complete inactivity of a musculotendinous unit for prolonged periods should be avoided.[22] Splinting the inflamed area for half of the day allows the patient to have limited use of the affected extremity.

The use of ice for acute inflammation is a widely accepted practice. The effects of ice include reduction in edema secondary to vasoconstriction and reduction in pain from decreased pain receptor conduction.[22,41] Gel packs, crushed ice in a damp towel, or simply ice in a paper cup are practical ways of application. The ice should be applied for no more than 10–15 minutes at a time. In chronic cases of tendinitis, ice may be applied to reduce discomfort after an aggravating activity.[22]

Heat, a commonly used modality in chronic tendinitis, is thought to reduce pain according to the gate control theory.[41] Heat is now commonly alternated with ice for chronic pain.

Ultrasound therapy is a form of deep heat. It is absorbed at a higher rate by tissues of higher protein content—e.g., muscles, tendons, ligaments. It results in increased musculotendinous distensibility and therefore is especially useful before beginning stretching exercises. Ultrasound is thought to increase blood flow (similar to local heat) and thus to break up inflammatory exudate.[41] It is the only safe "diathermy" with metallic implants. Ultrasound may also be used to drive hydrocortisone cream (10%) transcutaneously into the tendinous area, a process known as phonophoresis.[41,82] The disadvantage of ultrasound is that it requires considerable time of the clinician.

Transcutaneous electrical nerve stimulation (TENS) is becoming more popular for use in reducing painful conditions. However, this modality treats the pain without reducing the inflammation and therefore can be used only as an adjunctive treatment.

Stretching exercises, preceded by gentle warmth to relax muscles and tendons, should be done carefully, proceeding slowly.[54] The same caution applies to strengthening exercises. The axiom, "No pain, no gain," does not apply. These exercises should be done only in the pain-free range to avoid further trauma to damaged tissues.[41]

NSAIDs are now widely recommended in the treatment of tendinitis.[55] Full doses vary among the drugs.[8] Corticosteroid injections in inflammatory tendon conditions can be useful. However, the injections have an associated risk of tendon rupture, presumably owing to reduced collagen production, circulatory stasis, and atrophy. To reduce the risk of rupture, activity should be decreased for 2–3 weeks after injection.[22] The patient must be carefully instructed about permissible activity because the decrease in pain after the injection may stimulate a desire to resume full activity. In addition, the risk of rupture can be reduced by limiting the number of injections to two or three. Surgery is the last therapeutic measure that should be tried. Most cases of tendinitis respond to nonoperative modalities.

SHOULDER

Tendinitis of the shoulder most often involves the supraspinatus or the bicipital tendon. Although supraspinatus tendinitis may exist alone (especially as calcific tendinitis), it is most often part of the clinical condition known as impingement syndrome.[68] In this condition, the greater tuberosity of the humerus impinges upon the anterior acromion and coracoacromial ligament during shoulder flexion and abduction, causing inflammation and tenderness of the intervening structures (Fig. 1).

Bicipital tendinitis can present as an entity separate from impingement syndrome. The focal point of inflammation is at the tenosynovial sheath in the intertubercular groove.[50,82] Because its probable origin is at the sheath rather than the tendon, it is often referred to as bicipital tenosynovitis.

Impingement Syndrome

Impingement syndrome is a frequent cause of shoulder pain in people who regularly engage in overhead use of their arms.[10,31] Although both the bicipital and supraspinatus tendon may be inflamed, one may be more

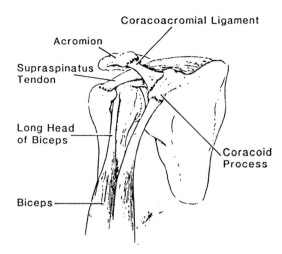

FIGURE 1. Normal anatomy of the shoulder. (Reprinted with permission from Ball GV, Koopman WJ: Clinical Rheumatology. Philadelphia, W.B. Saunders, 1986.)

Labels on Figure 1:
Coracoacromial Ligament
Acromion
Supraspinatus Tendon
Long Head of Biceps
Biceps
Coracoid Process

The combination of avascularity and impingement leads to inflammation and the eventual formation of osteophytes, which further irritate the area and lead to attrition of the tendon. Neer has divided the progression of this condition into three stages, each associated with a characteristic patient age. Stage 1 coincides with edema and hemorrhage when the patient is usually less than 25 years old, stage 2 with fibrosis and tendinitis between the ages of 25 and 40 years, and stage 3 with bone spurs and rupture at 40 years or later.[10,49]

The patient reports pain with overhead activities such as reaching up or combing hair and often has ceased to participate in recreational sports. There is generally pain over the greater tuberosity of the humerus.[10,31] Radiographs may show spurs and bony proliferation at the humeral tuberosity or the acromioclavicular joint.[68]

One method of testing for impingement syndrome is to observe the patient during abduction of the involved humerus. Impingement syndrome usually causes no pain between 0 and 45 degrees of abduction because there are no soft-tissue structures being pinched between the humerus and acromial structures. Between 45 and 60 degrees, the pain begins and continues until approximately 120 degrees (if pain does not preclude abduction before 120 degrees is reached).[25,50] Through this portion of the arc, the patient may begin to shrug in order to continue elevating the arm by scapular movement rather than by glenohumeral abduction, thus avoiding the painful impingement.[41] At about 120 degrees of abduction, the painful soft tissues will have passed through the pinch point and the pain recedes.[50] Pain may also occur with forward flexion at the shoulder, the severity depending on the relative involvement of the bicipital tendon. If the

severely involved than the other, depending on the amount of shoulder flexion relative to abduction during the aggravating activity. For instance, activities involving more forward flexion (underhand pushing, throwing) tend to have greater bicipital involvement, whereas those with greater abduction (swimming, or pulling boxes from overhead shelves) have more supraspinatus involvement.[22]

The proposed factors in the development of subacromial impingement lesions include trauma and mechanical wear, in combination with a relative avascularity in the supraspinatus at the point of impingement (Fig. 2).[31] The region of avascularity is postulated to be due either to pressure exerted upon the tendon as it curves over the humerus, which compresses blood out of the tendon in that region, or to a "watershed" zone stemming from the nature of embryological development of vascularity in the region.[10,31]

FIGURE 2. Relative avascularity in the areas of impingement of the supraspinatus. (Reprinted with permission from Ball GV, Koopman WJ: Clinical Rheumatology. Philadelphia, W.B. Saunders, 1986.)

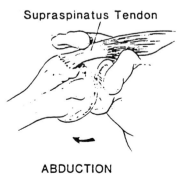

Supraspinatus Tendon

ABDUCTION

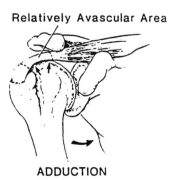

Relatively Avascular Area

ADDUCTION

supraspinatus tendon is the primary inflammatory site, the pain experienced during abduction is lessened with humeral external rotation owing to the posterior rotation of the greater tuberosity and decreased impingement (Fig. 2).[21,22] If the bicipital tendon is the principal site of impingement, the pain upon forward flexion is reduced by humeral internal rotation. Another provocative test for impingement syndrome is forcible flexion of the shoulder by the examiner with the patient's arm at approximately 40 degrees of horizontal adduction.

The supraspinatus tendon can be palpated at its insertion site, which is at the triangle bounded laterally by the acromion, anteriorly by the clavicle, and posteriorly by the spine of the scapula.[68,82] The contraction of this muscle can be felt if the patient is instructed to abduct the humerus against resistance while the examiner palpates the triangle. Tenderness that is increased by this maneuver indicates supraspinatus tendinitis, with or without an impingement syndrome.[82] If the diagnosis is still in question after these tests, pain relief after an injection of local anesthetic beneath the acromion is indicative of impingement syndrome. Injection of local anesthetic into the acromioclavicular joint helps to make the differential diagnosis in acromioclavicular joint disease.[10]

If a patient with impingement syndrome continues the aggravating activity, the inflammation may result in attrition and eventual tendon rupture (as indicated by Neer's stages) or in a frozen shoulder.[35]

Bicipital Tenosynovitis

The bicipital tenosynovium is a synovial membrane that extends as a long outpocketing from the glenohumeral joint into the intertubercular groove of the humerus, where it surrounds the long head of the biceps.[35] Bicipital tenosynovitis is most common in patients 45–65 years old and is more common in women.[35,39,50] It occurs as a result of mechanical stress created at the bicipital tenosynovium by chronic repetitive activity or by a singular traumatic incident. Examples of activities reported to result in bicipital tenosynovitis are lifting heavy items, tightening lids, and shoveling.[31,35] A sudden jar or pull of the arm is the usual form of trauma associated with this synovitis.[46]

Patients report pain, especially with overhead activities, of gradual or acute onset after vigorous activity.[35,68] The pain usually originates at the intertubercular groove, located at the anterior medial shoulder, but it may radiate to the elbow along the course of the biceps muscle.[35]

The most common finding is tenderness over the bicipital groove of the humerus.[8,41] In some cases, swelling of the biceps tendon sheath is detectable as the examiner simultaneously rolls his fingers across the biceps tendons of both arms for comparison. Passive range of motion is normal.[68]

Pain can be elicited over the humeral groove by resisted flexion and supination of the forearm (biceps contraction) or by extension at the elbow with internal rotation of the forearm (biceps stretching). The most widely known test for bicipital tenosynovitis is Yergason's. With the shoulder adducted, the elbow flexed at 90 degrees, and the forearm pronated, the patient attempts supination and external rotation, which the examiner resists. Pain at the intertubercular groove indicates bicipital tenosynovitis. Speed's test is sometimes considered superior to Yergason's because it results in movement of the humerus over the tendon in the groove. In Speed's test, the elbow is extended and the forearm supinated; when the examiner resists the patient's attempts to flex the shoulder, the patient feels pain at the groove.[50]

Another cause of bicipital tenosynovitis is chronic subluxation of the biceps tendon. Diagnosis can be made by palpating movement of the tendon from the bicipital groove as the arm is internally and externally rotated while abducted. Radiographs may show spurring or degenerative changes in the groove if subluxation is occurring.[64] In bicipital tenosynovitis without subluxation, the radiograph is usually normal.[35]

Differential Diagnosis of Shoulder Pain

The differential diagnosis of shoulder pain includes the following conditions, many of which are also part of the differential diagnosis in elbow, arm, and hand pain and will be referred to in later sections:

Bicipital tendinitis
Supraspinatus tendinitis
Impingement syndrome
Calcific tendinitis

Trapezius myalgia
Rotator cuff injuries
Acromioclavicular arthrosis
Bursitis
Adhesive capsulitis
Thoracic outlet syndrome
Brachial plexus injury
Cervical radiculopathy
Reflex sympathetic dystrophy
Referred pain
Osteonecrosis
Osteoarthritis
Rheumatoid arthritis
Gout
Cellulitis
Steroid arthropathy
Tumors
Shoulder dislocation
Fracture
Septic arthritis/bursitis

Calcific tendinitis

The supraspinatus tendon is the most common location of calcific tendinitis.[9,41] The most common area of calcification within the supraspinatus is the avascular zone described in the discussion of impingement syndrome.[31] The etiology of calcific tendinitis is not known, but vascular factors are considered significant.[9] The deposits are thought to occur at a site of focal necrosis or degeneration, probably secondary to overuse or subclinical injury in which recovery is impaired by the area's relative avascularity.[9,39]

The condition affects both sexes equally and usually occurs during the fifth and sixth decades.[9] Calcific tendinitis can exist in an acute, chronic, or mixed stage.[36] Calcific tendinitis of acute onset tends to reach maximum severity within several days and then rapidly improve as the calcium ruptures into the subacromial bursa.[68] In the acute stage, the pain is disabling and often described as red hot and throbbing; it is also constant instead of movement related, as in noncalcific tendinitis.[36,39,50] The signs are those of a chemical inflammatory reaction.[39]

A history of symptoms is an important part of the diagnosis of calcific tendinitis because calcific deposits are found on the radiographs of many asymptomatic patients.[12,50] On the other hand, deposits in patients with calcific tendinitis are often missed in singular views. Multiple radiographic views are required if this condition is being considered.[10]

Trapezius Myalgia

Trapezius myalgia is also known as regional myofascial pain syndrome, fibrositis, fibromyositis, and fibromyalgia. Trapezius myalgia is a disorder characterized by pain, tenderness, and stiffness of the trapezius muscle, its tendon insertions, and adjacent soft tissues. Because there is no histological evidence of cellular inflammation, the condition is more accurately called fibromyalgia than fibromyositis. This condition is most common in the type A, tense, anxious, striving, young, otherwise healthy woman. The patient reports a gradual onset of diffuse, achy shoulder pain aggravated by straining. Symptoms increase with mental or physical stress. Fatty-fibrous nodules, known as trigger points, can be found scattered throughout the shoulder. Diagnosis can be made by recognition of the personality and age noted above, nonrheumatic symptoms, and exclusion of connective tissue disorders.[8]

Treatment of Tendinitis at the Shoulder

The first step in successful treatment is accurate diagnosis of the condition causing pain in the shoulder. The importance of an accurate diagnosis is shown by a randomized, double-blind study of 77 patients with local shoulder pain.[68] In this study, one group of patients was diagnosed by provocative muscle testing and then given injections of corticosteroids into specific areas, such as the joint space, bursa, or tendon sheath. The second group was palpated about the shoulder and given injections at the most painful spot. After 1 week, 60% of the group injected on the basis of diagnosis improved, as opposed to only 20% of those injected on the basis of palpation.

Once the condition has been diagnosed as tendinitis, the treatment for the most part follows the principles outlined in general treatment. NSAIDs, ice or alternating heat and ice, and rest are advised initially. In generally, diathermy and ultrasound are not as effective as anti-inflammatory drugs in the treatment of shoulder tendinitis. "Rest" is a relative state, particularly for the shoulder, because it is the most frequently restricted joint after tendinitis.[15] Exacerbating activities should be avoided, but so should total inactivity, which may produce stiffness and adhesive capsulitis.[35] After the acute symptoms abate (often in 3–4 days), the patient should begin exercises in the passive range of motion (within the limits of pain) with assistance from the other arm.[82] The biceps and supraspinatus tendons can be stretched with wand and pendulum exercises, respectively.[68] If there is no satisfaction with these methods, injection with corticosteroids is advised. However, no more than two or three injections should be given in order to avoid the risk of tendinous degeneration.[10] A potential risk of tendon sheath injection is postinjection "flare," a form of synovitis, which occurs several hours after injection. This can be controlled with cold applications and short-term analgesics.[8]

If all of these measures fail, a rotator cuff tear should be ruled out with an arthrogram or MRI.[64] In general, stage 1 impingement lesions are reversible and respond well to rest and physiotherapy. Stage 2 response to these measures is questionable, and stage 3 usually requires surgery, consisting of anterior acromioplasty, rotator cuff repair, and arthroplasty of the acromioclavicular joint. The potential complications of impingement syndrome surgery include stiff shoulder (the most common postoperative complication), residual impingement, and, rarely, infection.[10]

ELBOW

Tendinitis at the elbow takes the form of inflammation of the tendinous origins of the forearm muscles at the lateral or medial epicondyles of the humerus. Cases of triceps tendon inflammation at the elbow have also been reported.[1]

The pathogenesis of epicondylitis has been argued for years. More than 20 processes have been postulated, including radiohumeral bursitis, traumatized synovial fringe, granulation tissue in the subtendinous fat pad, periostitis (possibly secondary to repeated tears from the bone), and degenerative changes in the annular ligament.[12,19,22,36,48] However, by far the most commonly accepted mechanism is that of inflammation due to multiple microtears occurring at the tendinous insertions to the epicondyles.[18,21,22] The involved tendinous origin at the lateral epicondyle is known as the common extensor tendon. It attaches wrist and digit extensors (including the extensor carpi radialis brevis, extensor digitorum communis, extensor digiti minimi, and part of the extensor carpi

ulnaris) to the humerus. Similarly, the wrist flexors (including the flexor carpi radialis and parts of the pronator teres, palmaris longus, flexor carpi ulnaris, and flexor digitorum superficialis) attach at the medial epicondyle by way of the common flexor tendon.[33] The tears in the common tendons are thought to occur most often in the extensor carpi radialis brevis origin at the lateral elbow and the flexor carpi radialis or flexor digitorum superficialis origins at the medial elbow.[71]

Epicondylitis usually results from activities that overstrain the muscles arising at the epicondyle, either in a singular mechanical event or in chronic repetitive motions.[82] Direct trauma to the epicondyle may also result in epicondylitis. Activities associated with lateral epicondylitis are twisting or rotating movements, the most publicized being those performed in tennis.[36] Medial epicondylitis has been associated with impact activities.[27] Lateral epicondylitis is frequently called tennis elbow, and medial epicondylitis, golf elbow. It must be remembered, however, that while lateral epicondylitis is more common in tennis players than in the general public,[22] fewer than 5% of those affected by "tennis elbow" play any sport at all.[19]

Epicondylitis is seven times more common on the lateral than the medial epicondyle.[19] It is more common on the right than the left elbow but not uncommonly is bilateral.[12,19] No significant difference between male and female incidence is found. Because lateral epicondylitis most often occurs in the fourth decade, degeneration of the tendon is postulated as an etiological factor. These patients also show an increased incidence in other soft-tissue degenerative processes (such as rotator cuff tears, bicipital tendinitis, de Quervain's disease, carpal tunnel syndrome, and medial epicondylitis).[12,71]

Lateral Epicondylitis

The patient with lateral epicondylitis typically reports pain over the lateral epicondyle and often with radiation distally along the extensor muscle mass.[48] The symptoms usually have a gradual onset and are exacerbated by vigorous activity. In the more severe states, symptoms occur regularly upon particular movements.[21] At the first consultation the symptoms may have been present for months.

The condition may have progressed to the point where turning a doorknob or picking up a cup is difficult because of pain.[27] Patients report that the pain is aggravated by forceful gripping, lifting with the palm down, throwing and wringing motions, and extension at the wrist.[22,35] The lateral epicondyle is tender to palpation. It is important that both sides be palpated because in the normal elbow palpation at the epicondyle produces discomfort that must be differentiated from the tenderness of epicondylitis. In general, pain is elicited at the epicondyle upon resisted wrist extension (extensor muscle mass contraction) or passive wrist flexion and pronation (extensor muscle mass stretching). There are three formal methods of testing for lateral epicondylitis.

1. Cozen's test: The patient's elbow is flexed at 90 degrees and stabilized with the examiner's thumb at the lateral epicondyle. The patient makes a fist and then attempts to pronate the forearm and to radially deviate and extend the wrist while the examiner resists the motion. Pain elicited at the lateral epicondyle is a positive result.[50]

2. Test two: The examiner pronates the patient's forearm, flexes the wrist fully, and extends the elbow. Pain at the lateral epicondyle is a positive result.[50]

3. Test three: The patient holds the shoulder flexed at 90 degrees and the wrist and fingers passively flexed. "Postural" discomfort and pain at the lateral epicondyle is a positive result.[48]

Range of motion at the elbow may lack the last few degrees of extension. Radiographs may show bone chips, lateral exostosis, or calcific deposits in the tendon. The x-rays may be normal.[55]

Medial Epicondylitis

Patients with medial epicondylitis present with pain at the medial epicondyle, and the onset and progression of symptoms are similar to those in lateral epicondylitis. Pain is elicited at the medial epicondyle with palmar flexion against resistance, or with supination of the forearm while the wrist and elbow are extended.[50]

Differential Diagnosis of Elbow Pain

The following list includes conditions that may lead to elbow pain and must be differentiated from a diagnosis of tendinitis. Some of these syndromes may also result in shoulder pain.

> Lateral epicondylitis
> Medial epicondylitis
> Radial tunnel syndrome
> Olecranon bursitis
> Septic bursitis
> Gout osteoarthritis
> Tumor
> Dislocation/fracture
> Traumatic myositis ossificans
> Osteochondritis dissecans
> Thoracic outlet syndrome
> Cervical radiculopathy
> Rheumatoid arthritis
> Ulnar nerve entrapment

Many conditions that lead to elbow pain can be differentiated from tendinitis without difficulty. Some factors that help in these diagnoses are:

Olecranon bursitis: swelling, location

Septic bursitis: bursal aspirate leukocyte count, Gram stain

Gout: crystals in the aspirate

Ulnar nerve entrapment: numbness, tingling, pain in the ulnar nerve distribution, reproduction of symptoms upon tapping the ulnar nerve at the cubital tunnel or upon sustained elbow flexion[49]

Dislocation or fracture: history, x-ray

Traumatic myositis ossificans: history, x-ray

Osteochondritis dissecans: swelling, restriction of motion at the elbow, x-ray

Tumor: history, x-ray

Differentiating lateral epicondylitis from radial tunnel syndrome can be difficult. Radial tunnel syndrome (RTS) results from compression of the posterior interosseous nerve (a branch of the radial nerve) as it passes under the arcade of Frohse, the fibrous arch between the two heads of the supinator muscle.[49,71] This is the site of pain in RTS. The location of the pain is important in differentiating RTS from lateral epicondylitis. In RTS, finger extension and ulnar wrist extension are often weak, but there is no sensory deficit.[48] Several provocative tests for RTS should not be positive in lateral epicondylitis:

1. Pressure over the supinator at the radial head produces the symptoms.[49]

2. With elbow extended and wrist neutral, the patient attempts to extend the middle finger against resistance and experiences pain at the supinator.[48]

3. With elbow extended, the patient attempts supination of the forearm against resistance and experiences pain at the supinator.[49]

If the differentiation is still in question, the lateral epicondyle area can be infiltrated with 1–2 ml of 1% lidocaine. Relief of symptoms is indicative of lateral epicondylitis.[8]

Treatment of Tendinitis at the Elbow

As with other tendinitis conditions, conservative measures such as rest, NSAIDs, ice, and alternating ice and heat are tried first, usually with good results.[8,12,71] The condition often spontaneously disappears without medical attention.[12,21,68]

If the initial measures are unsuccessful, the arm can be splinted in 90 degrees of elbow flexion, slight forearm supination, and slight wrist extension.[55] If the condition continues, an injection of 2–4 ml of corticosteroid-anesthesia mixture at the epicondyle down to the periosteum is advised.[8,21,27] A single injection is reported to cure approximately 60% of patients.[10] Injections may be repeated, but no more than three can be given to avoid the risk of tendon attrition.

After the acute symptoms subside, a strap encircling the forearm just distal to the elbow is recommended. It in effect transfers the origin of the affected muscles to the strap instead of the epicondyle.[8,27,68] The strap can be worn at all times, but it must be used during any aggravating activities, such as a sport, that the patient is reluctant to avoid. Strengthening (wrist curls) and stretching exercises should be initiated.[55] Patients should be educated to alter activities in order to avoid aggravating motions as much as possible. For instance, they should begin to lift with the palm up instead of down.

If conservative measures have been attempted for at least 1 year without results, surgery may be recommended.[19] However, fewer than 5% of patients require surgery. The multitude of postulated pathogenic mechanisms of epicondylitis is paralleled by the multitude of surgical techniques to remedy the condition, including excision of granulation tissue, decortication of the lateral exostosis, excision of tears and repair, and some combination thereof. The patient can expect splinting for approximately 2–4 weeks after surgery followed by deferment of vigorous activities for several months.[27,55]

WRIST AND HAND

Tendinitis of the wrist and hand may exist as inflammation of any of the tenosynovial sheath compartments in which the tendons of the extrinsic muscles of the hand traverse the wrist. These tendons are commonly grouped as the dorsal, or extensor, group and the volar, or flexor, group. Tendinitis of the digits is flexor tenosynovitis.

Extensor Tendinitis

On the dorsal side of the wrist are six fibro-osseous compartments through which tendons pass. Three compartments are formed by the carpal bones, the radius, and the extensor retinaculum (Fig. 3). The retinaculum is approximately 2–3 cm long (proximal end to distal

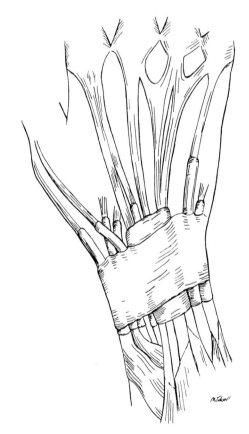

FIGURE 3. Illustration of the six dorsal compartments of the wrist formed by the retinacular ligament and the bones. Accessory tendons may be found in any of the six compartments. (Reprinted with permission from Kasdan ML, Romm S: Essentials of Plastic, Maxillofacial, and Reconstructive Surgery. Baltimore, Williams & Wilkins, 1986).

end). The retinaculum surrounds the dorsal and lateral sides of the wrist, running from the lateral radius to the medial ulnar styloid. Septa, or outgrowths, from the retinacular undersurface attach to the underlying bones and make up the sides of the six compartments. Sheaths cover the tendons as they run through the compartments. The sheaths begin slightly (10–15 mm) proximally to the retinaculum.[40]

In general, an elongated swelling may occur along the involved tendon on the dorsum of the lower forearm or hand.[73] Inflamed tenosynovium may collect and "heap up" at the distal margin of the extensor retinaculum upon extension of the fingers.[55] If the swelling of the sheaths is severe, it takes on an hourglass appearance owing to the restrictive nature of the retinaculum in the midportion of the tendon sheath.[73]

First Dorsal Compartment: de Quervain's Disease

Inflammation of the tendon sheaths of the abductor pollicis longus and extensor pollicis brevis at the first dorsal compartment is known as de Quervain's disease (Fig. 4) after Fritz de Quervain, a Swiss surgeon who reported the

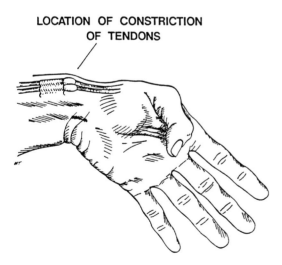

LOCATION OF CONSTRICTION OF TENDONS

FIGURE 4.   Area of constriction in the first dorsal compartment of the abductor pollicis longus and extensor pollicis brevis tendons creating de Quervain's disease (tenosynovitis). (Reprinted with permission from Karwowski W, Kasdan ML: The partnership of ergonomics and medical intervention in rehabilitation of workers with cumulative trauma disorders of the hand. In Mital A, Karwowski W (eds): Ergonomics in Rehabilitation. Philadelphia, Taylor & Francis, 1988, pp 35–53.)

first case in 1895. This is the most common tendinitis at the wrist.[22] The first compartment is formed by the bony groove in the radial styloid, which is covered by the fibrous extensor retinaculum. The predisposition of this compartment to tenosynovitis seems to be related to its highly restrictive, nonexpandable nature, the presence of an individual tunnel for the extensor pollicis brevis, and the multidimensional function of the thumb relative to the other digits.[17,74]

Like other mechanical tendinitides, the condition can occur from direct trauma or from overuse.[46,47,68] The synovitis results from the friction generated among the tendon, tendon sheath, bony groove, and retinaculum during thumb use.[17,22] It occurs three times more commonly in women than in men[47,80] and most commonly in the fifth or sixth decade.[47] The right hand is more commonly affected, but the condition becomes bilateral in 30% of patients.[47,55] It is more common in those who engage in activities requiring wringing motions, abduction of the thumb under stress, or ulnar deviation at the wrist, especially when combined with adduction of the thumb and grasping motions, such as in typewriting and working on a grinding or buffing machine.[46,47] Not uncommonly patients affected with de Quervain's disease later develop trigger finger or carpal tunnel syndrome.[55,71]

The primary pathohistological change in de Quervain's disease is usually in the tendon sheath, where there are thickening and loss of the normal pearly luster.[46] The tendon has increased vascularity.[17] The tendon sheath can be 2–4 times thicker than usual, the degree of thickening related to the chronicity of the disease. The tendons may be thinned and frayed within the canal and swollen at the canal limits.[46] As the inflammatory process continues, stenosis of the sheath increases.

Patients present with complaints of pain at the radial styloid. The pain often radiates up the forearm or down to the thumb.[16,46,47] Pain may increase with wringing motions of the wrist, unscrewing a jar lid, opening a car door, turning a key, or buttoning a shirt.[16,18] The pain is increased with thumb motion.[46,48] The most painful motion is severe adduction of the wrist or extreme abduction of the thumb.[46] The patient may report dropping things because pain makes the grip insecure.

If the condition is chronic, the patient may maintain the wrist in radial deviation owing to

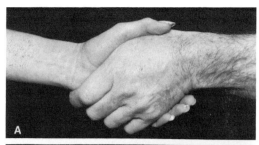

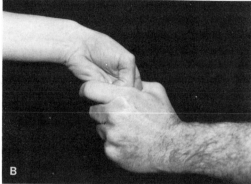

FIGURE 5. Finkelstein's test for de Quervain's disease. A, The patient's hand is grasped so that the thumb is abducted over the examiner's first web space. The wrist is brought into ulnar deviation. The patient usually experiences little or no pain. B, With the thumb adducted and folded into the palm, the wrist is passively deviated ulnarly. The patient usually feels excruciating pain in the area of the first dorsal compartment.

constriction in the compartment.[47] The first compartment groove at the radial styloid is tender upon palpation, and often there is an oval-shaped, soft-tissue swelling. Occasionally, the swollen area is erythematous.[42] Thickening of the compartment roof or ganglion cyst may be felt.[17]

The test often noted as pathognomonic of de Quervain's disease is Finkelstein's (Fig. 5). The patient's thumb is passively adducted into the palm, and the examiner deviates the wrist to the ulnar side. Pain at the radial styloid is a positive result. However, other conditions, such as intersection syndrome, neuritis of the sensory branch of the radial nerve, and basal thumb joint arthrosis, can give a false positive with this test.[48,49,80]

Radiographs of de Quervain's are almost invariably normal.[46]

Treatment of de Quervain's Disease

The principles of treatment follow those discussed in general treatment, such as NSAIDs,

rest, splinting (thumb spica), and one to three hydrocortisone injections into the tendon sheaths.[22,80] If the symptoms have been present only briefly, these methods may be successful, but they are less successful than they are in tenosynovitis of other compartments.[55,74,80] If the condition is chronic and there is stenosis at the canal, nonoperative treatment is usually ineffective.[80] If there are no results after 1–2 months of conservative treatment, surgery is indicated.[17,46] In surgery, the stenosed tendon sheath is partially excised. Care must be taken during the procedure to locate any anomalous compartments, which must also be decompressed for successful relief of symptoms.[17,47,48] Multiple insertions, which are common with the abductor pollicis longus, are another important consideration.[80]

The most common complications of this surgery are a tender, hypertrophied scar and neuritis of the sensory nerve.[48] Careful attention to dissection, gentle retraction of the nerve, and the use of a transverse incision can help prevent these problems. Another postoperative complication is subluxation of the tendons from the radial styloid groove upon volar flexion.[16] The risk can be reduced by preserving the anterior radial aspect of the ligament.[55]

Second Dorsal Compartment: Intersection Syndrome

In spite of widespread agreement that tenosynovitis of the extensor carpi radialis longus and brevis tendons in the second dorsal compartment of the wrist is intersection syndrome, the name of this condition is still much debated.[30,55] It is sometimes called abductor pollicis bursitis because the problem is inflammation of a bursa that develops from friction at the intersection of the abductor pollicis longus muscle belly and the extensor carpi radialis tendons.[48] Others call it peritendinitis crepitans or paratenonitis of the forearm.[74,79]

Intersection syndrome is generally attributed to repetitive extension and flexion of the wrist or to direct trauma.[55] Activities associated with the condition include wringing of laundry, handling a wrench or lever, and lifting weights (especially "curls").[13,18,30,79,80]

Pain, swelling, and crepitance are noted where the abductor pollicis longus and extensor pollicis brevis muscle bellies obliquely cross over the underlying tendons of the extensor carpi radialis brevis and longus (which continue distally through the second compartment). Therefore, the patient points to the intersection site as the location of the problem (Fig. 6). This site is somewhat dorsal and approximately 4–8 cm proximal to the painful site in de Quervain's disease.[30] The swelling does not adhere to the underlying skin. Distinct crepitance can often be felt.[48] At times, the crepitance may "squeak" upon palpation or with wrist motion.[13,80] Erythema may be present in severe cases. Finkelstein's test elicits pain at the intersection site.[30,48]

The most difficult entity to differentiate from an early intersection syndrome is de Quervain's disease. These two entities can be differentiated by the different locations of pain and swelling.

Treatment of Intersection Syndrome

Nonoperative measures such as rest, splinting in 15–20 degrees of wrist extension, NSAIDs, and ice may be attempted initially.[30] If necessary, hydrocortisone may be injected into the second dorsal compartment.[13,30,48,55,80] One report estimates that approximately 60% of patients obtain permanent relief without surgery.[30]

Surgery consists of incision or excision of the tenosynovium of the second dorsal compartment.[13,30] The wrist may be splinted in 15–20 degrees of extension with a palmar splint for about 2 weeks postoperatively. As in the surgical procedure for de Quervain's, the sensory

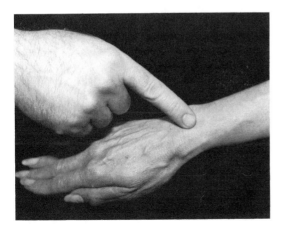

FIGURE 6. The area of the intersection syndrome is proximal to the examiner's index finger on the dorsal radial aspect of the patient's wrist.

branch of the radial nerve may develop a neuroma.[55]

Third Dorsal Compartment

The tendon of extensor pollicis longus occupies the third dorsal compartment. Tenosynovitis at this compartment is not common, but when it occurs, it often does so in combination with tenosynovitis of another compartment, especially the second.[16,71]

Extensor pollicis longus tenosynovitis is thought to be caused by repetitive extension and flexion of the thumb with ulnar and radial deviation of the wrist, as in drumming.[55] Hence, tenosynovitis of the third compartment is sometimes called "drummer boy's palsy." The condition is more common in those with a previous Colles fracture, especially if it is nondisplaced.[71] This tenosynovitis may result from degenerative changes at Lister's tubercle.[80] The extensor pollicis longus is one of the more commonly affected tendon sheaths in rheumatoid patients.[42]

Lister's tubercle is used as a landmark. It is a prominence just proximal to the radiocarpal articulation on the dorsum of the radius. The extensor pollicis longus tendon curves just ulnarly to Lister's tubercle. The second compartment tendons are radial to the tubercle.

The patient complains of pain at Lister's tubercle that may radiate proximally and distally. The pain is felt upon flexion and extension of the distal phalanx of the thumb.[16] The tubercle may swell.

The risk of tendon rupture secondary to extensor pollicis longus tenosynovitis is higher than in other compartments. This predisposition seems to be related to a region of avascularity in the tendon at Lister's tubercle.[71]

As with other tenosynovitis, nonoperative measures are tried initially to quiet the inflammation. Owing to the increased risk of rupture, operative measures are taken earlier.[80] The third dorsal compartment is incised, and the extensor pollicis longus tendon is transposed superficially to the ligament.[55]

Fourth Dorsal Compartment

The tendons of the extensor indicis proprius and extensor digitorum communis occupy the fourth dorsal compartment. This compartment is an uncommon site of tenosynovitis (from trauma)[16,80] but one of the more common sites of rheumatoid tenosynovitis.[42,61] It has been suggested that fourth compartment tenosynovitis is secondary to extension of the muscle belly of the extensor indicis proprius into the fourth compartment, which presumably reduces the compartmental space and thus increases friction generated with movement. One study showed 75% of cadavers with the muscle belly extended into the compartment.[65]

Usually pain is felt on the dorsum of the wrist and is exacerbated by vigorous finger and wrist movement.[16,65] There may be local tenderness over the fourth dorsal compartment. Nonoperative measures are tried initially; surgical decompression follows if these measures are unsuccessful.

Fifth Dorsal Compartment

The extensor digiti minimi tendon is ensheathed in the fifth compartment. Tenosynovitis at this location is rare[2,26,34] and is also postulated to be the result of a muscle belly that extends into the compartment.[2] The existence of multiple tendon insertion slips has been implicated, but in view of the high incidence of multiple tendon insertions (and rarity of the condition), this theory has lost favor.[34,66]

There is tenderness upon palpation and, in some, swelling of the tendon sheath just distal to the ulnar head.[16,34] The pain is aggravated with gripping.[34]

Treatment follows the same principles as for other compartments. If surgery is required, multiple insertion slips must be searched out and decompressed, much as with de Quervain's disease, to ensure relief of symptoms.

Sixth Dorsal Compartment

The extensor carpi ulnaris occupies the sixth compartment and is one of the most common areas of rheumatoid tenosynovitis, which, in this case, produces subluxation of the extensor carpi ulnaris tendon from the compartment. Forearm hypersupination and forced ulnar wrist deviation can produce the problem.[14]

Tenosynovitis at the sixth compartment results in pain and tenderness at the dorsal ulnar aspect of the wrist.[32] The tendon is palpable at the base of the fifth metacarpal. Swelling may be present. In some instances, the pain may be localized deep in the wrist, making the diagnosis difficult.[24] If subluxation of the tendon is occurring, the patient notes a recurrent "snapping" over the wrist that can be reproduced by active (but often not by passive) forearm supination with ulnar deviation of the wrist.[14] Often the tendon then snaps back into the compartment upon pronation. Pain in this compartment should be differentiated from tear of the triangular fibrocartilage and tear of the lunotriquetral joint.

If subluxation is the cause of the tenosynovitis and the history suggests that subluxation is acute, splinting of the wrist for 6 weeks is suggested.[14] If the subluxation is chronic, surgical reconstruction of the sixth compartment may be considered.[14,32,55] If the tenosynovitis is not secondary to subluxation, nonoperative measures should be attempted first.

Flexor Tendinitis

On the volar aspect of the wrist and hand, the tendons are ensheathed at two separate regions: once at the wrist and again in the digits (the digital sheaths). At the wrist, the digital flexor tendons run through the carpal tunnel.[40] Along the digit, the flexor tendons and their sheaths are constrained by fibrous ligaments to prevent bowstringing.[17] The ligaments consist of five annular pulleys (A1 and A5) and three or four cruciate ligaments (Fig. 7).[37]

The flexor carpi radialis tendon also has a narrow tendon sheath. It begins at the wrist joint and covers the tendon as it passes under the crest of the trapezium to its insertion on the second and third metacarpals.[67]

The term "flexor tenosynovitis" usually refers to digital tenosynovitis, although it is also used to refer to tenosynovitis of the palmocarpal sheaths (bursae) at the wrist. Tenosynovitis of the flexor carpi radialis sheath may also oc-

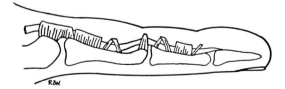

FIGURE 7. The annular and cruciate ligaments holding the flexor tendons within the digital sheath. (Reprinted with permission from Kasdan ML, Romm S: Essentials of Plastic, Maxillofacial, and Reconstructive Surgery. Baltimore, Williams & Wilkins, 1986.)

cur. Calcific tendinitis may affect the flexor carpi radialis and the flexor carpi ulnaris.[57]

Flexor tenosynovitis occurs most commonly in rheumatoid patients and often as the first symptom of the disease.[48] Therefore, anytime a patient presents with flexor tenosynovitis, the possibility of rheumatoid arthritis should be considered if the associated history is positive.

Swelling in flexor tenosynovitis is often not obvious, because, unlike the extensor aspect of the hand, the volar skin is thick.[73] In the wrist and forearm, the swelling is proximal to the transverse carpal ligament.

Flexor Carpi Radialis

Flexor carpi radialis tenosynovitis is thought to occur secondary to trauma, arthrosis deformans in the trapezioscaphoid joint, or chronic repetitive use.[67,76,80]

The condition is characterized by pain over the flexor carpi radialis tendon and tenderness along the tendon at the distal wrist crease (Fig. 8). The pain is aggravated by wrist extension and by wrist flexion against resistance.[67,77] Crepitus may be present.

Radiographs are helpful in identifying arthritic conditions or calcification of the tendon insertion.[48,76,77] The condition must be differentiated from Lindburg's syndrome, which also presents with volar and radial wrist pain. In Lindburg's syndrome, the patient complains of vague pain, a sensation of tightness, and thumb cramping. The pain is exacerbated by passive extension of the index finger. This entity is in part due to the existence of an anomalous tendon slip from the flexor pollicis longus usually to the flexor digitorum profundus of the index finger. Lindburg's sign is the inability to flex the thumb fully without simultaneously flexing the index finger.[80] The existence of the tendon slip, however, does not always lead to the syndrome; 25% of people have the anomalous tendon, but the syndrome is much less common.[71]

Initial treatment of flexor carpi radialis tenosynovitis consists of nonoperative measures, such as rest, ice, splinting in 20 degrees of wrist flexion, NSAIDs, and steroid injections if the initial treatment is unsuccessful.[80] These methods are successful in most patients,[67,77] but for the recalcitrant case, surgical decompression may be indicated.[48,77]

Flexor Carpi Ulnaris

Flexor carpi ulnaris tenosynovitis is associated with repetitive wrist motions. It may be bilateral.[80] Inflammation of the tendon usually occurs just proximal to its insertion on the pisiform. If untreated, the inflammation may lead to an ulnar neuritis at Guyon's canal. Calcifications may exist within the tenosynovium.[55]

Pain is present at the ulnar side of the wrist and is aggravated by wrist flexion and ulnar deviation against resistance.[80]

Treatment is basically the same as in flexor carpi radialis tenosynovitis.[80]

Digital Flexor Tenosynovitis of the Wrist

Tenosynovitis of the digital flexors of the wrist has been linked to repetitive flexion of the fingers and wrist, to hyperextension injuries, and to direct trauma.[55,80] Flexor tenosynovitis at the wrist is the most common reported cause of carpal tunnel syndrome.[20,28] All of the entities mentioned under "Systemic Disorders" (p. 405) should be considered as possible factors in flexor tenosynovitis. For example, patients with diabetes mellitus have an increased incidence of tenosynovitis of the digital flexors.[58]

In flexor tenosynovitis, pain over the volar wrist is increased with finger flexion and extension. There may be swelling at the wrist just proximal to the flexion crease.[80] Symptoms of carpal tunnel syndrome (neuritic pain in the radial three and one-half digits on the volar aspect) can be present. Occasionally, inflammation of the tendons at the tunnel may result in tendon rupture.[52]

Rest, splinting, ice, and NSAIDs are some-

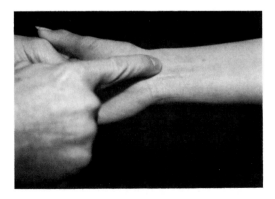

FIGURE 8. The examiner is pointing to the flexor carpi radialis tendon.

sionally necessary.[55] As with many other tendinitides, the degree of success with nonoperative measures is related to the severity and chronicity of symptoms at initial treatment.[28] Patient motivation and cooperation are essential. If steroid injections are necessary, the median nerve should be avoided; the canal should be entered just proximal to the wrist crease on the ulnar side of the palmaris longus.[71]

Surgical decompression is usually indicated for cases that do not respond to conservative treatment.[55] The recovery period for this tenosynovitis may be prolonged.[80]

Flexor Tenosynovitis of the Digits

Flexor tenosynovitis of the digits is often recognized only after the condition has progressed to the point of stenosis and triggering. The condition begins with inflammation. If the inciting factor is not reversed, it will progress to thickening of the tendon sheath, which eventually causes constriction and secondary enlargement of the tendon. The tendinous enlargement begins to catch at the first annular retinacular pulley of the digit. In the early stages of triggering, the finger may merely be "slow" to function. As the condition progresses, the finger begins to "catch" at the tendon nodule,

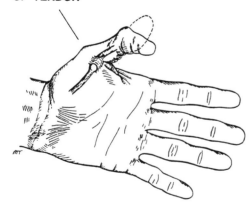

LOCATION OF CONSTRICTION OF TENDON

FIGURE 9. Flexor tenosynovitis. The bulbous deformity in the flexor pollicis longus catches under the first annular ligament, producing the snapping or "trigger" sensation. (Reprinted with permission from Karwowski W, Kasdan ML: The partnership of ergonomics and medical intervention in rehabilitation of workers with cumulative trauma disorders of the hand. In Mital A, Karwowski W (eds): Ergonomics in Rehabilitation. Philadelphia, Taylor & Francis, 1988, pp 35–53.)

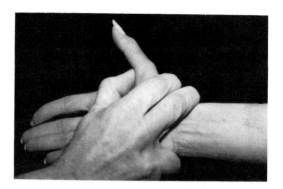

FIGURE 10.   Flexor tenosynovitis. The examiner's thumb is placed over the palmar digital crease and the patient is asked to actively extend and flex the interphalangeal joint. The snapping or triggering sensation is palpable.

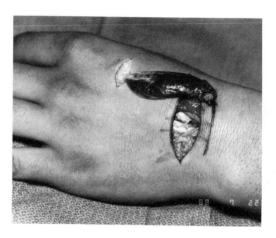

FIGURE 11.   An anomalous extensor digitorum brevis manus muscle is often mistaken for a soft-tissue tumor. Usually surgery is necessary for a definitive diagnosis.

hesitate for a moment, and then, with continued muscular contraction, snap past the catch, thereby simulating a "trigger" (Fig. 9).[48] The constriction usually occurs at the proximal annular pulley (the A-1 pulley). The dysfunctional motion usually occurs at the proximal interphalangeal joint. Because the finger flexors are relatively stronger than the extensors, the patient often flexes the finger past the nodule or constriction, but then can extend the finger only with difficulty or with the help of the other hand (Fig. 10).[35]

The most commonly affected digit is the thumb.[47] The ring finger is the next most commonly affected.[74] Multiple digit involvement occurs in 15% of patients and is more common in patients with rheumatoid arthritis.[42]

Tenosynovitis of the digital flexors has been associated with activities in which hard objects times successful; steroid injections are occa-press against the tendons in the palms while the digits are in motion; an example is the use of a wrench or pliers.[47] It also is apparently associated with some predisposition to teno-synovitis; more than two-thirds of patients manifest at least one other tenosynovitis.[55] The pain of flexor tenosynovitis is often explained as a discomfort at the flexor sheath rather than a severe pain.[47] Often a nodule can be felt if the tendon is palpated during finger motion (Fig. 9). Snapping and catching of the finger are more easily produced by applying pressure over the flexor sheath (Fig. 10).

Nonoperative measures should usually be at-tempted first.[55] Conservative management may involve splinting (see Chapter 33), activity re-strictions, or steroid injection. The accuracy of injection can be checked by palpating the op-posite end of the sheath to assure filling while injecting.[42] If these measures are unsuccessful, surgical release of the A-1 annular pulley and removal of exuberant tenosynovium and ten-don nodules may be necessary.[55] In cases of severe, stenosing tenosynovitis, surgery may be indicated as the primary treatment.

Anomalous muscles may become sympto-matic after a direct blow or overuse.[80] They are often mistaken for soft-tissue tumors and are accurately diagnosed only after surgery. The hand and wrist muscle most likely to be anom-alous is the extensor digitorum brevis manus (Fig. 11). The patient presents with a dorsal wrist mass that is firm with the fingers ex-tended but soft upon relaxation.[56]

Occupational tenosynovitis can interfere with function to the point that a productive worker is unable to continue in his or her usual job. Early diagnosis and treatment are important. The occupational physician and nurse must have a thorough understanding of the workplace and job design. Intervention by modifying the way a task is performed, rotation of work duties, and application of human factor engineering (ergonomics) may prevent some cases of ten-dinitis.

REFERENCES

1. Amadio PC: Tendon injuries in the upper extremity. In Dee R, Mango E, Hurst LC (eds): Principles of Orthopaedic Practice, vol 2. New York, McGraw-Hill, 1989, pp 699–718.
2. Ambrose J, Goldstone R: Anomalous extensor digiti minimi proprius causing tunnel syndrome in the dorsal compartment. J Bone Joint Surg 57A:706–707, 1975.
3. Armstrong TJ: Ergonomics and cumulative trauma dis-orders. Hand Clin 2:553–565, 1986.
4. Armstrong TJ, Fine LJ, Goldstein SA, et al: Ergo-nomic considerations in hand and wrist tendinitis. J Hand Surg 12A:830–837, 1987.
5. Armstrong TJ, Fine LJ, Radwin RG, Silverstein BS: Ergonomics and the effects of vibration in hand-in-tensive work. Scand J Work Environ Health 13:286–289, 1987.
6. Armstrong TJ, Radwin RG, Hansen DJ, Kennedy KW: Repetitive trauma disorders: Job evaluation and de-sign. Hum Factors 28:325–336, 1986.
7. Bammer G, Blignault I: A review of research on re-petitive strain injuries. In Buckle P (ed): Musculo-skeletal Disorders at Work. Philadelphia, Taylor & Francis, 1987, pp 188–223.
8. Berkow R, Fletcher AJ: The Merck Manual of Diag-nosis and Therapy, 15th ed. Rahway, NJ, Merck, 1987.
9. Bigliana LU: Rheumatologic and degenerative disor-ders. In Dee R, Mango E, Hurst LC (eds): Principles of Orthopaedic Practice, vol 1. New York, McGraw-Hill, 1989, pp 621–627.
10. Bigliani LU, Morrison DJ: Subacromial impingement syndrome. In Dee R, Mango E, Hurst LC (eds): Prin-ciples of Orthopaedic Practice, vol 2. New York, McGraw-Hill, 1989, pp 627–634.
11. Bluestone R: Symptoms and signs of articular disease. In Resnick D, Niwayama G (eds): Diagnosis of Bone and Joint Disorders, vol 2, 2nd ed. Philadelphia, W.B. Saunders, 1988, pp 822–843.
12. Boyd HB, McLeod AC: Tennis elbow. J Bone Joint Surg 55A:1183–1187, 1973.
13. Brooker AF: Extensor carpi radialis tenosynovitis. Or-thop Rev 6(5):99–100, 1977.
14. Burkhart SS, Wood MB, Linscheid RL: Posttraumatic recurrent subluxation of the extensor carpi ulnaris ten-don. J Hand Surg 7:1–3, 1982.
15. Burkman K, Tanner ED: Shoulder pain. In Kaplan PE, Tanner ED (eds): Musculoskeletal Pain and Dis-ability. Norwalk, CT, Appleton & Lange, 1989, pp 97–131.
16. Burman M: Stenosing tendovaginitis of the dorsal and volar compartments of the wrist. Arch Surg 65:752–762, 1952.
17. Cailliet R: Hand Pain and Impairment. Philadelphia, F.A. Davis, 1975.
18. Chuinard RD: The upper extremity: Elbow, forearm, wrist, and hand. In D'Ambrosia RD (ed): Musculo-skeletal Disorders: Regional Examination and Differ-ential Diagnosis, 2nd ed. Philadelphia, J.B. Lippin-cott, 1986, pp 395–446.
19. Coonrad RW, Hooper WR: Tennis elbow: Its course, natural history, conservative and surgical manage-ment. J Bone Joint Surg 55A:1177–1182, 1973.
20. Coyle MD: Nerve entrapment syndromes in the upper extremity. In Dee R, Mango E, Hurst LC (eds): Prin-ciples of Orthopaedic Practice, vol 2. New York, McGraw-Hill, 1989, pp 672–684.
21. Currey HL: Medical orthopaedics. In Mason M, Cur-rey HL (eds): Clinical Rheumatology. Philadelphia, J.B. Lippincott, 1970.
22. Curwin S, Stanish WD: Tendinitis: Its Etiology and Treatment. Lexington, MA, D.C. Heath, 1984.
23. Dick HM: Tumors of the hand and wrist. In Dee R, Mango E, Hurst L (eds): Principles of Orthopaedic

Practice, vol 1. New York, McGraw-Hill, 1989, pp 767–774.

24. Dickson DD, Luckey CA: Tenosynovitis of the extensor carpi ulnaris tendon sheath. J Bone Joint Surg 30A:903–907, 1948.

25. Dimberg L, Olafsson A, Stefansson E, et al: The correlation between work environment and the occurrence of cervicobrachial symptoms. J Occup Med 31:447–453, 1989.

26. Fry HJ: Overuse syndrome, alias tenosynovitis/tendinitis: The terminology hoax. Proc R Soc Lond 78:414–417, 1986.

27. Garroway RY, McCue FC: Ligament injuries of the wrist, hand and elbow. In Dee R, Mango E, Hurst LC (eds): Principles of Orthopaedic Practice, vol 1. New York, McGraw-Hill, 1989, pp 553–561.

28. Gelberman RH: Carpal tunnel syndrome: Results of a prospective trial of steroid injection and splinting. J Bone Joint Surg 62A:1181, 1980.

29. Goldstein SA, Armstrong TJ, Chaffin DB, Matthews LS: Analysis of cumulative strain in tendons and tendon sheaths. J Biomech 20:1–6, 1987.

30. Grundberg AB, Reagan DS: Pathologic anatomy of the forearm: Intersection syndrome. J Hand Surg 10A:299–302, 1985.

31. Guyton JM, Koopman WJ: Shoulder, hip, and extremity pain. In Ball GV, Koopman WJ (eds): Clinical Rheumatology. Philadelphia, W.B. Saunders, 1986, pp 330–356.

32. Hajj AA, Wood MB: Stenosing tenosynovitis of the extensor carpi ulnaris. J Hand Surg 11A:519–520, 1986.

33. Hollinshead WH, Rosse C: Textbook of Anatomy, 4th ed. Philadelphia, J.B. Lippincott, 1985.

34. Hooper G, McMaster MJ: Stenosing tenovaginitis affecting the tendon of extensor digiti minimi at the wrist. Hand 11(3):299–301, 1979.

35. Hume E: Disorders of the shoulder joint. In Gartland JJ (ed): Fundamentals of Orthopaedics, 4th ed. Philadelphia, W.B. Saunders, 1987, pp 218–240.

36. Hume E: The upper extremity. In Gartland JJ (ed): Fundamentals of Orthopaedics, 4th ed. Philadelphia, W.B. Saunders, 1987, pp 241–273.

37. Hunter JM: Anatomy of flexor tendons: Pulley, vincular, synovial vascular structure. In Spinner M (ed): Kaplan's Functional and Surgical Anatomy of the Hand, 3rd ed. Philadelphia, J.B. Lippincott, 1984.

38. Hurst LC, Nathan J: Infections in the upper extremity. In Dee R, Mango E, Hurst L (eds): Principles of Orthopaedic Practice, vol 1. New York, McGraw-Hill, 1989, pp 741–751.

39. Justis EJ: Nontraumatic disorders: In Crenshaw AH (ed): Campbell's Operative Orthopaedics, 7th ed. St. Louis, C.V. Mosby, 1987.

40. Kaplan EB, Milford L: The retinacular system of the hand. In Spinner M (ed): Kaplan's Functional and Surgical Anatomy of the Hand, 3rd ed. Philadelphia, J.B. Lippincott, 1984, pp 245–281.

41. Kaplan PE, Tanner ED: Tendinitis, bursitis, and fibrositis. In Kaplan PE, Tanner ED (eds): Musculoskeletal Pain and Disability. Norwalk, CT, Appleton & Lange, 1989, pp 1–24.

42. Kelly AP, Jacobson HS: Hand disability due to tenosynovitis. Ind Med Surg Aug 1964:570–574.

43. Knishkowy B, Lederman RJ: Instrumental musicians with upper extremity disorders: A follow-up study. Med Probl Perform Art 1:85–89, 1986.

44. Leach RE, Schepsis AA: Shoulder pain. Clin Sports Med 2:23, 1983.

45. Lederman RJ, Calabrese LH: Overuse syndromes in instrumentalists. Med Probl Perform Art 1:7–11, 1986.

46. Lipscomb PR: Chronic nonspecific tenosynovitis and peritendinitis. Surg Clin North Am 24:780–797, 1944.

47. Lipscomb PR: Tenosynovitis of the hand and the wrist: Carpal tunnel syndrome, de Quervain's disease, trigger digit. Clin Orthop 13:164–180, 1959.

48. Lister B: The Hand: Diagnosis and Indications, 2nd ed. New York, Churchill Livingstone, 1984.

49. MacKinnon SE: Nerve compression syndromes. In Marsh JL (ed): Current Therapy in Plastic and Reconstructive Surgery. Philadelphia, B.C. Decker, 1989, pp 166–173.

50. Magee DJ: Orthopedic Physical Assessment. Philadelphia, W.B. Saunders, 1987.

51. McKenzie F, Storment J, van Hook P, Armstrong TJ: A program for control of repetitive trauma disorders associated with hand tool operations in a telecommunications manufacturing facility. Am Ind Hyg Assoc J 46:674–678, 1985.

52. Millender LH, Nalebuff EA, Feldon PG: Rheumatoid arthritis. In Green DP (ed): Operative Hand Surgery, vol 2. New York, Churchill Livingstone, 1982, pp 1161–1262.

53. Neer CS: Impingement lesions. Clin Orthop 173:70–77, 1983.

54. Norris RN: Overuse injuries. Guitar Player, Sept 1989, pp 94–98.

55. Pruzansky M: Stenosing tenosynovitis. In Chapman (ed): Operative Orthopaedics, vol 2. Philadelphia, J.B. Lippincott, 1988, pp 1185–1197.

56. Reef TC, Brestin SG: The extensor digitorum brevis manus and its clinical significance. J Bone Joint Surg 57A:704–706, 1975.

57. Resnick D: Calcium and hydroxyapatite crystal deposition disease. In Resnick D and Niwayama G (eds): Diagnosis of Bone and Joint Disorders, vol 3. Philadelphia, W.B. Saunders, 1988.

58. Resnick D: Disorders of other endocrine glands and of pregnancy. In Resnick D, Niwayama G (eds): Diagnosis of Bone and Joint Disorders, vol 4, 2nd ed. Philadelphia, W.B. Saunders, 1988, pp 2286–2317.

59. Resnick D: Thyroid disorders. In Resnick D, Niwayama G (eds): Diagnosis of Bone and Joint Disorders, vol 4, 2nd ed. Philadelphia, W.B. Saunders, 1988, pp 2199–2218.

60. Resnick D, Niwayama G: Osteomyelitis, septic arthritis and soft tissue infection: The organisms. In Resnick D, Niwayama G (eds): Diagnosis of Bone and Joint Disorders, vol 4, 2nd ed. Philadelphia, W.B. Saunders, 1988, pp 2647–2754.

61. Resnick D, Niwayama G: Rheumatoid arthritis. In Resnick D, Niwayama G (eds): Diagnosis of Bone and Joint Disorders, vol 2, 2nd ed. Philadelphia, W.B. Saunders, 1988, pp 954–1067.

62. Resnick D, Niwayama G: Rheumatoid arthritis and the seronegative spondyloarthropathies: Radiographic and pathologic concepts. In Resnick D, Niwayama G (eds): Diagnosis of Bone and Joint Disorders, vol 2, 2nd ed. Philadelphia, W.B. Saunders, 1988, pp 894–953.

63. Resnick D, Niwayama G: Sarcoidosis. In Resnick D, Niwayama G (eds): Diagnosis of Bone and Joint Disorders, vol 6, 2nd ed. Philadelphia, W.B. Saunders, 1988, pp 4012–4032.

64. Riggins RS: The shoulder. In D'Ambrosia RD (ed): Musculoskeletal Disorders: Regional Examination and

Differential Diagnosis, 2nd ed. Philadelphia, J.B. Lippincott, 1986, pp 367–394.
65. Ritter MA, Inglis AE: The extensor indicis proprius syndrome. J Bone Joint Surg 51A:1645–1648, 1969.
66. Schenk RR: Variations of the extensor tendons of the fingers: Surgical significance. J Bone Joint Surg 46A:103–111, 1964.
67. Schmidt HM: Clinical anatomy of the m. flexor carpi radialis tendon sheath. Acta Morphol Neerl Scand 25:17–28, 1987.
68. Sheon RP, Moskowitz RW, Goldberg VM: Soft Tissue Rheumatic Pain: Recognition, Management, Prevention, 2nd ed. Philadelphia, Lea & Febiger, 1987.
69. Silverstein B, Fine L, Stetson D: Hand-wrist disorders among investment casting plant workers. J Hand Surg 12A:838–844, 1987.
70. Smith JW, Bellinger CG: The blood supply of tendons. In Tubiana R (ed): The Hand. Philadelphia, W.B. Saunders, 1981, pp 353–358.
71. Thorson EP, Szabo RM: Tendinitis of the wrist and elbow. Occup Med State Art Rev 4:419–431, 1989.
72. Tichauer ER, Gage H: Ergonomic principles basic to hand tool design. Am Ind Hyg Assoc J 38:622–634, 1977.
73. Tubiana R, Thomine JM, Mackin E: Examination of the Hand and Upper Limb. Philadelphia, W.B. Saunders, 1984.
74. Usoltseva EV, Mashkara KI: Surgery of Diseases and Injuries of the Hand. St. Louis, C.V. Mosby, 1979.
75. Verdan C: Lymphatic vascularization of tendons. In Tubiana R (ed): The Hand. Philadelphia, W.B. Saunders, 1981, pp 359–360.
76. Viegas SF: Atypical causes of hand pain. Am Fam Physician 35:167–172, 1987.
77. Walker L, Meals R: Tendinitis: A practical approach to diagnosis and management. J Musculoskel Med, May 1989:24–54.
78. White NB, et al: A method to determine blood flow in long bone and selected soft tissues. Surg Gynecol Obstet 119:535, 1964.
79. Williams JG: Surgical management of traumatic noninfective tenosynovitis of the wrist extensors. J Bone Joint Surg 59B:408–410, 1977.
80. Wood MB, Dobyns JH: Sports-related extraarticular wrist syndromes. Clin Orthop 202:93–102, 1986.
81. Young VL, Fernando B: Painful hand syndrome. In Marsh JL (ed): Current Therapy in Plastic and Reconstructive Surgery. Philadelphia, B.C. Decker, 1989, pp 237–242.
82. Zohn DA: Musculoskeletal Pain: Diagnosis and Physical Treatment, 2nd ed. Boston, Little, Brown, 1988.

Chapter 29

INFECTIONS OF THE HAND

Robert L. Reid, M.D., FACS

This chapter provides an historical perspective and general principles of management of hand infections. Specific hand infections and their management are also covered. The information is directed mainly toward the primary-care and occupational physician.

HISTORICAL PERSPECTIVES

Although infections of the hand have obviously occurred throughout human existence, their nature and extent were not featured prominently in early surgical literature. Allen Kanavel, of Chicago, made the first special study of hand infections. The first edition of his *Infections of the Hand*, published in 1912,[8] still makes fascinating reading. The 6th edition in 1933[9] presented the results of 25 years' experience in managing hand infections. Prior to his teachings, the management of hand infections had routinely been delegated to the least experienced house officer in the training program.

Kanavel described the minute anatomy of the hand, the boundaries of potential fascial spaces, and the correct locations for incisions—all at a time when hand infections often caused severe mutilation, residual deformity, and even death. He showed that with exacting diagnosis, properly placed surgical incisions, and comprehensive follow-ups, complete function could be restored in 95% of severe fascial space infections, even before the advent of antibiotics. In devastating tendon sheath infections, morbidity could be reduced by half if only the diagnosis were made early.

One of his most important concepts was that of placing the infected hand in the now well-known "position of function" (Fig. 1)—that is, with the wrist slightly extended, fingers flexed, and thumb abducted. This is the position in which maximum power can be exerted with least effort. It is also usually the most comfortable position and the one in which, when there is residual stiffness, the hand maintains some useful function. This position is now, to a great degree, replaced by the "safe position"[19] (Fig. 2), the "blade of the hoe" position,[3] which seems to better prevent contractures of the metacarpophalangeal and proximal interphalangeal joints of the fingers after the hand has been immobilized by disease or injury.

Kanavel treated early cases of hand infection with bed rest, elevation of the hand, and hot, moist compresses. Later, when the infection localized, he incised the area in a bloodless

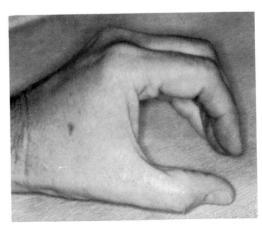

FIGURE 1. The position of function.

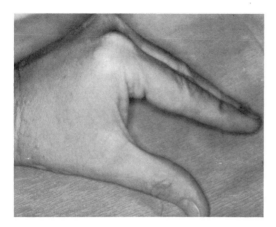

FIGURE 2. The safe position.

field with the patient under general anesthesia. He removed all drains within 48 hours of surgery and began the patient with hand and finger motion exercises with 48 hours of surgical drainage. Later, physiotherapy and exposure to sunlight seemed to improve his results.

In the preantibiotic days, patients often died from a streptococcal septicemia a few days after a simple finger prick with a contaminated object. Physicians and nurses were especially prone to these infections. Kanavel showed that conservative treatment of the acute hemolytic streptococcal cellulitis could be lifesaving. He advised immediate bed rest, immobilization, elevation of the entire area, and no incisions until pus was obvious and well localized.

Kanavel's basic principles have withstood the test of time even though some of them have been modified. Kanavel's classic incisions have now been generally replaced by a minimal incision[16] over the area of maximal tenderness.

Today, hand society meetings seldom include papers about infections of the hand; in fact, search of the literature in English for the past 10 years has revealed only a few publications on the subject. This might suggest that hand infections are less common and of less significance than previously. But there is no evidence that infections are less numerous, although the patterns and magnitude of infections have changed. Some types —e.g., fascial space infections—are less common, whereas new types—among them, genital herpes and atypical mycobacterial infections—are increasing in frequency. If infections are less significant, the standard of care may be improving. In any event, there is no doubt that the final result of a hand infection is directly related to

the primary treatment. Treatment cannot be correct unless the diagnosis is exact. Unfortunately, too many patients are still left with persistent and disabling residuals because primary care of a hand infection was inappropriate or inadequate.

The types of open hand injuries occurring in the modern workplace are common and diverse.[10] Each has the potential to result in an infection. The role of the occupational physician or nurse is early diagnosis and treatment, which is paramount for the outcome of the incident. Education concerning the reporting and treatment of even trivial injuries in the workplace is extremely important. The worker needs to feel comfortable and secure reporting "minor" hand injuries to the local treatment facility. The initial treatment plan may include documentation, evaluation, local treatment, tetanus prophylaxis, antibiotic therapy, or even incisions for drainage. Occupational medical personnel need to have a good working relationship with a hand surgeon so that the moment things do not appear to be going well a quick consultation can be obtained.

The remainder of this chapter discusses the basic treatment that may be afforded by occupational medical personnel and points out the types of infections for which prompt consultation might have a positive effect on outcome.

GENERAL PRINCIPLES

Most hand infections seem to result from some form of neglect, either in the prevention of contamination or in early treatment once contamination has occurred.[11] Tables 1 and 2 list the common and uncommon organisms responsible for the majority of hand infections.

Both general factors (Table 3) and local factors (Table 4) may influence the treatment and

TABLE 1.   Bacteriological Sources of 65% of Hand Infections

Staphylococcus aureus	.50%
β-Hemolytic streptococci	.15%
Aerobacter aerogenes	.10%
Enterococcus species	.10%
Escherichia coli	.5%
Multiple organisms	.70%

Reprinted with permission from Kilgore ES, Graham WP: The Hand: Surgical and Non-surgical Management. Philadelphia, Lea & Febiger, 1977, p 307.

TABLE 2.   Organisms Responsible for Less Common Hand Infections

1. Bacteria: Gram-negative *Pseudomonas*, *Proteus*, *Gonococcus*, *Pasteurella*, and *Brucella* species; *Mycobacterium* species that cause leprosy and tuberculosis; gram-positive clostridia and anthrax bacilli
2. Fungi may cause deep, but more commonly cause superficial, mycoses.
3. Viruses: herpes simplex, herpes zoster, and milker's nodule
4. Chlamydiae: the intracellular parasites of cat-scratch fever
5. Protozoa: an example are those that cause leishmaniasis.
6. Metazoa: worms that cause such diseases as cutaneous larva migrans, dracontiasis, filariasis, gnathostomiasis, loiasis, onchocerciasis, and trichinosis.
7. Miscellaneous: *Erysipelothrix rhusiopathiae* (*E. insidiosa*), which causes erysipeloid; *Pseudomonas mallei*, which causes glanders.

Reprinted with permission from Kilgore ES, Graham WP: The Hand: Surgical and Non-surgical Management. Philadelphia, Lea & Febiger, 1977, p 307.

TABLE 3.   General Factors Affecting Hand Infections

1. Diabetes mellitus
2. Anemia
3. Conditions or drugs affecting immunological status
4. Hypoproteinemia
5. Deficiency states
6. Existing infections at other sites
7. Skin conditions such as eczema and psoriasis
8. Present medications
9. Drug sensitivities

Reprinted with permission from Watson N, Smith RJ: Infections of the hand. In Methods and Concepts in Hand Surgery. London & Boston, Butterworth, 1986, p 98.

TABLE 4.   Local Factors Affecting Hand Infections

1. Unusual organisms such as those causing erisypeloid in butchers
2. Peripheral vascular disease
3. Occupational problems such as regular maceration of hand skin
4. Chronic lymphedema
5. Previous local radiation therapy
6. Undetected foreign body

Reprinted with permission from Watson N, Smith RJ: Infections of the hand. In Methods and Concepts in Hand Surgery. London & Boston, Butterworth, 1986, p 98.

outcome of hand infections. These factors need to be elicited at the time of the general medical history so that they may be included in the general medical plan.

In acute injuries, there is no agreement in the literature regarding the need and type of prophylactic antibiotics.[5] A study from the Mayo Clinic[7] offers some sensible guidelines for management of mutilating hand injuries. A degree of selectivity is recommended, especially in injuries associated with farm accidents. In principle, no prophylactic antibiotic treatment is justified, because the types of bacteria isolated are highly variable and susceptibility patterns require the administration of potentially toxic antibiotics. Reculture and treatment with a specific antibiotic as the wound flora clarifies are recommended.

In injuries sustained in the home or factory, the predominance of gram-positive organisms indicates that use of a semisynthetic penicillinase-resistant agent is justified, providing appropriate cultures are obtained before treatment is begun. The Mayo Clinic study stresses that the surgical dictums of the preantibiotic era must be meticulously followed. Careful initial surgical wound care followed by delayed primary or secondary wound closure seems to be the best guard against infection.

The occupational physician is not likely to provide definitive care for severe types of injuries. Careful handling at the injury site, wrapping the wound in a clean, moist dressing, and splinting and elevating of the part are all valuable adjuncts to prevent further contamination and to promote the preservation of viable tissue that the hand surgeon may use in the reconstructive process.[14]

Once a severe infection is established, consultation with an appropriate surgeon is indicated. Hospitalization may be required if the magnitude of the infection warrants it. Spiegel et al.[21] devised a protocol for hand infection management in a university setting that reduced readmission rates by 10%, incidents of arthritis from 10% to 3%, reoperation rate from 34% to 1%, the incidence of stiffness from 28% to 16%, and osteomyelitis from 6% to 1%. In addition, the average hospital stay decreased by 1 day. Their protocol prescribes incision and drainage of the infection in the operating room. In addition, when the patient is first seen, intravenous antibacterial therapy effective against anaerobic and aerobic bacteria is begun after obtaining anaerobic and aerobic cultures. Some hand surgeons prefer additional Gram stains at the time of the initial evaluation.[10] Incidentally, the results of Spiegel et al. confirm that nearly 30% of all cultures reveal a mixture of anaerobic and aerobic organisms.

GENERAL MANAGEMENT PRINCIPLES

An injured worker must report the injury so that treatment may be initiated. Abrasions, lacerations, blisters, and similar wounds need to be scrubbed, cleansed, and dressed. If the skin opening is jagged or contamination is suspected, debridement and cultures may be indicated. Tetanus prophylaxis must be considered.[6] If the patient has been fully immunized and the last dose of toxoid was given within 10 years, or if the wound is not tetanus prone, a booster dose of toxoid is not indicated. If the wound is tetanus prone and more than 5 years have elapsed since the last toxoid, 0.5 cc of adsorbed toxoid should be given. If prior immunization has been inadequate and the wound is not tetanus prone, 0.5 cc of adsorbed toxoid is given. For tetanus-prone wounds, the recommended dosage is 0.5 cc of adsorbed toxoid and, in another extremity, 250 units (or more) of human tetanus antitoxin. In addition, appropriate antibiotic therapy should be considered. Because many patients do not accurately recall prior immunizations, medical personnel need to attempt to document all boosters.

Antibiotics. For the routine minor hand wound or infection, antibiotics are not necessarily required, especially if the wound is clean and superficial.

Dressings. The skin of the hand is particularly susceptible to maceration, and daily dressing changes are valuable in preventing it.

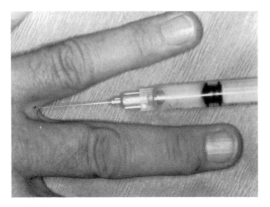

FIGURE 3. Metacarpal block anesthesia. A small amount of anesthetic agent is also injected on the dorsum of the involved digit near the metacarpophalangeal joint and in the web space on the opposite side of the digit.

A mixture of equal parts hydrogen peroxide and normal saline solution will make dressing removal easier and less painful. Daily dressing changes allow wound inspection to determine the presence of local signs of inflammation— rubor (redness), calor (heat), tumor (swelling), or dolor (pain)—together with loss of function of the part.

Splinting. The need for rest of the part in cases of early infection, injury, and inflammation has been recognized for centuries, but Koch[12] in 1946 reemphasized this principle. The position of "safe splintage"[19] is ideal and appears to be the best treatment in case a chronic infection does develop (see Fig. 2).

Elevation. To the splinting must be added elevation of the part. The more swelling and inflammation present, the longer the elevation should last. As a practical rule, the patient should keep the fingers elevated above the heart. To prevent elbow flexion and avoid impeding drainage outflow, I do not use a sling, but rather ask the patient to keep the hand elevated. The patient is encouraged to actively move all parts of the extremity, including nondamaged digits, elbow, and shoulders. I encourage the patient to establish a regular pattern of active motion during each waking hour.

Anesthesia. There is no place for local infiltration anesthetic techniques in hand infections. I prefer a metacarpal block (Fig. 3) for treating an infection occurring at or distal to the proximal interphalangeal joint of a finger or the interphalangeal joint of the thumb. An infection proximal to these areas can best be managed with a regional block, or even general anesthesia, depending upon the magnitude of the infection. Wrapping the infected area with an exsanguinating dressing before tourniquet elevation is clearly contraindicated. Simple elevation of the limb for a few minutes before tourniquet elevation usually suffices.

X-rays. Radiographs are absolutely essential in cases of hand infection to rule out underlying fractures, foreign bodies, tumor, or osteomyelitis. An initial normal baseline x-ray assists in determining whether osteomyelitis or septic arthritis later develops.[10]

SPECIFIC HAND INFECTIONS

Acute Paronychia. Usually presenting in a corner of the nail fold, when acute paronychia extends to the opposite corner of the fold, it is called a runaround. *Staphylococcus aureus* is

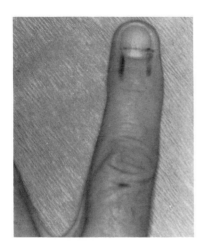

FIGURE 4. Paronychial incisions may include two dorsal flaps or removal of a portion of the nail base.

the predominant organism.[13] Treatment (Fig. 4) consists of lifting the nail fold and removing either a portion or all of the nail. Soaks and dressing changes usually complete the treatment.

A bacteriological study of paronychia in children[1] showed that the infections were a mixture of aerobic and anaerobic organisms. The predominant anaerobic organisms were *Bacteroides* species, gram-positive cocci, *Fusobacterium* species, and *Bifidobacterium* species. The predominant aerobic organisms were *Staphyloccus aureus*, hemolytic streptococci, *Eikenella corrodens*, and *Klebsiella pneumoniae*. Antibiotics may be useful in these infections, but the spectrum of coverage needs to be considered. The treatment of choice is surgical drainage. In view of the wide variety of organisms frequently found in paronychias, it is still wise to perform aerobic and anaerobic cultures at the time of drainage so that the results are available if serious consideration needs to be given to antibiotic therapy.

Chronic Paronychia. Workers whose jobs entail repeated and prolonged exposure of the hand to moisture or immersion in water frequently contract chronic paronychias. Pus is rarely formed with these infections, but frequent scaling and pitting of the nails are frequent. Surgery is rarely needed in this chronic condition, although the nail may need removal for fungal cultures, which may be followed by prolonged treatment with appropriate antifungal medications. It is frequently necessary to recommend a job change to work that is conducive to healing of this condition.

Conditions that May Mimic Nail Infections. Subungual melanoma produces a dark smudge under the nail. The nail needs removal, preferably under metacarpal block, for definitive biopsy and diagnosis.

A glomus tumor is rare. It causes exquisite pinpoint pain about the nail that may lead the unwary to recommend incision and drainage for infection.

A mucous cyst extending from an arthritic distal interphalangeal joint may resemble an infection, especially when it is associated with a flare-up of the local arthritic process. An x-ray and evaluation of adjacent distal interphalangeal joints with the findings of Heberden's nodes usually clarify the diagnosis. A mucous cyst frequently distorts the nail bed and puts pressure on the root of the nail. These cysts may become secondarily infected and may lead to osteomyelitis of the distal joint. An x-ray usually aids in making the diagnosis. Positive findings are narrowing of the joint space and dorsal osteophytes at the distal interphalangeal joint.

Pulp Space Infections. Collections of pus at the closed space at the ends of the fingers and thumb are pulp space infections (Fig. 5). They are nearly always due to a staphylococcal organism. Early incision and drainage usually resolves the problem quickly. The importance of a collection in the terminal pulp (Fig. 5, No. 3) is that when it becomes chronic it may lead to a pressure osteomyelitis of the tuft of the terminal phalanx. The incision and drainage (Fig. 6) can be accomplished under metacarpal block anesthesia. Care is taken to make the incision where a painful scar is unlikely to occur (Figs. 6 and 7) and to divide all septa in order to prevent chronic loculation of the pus. The danger of a felon (Fig. 5, Nos. 5 and 6) is that if it is not drained, infection may spread to the flexor tendon sheath, leading to a very serious complication. Military recruits develop blisters on their hands that frequently become infected from their own saliva. The infection may spread from subcutaneous areas (Fig. 5, No. 8) directly into the flexor tendon sheath, again leading to a serious problem.

Tendon Sheath Infection. In cases of tendon sheath infection, the primary physician should seek help from a hand surgeon. This is a most serious infection. The major role of the primary physician is diagnosis and prompt referral because of the propensity for stiffness and permanent impairment. For diagnosis, these

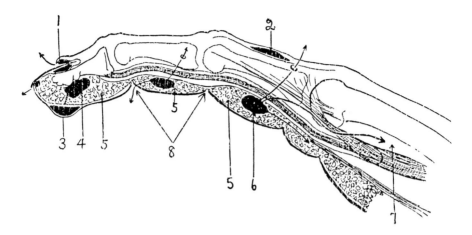

FIGURE 5. Diagram of locations of abscesses and where they point. (1) Paronychia. Perforates base of nail, preserves matrix. (2) Subcutaneous disk of septic necrosis. (3) Phlyctenular abscess indicative of felon beneath. (4) Felon. (5) Three fat pads of a finger separated from each other by the flexion creases, which act as barriers to pus. (6) Abscess in fat pad. May perforate posteriorly through skin, proximally to subcutaneous tissue in palm, or by lumbrical canal to palmar space. (7) Palmar space. (8) Puncture wounds in the flexion creases are dangerous because they lead directly into the tendon sheath. (Reprinted with permission from Boyes JH: Bunnell's Surgery of the Hand, 5th ed. Philadelphia, J. B. Lippincott, 1970, p 617.)

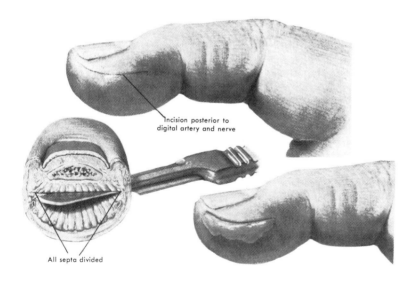

Incision posterior to
digital artery and nerve

All septa divided

FIGURE 6. An incision and drainage of felon. (Reprinted with permission from Milford L: Infections of the hand. In Crenshaw AH (ed): Campbell's Operative Orthopaedics, 7th ed. St Louis, C. V. Mosby Co., 1987, p 497.)

infections (Fig. 8) demonstrate the four cardinal signs of Kanavel:[9]

1. The involved finger is held in slight flexion.
2. The finger is uniformly swollen and red.
3. Intense pain is experienced on any attempted extension of the digit.
4. Tenderness is present along the entire course of the tendon sheath.

These infections require surgical drainage[17] and specific antibiotic administration.

Thenar and Palmar Space Infections. Puncture wounds or tense flexor tendon sheath infections may lead to thenar and palmar space infections (Fig. 9), which are serious occurrences. When the hand is extensively swollen and the patient has systemic signs, prompt referral to a hand surgeon is appropriate. These infections need immediate surgical drainage

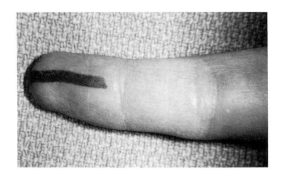

FIGURE 7. A central palmar longitudinal tuft incision may be used without fear of significant sensory loss or residual painful scarring.

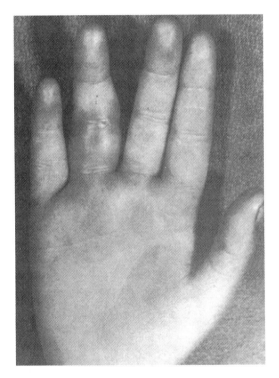

FIGURE 8. Tendon sheath infection. (Reprinted with permission from Lister G: The Hand: Diagnosis and Indications, 1st ed. Edinburgh, Churchill Livingstone, 1977, p 121.)

once localization has occurred. I prefer hospitalization and general anesthesia. An infection may occur in the deep flexor surface of the wrist from a **horseshoe infection** that spreads to Parona's space of the wrist via the thumb flexor sheath or the little finger flexor sheath into the ulna bursa on the flexor surface of the wrist. Some of the most important physical findings associated with these deep infections are lymphedema of the dorsum of the hand

and thumb infection with tenderness along the flexor pollicis tendon sheath associated with swelling and tenderness proximal to the flexion wrist crease and further tenderness along the flexor tendon sheath to the little finger. Frequently, the patient is febrile and has symptoms of toxicity.

UNCOMMON INFECTIONS

Pyogenic Granuloma. A chronically macerated area under a moist dressing is the usual site of a pyogenic granuloma[11] (Fig. 10). The tumor is overgrowth of chronic granulation tissue. Appropriate biopsies and cultures need to be performed, but these lesions usually respond to wound care, local excisions, and silver nitrate application.

Orf. A lesion that is somewhat flatter in appearance than pyogenic granuloma and has a surrounding halo of erythema is an orf.[22] A history of contact with sheep establishes the diagnosis because the responsible virus lives about sheep incisor teeth. The lesion is usually self-limiting, and only symptomatic treatment is indicated.

***Eikenella corrodens* Infections.** Smith et al.[2] pointed out that *Eikenella corrodens*, a gram-negative rod, can be a significant pathogen alone or in synergy with streptococci or other organisms. *Eikenella corrodens* is a facultative gram-negative rod that inhabits the human mouth and upper respiratory tract, and infections often occur in wounds associated with oral contamination. It is particularly important in hand or knuckle wounds where a tooth may have penetrated a joint. The infection usually responds to good surgical drainage and ampicillin and penicillin.

Pasteurella multocida. A cat bite may inoculate *Pasteurella multocida*, a gram-negative bacillus, into the tissues. Intravenous penicillin is the first-line drug. Septic arthritis or osteomyelitis may be a sequel to this infection.

Herpes simplex.[15,18] Herpetic lesions may occur anywhere in the body and typically appear as grouped blisters on an erythematous base. When they occur about the nail fold or distal fat pad in physicians, dentists, nurses, and dental hygienists, they may be confused with paronychias or felons. The pain in these lesions is often severe. The treating physician needs to avoid the temptation to incise and drain. There is no pus under pressure that needs

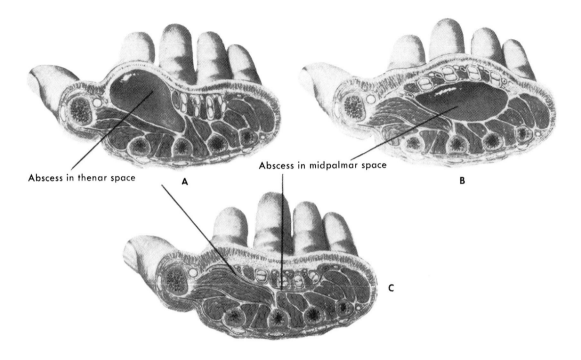

Abscess in thenar space   Abscess in midpalmar space
A   B

C

FIGURE 9. Boundaries of palmar spaces. (Reprinted with permission from Milford L: Infections of the hand. In Crenshaw AH (ed): Campbell's Operative Orthopaedics, 7th ed. St Louis, C. V. Mosby Co., 1987, p 500.)

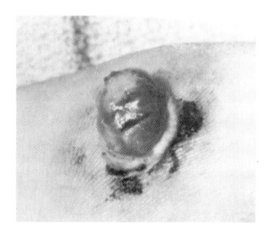

FIGURE 10. Pyogenic granuloma of the palm. (Reprinted with permission from Kilgore E, Graham WE: The Hand: Surgical and Non-surgical Management, 1st ed. Philadelphia, Lea & Febiger, 1977, p 312.)

to be released, and the likelihood that a secondary infection will develop is strong. Local treatment aimed at keeping the area dry is all that is needed; the lesion usually resolves in 17–21 days. Local pain is the distinguishing feature of this lesion. For the treatment of chronic herpes, one may consider acyclovir (Zovirax).[10]

Chronic Fungus and Atypical Mycobacterium Infections. Special media or cultural environments are required to diagnose chronic fungal and atypical *Mycobacterium* infections, which can be quite troublesome. These types of infections may be suspected when a chronic condition does not respond to the usual treatment.

Usually, when a fungus is suspected, the drainage material needs to be cultured on Sabouraud's medium.

When there is a history of wound contamination from soil or from handling fish, an atypical mycobacterial infection should be suspected. The laboratory needs to be alerted to culture the material at 32° C instead of 37° C, as is usual for *Mycobacterium* cultures.

CONCLUSION

All hand injuries have the potential of developing an infection. Early diagnosis and treatment are critical to obtaining a satisfactory result when infection occurs. Early referral to a hand surgery specialist is indicated in infections associated with high morbidity. When patients fail to respond to appropriate conservative management, referral to the appropriate specialist should be considered.

REFERENCES

1. Brook I: Bacteriologic study of paronychia in children. Am J 141:703–705, 1981.
2. Brooks GF, O'Donoghue JM, Rissing JP, et al: *Eikenella corrodens*, a recently recognized pathogen. Medicine 53:325–341, 1974.
3. Bunnell S: Surgery of the Hand, 3d ed. Philadelphia, J. B. Lippincott, 1956.
4. Byrne JJ, Boyd TF, Daley AK: Pasteurella infections from cats. Surg Gynocol Obstet 103:53, 1958.
5. Carter S, Mersheimer W: Infections of the hand. Orthop Clin North Am 1:455–466, 1979.
6. Committee on Trauma of the American College of Surgeons: A Guide to Prophylaxis against Tetanus in Wound Management. Chicago, American College of Surgeons, 1979.
7. Fitzgerald RH, Cooney WP, Washington JA, et al: Bacterial colonization of mutilating hand injuries and its treatment. J Hand Surg 2:85–89, 1977.
8. Kanavel AB: Infections of the Hand. London, Bailliere Tindall & Cox, 1912.
9. Kanavel AB: Infections of the Hand, 6th ed. Philadelphia, Lea & Febiger, 1933.
10. Kasdan ML, Rogers JH: Hand infections seen in the industrial clinic. Occup Med State Art Rev 4:463–471, 1989.
11. Kilgore ES: Hand infections. J Hand Surg 5:723–726, 1983.
12. Koch SL: Inflamed and injured tissues need rest. Surg Gynocol Obstet 82:749, 1946.
13. Leddy JP: Infections of the upper extremity. J Hand Surg 11A:294–297, 1986.
14. Linscheid RL, Dobbyns JH: Common and uncommon infections of the hand. Orthop Clin North Am 6:1063–1104, 1975.
15. Louis DS, Silva J: Herpetic whitlow: Herpetic infections of the digits. J Hand Surg 4:90–93, 1979.
16. Milford L: Infections of the hand. In Crenshaw AH (ed): Campbell's Operative Orthopaedics, 7th ed. St Louis, C. V. Mosby, 1987, pp 495–506.
17. Neviaser RJ: Closed tendon sheath irrigation for pyogenic flexor tenosynovitis. J Hand Surg 3:462–466, 1978.
18. Redfern AB: Herpetic hand infection. Am Soc Surg Hand Newsletter, June 1, 1989.
19. Reid RL: Position of immobilization for the hand. Milit Med 143:626–628, 1978.
20. Reid RL: Selected upper extremity infections. Paper presented at American College of Surgeons meeting, Kentucky chapter, Lexington, KY, Apr 4, 1981.
21. Spiegel JD, Szabo RM: A protocol for treatment of severe infections of the hand. J Hand Surg 13A:254–259, 1988.
22. Watson N, Smith RJ: Infections of the hand. In: Methods and Concepts in Hand Surgery. London & Boston, Butterworth, 1986, pp 97–113.

Chapter 30

POSTOPERATIVE CARE

Lois E. Thompson, R.N.

In no other field of surgery does the postoperative management of the patient play so critical a role as it does in hand surgery. At the risk of sounding a bit trite, it is axiomatic that the postoperative care of the hand is at least as important as the operation itself.

David P. Green, 1987

Postoperative care of the upper extremity provides patient comfort, protection of the surgical repair, enhancement of rehabilitation, and prevention of complications that may result from inappropriate attention after surgery. Patients require different regimens according to the wishes of the surgeon and the nature of the procedure. The majority have an uncomplicated recovery, but if their injury and surgery have been sufficiently serious to require hospitalization, they need quality postoperative care.

GENERAL CARE

Patients should be informed of any postoperative instructions, including restrictions of diet or activity and specific care of the injured extremity. They should be advised of the severity of pain to expect from the procedure and should be assured that medication for pain has been prescribed and at what intervals it is to be given. Except for the more severe injuries, such as amputation, severe crush injuries, and large soft tissue defects, oral medications are often sufficient to control pain. Healthy patients can be active early and should be encouraged to be so. They are able to bathe and feed themselves and take charge of their toilet activities and, again, they should be encouraged to do these things. Independence, however, carries the risk of serious oversights in the care of the injured limb, especially if these patients are part of a ward population that is less well and is attended by staff with only marginal knowledge of the upper extremity. From the moment of admission hand patients should strive for personal independence and early discharge. Keeping them fully informed of their progress pushes them in this direction. The more you educate patients, the more helpful they are. It is important to include family members in this process, because the family unit may well be threatened by work-related accidents. The family should learn how best to assist after discharge.

LOCAL CARE OF THE INJURED LIMB

When the patient is admitted to the unit, the wounds should be checked and the patient reassured that all is well at that time. A forewarning that frequent monitoring is necessary should be given. Otherwise, you sometimes hear, "What's wrong?" as you look repeatedly at the injured limb.

The dressings should be kept clean and dry. Any exposed wound showing drainage should be cleansed, both for the patient's comfort and for ease of inspection by the nurse. This is done with sterile water or saline solution. Regular cleansing also ensures frequent observation of the patient and the extremity and thus allows early detection of any complications that develop.

Fractures

When fractures have occurred, additional care may be required. The fracture that has been splinted or casted requires elevation of the extremity until edema subsides. The circulation to the fingertips must be checked. The nurse must also check for the presence of any paresthesia; nerve damage may have occurred from entrapment of the nerve in the fracture line or from bruising of the nerve at the time of injury. Surgery may be necessary to determine the source of major persistent paresthesia.

When percutaneous pinning is used, the pin may be cut and an end of it left outside the skin. These pins may be covered with a dressing initially, but if they are exposed, observation and regular care are necessary to prevent infection. The pin entry site must be kept clean and dry until the pin is removed. Cleansing may be needed five or six times a day initially; later two times daily probably suffices. Sterile water, saline solution, or half-strength peroxide may be used to clean the wound in the immediate postoperative period. When the patient is discharged, tap water and a clean cloth are sufficient. To prevent a pin tract infection, it is essential to keep the tissue mobile around the exposed pin, which can be accomplished by gently pressing the tissue proximally along the pin. This is normally not painful to the patient and allows for drainage along the pin tract. Antibacterial ointment may be used around the pin, but it is not necessary. If used, it must be applied in a thin layer and

must be *completely* removed before more ointment is applied. It is helpful to explain to the patient how the pins are removed. Patients often imagine that additional surgery is needed. In order to alleviate fear, the nurse should explain that the pins are normally taken out in the clinic or office.

External fixators are cared for in a similar fashion to pins. Some surgeons follow elaborate rituals in caring for entrance sites of external fixators, including the use of various potions and dressings. These practices may serve equally well to prevent pin tract infections, but they are more difficult for the patient and require expensive supplies. It is important to keep care as simple as possible to assure that the patient will comply.

Elevation

With certain specific exceptions (see "Compartment Syndrome" below), all injured limbs benefit from elevation, which should be part of routine management. Elevation can be accomplished by positioning the limb on pillows or by suspending it. Special products are available to support the extremity and make suspension easier. However, because these aids are not available in all institutions, the nurse should be able to produce effective, safe elevation with available materials. Stockinette may be used. The length of stockinette needed is twice as long as the distance from the elbow to the point at which the stockinette will be suspended, plus approximately 8 inches. The width of stockinette should just exceed half the circumference of the dressed operative area. The stockinette is folded in half lengthwise, and the elbow is placed in the fold. The side edges are pulled around the arm and secured with safety pins on both sides beyond the fingertips. The free ends can then be tied together or connected with safety pins and the arm suspended from an IV pole. This system can only work if the elbow is kept flexed at 90 degrees.

Stockinette suspension requires close observation by the nurse and assistance from the patient and family members. If the arm is allowed to extend and thus lose support at the elbow, the stockinette slips onto the forearm, pulls the cast or splint distally, and causes constrictive pressure, which will then *increase edema*. Care must be taken if the extremity is suspended to give additional support by allowing the suspended elbow to rest on a pillow. When the patient is ambulatory, the operated extremity must be elevated in a sling. Elevation provided by a sling is less effective but is adequate for a limited period soon after surgery and for longer periods after the danger of edema has abated.

Exercise

Regardless of the elevation system used, it is imperative for healing purposes that the patient exercise all joints of the injured extremity that are not immobilized. General exercises should be performed several times daily and the nurse caring for the patient has the responsibility of supervising them. Shoulder mobilization is of particular importance; a frozen shoulder develops insidiously, especially if an arm is suspended in a sling. The arm should be raised above the head and the hand placed between the shoulder blades by both internal and external rotation at hourly intervals when the patient is awake.

Specific exercises are required after certain procedures, such as flexor tendon repair, replantation, tenolysis, and capsulectomy. These exercises are usually performed on an hourly basis. The nurse needs to cooperate with the therapist, who gives specific instruction but is often available only during normal working hours. In the absence of a therapist, the nurse assumes responsibility for supervising these exercises, which are detailed in Chapter 33.

It is appropriate here to emphasize two points. The first is that exercises may be passive or active. Passive exercises are controlled by someone other than the patient, or by the patient's opposite hand. Passive exercises are somewhat more hazardous than active ones.

The second point is that pain may be "good" or "bad." Exercise generally causes "good" pain. Passive exercise is more likely to progress from "good" pain to "bad" pain. The extent to which pain should be tolerated in exercise is indicated by the surgeon and monitored by the patient, the only person who can monitor it. Several facts will be evident once that is realized:

1. The patient must clearly understand that the pain in question is indeed "good" and is *not* indicative of damage, as is usually the case.

2. Passive exercise is more likely to move from "good" to "bad" pain than is active.

3. In order to "monitor" the process, the patient should be helped with pain medication that in no way impairs his or her perception or thought processes.

Donor Sites

Donor sites require additional care. The donor site of a split-thickness skin graft may be dressed with any one of a variety of gauzes, nonstick dressings, and impregnated materials. Some small donor sites may be hidden by casts. If not, the dressings should be removed the morning after surgery *down to* any impregnated gauze. Dressing removal is painful to the patient and should be preceded by analgesia. It is further eased if the sponges placed over the innermost layer of gauze are soaked in mineral oil at the time of application in surgery. After exposure, the wound is then left to dry. Heavy-duty hair dryers that stand independently are helpful in speeding the process. Heat lamps carry the danger of burning the area and are best avoided. Donor sites may take 2–3 days to dry completely and should be shielded from bedclothes to prevent them from sticking to the wound. The patient must be instructed that skin at a donor site takes time to mature. Heavy clothing, such as denim, may rub against the donor site and cause bleeding in the first 2 weeks. For this reason, the wound may need to be dressed with two or three thicknesses of gauze for protection when the patient wears clothes, particularly when the thigh is the donor site. For optimal results, donor sites must be protected from the sun for 1 year after surgery. If the site is allowed to become sunburned, it has less chance of returning to its normal color.

Donor sites for full-thickness grafts, pedicle flaps, free flaps, and bone are usually closed primarily. If this is not possible, a split-thickness graft may be used alone or in combination with primary closure. If a split-thickness graft has been used, a bolus is usually applied. The marginal wounds should receive routine care as discussed above.

COMPLICATIONS

As in all surgical situations, complications may arise that are a result not of the surgery itself but rather of preexisting disease, the use and duration of anesthesia, or other injuries that may or may not have been detected. Nurses, however specialized their training and assignment, must be constantly vigilant for complications outside their area of immediate responsibility.

Usually, troubles in the postoperative extremity are due to three events: edema, hemorrhage, and ischemia. These may occur alone or in any combination to produce the symptoms and signs that alert the informed nurse to their existence.

Edema.   Edema follows all tissue injury. It results from increased capillary permeability provoked by local humoral agents. This permeability permits passage into the extravascular compartment not only of tissue fluid but also of serum proteins that serve to increase the outflow of fluid. The increased volume of extracellular fluid gathers where space is most available—for example, on the dorsum of the hand and in relaxed joints. The resulting joint posture is less than optimal, because shortening of the relaxed ligaments will later produce limitation of motion. If severe, the edema can cause pressure with dire consequences to the circulation in the entire limb, but especially in muscle, where a compartment syndrome may result. If edema persists, the protein content causes fibrosis, which promotes tendon adhesions and fixed joint contractures.

Hemorrhage.   Hemorrhage may be evident and brisk enough to require emergency attention to avoid shock. Concealed hemorrhage may be equally serious. The resulting hematoma may not only lead to scar but may also cause embarrassment of circulation or serve as a nidus for infection, which may be systemically disturbing and locally disastrous with respect to the success of repair.

Ischemia.   Ischemia may be of the limb, of the part operated upon, of a vital flap, or of a wound margin. It may result from either of the first two basic problems, edema or hemorrhage. It may be total, resulting in necrosis, infection, and tissue loss, or partial, causing fibrosis of functionally significant tissues.

These three basic postoperative events, the first unavoidable to some degree, the others common but almost always preventable, lead to a number of complications that can severely compromise the surgical outcome. Nurses caring for the upper extremity must know the symptoms and signs of these complications.

Specific Problems

Swelling.   "Swelling" and "edema" are often, somewhat incorrectly, used interchangeably. Swellings may arise from many causes other than the abnormal collection of tissue fluid, which is edema. Swelling is perhaps best considered as occurring in two forms, local and general, the latter almost invariably due to edema. Localized swellings that occur postoperatively are limited to hematoma from hemorrhage and infection, which are dealt with separately below.

Generalized swelling due to edema is, as emphasized above, a normal tissue response to any invasion and contributes to scar and adhesion formation. It can cause neurological and vascular problems. The degree of edema varies greatly, depending upon the preoperative trauma and the surgical procedure. Significant edema is recognized by the development of increased pain, shiny skin showing loss of normal creases, and firm, puffy tissue that pits on pressure. Edema can make tight a dressing or cast that was correctly applied initially and create the need for splitting it.

Splitting the Dressing or Splint.   The dressing, which was applied in surgery with great care to avoid any constriction, becomes, as a result of even normal postoperative edema, inevitably too tight. If ignored, it progressively becomes the cause of discomfort, further swelling distally, and eventually of compartment syndrome (see below). Confirmation of unacceptable swelling is not always simple. The patient may immediately endorse your suspicions or may be unaware that the dressing is tight. Numbness due to the injury, the surgical procedure, or anesthesia may make the patient unaware of a gathering problem. A nurse cannot determine that a dressing is tight simply by looking at it. For this reason, it is safest to split the dressing or splint as soon as a problem is suspected, provided that standing or specific orders permit that action. If they do not, permission should be sought with urgency. The nurse should discuss with the surgeon in advance the establishment of a standard policy regarding release of dressings, splints, and casts.

The dressing must be cut from end to end, down to skin. Care must be taken to avoid dislodging drains or pins. A common mistake is to cut the dressing only until the patient expresses relief. This is often followed hours later by recurrent pain, at which juncture the nurse falsely believes that a tight dressing has been eliminated as the cause of pain. The constriction tends to relocate to the point beyond which the dressing was not split. A splint is treated in the same manner as a dressing, and the cut is made through the soft dressing portion of the splint. If the plaster portion of the splint encompasses an area such as the thumb, then a cast saw is needed to obtain complete release of the plaster.

A tight cast must be cut on both sides from end to end. Once the plaster is released, the soft dressings must be cut from end to end down to skin on one side only. The cast can then be taped to continue support. Strips of tape must be made long enough to encircle the cast and then stick to themselves; it is often impossible to make the tape adhere firmly to the plaster. The cast usually is replaced when major edema has subsided. Some nurses are misled in believing that the detection of a strong distal pulse ensures that a dressing is not tight. This is absolutely *not* true; ignoring a tight cast can lead to severe and permanent complications. The most immediate gain, and the one most appreciated by the patient, from releasing a dressing or cast, is relief of pain along with reduction or elimination of the need for analgesia.

Further treatment of swelling requires a search for, and correction of, any cause that can be eliminated, such as hematoma, seroma, sepsis, or proximal constriction.

Compartment Syndrome. Compartment syndrome is a postoperative emergency caused by edema in one or more muscle compartments that advances to such a degree that blood supply to the muscle is obliterated. It leads to muscle necrosis, scarring, and a severely impaired extremity. Compartment syndrome is preventable with vigilant observation and prompt surgery when needed. The hand has intrinsic compartments, and the forearm has anterior and posterior compartments. Compression can occur in any of these, but it most commonly involves the anterior forearm compartment, where the untreated outcome is Volkmann's ischemic contracture.

Compartment syndrome occurs most commonly after roller injuries, burns, and supracondylar fractures. Because the primary cause of the syndrome is lack of perfusion of the muscles of the forearm, any fall in blood pressure increases its likelihood. It is, therefore, particularly important after injuries commonly associated with compartment syndrome that nor-

movolemia be maintained. In addition, because elevation (see above) reduces pressure in the limb, extremities likely to develop compartment syndrome should be kept flat and not elevated. Because the fascial envelope enclosing the muscles of the forearm is relatively inexpansible, the rise in fluid volume provoked by gathering edema causes the envelope to attempt to assume a spherical shape to best contain the fluid. The result is flexor tendon retraction. Thus, passive traction on the tendons increases the already elevated pressure in the compartment and causes severe pain, which can also be elicited by direct pressure exerted over the appreciably tense compartment. Do not make the mistake of assuming that a good pulse and good sensation mean that a compartment syndrome is not present. Muscle ischemia occurs before nerve compression is sufficient to cause numbness and long before the elevated compartment pressure occludes the major vessels. Any patient complaining of severe pain or having an appropriate injury should be tested for compartment syndrome every hour without fail. If you have the slightest suspicion of a compartment syndrome, notify the surgeon immediately.

Compartment pressures are rarely taken because the clinical signs are clear, even in the unconscious patient, in whom passive finger extension in the presence of the syndrome is clearly more restricted than in the opposite limb. Treatment for suspected compartment syndrome is fasciotomy. This is a surgical procedure in which an incision is made in the skin and fascia overlying the compressed compartment. It allows the skin and fascia to separate significantly and permits normal circulation to the muscle. The exposed tissue may be left for secondary closure or covered with a skin graft.

Hemorrhage. Hemorrhage may be slow or rapid, evident or concealed. Rapid bleeding usually arises from an artery, except in the rare instance where venous bleeding is accelerated by proximal constriction. Even arterial bleeding is minimal, provided that the vessel is divided completely. Copious, continuous, and therefore potentially fatal bleeding only occurs in the extremity with *partial* arterial injury. In that circumstance, the usual hemostatic mechanisms of vessel constriction and retraction are inefficient, because retraction *widens* the hole in the vessel, *increasing* the blood loss. Such circumstances may infrequently arise after surgery for major trauma. The partially injured vessel may not have bled noticeably at an earlier juncture owing to hypovolemic vasoconstriction. More commonly, as the blood pressure rises postoperatively, ligatures may yield or repairs may leak, either in the vessels of the limb or at anastomoses to free tissue transfers. Such rapid hemorrhage is initially concealed and may remain so, forming a false aneurysm. More commonly, once a significant hematoma has accumulated, the wound closure proves inadequate to conceal the loss and external evidence appears, usually in the form of rapidly spreading stains on the dressings. If these go unnoticed and the hemorrhage is rapid, the bedclothing is also saturated. In such rare cases, the patient probably is in hypovolemic shock. Essential circulation is maintained by vasoconstriction, most noticeably of the vessels of the skin and the kidney, mediated by the sympathetic nervous system. Thus, the patient who has hemorrhaged to the point of shock is restless and has cold, sweaty skin. The pulse increases as the heart attempts to keep blood supplied to the tissues. If a catheter is in place for monitoring urinary volume, it is evident that the output has diminished because the body strives to conserve all possible fluids. The blood pressure falls but at a *much* later stage; the nurse should not assume that a normal blood pressure reading means that the patient is not bleeding. Once the presence of severe bleeding is suspected, surgical help must be summoned immediately.

Control of bleeding and resuscitative measures should then be taken. If the patient is breathing freely, first lower the head of the bed to diminish blood volume in the lower extremities and force more blood to the brain and heart. This can be further enhanced by flexing the patient's knees, which compresses the viscera. Intravenous fluids must be started immediately. Plasma expanders are preferable, but if they are not readily available, any crystalloid solution serves the urgent purpose. Because the peripheral vessels are constricted in the attempt to keep the available blood supplied to vital organs, the longer the delay in starting the intravenous infusion, the greater the difficulty; the nurse should not hesitate to seek assistance.

While one nurse is starting the IV, another must act quickly to arrest the bleeding. Firm, direct pressure should be applied over any apparent hemorrhage. If this does not stop the bleeding, a *tourniquet* should be applied. Many nurses are taught that a tourniquet might harm the limb. This is highly unlikely and irrelevant to the emergency at hand. The tourniquet is routinely used for up to 2 hours in extremity surgery with entirely reversible consequences. The nurse should apply the tourniquet (a blood pressure cuff should be used) at a pressure above the patient's systolic pressure, and it should be adjusted as hypotension is corrected, noting the time the tourniquet was applied and staying with the patient until the tourniquet is removed. It is sometimes easier to remember the needed responses if the hemorrhaging patient is thought of as a bathtub that was full but is draining because the plug has been pulled. Rapid intravenous infusion is like opening the faucet—only a partial solution. The drain must be plugged—the hemorrhage arrested—for the water level to return to normal. In all cases of rapid, significant hemorrhage, definitive control is achieved in surgery, where the source can be clearly visualized and eliminated. Where significant loss has occurred, the hematocrit is observed for several days to ensure that later hemodilution does not result in chronic anemia, which, aside from its other effects, may delay recovery in the injured limb.

In contrast to rapid hemorrhage, which constitutes an emergency, slow bleeding is less dramatic but may nonetheless be very important. It may be venous or arteriolar and may be due to the use of anticoagulant therapy, which is employed in some centers after microvascular work. When such agents are in use, or when the initial injury has required copious transfusion, a coagulation screen should be sought. Slow hemorrhage is rarely external but causes the accumulation of a hematoma within the wound.

Hematoma. A hematoma is a collection of blood within the tissues that may cause increasing pressure and therefore pain. On inspection of the wound, swelling may or may not be evident. If present, the swelling may or may not be fluctuant, depending upon whether the blood has clotted or not. If it communicates with the suture line, it may produce a dark red, serosanguineous discharge. Any hematoma is important, both immediately and in the long term. Its presence beneath free skin grafts results in their total loss. Under wound margins, and especially flaps, a hematoma may cause sufficient ischemia to produce necrosis. If left, the collection of blood forms an excellent medium for bacterial multiplication and is a major cause of wound sepsis. If infection does not ensue and healing progresses, the hematoma becomes organized and forms scar tissue that is often crippling to the injured hand. For all of these reasons, the surgeon usually drains a hematoma. This may be done by suture removal on the ward, or it may require surgery. If the surgeon expects further bleeding after evacuation, he often inserts a drain to prevent accumulation within the tissues.

Ischemia. Ischemia, if complete, results in necrosis. If partial, it increases the likelihood of infection, as does a hematoma. Also like the hematoma, if infection does not follow, reduced vascularity, scarring, and diminished function do. For these reasons, the role of the nurse in inspecting the limb for vascular compromise is of paramount importance.

The first observations immediately after upper extremity surgery are to ensure that there is adequate blood flow to all fingertips and flaps. Viability of any area is dependent upon oxygenation of tissues. Therefore, circulation is a concern after any surgery to the upper extremity. Vascular compromise is a postoperative emergency. It can be due to arterial insufficiency or to venous occlusion.

Circulation checks are necessary to assure that good blood flow is present. The frequency of such observations is determined by the surgeon and is greater after replantation or free-tissue transfer. To assess blood flow, a sufficient area must be visible to allow adequate inspection. It has been my experience that nurses are more easily misled to believe that a poorly perfused area is healthy when they are able to see only a small portion of the area. Adequate access can be achieved, while maintaining immobilization and protection of the part, by constructing a bolus cast similar to that described under "Infection" (see below). Secondly, the skin must be clean. Thirdly, good lighting is essential. With inconsistent or poor lighting, it is impossible to assure that flow is adequate and that color has not changed. Different types of lighting supply different colors and may falsely enhance or diminish the patient's skin tone. The light used may lead the nurse to believe falsely that an operative area is well or is in trouble. The nurse must use the best lighting available. However, aware of the limitations of lighting, the nurse includes other clinical checks to enhance her judgment. To assist in assessing color, the operative area should be compared with an untraumatized area. For fingers, this would be an uninjured finger on the same or opposite hand. In the case of microvascular flaps, the flap color must be compared with the donor site, which sometimes bears no resemblance to the color of the recipient area. Some nurses hesitate to use bright lighting at night out of concern for the patient.

In addition to color, the presence and rate of capillary refill must be observed. Capillary refill should be checked at the most distal point of the digit or flap. In a digit, the pulp is usually the point of choice in detecting refill. If refill cannot be detected at the pulp, the point immediately adjacent to the nail or the nail bed itself should be tried. This is usually necessary in traumatized tissue and very dark-skinned people. Refill that is faster than in the control area denotes venous congestion. In the early stages, this is generally accompanied by a brighter color of the operative area. Venous congestion of mild degree is of little consequence, but in an advanced form it can lead to vascular insufficiency. Refill that is slower than the control denotes arterial insufficiency and is generally accompanied by a color paler than the control.

It is difficult to decide at what point mild venous congestion or slowing of arterial flow becomes a serious matter. The nurse must realize that any change can be a threat to the part. Therefore, all patients must be checked hourly for vascular status for the first 24 hours postoperatively. This is essential in all trauma-related cases. To assist in determination of healthy vascularity of fingers, an external temperature probe is helpful in measuring skin temperatures of the fingers in question for comparison with a control. Adjacent uninjured fingers on the same hand are best used, if available, as controls. The opposite hand is free to grasp cold drinks, to be kept warm under bedclothes, or to engage in other activities that make the skin temperature fluctuate to such a degree as to make it an unreliable control. The lowest acceptable postoperative temperature is 30° C at the most distal point of a limb.

Skin temperatures naturally vary but if the temperature should drop below 30° C, there is reason for concern. A fall in the temperature that is not mirrored in the control is a clear indication to inform the surgeon and to increase observation checks to every 15 minutes until it can be determined whether the change is temporary and will return to normal or a warning of impending vascular compromise.

When deterioration is suspected, it is wise to check for any external causes such as tight dressings or casts. Circular dressings on the fingers and dressings in the web spaces can cause vascular problems, especially if there is edema. Finger dressings that have become blood soaked and allowed to dry are especially hazardous, because they become rigid and apply pressure to swelling tissue.

Transient vascular spasm is not uncommon. It is evident when an area that was previously well perfused shows sudden change, as evidenced by pallor. Like any change in vascular status, it should be monitored every 15 minutes until circulation returns to normal or exhibits further deterioration. The fact that a spasm was present is verified only when the original healthy flow returns to the embarrassed tissue. The nurse should never hesitate to inform the operating surgeon of a change in color, refill, or temperature. The surgeon may use other tests, such as stabbing the part with a blade or needle. He may change the position of the limb, remove sutures, substitute for venous drainage by encouraging bleeding of the part, or otherwise attempt to improve flow. He may elect to return the patient to the operating room; the situation is commonly worse than suspected.

Infection. Infection, with specific exceptions, almost always arises as a result of hemorrhage-produced hematoma or ischemia. Bacteria play a secondary, opportunistic role in these conditions. In patients in whom the defense mechanisms are diminished, such as diabetics, those on long-term steroids, and those in whom the immune response has been suppressed by advanced years, disease, or medication, symptoms usually associated with developing sepsis may be diminished. These systemic factors should be known to the nurse, who should be especially alert to the possibility of infection in these patients. Many infections arise because of inadequate perfusion with blood, which is the source of most host defenses. Such circumstances can be enumerated:

1. The presence of inanimate objects
   a. Those inserted by the surgeon, including pins, plates, joint replacements, and rods to permit later tendon grafting.
   b. Those inserted by the injury, including glass, metal, and wooden fragments, road dirt, oil and grease, paint—indeed all substances the patient may have come in contact with before or during the surgery.

2. Tissues devitalized by the injury
   a. Well-defined—any part to which the sole blood supply has been arrested and not restored.
   b. Ill-defined—skin, muscle, bone, and other soft and hard tissues that have been crushed and thereby deprived of circulation by thrombosis, vessel avulsion, or local edema.
3. Tissues devitalized by post-traumatic edema
4. Hematoma
5. Tissues devitalized by post-traumatic ischemic events
   a. Wound margins
   b. Skin grafts and flaps
   c. Muscle compartments
   d. Parts, be they individual digits or the entire limb.

The surgeon carries the major responsibility for avoiding infection in such circumstances by prescribing appropriate antibiotics when he has inserted inanimate objects, by detecting and removing all foreign material, by radically debriding all devitalized tissue, by ensuring perfect hemostasis, and by achieving successful and lasting revascularization. The nurse should be aware of these conditions and increase her vigilance. Soft tissue sepsis develops more rapidly than bone sepsis, streptococcal infections develop more rapidly than staphylococcal ones, and staphylococcal infections develop much earlier than the rare mycobacterial infections, such as *M. marinum*, which is associated with injuries occurring in certain waters. Most commonly in the postoperative phase, the nurse is confronted with wound infections that are localized or rapidly spreading—an important distinction. The importance of this difference is that swiftly spreading infection affects the patient systemically much sooner and more seriously than localized sepsis does. Whether or not the infection remains localized in the otherwise healthy patient is determined by the organism that causes it.

Rapidly Spreading Sepsis. *Streptococcus* species spread rapidly on account of their intrinsic enzymes and produce cellulitis and lymphangitis. *Clostridium* species, though rare, swiftly extend along muscle planes, producing the gas that can be seen on standard x-rays. In all patients with unconfined infection, systemic symptoms and signs are uppermost. They show general malaise, often to the point of disorientation. There may be evidence of circulatory disturbance similar to hypovolemic shock, with cold, sweating extremities and hypotension. The temperature may exceed 103° F or may be below normal. Although it should be emphasized that the diagnosis is clinical and requires emergency surgical care, blood cultures are taken, optimally at the height of systemic symptoms and signs, which frequently fluctuate.

Local Sepsis. Though less hazardous to the patient's survival and therefore less dramatic, local wound infection is more common and has serious implications for the function of the injured limb. The patient reports an increase of pain, which may be throbbing in nature, reflecting increased tissue tension. The patient also reports inability to sleep due to the pain, despite the use of analgesics and hypnotics. This is a cardinal sign of pus in the hand. There may be systemic complaints of fever, chills, and rigors, but these occur in a minority of localized wound infections. On examination, the dressing may be stained and malodorous. The experienced nurse may draw some accurate conclusions regarding the nature of the infection from the color of the staining and the distinctive odor of the discharge. For example, *Pseudomonas* species may cause a greenish blue stain with the smell of rotting vegetation. The part will be swollen. Wound erythema, which normally diminishes steadily after surgery, is more evident and extensive. The area is tender, especially over an accumulation of pus.

Treatment of Infections. Treatment of a *threatening* infection starts with elimination of any identifiable cause among those enumerated above. To this are added rest, elevation, and antibiotics, selected on an educated guess as to the infecting organism and its sensitivity.

An *established* infection is managed by drainage and culture of all pockets of pus, often the insertion of irrigation catheters, and, again, rest, elevation, and antibiotics. Irrigation of a wound can be a problem for both the patient and the nurse. If force is required to achieve it, the patient experiences pain and may not permit further attempts. If egress of the fluid is uncontrolled, the dressing and bedding rapidly become saturated, which is uncomfortable for the patient, inconvenient for the nurse, and, most important, may affect wound management adversely. These difficulties can be avoided if, at the time of drainage in the operating room, the surgeon ensures free flow of the irrigation and applies a dressing that ensures efficient, controlled irrigation. Our method of achieving this is to place a bolus over the point at which the irrigating fluid exits—usually a drain. The bolus is made by placing sponges in a glove turned inside out to remove the fingers. A full cast is then applied, incorporating the irrigating catheters with only the connector exposed. When the cast is dry, the plaster over the bolus is cut away and the bolus removed. The cavity that remains in the cast is then packed with sponges. The wound is irrigated every hour with a selected volume of Ringer's lactate. The sponges in the cavity, now wet, are removed and fresh, dry sponges inserted. In this manner, irrigation can be continued efficiently for several days without destruction of the cast.

Pain and Numbness. Pain is a normal physiological response to any injury. Pain may become apparent in many ways. The patient may report feeling pain, or the nurse may recognize restlessness, guarding, or grimacing as evidence of discomfort. It is important to know all the characteristics of the pain. Is it mild, moderate, or severe? Is it constant or sporadic? Is it dull or sharp? Does it radiate? What precipitates it, and what, if anything, decreases it? Is it accompanied by numbness or tingling? A legitimate reason for the pain should be sought, rather than simply resorting to medication. Before any analgesia is given, the nurse must be certain that the pain is from the injury and the surgery. The nurse who knows what surgery was performed can better determine the level of pain the patient can expect. Pain resulting from other causes requires action other than the administration of drugs, the use of which may mask important changes and delay essential care. Most of these other causes and their management have already been detailed above: tight dressings, compartment syndrome, hematoma, ischemia, and infection.

Irregular Casts or Splints. In addition to casts and slings that are generally tight, the primary cause of pain commonly is a sharp edge, a curved edge that compresses tissue even after a splint is cut, or a pressure point produced during the application of the cast or splint. In each case, appropriate action must be taken to alleviate the pain.

Occasionally a staple or suture is placed in such a manner as to cause undue tension. These can usually be removed, but it is unwise to do so before communicating with the surgeon.

The tourniquet is used in most hand surgery. Even with careful use, injury can occur. Injury may be due to incorrect pressure in the cuff or inflation for too long. It is recognized by localization of the pain to the cuff site and is sometimes accompanied by generalized numbness and tingling in the limb. The tourniquet pain usually resolves itself but may last for several weeks. There is no specific treatment for this problem other than explanation and reassurance. Proper documentation and notification of operating room personnel are important when tourniquet complications arise so that appropriate action is taken. This involves a review of routines, which should include daily calibration of tourniquet pressure and regular, clear statements to the surgeon of tourniquet inflation time.

Axillary Block Injection. The patient undergoing regional anesthesia by axillary block may have additional pain in the area of injection of the anesthetic agent. This pain is characterized by its dull, aching nature throughout the limb and is associated with acute tenderness upon palpation in the axilla and with paresthesias passing down the limb. Hot packs may help, but the treatment is otherwise the same as for tourniquet injury.

Other Causes of Pain. It is important to listen to the patient and to look for any other external cause of the discomfort. The patient is frightened by pain that seems unrelated to the surgery, even if it is of a mild nature. Such culprits as razor burns from preoperative shaves, rashes from the surgical scrub, and elbows resting on the patient during surgery are often causes. Burns and rashes should be treated as directed by the surgeon.

Some patients have discomfort related to prolonged pressure to a specific area or due to positioning of a limb during surgery. This pain is best treated by exercise of the involved part if permissible, avoidance of further pressure on the area, and mild-to-moderate pain medications.

Pressure sores are rare after upper extremity surgery, but they occur. The conscious patient reports discomfort caused by these injuries. Generally the skin is not broken but exhibits discoloration, which may or may not lead to necrosis. These areas *must* be kept pressure-free until healing has taken place, which may take months. They can usually be avoided by proper positioning and protection during surgery.

Some numbness is normal after many operative procedures, and patients are often surprised by it, even though they have been in-structed of this preoperatively. Numbness after regional anesthesia is the most significant numbness that was not present preoperatively. It is sometimes described as tingling or needles and pins. Recovery from regional anesthesia can take up to 24 hours, depending upon the agent used. The discomfort of numbness can be minimized by oral medications.

Numbness is normal in the area immediately adjacent to the incision, because the surgical incision disrupts nerve endings that supply sensation to the skin. This numbness usually subsides in approximately 3 months as the nerve endings regenerate. The presence of any numbness should be monitored. Any unexpected numbness should be documented, reported to the surgeon, and discussed with the patient. Long-term follow-up may be required.

The patient's psychological status plays a major part in his response to trauma and surgery. It can be difficult to assess the degree of pain and to determine whether the amount of pain is normal or abnormal. The nurse must listen to all reports of pain and take appropriate precautions to assure that proper care is given. The nurse must be sure the patient's discomfort is not a sign of a worsening condition. In addition to the discomfort, disfiguration, and loss of function, the patient has the added worry of the possible loss of income. These patients can be assisted by referrals to social workers, clergymen, psychologists, and support groups as necessary. In work-related injuries, there is the added responsibility of assessing whether the injured party is hoping to receive financial benefit based on the degree of "suffering."

SUGGESTED READINGS

1. Friedman CM: The nurse and hand surgery. In Hunter JM, Schneider LW, Macken EJ, et al (eds): Rehabilitation of the Hand, 2nd ed. St. Louis, C.V. Mosby, 1984, pp 952–957.
2. Kasdan AS: The role of the nurse in the plastic surgery office. Plast Surg Nursing 6(4):146–147, 1986.
3. Kasdan AS, Kasdan ML, Janes C: Taking the extra step: The nursing role in same day surgery. Today's OR Nurse 6(12):18–20, 1984.
4. Kasdan A, Kasdan ML: The RN assistant in hand surgery. Today's OR Nurse, 9(5):28–32, 1987.
5. Landers AF, Kasdan A: Postoperative care of hand injuries. Hand Clin 2(3): 1986.
6. Whaley N, Kasdan ML: Nursing role in office hand surgery. Today's OR Nurse 2(12):11–14, 1981.

Chapter 31

OCCUPATIONAL CONTACT DERMATITIS OF THE UPPER EXTREMITY

Chester L. Davidson, M.D.

The physician caring for patients in an industrial environment is apt to see a wide variety of occupational diseases. However, more workers suffer from occupational skin diseases than from any other single category of work-related disorder.[39] Mathias[23] reported that approximately 40% of all work-related conditions involve the skin. Between 90 and 95% of occupational skin diseases are contact dermatitis in origin, and more than one-third of them involve the hand and upper extremity.

About 25% of workers with occupational skin disease lose time from work. Each worker affected misses an average of 10–12 workdays because of such a disease.[23] The consequences of occupational contact dermatitis to the worker can be even more serious than loss of time from work. Contact dermatitis may force the employee to lose a seniority position or even to change careers.

Once the physician determines that the worker's dermatitis is of contact origin, whether or not the causation is occupational must be established by determining whether the worker was exposed to the offending agent in the workplace. Both the employee and the employer benefit from these determinations. If the causation is occupational, frequently the problem can be eliminated. The employee can reduce the number of workdays missed, and the employer can decrease the amount of production lost due to occupational illness. Once an occupational basis of the worker's dermatitis is established, the employer must address the additional issue of safety in the workplace and

may be required to assume additional financial responsibilities.

A comprehensive review of occupational skin diseases is beyond the scope of this chapter and can be found in texts[2,9,13] and periodicals dedicated to this subject (e.g., *Contact Dermatitis* and the *American Journal of Contact Dermatitis*.) General emphasis here will be placed on irritant, allergic, and urticarial contact dermatitis. Recent findings will be related to specific occupations whose workers are at increased risk of developing contact dermatitis of the hand and upper extremity. Harmful materials to which the worker is exposed will be enumerated, and methods useful for preventing or reducing contact with noxious substances in the workplace will be detailed. A section on workers' compensation will delineate criteria useful in determining whether the worker's contact dermatitis is of occupational origin.

TYPES OF DERMATITIS

Contact with chemicals constitutes the major dermatological hazard in the working population. Each year the introduction of new compounds and processes broadens the hazardous potential.[6] Contact with many chemical substances, both organic and inorganic, causes various types of dermatitis. Most of these substances produce irritant contact dermatitis; some cause allergic contact dermatitis; and contact with a few causes contact urticaria.

Contact dermatitis is a reactive inflammation in the skin provoked by direct contact with environmental chemicals or substances.[24] The morphology of irritant and allergic contact dermatitis is mostly nonspecific, but eczematous changes are typically found. There are no morphological or histological features that reliably allow the clinician to distinguish between irritant and allergic origins of the worker's dermatitis. Patch testing may be required to differentiate these types of contact dermatitis.

Hand dermatitis can be seriously disabling and is often chronic. Its management can be frustrating even to the most experienced physician. Regardless of the etiology of hand dermatitis (allergic or irritant contact dermatitis, atopic eczema, psoriasis, or other), nonspecific irritation, both in the work environment and at home, is frequently a factor in aggravating and continuing the dermatitis. For example, once the skin's barrier function has been compromised by overuse or improper use of skin cleaning agents, exposure to solvents, or other cause, the skin is susceptible to the effects of these and many other environmental materials.

Irritant contact dermatitis (Figs. 1–3) is produced by materials that act directly on the skin via nonimmunological mechanisms.[2] The application of chemical substances produces irritant dermatitis initially by disrupting the skin's barrier. Irritation develops predominantly or

exclusively on skin surfaces that come into obvious, frequent, or repeated contact with the causal agent. The distribution of the dermatitis depends somewhat on the physical form of the causal agent and the manner in which exposure occurs. Contact with solids and liquids causes an eruption on the exposed areas, commonly the hands and the upper extremity; contact with fumes, vapors, or mists, on the other hand, causes an eruption on all exposed areas such as the face, ears, neck, and upper extremity.[11] Because the palmar surfaces are relatively resistant to irritant dermatitis, the site of initial hand involvement may be the finger webs or the dorsal surfaces of the hands. The dermatitis may progress to involve the entire hand and upper extremity.

A diagnosis of irritant dermatitis is based on a clinical history of exposure to a known potential irritant and on physical findings of appropriate skin changes in expected locations. The clinical appearance of dermatitis varies considerably depending on the type and duration of the exposure. Only slight erythema may result from contact with a mild irritant. Moderately irritating substances produce an eczematous reaction characterized by erythema, vesiculation with subsequent oozing, crusting, and scaling.[2] Large bullae with necrosis and ulceration may result from contact with a strong irritant.

Weaker irritants, such as detergents or sol-

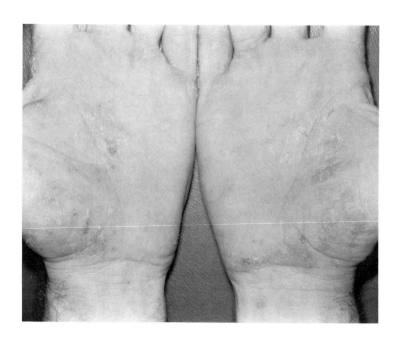

FIGURE 1. An irritant dermatitis on the hands of a furniture finisher resulting from cleanup with solvents

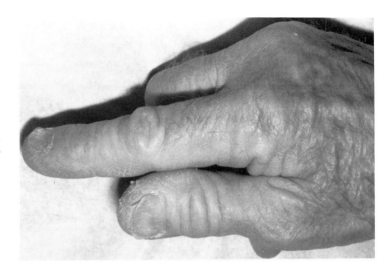

FIGURE 2. Xerotic irritant dermatitis and occupational koilonychia (spoon nail) in a painter who used mineral spirits for cleanup

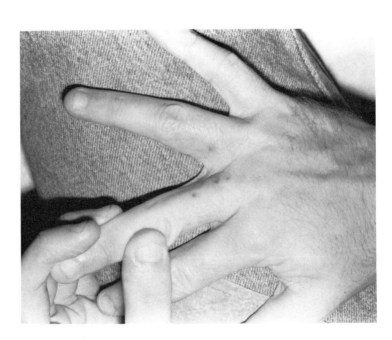

FIGURE 3. The hands of a slaughterhouse worker who developed macerated irritant dermatitis from wet work while processing picnic hams.

vents, may produce dermatitis only after repeated or prolonged exposures. A strong irritant such as battery acid, however, rapidly causes a demonstrable reaction in the majority of people on first exposure. The patient with irritant dermatitis may report stinging and burning sensations. Pruritus is variable and not usually as severe as in the vesicular stages of allergic contact dermatitis.[2]

Given the necessary environmental conditions and exposures, any chemical or substance may be a potential irritant. Many factors cause a substance to become an irritant, including inherent chemical properties, application site, and duration of exposure. Friction, occlusion, local trauma, heat, humidity, and ultraviolet light are important factors contributing to the production of irritant contact dermatitis. Some common agents capable of causing irritant contact dermatitis in the workplace are shown in Table 1.

The most important risk factors predisposing the worker to irritant dermatitis are considered to be atopy and other preexisting skin disease.[23] Several studies demonstrate that atopic persons are at higher risk for developing irri-

TABLE 1.   Common Industrial Irritants[23]

Detergents
Solvents
Petroleum oils and grease
Machining (cutting) fluids and lubricants
Food substances
Plants
Fiberglass and other particulate dust

tant contact dermatitis.[21,31] Individuals with existing allergic or irritant dermatitis also have a lowered threshold for further irritation probably because of disruption of the skin's barrier.[7] The importance of the worker's preexisting or underlying dermatitis is discussed in the section on workers' compensation.

Allergic contact dermatitis (ACD) is an acquired immunologically mediated (delayed) inflammatory response in the skin to contact with environmental allergenic substances (Fig. 4). Of the thousands of chemicals in commercial use today, only about 200 are commonly recognized as allergic contact sensitizers.[2] Table 2 lists the most common allergens to which workers are exposed. Only a small percentage of people develop sensitivity to the many allergenic substances in the environment. In addition to personal susceptibility to allergy, the antigen itself may determine the sensitization rate. *Rhus* oleoresin (the exudate causing poison ivy and oak), for example, is able to sensitize about 70% of people exposed.[2]

In contrast to the rapidly evolving eruption resulting from contact with a potent irritating substance, skin lesions in a sensitized individual may not appear for several days to a week after exposure to the offending allergen.[6] Typically ACD begins with erythema, which is followed by papules and vesicles that often rupture and ooze. Interdigital and palmar surfaces initially show multiple pruritic vesicles in groups and clusters.

As with irritant dermatitis, the skin surfaces affected depend on the physical form of the allergen and the manner in which exposure occurs. The distribution of the skin eruption corresponds with that of the antigenic exposure. Involvement of additional skin surfaces without obvious contact, however, is much more likely to occur with contact allergy than with irritant dermatitis.[23] New lesions may appear at distant, unrelated sites owing to inadvertent transfer of the allergen by the hands or through autosensitization "id" type phenomena.[2]

A positive patch test confirms the clinical diagnosis of ACD. Once the presence of the offending allergen is demonstrated in the workplace, employee protection and antigen replacement efforts can begin. Adams and Fisher[4] outline safe and practical alternatives for common and important antigens currently encountered industrially. The interested reader will find their comprehensive and detailed treatise invaluable in helping remove the worker from industrial exposure to antigenic substances.

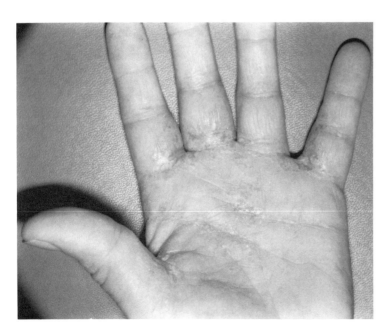

FIGURE 4. Allergic contact dermatitis from lacquer on a cabinetmaker's hands

TABLE 2. Common Industrial Allergens[11,13,23,35,39]

Rhus and Compositae plant species
Metallic salts and compounds of nickel, chromate, cobalt, and gold
Various accelerators and antioxidants used in rubber
Uncured epoxy, acrylic, and phenoformaldehyde resins (including hardeners and curing agents)
Organic dyes (PPDA and like compounds)
Biocides and germicides

Contact urticaria is a local skin response that occurs at the sites of primary contact with various materials.[23] The reaction generally begins less than 1 hour after exposure. The mode of action of chemical urticariogens is unknown. Both immunological and nonimmunological factors have been implicated.[20,41]

Contact urticaria is usually characterized as a wheal-and-flare response at the site of contact. Taylor,[38] however, found that this response occurs only in some cases and that erythema predominates. Most patients have various transient sensations such as itching, burning, and stinging. Kligman[20] reported that these suburticariogenic responses are often related to the concentration of the offending urticariogen. He found that patients who develop contact urticaria from a specific concentration of an offending substance generally develop only erythema from contact with a diluted amount of the substance and that further dilution variably produces pruritus alone.

Some patients may develop a more generalized reaction with distant or widespread urticarial lesions, perhaps owing to percutaneous absorption. Only rarely is the reaction severe enough to lead to anaphylactic shock.[23,38] In addition to the contact urticarial reaction, many patients also experience irritant or allergic contact dermatitis.

It is likely that contact urticaria occurs more commonly than reports suggest. The transient nature of the eruption makes observation difficult. Likewise, patients who experience only pruritus or erythema at the site of contact with urticariogenic substances may not seek diagnostic evaluation. Nethercott and Holmes[29] established only one case of contact urticaria (in a cook who was sensitive to shellfish) among the 1,346 patients assessed and patch-tested between 1981 and 1988.

Hazardous Occupations

Because the National Institute for Occupational Safety and Health lists dermatological disorders as one of the most common occupational-related conditions, Mathias and Morrison[25] sought to identify current high-risk industries for the development of occupational skin disease. They reviewed the overall rates, numbers, and proportions of occupational skin disease recorded in the Bureau of Labor Statistics Annual Survey of Occupational Injuries and Illnesses from 1973 to 1984. Industries with the highest incidences of contact dermatitis are listed in Table 3. Manufacturing (especially of rubber and plastic products) and agricultural industries consistently reported the highest incidences and largest total numbers of workers with contact dermatitis. In fact, skin disease accounted for nearly two-thirds of all occupational illness within the various agricultural industries.

Hazardous Exposures

Storrs et al.[37] compiled the results of patch testing carried out by the North American Contact Dermatitis Group for the years 1984 and 1985. The most common sensitizers identified were nickel, paraphylenediamine (PPDA), quaternium-15, neomycin, thimerosal, formaldehyde, cinnamic aldehyde, and thiuram compounds. Because these substances are found both in the home and the workplace, the results are applicable to patients with both occupation- and nonoccupation-related allergic contact dermatitis. In one-third of patients (398 of 1,199) who reacted, the hand was the primary site of dermatitis. Table 4 lists industrial agents that most frequently cause irritant or allergic contact dermatitis.

TABLE 3. Industries and Products Associated with High Incidences of Contact Dermatitis.[23]

Landscaping and horticulture
Forestry
Poultry dressing and processing
Fresh and frozen packaged fish
Beet sugar
Miscellaneous agricultural chemicals
Surface active agents and penetrants (emulsifiers, wetting agents, finishing oils, etc.)
Adhesives and sealants
Leather tanning and finishing
Abrasive products
Plating and polishing operations
Storage batteries
Boat building and repairing
Ophthalmic goods
Miscellaneous sporting and athletic goods

TABLE 4. Substances and Conditions Frequently Causing Occupation-related Contact Dermatitis[1,12]

Poison ivy and oak
Detergents and cleaning agents
Solvents
Machining oils and coolants
Petroleum oil, greases, and lubricants
Food products
Inedible plants or animals
Agricultural chemicals
Metals and metalic salts
Fiberglass and particulate dust
Plastics and resins
Textiles, fabrics, and related materials
Infectious agents
Rubbish, dirt, and sewage
Environmental conditions (heat and humidity)

EXAMPLES

Contact Urticaria

Because contact urticaria is most frequently caused by foods (e.g., dairy products, fish, citrus, fruits, nuts, spices, grains, meats, and vegetables) containing allergens and vasoactive substances, food handlers are at particular risk of developing it.[23] Other occupations at risk include veterinarians and slaughterhouse workers (animal hair and tissue), gardeners (plants and grasses), hairdressers (henna dye[30] and ammonium persulfate[16,19]), and health care workers (medicinals, rubefacients, and allergenic antibiotics[23]). Taylor[38] cited examples including a physician and several patients, one a newborn, who developed contact symptoms of urticaria after exposure to latex gloves. Symptoms of contact urticaria from latex glove exposure range from local itching and redness to alarming and potentially serious systemic reactions such as generalized urticaria, rhinitis, asthma, and even anaphylaxis.[15]

Irritant and Allergic Contact Dermatitis

Because they handle many irritating and allergenic substances, workers in certain occupations are at particular risk of developing contact dermatitis of the hand and upper extremity. Food handlers, hairdressers, and various horticulturists will be discussed here with particular reference to recently published findings.

Food Handlers

Fisher[13] categorizes dermatitis resulting from contact with foods into five varieties: (1) irritant dermatitis, (2) allergic contact dermatitis, (3) immediate urticarial type of dermatitis (contact urticaria), (4) immediate vesicular eruption, and (5) phototoxic dermatitis. Foods such as citruses are capable of producing all these reactions. Other foods are notorious for causing a particular reaction; contact with celery and limes, for example, causes phytophototoxic dermatitis.

Certain plants contain light-sensitizing compounds that cause irritant dermatitis upon skin exposure to certain wavelengths of ultraviolet light (phytophototoxic dermatitis).[5] Furanocoumarin compounds, for example, are found in the *Umbelliferae* family (celery, parsley, carrots, and coriander), the *Moraceae* family (common figs), and the *Rutaceae* family (limes, common rue, burning bush, hog-wood plant, among others). These phytoalexins are produced by the plant in response to disease or injury, and they probably contribute to the plant's disease resistance. Exposure to these plant families commonly causes blistering erythematous lesions with or without postinflammatory hyperpigmentation.

Celery is one of the major causes of phytophotodermatitis in farmers who harvest it and in industrial workers who process the plant stalks and leaves. Berkley et al.[5] described 30 grocery store workers who developed a phytophototoxic dermatitis from celery. The eruption was vesicular and scaly and occurred mostly on the dorsum of the hands, interdigital areas, and inner aspect of the forearms. It was often linear as a result of brushing contact with the plant, which streaked the furanocoumarin across the skin.

Bartenders commonly develop vesicular phytophotodermatitis on the first and second fingers from squeezing limes while making cocktails outdoors in the summer months. Workers engaged in collecting figs and bergamot fruit commonly develop hyperpigmentation of the hands without antecedent dermatitis.[5]

Exposure to citrus fruit is increased in certain occupations, including the citrus growing and packaging industries, food and beverage preparation (such as cooks, bakers, and bartenders), and retail food sales. Citrus handlers develop allergic contact reactions to peel oil

(D-limonene, geraniol, and citral) and irritant dermatitis from contact with fruit juices.[8] Other contact dermatitis reactions are seen in workers exposed to extraneous allergens and irritants applied to the fruit. These substances include dyes, wax coatings, fertilizers, and mold-retarding agents.[8] The hands are most often the site of citrus allergic or irritant dermatitis.[9]

Hand dermatitis from chromates is a frequent problem among cement workers, foundry workers and welders, sheet metal workers, those who work in offset printing, and, recently, workers in the milk-producing industry.[17] Potassium dichromate is used to preserve a milk sample for transportation from the farm to the quality control laboratory for assay for protein, butterfat, and white blood cells (an indicator of bovine mastitis). In a Pennsylvania quality control laboratory that examines 300,000 samples of milk monthly, Herzog et al.[17] found that the use of chromates as preservatives places laboratory workers exposed at considerable risk for developing allergic contact dermatitis. Antigen substitutions with bronopol and Kathon CG (methylisothiazolinone) are recommended in order to reduce the incidence of allergic contact dermatitis among workers in milk-testing laboratories.

Hairdressers

The principal occupational cutaneous hazard for hairdressers is contact dermatitis. Hairdressers repeatedly come into contact with a variety of substances, including hair tonics, permanent wave solutions, dyes, and shampoos. Exposure to these chemicals while doing their usually wet work makes the occurrence of irritant, allergic, and urticarial contact dermatitis a well-recognized occupational disease among hairdressers.[30] Hairdressers' contact dermatitis is most often of an irritant nature.[18] In some cases, hand dermatitis improves merely by virtue of the beautician's being promoted out of frequent hair washing.

The most common sensitizers that hairdressers are exposed to are PPDA (hair dyes), nickel (metal accessories), thiuram compounds (rubber gloves), formaldehyde (shampoos), thioglycolates (permanent wave solutions), and ammonium persulfate (bleaches).[13,14,16,18,19] Nethercott et al.[30] patch-tested 18 hairdressers who had hand dermatitis and confirmed that PPDA compounds in hair dyes are by far

the most common sensitizers. Typically, the ACD that results from contact with these dyes begins on the medial aspect of the index and middle fingers used to hold the hair to be dyed.

Many hairdressers have been forced to change occupations because of PPDA allergy. In one series only 37.5% of the hairdressers with PPDA allergies were able to continue work in the trade.[30] It is possible, however, that advising a hairdresser who is sensitive to PPDA to seek other employment is ill advised. Reiss and Fisher[33] found that hair properly dyed with PPDA is not allergenic. PPDA-sensitized hairdressers can handle PPDA-dyed hair and can usually apply PPDA dye to their clients' hair without being subject to hand dermatitis if they wear gloves. Vinyl gloves are preferred because of the hairdresser's increased risk of becoming sensitized to rubber gloves.[13] Hairdressers and others who are known to be allergic to PPDA should be informed about possible allergic cross-reactions with benzocaine, procaine, sulfonamides, and sunscreens containing para-aminobenzoic acid (PABA).[13]

Glyceryl monothioglycolate (GMTG), a common sensitizer of both hairdressers and their clients,[42] is a reducing agent used in "acid" or "hot" salon permanent waves.[36] Ammonium thioglycolate is used under alkaline conditions for "cold" permanent waves. It is considered an irritant and, rarely, a sensitizer.[13,18] Morrison and Storrs[27] demonstrated the persistence of GMTG antigen in hair at least 3 months after the use of permanent wave solutions. The persistence of this compound may explain the long-lasting dermatitis that occurs in hairdressers and clients sensitive to GMTG.

The use of heavy rubber gloves while administering a "hot" salon permanent has been shown to protect sensitized hairdressers from reacting while applying GMTG to the hair. These gloves, however, are often too cumbersome to be of practical use.[36] Until a lightweight effective barrier glove is introduced, it would be best for sensitized hairdressers to avoid applying permanent wave solutions or to use "cold" hair permanents, if they are not also allergic to ammonium thiglycolate. Because of the persistence of GMTG antigens in the hair, GMTG-sensitive hairdressers should wear protective gloves when shampooing or otherwise handling hair that has been treated with GMTG.

Ammonium persulfate is used in hair bleaches as an oxidizer to boost peroxide bleaches and accelerate the bleaching process.[18] It is known to cause irritant dermatitis, ACD, and contact urticaria in hairdressers. Because Kellett and Beck[19] found positive patch tests to ammonium persulfate in 25% of hairdressers (12 of 49) who presented with hand dermatitis, it appears that ammonium persulfate is also a relatively common sensitizer of hairdressers.

Hairdressers' occupational health and safety can be improved by making them aware of their potential for allergy and by changes in their work habits. They should be encouraged to eliminate as many allergens as possible from the workplace and to use gloves when working with various chemicals. Hairdressers need to wash and rinse their hands more often and to use emollients frequently.

Horticulturists

In the United States contact dermatitis due to wild vegetation is caused most commonly by plants of the *Compositae* (daisy) and *Rhus* (poison ivy) families.[26] Although poison ivy remains the most frequent and important cause of phytodermatitis, the investigator should be aware of the important role other plants play in producing contact dermatitis.

Menz and Winkelman[26] patch-tested 74 patients suspected of having dermatitis to wild vegetation other than to *Rhus*. The eruption produced was typically similar to the acute ACD resulting from *Rhus* exposure. About three-quarters of cases were localized, and more than 90% affected an extremity. Dog fennel and cocklebur gave the most frequent positive patch-test results. Less frequent reactions were found with cedar, juniper, wild feverfew, fleabane, and burweed marsh elder. Gardening was the most common source of exposure to weeds.

Hand dermatitis represents a significant problem in the floral industry; about 45,000 workers are at risk in the United States.[40] Contact dermatitis in floral workers results from exposure to soaps, detergents, water, fertilizers, herbicides, and irritating or allergenic plants.[1] *Alstroemeria* (Peruvian or Inca lily) and *Chrysanthemum* are probably the most common plants causing ACD among flower shop workers.[40] *Alstroemeria* was introduced into floral design in the United States in about 1981 and is a particular favorite of florists because of its longlasting beauty. The hand dermatitis produced is often chronic and associated with scaling and fissuring of the tips of the fingers, which come into prolonged or repeated contact with the stems and petals. The eruption is similar to the ACD (*tulip fingers*) that involves the forefinger and thumbs of tulip bulb workers. *Alstroemeria* and tulips share a common antigen (tuliposide A).[3,40]

Wearing gloves when exposed to *Alstroemeria* may offer protection, but Marks[22] noted that tuliposide A penetrates vinyl, but not nitrile latex, gloves. However, the presence of the juice of the plant on scissors, clippers, table tops, vases, and other work surfaces makes contact with tuliposide A almost impossible to avoid. In many cases, the dermatitis is so severe that the worker has to change jobs.[3]

PREVENTING CONTACT DERMATITIS

General Measures

The effects of extrinsic environmental factors on the skin are mostly preventable through recognition, education, and avoidance of provocative agents.[43] Contact dermatitis is mostly prevented by protection from, or removal of, potential irritants and allergens from the work environment. The employee's work surfaces should be kept clean to avoid contamination of these areas. Irritants, allergens, or other noxious agents should be removed from the skin as soon as possible after contact occurs.

Educating the worker in the proper use of potential irritants found in the workplace will help the employee avoid dermatitis. For example, abrasive cleaners strip off superficial layers of the skin. Because continued use may adversely affect the skin's barrier function, abrasive cleaners should be restricted to thick palmar skin.[23] Waterless cleaners contain solvents that dissolve oily substances that soil the skin. Overuse leads to defatting the skin, which makes the skin more susceptible to dermatitis. The use of waterless cleansers should be followed by gently washing with a mild hand soap and water to remove any residual film. Repeated applications of a skin moisturizer may be helpful to retard any irritating effects of repeated washings with relatively harsh workplace cleaners.

Certain environmental conditions should be avoided in the workplace because exposure to them adds to the disruption of the skin's barrier function and increases the incidence of irritant dermatitis. Included are low relative humidity, friction, pressure, traction, and localized trauma, such as abrasion.[34,43] Combining the drying effects of low ambient air, low water temperature, and low relative humidity may result in chapping and dermatitis. Overhydration of the skin during wet work not only creates problems of maceration and irritation but also predisposes the skin to infections with bacteria, yeasts, and fungi.[43]

Protective Clothing

Efforts should be directed to ways, such as the use of protective clothing and devices, of preventing exposure of the worker to industrial substances.[43] Protective clothing must be properly designed for the task to be performed and fitted to the individual. Clothing and devices used for worker protection may themselves cause ACD. Included are gloves, fingerstalls, boots, safety shoes, masks, safety spectacles, helmets, and aprons.[15] Because the clothing may aggravate as well as cause a dermatitis, care must be taken to reduce heat entrapment and frictional irritation of the skin. Clothing may trap moisture and occlude potentially damaging substances next to the skin for prolonged periods and increase the likelihood that dermatitis will develop (Fig. 5).

Workers can usually protect their hands from direct contact with various industrial chemicals by wearing waterproof, heavy-duty vinyl gloves. In order to adequately protect the worker, gloves must have appropriate chemical and physical resistance and sufficient flexibility for the job task to be performed.[23] Gloves can provide effective protection from contact with irritants and from most allergens, but care must be taken to ensure that allergens do not pass through various glove materials in sufficient amounts to provoke an allergic contact dermatitis.[28,40] Vinyl gloves are often recommended for worker protection because of the smaller incidence of sensitization to vinyl.[13] The use of rubber gloves to protect workers who currently have dermatitis is potentially a therapeutic nightmare. Because the skin's barrier is disrupted, the worker's dermatitis can be complicated by the development of a secondary allergic contact dermatitis from various allergenic rubber compounds in the gloves.

Barrier Creams

The effectiveness of barrier creams for skin protection is controversial and unsupported by clinical trials.[1,23,32] To provide the worker with good protection, the barrier cream should increase the skin's barrier function and make it impossible for allergens or irritating substances

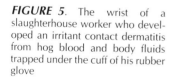

FIGURE 5. The wrist of a slaughterhouse worker who developed an irritant contact dermatitis from hog blood and body fluids trapped under the cuff of his rubber glove

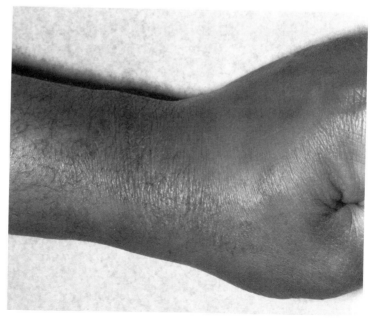

to penetrate the skin. At most, the cream's effects last only minutes, and the worker needs to reapply the cream frequently to ensure continued protection. If no other means of protection is available, a barrier cream may be used, but its composition must match the job to be done. A water-repellent type should be chosen for defense against acids, alkalies, water-soluble substances, soaps, and detergents. An oil-repellent cream is needed to protect against oils and organic solvents.[2] Because the skin usually tolerates barrier creams well, the creams are often very useful to facilitate the removal of oils and greases from the skin.[23] However, cost considerations usually prevent routine use except in workers with sensitive skin.

WORKERS' COMPENSATION

Contact dermatitis accounts for more than 90% of all workers' compensation claims from occupational skin diseases. About 80% of these claims are attributed to cutaneous irritation. Contact allergy accounts for most of the remainder.[13]

Workers' compensation laws in all states require only reasonable probability (more than 50% likelihood) that the employee's dermatitis resulted directly from occupational exposure. Mathias[24] modified general criteria used to determine probable occupational causation of any skin disease and applied them to contact dermatitis (Table 5). Reasonable probability can be determined by the examining physician after finding positive correlation of the worker's medical history and cutaneous findings with at least four of the seven criteria presented in Table 5.

TABLE 5.   Criteria for Evaluating Probable Occupational Causation in Contact Dermatitis[24]

1. The clinical appearance of the worker's dermatitis is consistent with that of a contact dermatitis.
2. The worker is exposed at the workplace to potential cutaneous irritants or allergens.
3. The anatomic distribution of the worker's dermatitis is consistent with cutaneous exposure in relation to the job task.
4. The temporal relationship between exposure and onset is consistent with contact dermatitis.
5. Nonoccupational exposures are excluded as probable causes.
6. The dermatitis improves when the worker is not exposed to the suspected irritant or allergen.
7. Patch tests identify a probable causal agent.

Discussion of Criteria

Criterion 1. Contact dermatitis is clinically an inflammatory eczematous process. As the worker's dermatitis progresses from acute to chronic stages, the clinical findings change from acute vesiculation to subacute serous exudation, from scaling and early lichenification to chronic scaling and predominant lichenification.

Although the skin biopsy demonstrates an eczematous inflammatory response, it is important to realize that the histological findings do not demonstrate the actual cause of the eczematization or whether it is related to an occupation.

Criterion 2. In obtaining a history of the evolution of the dermatitic process, important data must be documented concerning the employee's current job and how he does it. The history should also include:

1. Determination of the employee's exposure to industrial substances
2. Cleanup procedures, including materials used (soaps, solvents, soapless cleaners, abrasives, and so forth)
3. Previous treatment used by the worker (By determining preparations used to treat the dermatitis the examiner may be able to identify a secondary allergic contact dermatitis.)
4. Availability and use of protective clothing such as gloves, sleeves, and aprons.

Criterion 3. Skin surfaces that are maximally exposed develop the most contact dermatitis. For example, dermatitis from industrial liquids occurs on the hands and upper extremities, where direct contact is most frequent. If the distribution of the employee's dermatitis does not match the industrial exposure, a relationship cannot be formed. An example of a negative relationship would be the development of psoriasis in areas free from industrial mechanical trauma or the development of tinea pedis in a factory worker whose feet remain dry on the job.

Criterion 4. With the exception of skin exposures to strong irritants, a lag period is usually seen from beginning an exposure to a substance to erupting with either an allergic or irritant contact dermatitis. Sufficient time is needed for the irritant to interrupt the skin's barrier or the antigen to induce an allergic reaction. The lag period extends from a few weeks to several months and generally does not exceed 6 months.

Criterion 5. Nonoccupational causes of the employee's dermatitis must be excluded by means of the worker's history and by patch testing when indicated or appropriate.

Criterion 6. A weekend away from work or even a few days off from work are usually insufficient for contact dermatitis to heal. In order to use this criterion, either longer periods away from work or modification of the employee's job is generally necessary to allow the dermatitis time to resolve and the skin's barrier time for repair.

Criterion 7. Patch tests establish that an allergic contact dermatitis exists. Clinical relevance is established when it can be shown that the employee was exposed to that antigen at work. Patch testing should be performed according to standard procedures outlined in several texts concerning contact dermatitis.[2,9,13] Correct concentrations of antigens must be used in order to minimize false-positive or false-negative reactions. False-positive reactions may occur with the inappropriate use of irritating substances or as part of the excited skin syndrome.[7] False-negative patch test reactions occur when inappropriately low concentrations of test substances are used, when inappropriate vehicles for patch test substances are used, and when the patient is being treated with insufficiently high dosages of systemic steroids.

Preexisting Conditions

Workers' compensation laws also allow an employee to be compensated because the workplace caused a substantial aggravation of a preexisting dermatitis. When there is a reasonable probability that the dermatitis was aggravated by the job, the employee is compensable until the dermatitis has completely reverted to its clinical status before it was aggravated. Determining that the dermatitis is clinically more severe is aided subjectively by the patient's historical need to use more medication in the involved areas or objectively by the examiner's comparison with a previous clinical examination, if available. The spread of the preexisting dermatitis to previously uninvolved skin sites favors work-related aggravation of the dermatitis.

CONCLUSION

Industrially related contact dermatitis presents as an irritant reaction, a contact allergy, or an urticarial dermatitis. A workman's contact dermatitis would be considered work related if it can be proved that the employee was exposed to the antigen or irritant in the workplace. In addition to causing dermatitis, environmental substances found in the workplace may aggravate occupational dermatitis. Repeated episodes of dermatitis burden the worker with disability and discomfort and the employer with expense and lost production. In order to prevent occupational hand dermatitis, exposure of the worker to allergens and irritants must be controlled. Various articles of protective clothing are available to shield the employee from those hazardous industrial materials that cannot be removed or replaced. Cooperation among employee, employer, and health team is necessary to reduce and minimize the occurrence of occupation-related contact dermatitis.

REFERENCES

1. Adams RD (ed): Occupational skin diseases. Occup Med State Art Rev 1:1–360, 1988.
2. Adams RM: Occupational Skin Disease. New York, Grune & Stratton, 1983, pp 1–477.
3. Adams RM, Daily AD, Brancaccio RR, et al: Alstroemeria: A new and potent allergen for florists. Dermatol Clin 8:73–76, 1990.
4. Adams RM, Fisher AA: Contact allergen alternatives: 1986. J Am Acad Dermatol 14:951–969, 1986.
5. Berkley SF, Hightower AW, Beier RD, et al: Dermatitis in grocery workers associated with high natural concentrations of furanocoumarins in celery. Ann Intern Med 105:351–355, 1986.
6. Birmingham D: Occupational dermatology. In Demis DJ (ed): Clinical Dermatology. Philadelphia, J.B. Lippincott, 1989, pp 1–25.
7. Bruynzeel DP, Maibach HI: Excited skin syndrome (angry back). Arch Dermatol 122:323–328, 1986.
8. Cardullo AC, Ruszkowski AM, DeLeo VA: Allergic contact dermatitis resulting from sensitivity to citrus peel, geraniol, and citral. J Am Acad Dermatol 21:395–397, 1989.
9. Cronin E: Contact Dermatitis. Edinburgh, Churchill Livingstone, 1980, pp 1–915.
10. Cronin E: Clinical patterns of hand eczema in women. Contact Dermatitis 13:153–161, 1985.
11. Dooms-Goossens AE, Debusschere KM, Gevers DM, et al: Contact dermatitis caused by airborne agents. J Am Acad Dermatol 15:1–10, 1986.
12. Edman B: Sites of contact dermatitis in relationship to particular allergens. Contact Dermatitis 13:129–135, 1985.
13. Fisher AA: Contact Dermatitis, 3rd ed. Philadelphia, Lea & Febiger, 1986, pp 1–954.
14. Fisher AA: Management of hairdressers sensitized to hair dyes or permanent wave solutions. Cutis 43:316–318, 1989.
15. Foussereau J, Tomb R, Cavelier C: Allergic contact

dermatitis from safety clothes and individual protective devices. Dermatol Clin 8:127–132, 1990.

16. Heacock HJ, Rivers JK: Occupational diseases of hairdressers. Can J Public Health 77:109–113, 1986.

17. Herzog J, Dunne J, Aber R, et al: Milk tester's dermatitis. J Am Acad Dermatol 19:503–508, 1988.

18. Holness DL, Nethercott JR: Dermatitis in hairdressers. Dermatol Clin 8:119–126, 1990.

19. Kellet JK, Beck MH: Ammonium persulphate sensitivity in hairdressers. Contact Dermatitis 13:26–28, 1985.

20. Kligman AM: The spectrum of contact urticaria. Dermatol Clin 8:61–66, 1990.

21. Lammintausta K, Kalimo K: Atopy and hand dermatitis in hospital wet work. Contact Dermatitis 7:301–308, 1981.

22. Marks JG: Allergic contact dermatitis to *Alstroemeria*. Arch Dermatol 124:914–916, 1988.

23. Mathias CGT: Occupational dermatoses. J Am Acad Dermatol 19:1107–1114, 1988.

24. Mathias CGT: Contact dermatitis and workers' compensation: Criteria for establishing occupational causation and aggravation. J Am Acad Dermatol 20:842–848, 1989.

25. Mathias CGT, Morrison JH: Occupational skin disease, United States: Results from the Bureau of Labor Statistics annual survey of occupational injuries and illnesses, 1973 through 1984. Arch Dermatol 124:1519–1524, 1988.

26. Menz J, Winkelmann RK: Sensitivity to wild vegetation. Contact Dermatitis 16:169–173, 1987.

27. Morrison LH, Storrs FJ: Persistence of an allergen in hair after glyceryl monothioglycolate-containing permanent wave solutions. J Am Acad Dermatol 19:52–59, 1988.

28. Moursiden HT, Faber O: Penetration of protective gloves by allergens and irritants. Trans St John's Hosp Dermatol Soc 59:230–234, 1973.

29. Nethercott JR, Holmes DC: Occupational dermatitis in food handlers and bakers. J Am Acad Dermatol 21:485–488, 1989.

30. Nethercott JR, MacPherson M, Choi BCK, Nixon P: Contact dermatitis in hairdressers. Contact Dermatitis 14:73–79, 1986.

31. Nilsson E, Mikaelsson B, Andersson S: Atopy, occupational and domestic work as risk factors for hand eczema in hospital workers. Contact Dermatitis 13:216–223, 1985.

32. Orchard S: Barrier creams. Dermatol Clin 2:616–629, 1984.

33. Reiss F, Fisher AA: Is hair dyed with para-phenylenediamine allergic? Arch Dermatol 109:221–222, 1974.

34. Rycroft RJG: Low humidity dermatoses. Dermatol Clin 2:553–559, 1984.

35. Schuman SH, Dobson RL: An outbreak of contact dermatitis in farm workers. J Am Acad Dermatol 13:220–223, 1985.

36. Storrs FJ: Permanent wave contact dermatitis: Contact allergy to glyceryl monothioglycolate. J Am Acad Dermatol 11:74–85, 1984.

37. Storrs FJ, Rosenthal LE, Adams RM, et al: Prevalence and relevance of allergic reactions in patients patch tested in North America—1984 to 1985. J Am Acad Dermatol 20:1038–1045, 1989.

38. Taylor JS: Allergic reaction to latex can be life-threatening. Skin Allergy News 20:2, 1989.

39. Taylor JS, Parrish JA, Blank IH: Environmental reactions to chemical, physical, and biologic agents. J Am Acad Dermatol 11:1007–1021, 1984.

40. Thiboutot DM, Hamory BH, Marks JG Jr: Dermatoses among floral shop workers. J Am Acad Dermatol 22:54–58, 1990.

41. von Krogh G, Maibach HI: The contact urticaria syndrome—An updated review. J Am Acad Dermatol 5:328–342, 1981.

42. Warshawshki L, Mitchell JC, Storrs FJ: Allergic contact dermatitis from glyceryl monothioglycolate in hairdressers. Contact Dermatitis 7:351–352, 1981.

43. Weary PE: Prevention of skin disease. J Am Acad Dermatol 11:1022–1024, 1984.

Chapter 32

ARTHRITIS OF THE HAND AND UPPER EXTREMITY IN THE WORKPLACE

Gary L. Crump, M.D. and Paul D. Schneider, M.D.

An understanding of arthritis and related conditions is essential to the occupational health professional. A recent well-designed survey in Kentucky found that 17.2% of the working population (ages 16–64) reported some form of arthritis or rheumatism. Rheumatic conditions were the most frequently reported causes of disability, exceeding cardiovascular diseases, kidney diseases, diabetes, and all other causes. Because of the type of work done, it is not surprising that "blue collar" households report a greater incidence of physical impairment.[16]

This chapter presents a general overview of the patient with musculoskeletal complaints and possible arthritis. It then describes several of the more common forms of arthritis and connective tissue disease. Clinical findings, initial evaluation and management, and the appropriate timing of referral to a rheumatologist are emphasized.

Although we are rheumatologists, we present the material in a practical manner so that it is readily usable by the reader. It is beyond the scope of this chapter to discuss all recognized rheumatic diseases that affect the upper extremities. Fortunately, many of these are rare. There are, however, a relatively small number of fairly common forms of arthritis with which the occupational physician should be familiar. These are discussed from a purely clinical viewpoint. The reader is referred to any one of the standard textbooks of rheumatology for more detailed information.[4,17]

With the exception of degenerative and traumatic disorders, the bona fide rheumatic diseases that occur in the workplace happen by chance. Nonetheless, the occupational physician should be familiar with them in a general way because rheumatic disorders are common in the working population.

Arthritis is frequently used generically to describe any musculoskeletal pain. For the purpose of the present discussion, inflammation at the level of the joint manifested by *calor* (heat), *rubor* (redness), *dolor* (pain), *tumor* (swelling), and *loss of function* will serve to define "arthritis." Soft tissue and nonrheumatic upper extremity problems are discussed elsewhere in the text.

CATEGORIES OF MUSCULOSKELETAL PATHOLOGY

All too often the classic signs and symptoms of arthritis are not immediately obvious, and the treating physician must attempt to define the pathophysiology of the problem in order to formulate rational treatment plans. Fries[7] has suggested eight broad categories of musculoskeletal pathology that serve this end.

Chronic Synovitis. Indolent but obvious inflammation of the joints in the form of palpably thickened, warm synovium marks chronic synovitis, which typically involves multiple joints and is present for several weeks before treatment is sought. Constitutional symptoms such as low-grade fever, malaise, weight loss, and fatigue are common. A comprehensive history and physical examination are required to identify specific diagnostic findings—for example, a small patch of psoriasis or the nodules of rheumatoid arthritis. Therapy is likely to involve both nonsteroidal anti-inflammatory drugs (NSAIDs) and long-acting antirheumatic drugs (e.g., hydroxychloroquine, gold salts, penicillamine, methotrexate, azathioprine, sulfasalazine).

Spondyloarthropathy or Enthesopathy. Inflammation at the sites of the insertions of ligaments and tendons on bone, as well as the joints and surrounding structures, marks spondyloarthropathy or enthesopathy. The category includes ankylosing spondylitis and all its variants. Although the upper extremity joints are less frequently affected by overt synovitis than those of the lower extremity, recurrent tendinitis and bursitis of the upper extremities in a young man (ages 18–40) should prompt a careful history and physical examination. Symptoms include axial skeletal (neck and back) morning stiffness, asymmetric oligoarthritis, lower extremity periarthritis (in the form of sausage digits, Achilles tendinitis, plantar fasciitis), inflammatory eye symptoms (iritis, conjunctivitis), inflammatory genitourinary symptoms (urethritis, prostatitis), mucositis (painless oral ulcers, circinate balanitis), and skin lesions (keratoderma blennorrhagicum, nail dystrophy).

These disorders are frequently associated with the genetic marker HLA-B27. Even when the "complete" clinical picture of ankylosing spondylitis or Reiter's syndrome is not present, a greater frequency of HLA-B27 positivity is found in patients with isolated, single symptoms (e.g., Achilles tendinitis, plantar fasciitis, sausage digits).[3] This group of disorders exhibits greater responsiveness to phenylbutazone, indomethacin, naproxen,[15] and diclofenac sodium over the other NSAIDs.

Cartilage Destruction. Among the many etiologies that may lead to cartilage destruction are the repetitive trauma of the workplace, a single fracture extending through the joint, enzymatic dissolution of cartilage from a primary inflammatory process, and inherited biochemical instability of articular cartilage. Once established, the process is mechanically driven regardless of etiology. Symptoms develop as a consequence of continual mechanical abrasion of the joint surfaces and the secondary inflammation that results. Subchondral bone normally remodels in accordance with biome-chanical forces received from adjacent articular cartilage. When the cartilage is abnormal, the transmitted forces are aberrant and bone remodeling is abnormal. The result is the classic radiographic findings of osteoarthritis: subchondral cyst formation, osteophytes, sclerosis of bone, loss of joint space, and derangement (instability).

Because articular cartilage does not regenerate, therapy is invariably suboptimal. It is directed at (1) reducing the pain and secondary inflammation, usually with NSAIDs, (2) changing or reducing the physical stresses to which the damaged joint is exposed, and (3) strengthening the supporting muscles and connective tissues through appropriate exercise.

Crystal-induced Synovitis. The hallmark of crystal-induced synovitis is intense inflammation generated by the occurrence of inorganic crystals in the joint space either by shedding of preformed crystals (as in calcium pyrophosphate deposition disease) or de novo crystal formation (as in some instances of gout). The intensity of the clinical response to intra-articular crystals often causes diagnostic confusion with infection, cellulitis, or phlebitis. Definitive diagnosis depends upon the identification of intracellular crystals from the synovial fluid with the use of polarizing light microscopy. Therapy can often be specific and definitive as in the case of allopurinol for gout. Initial therapy consists of ample doses of NSAIDs, which are of benefit regardless of crystal type. Cochicine, which has only limited benefit in most other rheumatic diseases, is also an effective first-line agent as well as beneficial adjunctive therapy in microcrystalline disorders.

Infection. The only process besides microcrystalline disease to cause an exquisitely intense inflammatory response is joint infection, which occurs by either direct inoculation or hematogenous dissemination. Inoculation is more likely in a work setting in which injuries are common, and the infected joint should be carefully examined for possible sites of inoculation—e.g., abraded skin or puncture wounds. Even when an obvious portal of entry is identified, however, a more distant origin should be carefully screened out. Examples of such inconspicuous origins include intravenous drug use, urinary tract infection (UTI), and recent dental work in a patient with a heart murmur.

The appropriate diagnosis is made by joint aspiration and culture, but a comprehensive history and physical examination are mandatory and may well reveal a murmur, needle tracks, an asymptomatic UTI, cutaneous abscesses, or other sites of infection. Therapy consists of (1) appropriate antibiotics based on synovial fluid cultures, (2) drainage (either open surgical or repetitive needle), and (3) eradication of the primary source of the dissemination, if present.

Rapid diagnosis and therapy are essential for an optimal outcome because virulent organisms (e.g., *Staphylococcus aureus*) may cause significant articular cartilage damage in as short a time as 48 hours.[8] Adequate drainage minimizes this problem by removing the white blood cells (WBCs) and their proteolytic enzymes from the joint space and reducing intra-articular pressure.[9]

Focal Conditions. Bursitis, tendinitis, ligamentous strains, and overuse syndromes are focal conditions that involve the periarticular tissues and do not represent true joint pathology *per se*. They must, however, be considered in the differential diagnosis of joint symptoms because they frequently suggest joint disease on cursory screening.

Functional Conditions. Depression, fibromyalgia, psychogenic rheumatism, and malingering are none-too-rare functional conditions in the workplace that at first might suggest joint disease. However, despite terminology descriptive of inflammation (redness, heat, swelling) or hyperbolic descriptions of associated pain and disability, a paucity of objective abnormalities is revealed on examination and in the laboratory.

Myopathy. In the differential diagnosis of joint disease, myopathy rarely causes confusion. It is included for completeness. Inflammatory myopathies (dermatomyositis, polymyositis) are rare; they cause weakness that affects the proximal much more than the distal musculature. Hereditary myopathies and storage diseases are also rare and are likely to cause proximal weakness or exertional myalgias. None of these symptoms is likely to suggest joint disease to the observant clinician.

DIAGNOSTIC PROCEDURE

Armed with the above differential diagnosis of musculoskeletal pathology, and the knowledge that most minor musculoskeletal problems spontaneously resolve within 2–6 weeks, the clinician must decide when to investigate a problem aggressively and when simply to attend to the symptoms. Proposed indications[7] for aggressive investigations include but are not limited to (1) persistent synovitis of 6 or more weeks in duration; (2) acute, intense synovitis, particularly monarticular; (3) synovitis associated with constitutional symptoms; (4) conditions associated with significant trauma; and (5) conditions associated with neurological deficits. The last two circumstances are addressed elsewhere in this text and will not be included in the following discussion.

The physical findings at the joint of warmth, synovial thickening, effusion, crepitus on motion, deformity, and tenderness all identify the presenting problem as arthritis. The next step is a comprehensive history.

Medical History

The history of the present illness should be obtained in chronological order even though the current complaint is the most pressing to the patient. Diagnosis of the present problem may well depend upon the discovery of prior joint symptoms, as in the patient with an acutely inflamed wrist who reveals prior episodes of podagra (gouty pain in the great toe). The tempo of onset (acute, subacute, chronic) and intensity of inflammation (exquisite, indolent) help to separate microcrystalline disorders and bacterial infections from the more chronic systemic rheumatic diseases. The pattern of involvement over time (migratory or additive), distribution (small or large, upper or lower, symmetric or asymmetric, axial or central or peripheral) and absolute number of involved joints (monarticular, oligoarticular, polyarticular) are all data of diagnostic importance. Examples include rheumatoid arthritis (RA), which is a symmetric, chronic, additive polyarthritis involving hands and feet; Reiter's syndrome, which is typically an asymmetric, subacute oligoarthritis predominating in large lower extremity joints with frequent axial skeletal involvement; systemic lupus erythematosus (SLE) and acute rheumatic fever, which are migratory polyarthritides; and gout, which commonly presents with acute, intense monarticular (first metatarsal phalangeal joint) inflammation. Chronic monarticular arthritis suggests the possibility of an unusual infection such as fungus or tuberculosis. Gonococcal (GC)-

arthritis is usually migratory at onset and then "settles" into a few joints after 2–3 weeks. Distal interphalangeal joint involvement narrows the list of diagnostic possibilities to primary osteoarthritis, psoriatic arthritis, and much more rarely, gout, RA, and multicentric reticulohistiocytosis.

The patient is also an important variable in the diagnostic equation. For example, the peak incidence of rheumatoid arthritis is in women in the fifth decade. Women rarely present with spondyloarthropathies, which are most likely to be seen in young men. Gout is unusual in women before menopause. Men usually do not get GC arthritis, whereas a young sexually active woman is a good candidate. Systemic lupus is a disease that predominates in women of childbearing age. Proximal symptoms (shoulder and hip) in a woman past 50 in the absence of more significant distal complaints suggest polymyalgia rheumatica.

The host's occupation or avocation may be of major diagnostic import. A nurse in a dialysis clinic has a much higher risk of hepatitis B infection, which may present with a serum-sickness-like prodrome, including polyarthritis weeks before liver enzymes are elevated. Assembly-line workers doing frequent repetitive grasping are likely candidates for degenerative changes at the first carpometacarpal joints. Intravenous drug abusers have a particular diathesis for infection in the sternoclavicular and sacroiliac joints. Gardeners present with sporotrichosis synovitis after getting thorns in their fingers. Moonshiners get saturnine gout. Cigarette smokers may develop cancer or chronic obstructive pulmonary disease (COPD) and present with hypertrophic pulmonary arthropathy.

Attention should be devoted to the past medical history as well. Prior transfusions raise the specter of hepatitis B and acquired immune deficiency syndrome (AIDS). Current medications may be very important: steroids and chemotherapy increase susceptibility to bacterial and opportunistic infections; long-term steroid therapy may result in osteonecrosis, which frequently affects the shoulders and hips; diuretic therapy predisposes to gout, and anticoagulation to hemarthroses. Procainamide hydrochloride most often, but hydralazine, isoniazid, and phenytoin may all be associated with drug-induced lupus. Almost any drug can be associated with a serum sickness reaction that includes a polyarthritis.

Review of Systems

Recent illness must also be reviewed as part of the general review of systems. A recent bout of diarrhea or urethritis can trigger a spondyloarthropathy, a recent sore throat can trigger acute rheumatic fever, a recent sexual encounter may cause disseminated GC arthritis, and recent dental work may cause bacteremia eventuating in subacute bacterial endocarditis (SBE).

Next, each individual organ system should be systematically reviewed to discover the extra-articular manifestations of the many disorders associated with joint inflammation that may have escaped attention. Complaints referable to the skin may yield diagnostic information about SLE (alopecia, photosensitivity, mucosal ulcers), psoriatic arthritis, Lyme disease (erythema chronicum migrans), rubella (transient pruritic maculopapular centrifugal rash), gonorrhea (pustules), SBE (splinter hemorrhages, Osler's nodes, Janeway lesions), rheumatic fever (nodules, erythema marginatum), sarcoidosis (erythema nodosum), rheumatoid arthritis (nodules, vasculitis), gout (tophi), and other conditions. Inflammatory eye complaints are frequently, although not exclusively, associated with the spondyloarthropathies. Dry eyes (xerophthalmia), dry mouth (xerostomia), and parotid enlargement are often seen in the immunologically mediated systemic rheumatic diseases such as RA, SLE, and primary Sjögren's syndrome. Pleuropericardial complaints are associated with these disorders as well. An established heart murmur may suggest SBE, SLE, or ankylosing spondylitis. Colitic symptoms raise the question of ulcerative colitis, Crohn's disease, or Whipple's disease. Genitourinary symptoms can be seen with Reiter's syndrome, GC, and gout (stones). Neurological dysfunction may suggest Charcot-like joint destruction on the basis of loss of pain and proprioceptive function as seen in tabes dorsalis, diabetes mellitus, and syringomyelia.

The family history should identify diseases that are strongly inherited such as primary osteoarthritis and the HLA-B27-related disorders, as well as those with moderate familial tendencies such as gout, RA, SLE, and inflammatory bowel disease.

Physical Examination

A comprehensive physical examination is obviously an integral part of the diagnostic evaluation of an arthritis. As suggested above, all organ systems should be examined for evidence of underlying pathology. The musculoskeletal examination should include active and passive range of motion testing of all the peripheral joints, range of motion of the axial skeleton, measurement of chest expansion, and percussion of the spinous processes and sacroiliac (SI) joints for tenderness. Each peripheral joint needs to be individually evaluated for signs of inflammation (rubor, calor, tumor, dolor) and mechanical derangement (crepitus, instability, deformity).

During the general physical examination special consideration should be given to specific diagnostic features such as vasculitic changes, patches of psoriasis, nail dystrophy, oral and genital ulcers, funduscopic abnormalities, murmurs, bruits, pulses, and neurological deficits.

DIAGNOSTIC STUDIES

Synovial Fluid Analysis.[14] Synovial fluid analysis rapidly addresses both the general issue of whether the problem is mechanical or inflammatory and the particular one of infection and microcrystalline disease. In general, a white blood count on joint fluid of <2,000 suggests a noninflammatory process. WBC counts of >50,000 are highly suspect for infection and crystals. Enough overlap exists in the interpretation of joint fluid WBC counts that fluid should always be sent for routine culture, as well as culture on Thayer-Martin medium if gonococcal infection is a possibility.

The finding of increased numbers of red blood cells (RBCs) in the joint fluid suggests trauma. Trauma induced by the aspiration itself usually yields blood-tinged fluid that is nonxanthochromic and often clears. Grossly bloody fluid can be seen in pigmented villonodular synovitis, hemophilia, anticoagulation, and severe trauma. The appearance of fat globules in the bloody aspirate suggests a fracture that has extended from the marrow through the subchondral bone and articular cartilage.

The examination of the synovial fluid for crystals is ideally done with a polarizing light microscope. Monosodium urate crystals (gout) are typically needle shaped and negatively birefringent, so that the crystal appears yellow when its axis is parallel to the red compensator and blue when its axis is perpendicular to it.

Calcium pyrophosphate crystals (pseudogout) appear more rhomboid in shape and cause the opposite color change—i.e., yellow when the axis of the crystal is perpendicular to the red compensator, and blue when parallel. Hydroxyapatite crystals are more amorphous in appearance and can often be overlooked or dismissed as debris unless the preparation is stained for calcium with alizarin red.

A Gram stain of the joint fluid reveals the infecting organisms in a septic arthritis about half the time. This stain is invaluable in facilitating the initial choice of antibiotics until full culture and sensitivity data are available.

Joint fluid glucose and protein determinations are routinely ordered but are rarely of any value. It is possible to make the diagnostic differentiation between the systemic rheumatic diseases that consume complement (e.g., SLE, RA, juvenile rheumatoid arthritis) and the spondyloarthropathies on the basis of synovial fluid complement levels, but the complement levels need to be related to the total protein in the synovial fluid to be accurate.[2]

If amyloidosis is a consideration, the specimen can be spun and stained with Congo red.

Lupus erythematosus (LE) preparations, antinuclear antibodies (ANAs), and rheumatoid factors on synovial fluid generally add little diagnostic information and are rarely performed.

It should be obvious from the above discussion that there is no "standard" joint fluid evaluation. It is our practice always to send fluids for cell counts, crystal analysis, and bacterial culture in addition to whatever other studies the clinical situation may warrant.

Cultures. Because joint sepsis occurs only by direct inoculation or dissemination from another source, for all patients in whom joint sepsis is either documented or entertained the blood, urine, and any other potential source of dissemination should be cultured. If gonococcal infection is suspected, cervical, urethral, rectal, and pharyngeal cultures should be obtained.

Radiography. Plain radiographs of the joints are mandatory in virtually all circumstances of suspected joint pathology. Unfortunately, their diagnostic usefulness is limited mostly to mechanical derangements (fractures, dislocations) and noninflammatory conditions such as osteoarthritis. Primary inflammatory joint disease, including bacterial infection, rarely causes significant radiographic abnormalities before 7–10 days, and most systemic rheumatic diseases such as rheumatoid arthritis and psoriatic arthritis take months to years to cause diagnostic change.

Nonetheless, radiographs can be particularly helpful in several circumstances. Abnormalities of the sacroiliac joints (even when clinically silent) often help to diagnose a spondyloarthropathy with peripheral involvement. The presence of chondrocalcinosis may suggest that the process under investigation is related to calcium pyrophosphate deposition disease. Tumors of the bone and bone marrow, metastatic disease, osteomyelitis, and Paget's disease can be identified with plain films.

It is generally prudent to perform bilateral radiographs for purposes of comparison. Over time these films will serve as a baseline for monitoring the progression of any systemic disease that may be present.

Nuclear Medicine. The utility of the bone scan relates to its sensitivity. In septic arthritis the bone scan may be helpful in identifying the initial source of the infection. It can also detect involvement of joints such as the sacroiliacs that are otherwise difficult to "see" clinically. The bone scan offers a more complete picture of an undiagnosed polyarthritis in terms of symmetry, as well as number and full distribution of joints involved.

Newer technology such as three-phase scanning enables better localization of the inflamed tissue. This is often helpful in separating osteomyelitis from arthritis or soft tissue infection. Gallium and indium scans are even more specific than routine technetium studies in localizing foci of infection.

Magnetic Resonance Imaging (MRI). The ability of MRI to visualize the soft tissues has made it an ideal noninvasive modality for studying ligament and tendon abnormalities. Its great utility in the diagnosis of internal derangements of the knee has led to its increased use in the diagnosis of wrist and shoulder disorders. It is the study of choice for diagnosing avascular necrosis and is of great value in the identification of osteomyelitis and tumor of subchondral bone and marrow.

Synovial and Bone Biopsy. Synovial biopsy is most useful in the investigation of chronic monarticular arthritis. In this setting it is obligatory to rule out chronic infection with tuberculosis, fungi, and other unusual opportunistic organisms. Synovial biopsy similarly identifies pigmented villonodular synovitis and other metastatic and infiltrative diseases of the synovium. A bone biopsy occasionally must be performed to rule out osteomyelitis.

Other Diagnostic Studies. Specific serological testing is reviewed in the discussion of the individual disease entities that follows. Nonspecific laboratory evidence for a systemic inflammatory process is frequently found in routine studies. The acute phase reactants [erythrocyte sedimentation rate (ESR), fibrinogen, α_2-globulins, C-reactive protein] are all commonly elevated. The complete blood cell (CBC) count may show a normochromic, normocytic anemia consistent with the anemia of chronic disease. It may also show a mild thrombocytosis or leukocytosis, suggesting inflammation. The routine chemistry profile may show elevated globulins and decreased albumin, supporting the same conclusion.

SPECIFIC DISEASES

Rheumatoid Arthritis

Rheumatoid arthritis (RA) is the hallmark inflammatory arthritis. It is a chronic, systemic inflammatory disease whose earliest and principal manifestation is a proliferative synovitis. Extra-articular features, including rheumatoid nodules, pulmonary disease, ocular inflammation, vasculitis, and hypersplenism usually occur after several years of established joint disease. RA has a prevalence of 1–2%. It is at least twice as common in women as in men. The peak incidence is in the fourth through sixth decades, but it can occur at any age. As more women enter (and re-enter) the workforce, RA will become an increasingly frequent diagnosis in the occupational medicine practice.

The etiology of RA has been intensely studied yet remains incompletely understood. An environmental factor (perhaps an arthrotropic virus) in a genetically susceptible host (HLA-DR4) has been postulated. Numerous other factors are likely involved, including endocrine status, nutrition, and stress.[17]

The onset of symptoms is generally gradual, although a minority of patients may have an abrupt onset of joint pain, swelling, and stiffness. Many patients note mild constitutional symptoms of malaise, fatigue, anorexia, and weight loss. In general, the initially involved joints include the wrists, metacarpophalangeal (MCP) joints, and proximal interphalangeal joints (PIP). A few cases begin with an oligoarticular arthritis involving a large joint such as a knee or asymmetrically in the hands. Most cases cause symmetric polyarthritis of the hands and wrists within 6 months. As in any inflammatory arthritis, the patient reports morning stiffness lasting more than 30 minutes and up to several hours.

Examination of the patient with early RA typically reveals a doughy or rubbery soft tissue swelling of the small joints of the hand and wrist (Fig. 1). The joints are often quite tender and may be warm. Most striking is the marked pain on motion and limited motion and the decreased grip strength seen in many patients. Later, deformities characteristic of RA may be seen (Fig. 2). Frequently ulnar deviation and subluxation of the MCP joints are seen. "Swan neck" deformity is hypertension of the PIP joint with flexion of the distal interphalangeal (DIP) joint. Boutonnière deformity is a flexion deformity of the PIP joint with hypertension of the DIP joint. Rheumatoid nodules are found in about one-third of patients, usually in the olecranon bursa or along the extensor surface of the ulna.

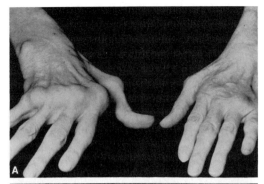

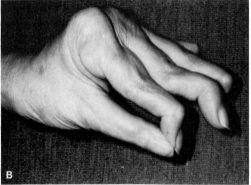

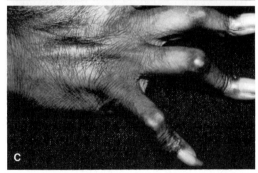

FIGURE 2. Rheumatoid arthritis. *A,* Ulnar deviation and subluxation of the metacarpophalangeal joints. *B,* Swan-neck deformities. *C,* Boutonnière deformities. Reprinted from the Revised Clinical Slide Collection on the Rheumatic Diseases, copyright 1981. Used by permission of the American College of Rheumatology.

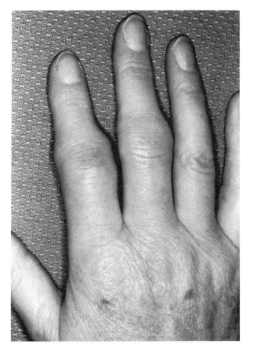

FIGURE 1. Early rheumatoid arthritis: Fusiform swelling of the proximal interphalangeal joints. Reprinted from the Revised Clinical Slide Collection on the Rheumatic Diseases, copyright 1981. Used by permission of the American College of Rheumatology.

The diagnosis of rheumatoid arthritis is based primarily on a history of an additive, symmetric, small-joint inflammatory polyarthritis, with physical findings confirming the presence of inflammatory synovitis. The symptoms should be present for at least 6 weeks. Diagnostic exclusions are other recognized forms of chronic polyarthritis such as psoriatic arthritis or systemic lupus erythematosus.[1] Laboratory studies in early RA may reveal a slight leukocytosis, thrombocytosis, or normochronic anemia. Acute phase reactants, such as ESR, are often elevated. Less than half of the patients have a positive test for rheumatoid factor at initial presentation, and up to 15% remain seronegative for the duration of their illness. Some of these patients may have a positive sensitized sheep cell agglutination test, which is a more specific and occasionally more sensitive test for rheumatoid factor activity. An appropriate screening laboratory workup for suspected RA includes a CBC count, Westergren ESR, rheumatoid factor by latex agglutination, and an ANA. Radiographs in early RA may be negative or may show soft tissue swelling around the involved joints. Later in the disease, cartilage loss, periarticular demineralization, and characteristic marginal erosions are seen (Fig. 3).

While the course of rheumatoid arthritis may be variable, the vast majority of patients eventually develop chronic joint damage and deformities. There is in fact a greater mortality in RA patients than among the population in general.[13] A growing consensus in rheumatology is that early use of second-line antirheumatic drugs is essential if the disease course is to be altered. Second-line drugs include gold salts, hydroxychloroquine, methotrexate, azathioprine, and sulfasalazine. Once the diagnosis of RA is suspected or established, therapy should be instituted with optimal doses of an NSAID. If the symptoms are not well controlled, the patient should be referred promptly to a rheumatologist.

Psoriatic Arthritis

While less prevalent than rheumatoid arthritis, psoriatic arthritis is still a rather common form of inflammatory arthritis. Estimates of the incidence of arthritis in patients with psoriasis vary widely, but the best estimates are in the range of 7–10%.[12] Case definition may be difficult because the arthritis may precede the detection of cutaneous psoriasis or may occur after many years of psoriasis. The several recognized patterns of joint involvement may overlap:

1. primary involvement of the DIP joints
2. a single joint or asymmetrical oligoarticular involvement in the hands
3. a severely deforming arthritis of the hands and feet with marked dissolution of bone and consequent "telescoping" of the digits (Fortunately, this "arthritis mutilans" form is infrequent, comprising 5% of cases or less.)
4. a clinical pattern indistinguishable from rheumatoid arthritis, but with a negative rheumatoid factor
5. an axial form similar to ankylosing spondylitis

Men and women are affected equally. The peak age at onset is the fourth and fifth decades as in RA. The clinical presentation is also similar to that of RA, with morning stiffness, pain, and swelling of joints.

Physical findings are also typical of a proliferative synovitis. The pattern of joint involvement may be helpful in distinguishing psoriatic from rheumatoid arthritis, especially if there is DIP joint involvement. These joints are rarely affected in RA (Fig. 4).

A thorough evaluation of the skin and scalp is mandatory. Not uncommonly, the patient is

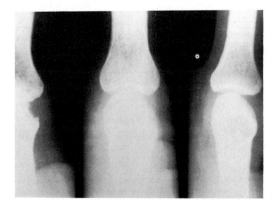

FIGURE 3. Rheumatoid arthritis: Radiographs showing progressive cartilage loss and development of marginal erosion, right to left. (Reprinted from the Revised Clinical Slide Collection on the Rheumatic Diseases, copyright 1981. Used by permission of the American College of Rheumatology.)

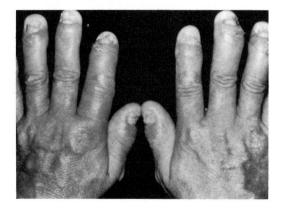

FIGURE 4. Psoriatic arthritis: Note the predominant distal interphalangeal joint involvement, nail dystrophy, and cutaneous changes of psoriasis. (Reprinted from the Revised Clinical Slide Collection on the Rheumatic Diseases, copyright 1981. Used by permission of the American College of Rheumatology.)

unaware of having psoriasis. The search must include not only the scalp and the usual sites, such as the extensor surfaces of the knees and elbows, but also the external ears, umbilicus, and gluteal crease. Nail changes including nail dystrophy (onycholysis) and nail pitting are more common in psoriasis patients with arthritis (63%) than in those without arthritis (37%).[13]

Laboratory tests are of little help in the evaluation of psoriatic arthritis. A mild elevation in the ESR may be seen. Rheumatoid factor is usually negative. If positive, it may well indicate coincident RA and psoriasis. A variety of HLA antigens have been associated with the various patterns of psoriatic arthritis but are not of any diagnostic utility. Radiographic features may be quite helpful. Psoriatic arthritis results in a rather characteristic "pencil-in-cup" erosion, especially at the DIP joint (Fig. 5). This erosion is characterized by marked destruction of the distal end of the middle phalanx down to a point, with widening and a large cuplike erosion of the base of the distal phalanx. Periosteal reaction is also frequently seen along the phalanges.

Psoriatic arthritis is said to result in less frequent and less severe disability than rheumatoid arthritis. However, in a minority of cases, especially of the arthritis mutilans form, the disease can be very destructive. Initial treatment is with NSAIDs. In particular, indomethacin, tolmetin, and meclofenamate seem to be effective. Any of the other nonsalicylate NSAIDs can also be tried. Salicylates seem relatively less effective in psoriatic arthritis. Because of the potentially destructive nature of psoriatic arthritis, early referral to a rheumatologist should be considered, especially if there are radiographic signs of erosive bony changes or if the NSAID is ineffective. Several second-line drugs, such as methotrexate and azathioprine, may modify the disease. These therapeutic decisions are best made and monitored by a rheumatologist.

Reiter's Syndrome

Reiter's syndrome is part of the spectrum of HLA-B27-associated diseases and is clearly related to psoriatic arthritis, ankylosing spondylitis, and inflammatory bowel disease. Reiter's syndrome may be defined as an inflammatory arthritis lasting more than 1 month and associated with urethritis or cervicitis. The classic triad of urethritis, conjunctivitis, and arthritis is not always seen. A group of mucocutaneous conditions are associated with Reiter's syndrome, including urethritis or cervicitis, inflammatory eye disease, oral ulcers, balanitis, and keratoderma blenorrhagicum. The last two are clinically and histologically indistinguishable from psoriasis. Reiter's syndrome is strongly associated with HLA-B27. The illness is most common in young men and usually follows an infection with an enteric pathogen such as *Salmonella*, *Yersinia*, *Shigella*, or *Campylobacter* or a venereal infection with *Chlamydia*. The relationship between the infection and the arthritis is incompletely understood on an immunological basis, but it is clinically striking. For this reason, the syndrome is also called "reactive arthritis."[4]

Clinically a young man usually presents with a rather intense, acute-onset oligoarthritis several weeks after an episode of urethritis or conjunctivitis. The arthritis has a predilection for the lower extremities, especially the knees, ankles, and metatarsophalangeal joints. Findings of enthesopathy such as Achilles tendinitis or heel pain may also be present. Fusiform swelling of the toes may result in "sausage toes." Rarely is the ocular inflammation serious, but it should always be examined by an ophthalmologist.

Laboratory tests are of limited utility, and the diagnosis is made primarily by clinical features. The ESR is often elevated significantly. The rheumatoid factor and ANA are negative in Reiter's syndrome. The HLA-B27 antigen

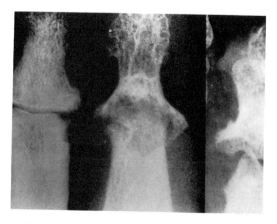

FIGURE 5. Psoriatic arthritis: Radiographs showing progression of distal interphalangeal joint involvement, left to right. Note the "pencil-in-cup" erosion. (Reprinted from the Revised Clinical Slide Collection on the Rheumatic Diseases, copyright 1981. Used by permission of the American College of Rheumatology.)

is found in 80% of cases, but it is also positive in 8–10% of the Caucasian population and so is of limited specificity. The test is very expensive and should be ordered only when the result will affect the diagnosis and treatment. Early radiographs reveal only soft tissue swelling; later, characteristic erosions (identical to psoriatic arthritis), periostitis, or asymmetric sacroiliitis may be seen.[4]

While most patients with Reiter's syndrome have only one or a few episodes of nonerosive arthritis, some develop chronic arthritis, which, like psoriatic arthritis and ankylosing spondylitis, can be destructive. A careful history, including a sexual history and complete physical examination are the best diagnostic tools. If Reiter's syndrome is suspected, initial therapy with indomethacin or tolmetin is indicated. Several other NSAIDs are also effective, including naproxen and diclofenac. Because of difficulty in diagnosis and the potential severity, suspected cases should be seen by a rheumatologist for confirmation, therapy, and monitoring.

Osteoarthritis

Osteoarthritis (OA) is the most common joint disease and is the single greatest cause of loss of time from work.[11] It occurs more frequently in the elderly; more than 80% of persons past 55 show radiological evidence of OA.[11] The term osteoarthritis is misleading because the initial pathology is a metabolic derangement and subsequent degeneration of articular cartilage. Only after degeneration is well established do some of the more clinically familiar findings occur, such as joint effusion (with usually mild inflammation), marginal bony hypertrophy, instability, and limitation of motion. The factors involved in the initiation of OA are not fully understood, but trauma, preexisting mechanical instability, and genetic factors are implicated. In contrast to RA and other forms of inflammatory arthritis, there is no evidence of systemic inflammation in OA.

Joints involved in OA typically include the weight-bearing joints (hips and knees), along with the spine and the DIP, PIP, and first carpal metacarpal joints of the hand. In the spine involvement manifests as degeneration of the intervertebral discs and marginal osteophytes arising from the vertebrae. The apophyseal joints are also frequently involved.

Greatest involvement is seen in the lumbar and cervical segments of the spine. In the upper extremities, primary osteoarthritis of the hands is especially common in older women. The typical complaint is aching or pain in the affected joints. The DIP or PIP joints may be involved selectively, or together in some patients (Fig. 6). The metacarpophalangeal joints and wrist are spared. Hand involvement in OA is very common in typists, pianists, and others who perform repeated motions of the hands. Patients may have morning stiffness of less than 15 minutes duration, but stiffness is seldom as striking or as long lasting as in rheumatoid arthritis. The pain tends to be aggravated with use of the hands. Many patients report worsening of pain during damp weather or changes in weather.

Physical examination reveals bony enlargement of the involved joints with decreased range of motion and pain. The joints may be slightly or markedly tender, but significant synovial membrane hypertrophy like that of RA is rarely seen. The enlarged DIP joints (or Heberden's nodes) may have painful mucous cysts, which may become infected. The enlarged PIP joints are called Bouchard's nodes.

Unlike RA, OA seldom yields specific laboratory abnormalities. Conversely, OA is readily established with radiographs. In the hands, the findings on x-ray are loss of cartilage and narrowness of the joint space, along with subchondral sclerosis and marginal osteophytes (or spurs) (Fig. 7). The disease progresses slowly, but symptoms may have a rather abrupt onset,

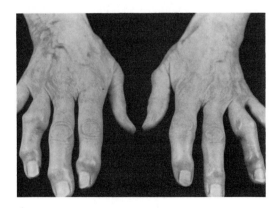

FIGURE 6. Osteoarthritis: Bony enlargement of the distal interphalangeal joints (Heberden's nodes) and of the proximal interphalangeal joints (Bouchard's nodes). (Reprinted from the Revised Clinical Slide Collection on the Rheumatic Diseases, copyright 1981. Used by permission of the American College of Rheumatology.)

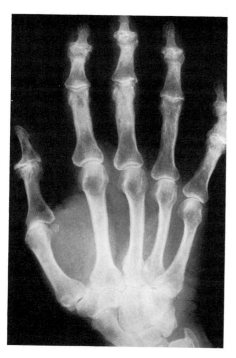

FIGURE 7. Osteoarthritis: Radiograph showing marked loss of cartilage at the interphalangeal joints with subchondral sclerosis and marginal osteophytes. (Reprinted from the Revised Clinical Slide Collection on the Rheumatic Diseases, copyright 1981. Used by permission of the American College of Rheumatology.)

to secondary OA. Osteoarthritis in the wrists or elbows of a jackhammer operator, for example, may point to occupationally related problems. Involvement of the MCP joints may reflect undiagnosed hemochromatosis. Radiographic calcifications within articular cartilage, or chondrocalcinosis, should prompt an evaluation for endocrine or metabolic diseases. Chondrocalcinosis renders the cartilage structurally unsound and therefore prone to osteoarthritis. It is frequently seen in the triangular fibrocartilage complex of the wrist on x-ray. Conditions associated with chondrocalcinosis include diabetes mellitus, hyperparathyroidism, hypothyroidism, hemochromatosis, Wilson's disease, and gout. Diseases such as Paget's disease of bone and acromegaly may also cause secondary OA. The laboratory evaluation in a patient with suspected secondary OA should include a thyroid profile with a thyroid-stimulating hormone (TSH) level and an automated chemistry profile, which gives information on liver function, calcium, metabolism, glucose level, renal function, uric acid level, and iron storage state (via the serum iron or ferritin level). Patients discovered to have a potential metabolic disease should be referred to the appropriate specialist.

Raynaud's Phenomenon and Related Connective Tissue Diseases

First described by Maurice Raynaud in 1862, Raynaud's phenomenon is a cold-induced vasospasm of the digits. The vasospasm results initially in pallor of the involved digits, then cyanosis, and finally rubor, particularly when the hand is rewarmed (Fig. 8). Many patients manifest only the pallor or a biphasic pattern. Diagnosis is based primarily upon a history of cold-induced episodes of digital cyanosis. Some patients have no reaction to a cold challenge, even with a typical history. In most but not all patients, the episodes are painful. Surveys have estimated the prevalence of Raynaud's phenomenon to be 5% of women and 4% of men.[5] While most patients with this syndrome have primary Raynaud's phenomenon, some have connective tissue diseases or other medical conditions or reactions to drugs or other environmental or occupational stimuli. When no underlying connective tissue disease or other secondary cause can be found, the term "Raynaud's disease" is sometimes used. When an

perhaps with a change in the occupational use of the hands. Therapeutic measures include rest of the joints and, where possible, reduction of the aggravating activities. The NSAIDs generally are effective at reducing symptoms, but they do nothing to retard the progression of the arthritis. Referral to a rheumatologist is not generally necessary but may be useful if the diagnosis is in question or if therapeutic difficulties arise. Remember that the other chronic arthritis affecting DIP joints—psoriatic arthritis—may be difficult to distinguish from primary osteoarthritis affecting the DIP joints.

This discussion has focused on primary osteoarthritis, a disease in which, by definition, there is no underlying or predisposing trauma or disease. There are, in addition, secondary forms of osteoarthritis. Causes of secondary OA may be broadly divided into those stemming from trauma or overuse of affected joints, those from preexisting or congenital structural abnormalities of the joints, and forms related to metabolism or endocrinology. An atypical pattern of joint involvement is the single best clue

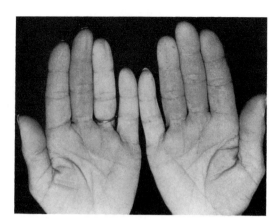

FIGURE 8. Raynaud's phenomenon: Pallor of three digits during an attack. (Reprinted from the Revised Clinical Slide Collection on the Rheumatic Diseases, copyright 1981. Used by permission of the American College of Rheumatology.)

underlying disease or external agent is implicated, the term "Raynaud's phenomenon" is applied. Well-documented occupational-related causes of Raynaud's phenomenon include exposure to vinyl chloride or silicotic dusts, or the use of vibratory machinery. Medical causes of Raynaud's phenomenon besides connective tissue diseases are rare; they include large vessel disease such as atherosclerosis, thromboangiitis obliterans, thoracic outlet syndrome, carpal tunnel syndrome or vasculitis, hyperviscosity syndromes or polycythemia and various drugs including beta blockers, ergotamines, bleomycin, cisplatin, estrogens, nicotine, and methylsergide.

The critical issue in the evaluation of a patient with Raynaud's phenomenon, especially that of recent onset, is determining the presence or likelihood of an underlying connective tissue disease. The connective tissue diseases in which Raynaud's phenomenon is most common are systemic lupus erythematosus (SLE) and systemic sclerosis or scleroderma. The prevalence of SLE is 4–20 per 100,000, and systemic sclerosis is perhaps one-tenth as common. The likelihood is therefore quite low that a patient who develops Raynaud's phenomenon will develop one of these diseases. Certainly a positive ANA or other features of connective tissue disease, including skin changes, are a strong clue. A recent study prospectively followed 58 patients with primary Raynaud's phenomenon for a mean of 2.7 years. Eleven patients (19%) developed a connective tissue disease, 3 developed systemic sclerosis, and 8

developed the more benign CREST (calcinosis, Raynaud's, esophageal dysmotility, sclerodactyly, and telangiectasis) variant. The best predictor of a connective tissue disease was an abnormal nailfold capillary pattern.[6] Beyond a thorough history and physical examination, evaluation should include a CBC count, ESR, chemistry profile, urinalysis, and ANA. A nailfold capillary examination is a relatively simple procedure, but some experience with the technique is necessary. Briefly, the nailfold is examined after applying a small amount of immersion oil under a low-power, wide-field microscope.

The treatment of Raynaud's phenomenon obviously includes removal of the offending drug or environmental factor and cessation of smoking. Environmental measures such as adequate heat in the home or workplace, are helpful. A change of job may be necessary if, for example, the patient works as a meat cutter. The use of gloves or mittens, and keeping the body core warm, are important. Finally, some patients require drug therapy. Calcium-channel antagonists are the most useful, especially nifedipine and the recently released nicardipine. Other options include α-adrenergic blockers such as guanethidine, vasodilators such as prazocin, topical nitrates, and pentoxifylline. These may be combined if needed in difficult cases.

A detailed discussion of the various associated connective tissue diseases is beyond the scope of this chapter, but a few important features should be mentioned. Systemic sclerosis (scleroderma) is an autoimmune disease characterized by hidebound fibrosis of the skin. A multisystem disorder, it may involve the lungs, gastrointestinal tract, kidneys, and even the heart. A very specific autoantibody, SCL-70, is detected in 20% of patients. This disease may be rapidly progressive and fatal. A related disorder is known as the CREST syndrome, which stands for calcinois, Raynaud's phenomenon, esophageal dysmotility, sclerodactyly, and telangiectasis. This disorder is characterized by skin involvement limited to the digits and milder and more indolent visceral involvement. Anticentromere antibody is specific for the CREST syndrome. The management of these disorders should always be supervised by a rheumatologist.

THERAPEUTIC CONSIDERATIONS

In diseases such as psoriatic arthritis and Reiter's syndrome, certain NSAIDs appear to be more effective than others, whereas in diseases such as osteoarthritis, the response to drugs appears to be individual to each patient. NSAIDs are the single most frequently prescribed class of drugs in arthritis. They are very effective. They also have many potentially serious side effects. A general discussion of these agents, which are listed by class in Table 1, is warranted.

All NSAIDs inhibit the production of inflammatory mediators—prostaglandins—by inhibiting the enzyme cyclooxygenase. Inhibition of prostaglandins accounts for certain side effects inherent to all these agents, namely gastric mucosal irritation and bleeding, and impairment of renal function. All NSAIDs are at least partly excreted by the kidneys. If there is pre-existing renal insufficiency, or if the patient has congestive heart failure, is on diuretics, or is elderly, dosage should be decreased and the patient's electrolytes and renal function should be carefully monitored.

The gastric mucosal side effects are even more complex. The risk of developing them increases with age and smoking. Among the NSAIDs, certain agents are relatively more likely to cause gastrointestinal distress or bleeding, but any of the agents can do so. Aspirin is undoubtedly the worst offender. The nonacetylated salicylates are the most innocuous in this respect and probably also least effective as anti-inflammatories. Between these extremes are the rest of the nonsalicylate NSAIDs, among which differences are small and individual to particular patients. Indomethacin may be somewhat more irritating, and diclofenac may be slightly more benign. New Food and Drug Administration prescribing information for all NSAIDs includes a warning to all patients of potentially fatal gastrointestinal bleeding.

Another problem recently reported is elevation of liver enzymes by NSAIDs. Diclofenac, in particular, is required to recommend liver enzyme measurement 8 weeks after starting therapy. Again, this problem may occur with any NSAID, and measurement of liver function tests two to three times per year is appropriate. Nevertheless, in our experience, transaminitis is rarely serious.

A review article[10] presents a detailed discussion of NSAIDs. A few of its main findings can be summarized here. All NSAIDs should be taken with food. In patients on warfarin (Coumadin), tolmetin (Tolectin) will not prolong the prothrombin time. Because sulindac (Clinoril) is less likely than other NSAIDs to impair renal function, it may be useful in patients with impaired renal function who require NSAIDs. All NSAIDs except piroxicam (Feldene) should be given a therapeutic trial of 2 weeks. Because of its long half-life, piroxicam should have a 3-week trial. Adequate dosing to achieve anti-inflammatory levels is essential with NSAIDs.

TABLE 1.   Chemical Classes of Nonsteroidal Anti-Inflammatory Drugs

Salicylates
  Aspirin
  Nonacetylated salicylates
    Choline magnesium trisalicylate (Trilisate)
    Salsalate (Disalcid, Mono-Gesic)
  Diflunisal (Dolobid)
Nonsalicylates
  Propionic acid
    Fenoprofen (Nalfon)
    Ibuprofen (Motrin, others)
    Naproxen (Naprosyn)
    Ketoprofen (Orudis)
    Flurbiprofen (Ansaid)
  Indolacetic Acid
    Indomethacin (Indocin)
    Tolmetin (Tolectin)
    Sulindac (Clinoril)
  Enolic Acid
    Piroxicam (Feldene)
  Phenylacetic acid
    Diclofenac (Voltaren)
  Mefenamic acid
    Meclofenamate (Meclomen)
  Pyrazole
    Phenylbutazone (Butazolidin, Azolid)

CONCLUSION

As long as people work with their hands, occupational physicians will see employees with complaints of pain in the upper extremities. A good history and physical examination should reveal whether the complaint is due to arthritis or to some other nonarticular cause of pain, and whether the symptoms are occupational or nonoccupational, or a combination. With the recognition of arthritis, the clinician should already have a reasonable suspicion of which form or forms the patient has. Often a rather simple laboratory investigation will help confirm the diagnosis. The clinician is urged to order tests selectively based on a differential diagnosis. The "arthritis profile" is a battery of tests available from most commercial laboratories. This "shotgun" approach often yields confusing and unnecessary information. If the patient is a young woman suspected of having rheumatoid arthritis, the uric acid level is irrelevant. Similarly, a (false) positive ANA in an older man suspected of having gout may result in needless concern that the patient has lupus.

Whenever possible, the patient's job task should be altered to reduce mechanical stress on the affected joints. In nearly all arthritis, the initial therapy is an NSAID. The physician should be familiar with one or two NSAIDs in each class, including the side effects. When the diagnosis is in question or when the response to therapy is poor, the patient should be referred to a rheumatologist. Early and effective treatment can enable the employee to remain functional on the job.

REFERENCES

1. Arnett FC, Edsworthy SM, Bloch DA, et al: The American Rheumatism Association 1987 revised criteria for the classification of rheumatoid arthritis. Arthritis Rheum 31:315–324, 1988.
2. Bunch TW, Hunder GG, McDuffie FC, et al: Synovial fluid complement determination as a diagnostic aid in inflammatory joint disease. Mayo Clin Proc 49:715–720, 1974.
3. Calin A: Reiter's syndrome. In Calin A (ed): Spondyloarthopathies. Orlando, FL, Grune and Stratton, 1984, pp 119–149.
4. Calin A: Reiter's syndrome. In Kelley WN, Harris ED Jr, Ruddy S, Sledge CB (eds): Textbook of Rheumatology. Philadelphia, W.B. Saunders, 1989, pp 1038–1052.
5. Campbell PM, Leroy EC: Raynaud phenomenon. Semin Arthritis Rheum 16:92–103, 1986.
6. Fitzgerald O, Hess EV, O'Conner GT, Spencer-Green G: Prospective study on the evolution of Raynaud's phenomenon. Am J Med 84:718–726, 1988.
7. Fries JF: Assessment of the patient with rheumatic disease. In Kelley WN, Harris ED Jr, Ruddy S, Sledge CB (eds): Textbook of Rheumatology. Philadelphia, W.B. Saunders, 1989, pp 417–424.
8. Goldenberg DL: Bacterial arthritis. In Kelley WN, Harris ED Jr, Ruddy S, Sledge CB (eds): Textbook of Rheumatology. Philadelphia, W.B. Saunders, 1989, pp 1567–1585.
9. Goldenberg DL, Brandt KD, Cohen AS, Cathcart ES: Treatment of septic arthritis. Arthritis Rheum 18:83–90, 1975.
10. Hochberg MC: NSAIDs: Patterns of usage and side effects. Hosp Pract 24:167–174, 1989.
11. Mankin HJ: Clinical features of osteoarthritis. In Kelley WN, Harris ED Jr, Ruddy S, Sledge CB (eds): Textbook of Rheumatology. Philadelphia, W.B. Saunders, 1989, pp 1480–1500.
12. Michet CJ, Conn DL: Psoriatic arthritis. In Kelley WN, Harris ED Jr, Ruddy S, Sledge CB (eds): Textbook of Rheumatology. Philadelphia, W.B. Saunders, 1989, pp 1053–1063.
13. Scarpa R, Oriente P, Pucino A, et al: Psoriatic arthritis in psoriatic patients. Br J Rheumatol 23:246–250, 1984.
14. Schumacher HR: Synovial fluid analysis and synovial biopsy. In Kelley WN, Harris ED Jr, Ruddy S, Sledge CB (eds): Textbook of Rheumatology. Philadelphia, W.B. Saunders, 1989, pp 637–649.
15. Wasner C, Britton MC, Kraines RG, et al: Nonsteroidal anti-inflammatory agents in rheumatoid arthritis and ankylosing spondylitis. JAMA 246:2168–2172, 1981.
16. Weir IL, Bonham GS, Hunter-Manns J: Kentucky Statewide Study of Persons with Disabilities. Stage 1 Report. Louisville, Urban Studies Center, College of Urban and Public Affairs, University of Louisville, 1989, pp 13–33.
17. Zvaifler NJ: Etiology and pathogenesis of rheumatoid arthritis. In McCarty DJ (ed): Arthritis and Allied Conditions. Philadelphia, Lea & Febiger, 1989, pp 659–673.

Chapter 33

HAND THERAPY FOR OCCUPATIONAL UPPER EXTREMITY DISORDERS

Connie Lane, P.T.

In recent years an increased understanding of the physiology and pathomechanics of hand and upper extremity function has led to the development of specialization in hand rehabilitation. Hand surgeons and therapists across the country have developed postoperative protocols and management techniques that have greatly improved surgical outcomes. The educational background and experience of the hand therapist have also led to understanding and expertise in the rehabilitation of many nonsurgical upper extremity conditions first seen by the occupational physician or nurse. Some of the conditions for which referral to a hand therapist is indicated and the appropriate therapeutic management are discussed here.

The referring physician, surgeon, or occupational nurse should recognize that, just as hand surgery has become a specialized area of medicine, so has rehabilitation. Detailed, indepth study of the hand and related treatment protocols are beyond the scope of the formal educational process for both occupational and physical therapists. The general therapist in a hospital or clinical setting rarely has the opportunity to see significant numbers of hand patients. In addition to being intensely interested in hand rehabilitation, the treating therapist should have pursued a course of continuing education in hand therapy and have had an opportunity to work closely with specialists in hand surgery.

Too often the referring physician sees patients with hand or upper extremity problems that appear insignificant or minor, and assumes that the condition will improve with time. Only upon the return visit, when joints are stiffer and pain patterns increased, is the patient referred to a hand therapist. Far less therapy is generally required when a patient is referred early and an appropriate home program is initiated. Referral after joint fibrosis has developed or long-term pain pathways have been established always necessitates a longer, more complicated treatment regimen, and outcomes are usually less than optimal.

CARPAL TUNNEL SYNDROME

One of the primary conservative measures in the management of this condition is splinting. Splinting, particularly during sleep, prevents the inevitable flexed posture of the wrist that compromises the median nerve. Splinting during the day, because it can become a "crutch" to the patient, is often not recommended but is occasionally necessary because of the patient's work duties or attitude.

An effective splint supports the wrist in neutral position. Extending the splint beyond the distal palmar crease should be avoided because it inhibits flexion of the metacarpophalangeal joints, thereby limiting the making of a fist and causing pinching in the palm. The splint should allow for adduction and opposition of the thumb so that the patient can continue to use the hand in a normal manner. However, forceful pinching should be discouraged, because forceful pinching can contribute to the development of carpal tunnel syndrome.[9] If the splint is not washable, cast stockinette is usually worn under it for perspiration absorption and comfort.

Unfortunately, most manufacturers of prefabricated splints do not appreciate these important splinting features. Splints often support the wrist in excessive extension, putting the contents of the carpal tunnel on stretch. Small, medium, and large size designations do not cover the wide variety of patient hand sizes. In addition, with prefabricated splints the metal insert used for support of the wrist tends to slip proximally with repetitive use of the hand and thus pinches the forearm. This problem can be easily remedied by shortening the metal insert, beveling the edges, and taping the opening for the insert.

The Liberty wrist support is generally comfortable and well tolerated by most patients (Fig. 1). The thermoplastic insert molded to the hand with the wrist in a comfortable neutral position also does not interfere with motion of the thumb and fingers.

Any patient who is wearing a splint 24 hours a day for conservative management of carpal tunnel syndrome should be on a stretching program, done once or twice daily to prevent joint stiffness.[11] In addition, isometric strengthening of the wrist in a neutral position does not irritate the median nerve and aids in the prevention of forearm weakness.

Another important aspect of conservative management is patient education. Patients who understand the pathogenesis of carpal tunnel syndrome appreciate the importance of limiting repetitious wrist motion and simultaneous wrist flexion with pinching.[1] Task analysis sometimes reveals excessive wrist motion or deviation. Use of excessive force is also sometimes observed. For instance, during a tour of a large computer operation, it was noted that many key operators pressed the keyboard unusually hard, with much greater force than necessary to produce a character. Pointing out this problem and instruction in relaxation techniques are sometimes helpful.

A review of non-work-related activities is also included in patient education. Often a patient with carpal tunnel syndrome reports increased symptoms while driving. It should be pointed out that hanging the hand over the top of a steering wheel for a prolonged period of time is indeed likely to bring on symptoms. This posture combines acute flexion of the wrist and pressure over the carpal tunnel with vibration, which is sometimes a contributing factor.[3] Patients who report an onset of symptoms after prolonged periods of knitting, crocheting, or some other hobby need to be told to reduce the time spent in these activities. Normal activities of daily living sometimes bring on annoying symptoms. Simple modification of techniques such as holding a hair dryer may eliminate some of the patient's discomfort.

Proper use of ergonomically designed equipment should also be explored by the therapist. For instance, the tour of the large computer

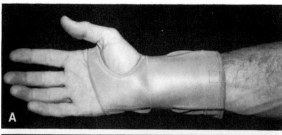

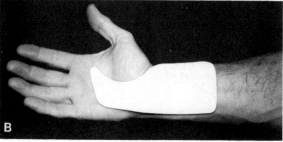

FIGURE 1. *A*, The Liberty wrist support does not interfere with thumb and finger motion. *B*, The splint has a thermoplastic insert that is molded to the patient's hand. (Distributed by North Coast Medical, Inc., Campbell, California.)

operation revealed that, though the company had provided expensive, ergonomically designed chairs, many employees sat on the chair with one leg crossed under the other and leaned on an elbow. This posture completely eliminated the ergonomic support and enhanced the likelihood of musculoskeletal problems. Proper posture of the back and neck affects the position of the wrist and hand while using hand tools or computers.

TENDINITIS

Tendinitis, a common diagnosis in the upper extremity, is often quite disabling. Armstrong has demonstrated that people who are involved in highly repetitive, forceful activities are significantly more likely to develop tendinitis than those in jobs with low repetition and force.[2] Every tendon in the hand and wrist has been reported to develop tendinitis, and specific symptoms for each have been described.[23] Exact diagnosis by means of a thorough history and careful physical examination is important in order to plan an effective treatment approach.

Physicians usually treat acute tendinitis with rest, either casting or splinting, and often nonsteroidal anti-inflammatory drugs.[7] If splinting is chosen, ice applied to the involved area may provide some relief of symptoms. After casting, joints are usually stiff and surrounding soft tissue tight. Application of heat before the exercise, provided acute tenderness and swelling have resolved, decreases stiffness and allows for more effective stretching. The therapist should have a thorough understanding of the factors that precipitate pain in order to plan a treatment regimen without restarting a vicious cycle of pain and inflammation.

Curwin describes a successful treatment approach with an eccentric exercise program that consists of icing, warm-up stretching, and eccentric strengthening of the affected muscles, followed by a repeat of stretching and icing.[8] As the program progresses, both speed of repetition and resistance of eccentric exercise are recommended.

Other authors report successful treatment with iontophoresis and application of a steroid or noncortical steroid medication.[22] Ultrasound is commonly used by some therapists, but in at least one study it was found to have no appreciable benefit over a placebo treatment.[17] The occupational physician and nurse, as well as workers' compensation carriers, are probably aware of therapists who routinely practice "modality loading," either deliberately or unconscientiously adding unnecessary charges to the patient's treatment. A hit-or-miss approach seldom produces satisfactory results and lacks a sound physiological basis. In my experience rest through immobilization and avoidance of aggravating activities followed by an effective stretching and strengthening program usually leads to the resolution of tendinitis.

As the condition improves, generalized upper extremity strengthening may be added to the exercise program. It may be combined with a work hardening program in the clinic and with home exercises. Gradual return to normal activities, both work and recreational, is recommended.

JOINT INJURIES

Interphalangeal joint strains and incomplete ligamentous tears are usually treated initially with immobilization. Following this period of immobilization the patient is referred for initiation of therapy. Assessment usually reveals joint swelling, tenderness, and decreased active motion. Heat is often applied before an active range of motion exercise program is initiated. The patient is taught to carry this program out at home on a regular basis, 8–10 times a day. The patient is also taught to avoid strenuous activities such as heavy lifting or gripping and passive range of motion, which may increase inflammation and stress incompletely healed structures. The compliant patient notes improvement in active range of motion almost immediately. A thorough questioning of patients who have not improved after a few days on a home program generally reveals a lack of understanding of the program or noncompliance. Occasionally the overzealous patient carries out the exercise program excessively and develops increased stiffness and swelling as well as pain. Buddy taping or splinting is often used to prevent reinjury during the early mobilization period (Fig. 2).

After approximately 6 weeks, progression to some form of dynamic splinting to regain any limited passive range of motion may be necessary. Resistive exercise to regain grip strength is also usually initiated at this time.

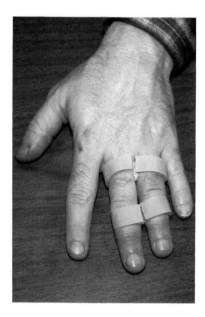

FIGURE 2.   Buddy splints or taping can be used to prevent lateral stress to injured interphalangeal joints.

It is important to educate the patient as to what to expect from joint injuries. The patient is told that any time a joint capsule or joint surface is violated, permanent joint enlargement with some residual joint stiffness can be expected. The implications of this can vary according to the patient's age and occupation.

STENOSING TENOSYNOVITIS

Trigger finger is sometimes seen in the manual laborer whose job requires repetitious or prolonged forceful gripping. Treatment of this annoying and painful condition in the past has been limited to cortisone injections, rest, and pulley resections. Recently, Evans et al. described a new approach in the conservative management of this problem.[10] In their study, 52% of patients had excellent results and 21% had good or improved results with no additional type of treatment. This treatment program includes static splinting of the involved finger with the metacarpophalangeal joint in 0 degrees of extension, combined with active "hook fist" exercise in the splint every 2 hours throughout the day (Fig. 3). Periodic passive, full-fist exercises are done to maintain the metacarpophalangeal joint range of motion.

Although this treatment approach is not adequate in every case, amazing success with complete resolution of symptoms has been achieved with it. Even severe cases can improve, if not completely resolve, with time in this conservative program.

Frequently joint stiffness and pain are associated with this diagnosis, particularly if the condition has persisted for several weeks. Prior application of heat helps reduce joint discomfort and increases soft tissue extensibility, thus improving the effectiveness of the exercise program in the splint.[16]

SCARS AND NEUROMAS

Even superficial hand injuries can result in hypersensitive scarring. It is not uncommon for the patient with this type of injury to return to his physician several weeks later with complaints of extreme hypersensitivity, inability to use the involved finger, and often decreased range of motion and strength of the affected hand. The problem can be particularly annoying in hand areas that are commonly in contact with tools or materials. The patient often develops extensor habitus of the involved finger (Fig. 4).

Treatment consists of progressive desensitization. The patient often cannot tolerate any pressure whatsoever and must start desensitization with rubbing the sensitive area with cotton or working the hand through sand. Generally continuation leads to tolerance of more varied contact media.[4] The patient is instructed in a home program of progressive contact with materials such as cotton, rice, and terry cloth. The patient is instructed to do scar massage several times a day to decrease tenderness and adherence. In some instances vibration is used as well to help increase tolerance of normal daily use of the hand.

In cases of joint stiffness and decreased grip strength, exercises to correct these conditions are included in the home program.

It is important to educate the patient that normal scar maturation takes 6–12 months from the time of injury.[12,18] The patient must be reassured that improvement will come in time.

Painful neuromas, particularly following digital amputation, usually respond well to the same treatment regimen. However, in some cases, surgical follow-up to bury the neuroma is sometimes necessary.[24]

Injury to the dorsal sensory branch of the radial nerve is particularly prone to the de-

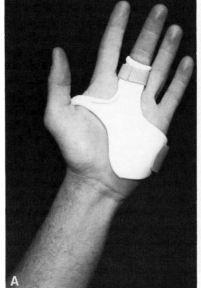
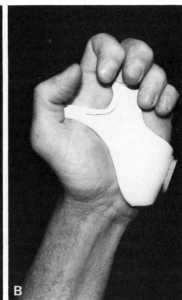

FIGURE 3. *A,* Palmar splint for stenosing tenosynovitis or "trigger finger." The splint supports the metacarpophalangeal joint of the affected finger in 0 degrees of extension. *B,* "Hook fist" exercise in the splint.

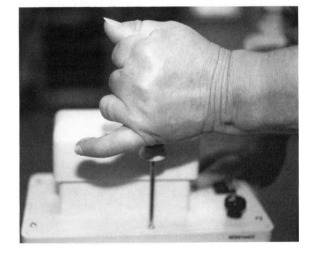

FIGURE 4. Tenderness of a fingertip after an injury can lead to avoidance of contact during daily use.

velopment of hypersensitivity. Contusions or lacerations in this area may cause severe symptoms. Transcutaneous nerve stimulation has occasionally been used in this area in addition to progressive desensitization for temporary relief of hypersensitivity. Fortunately, with time, this condition usually improves and the use of nerve stimulation can be discontinued.

ARTHRITIS

The first carpometacarpal (CMC) joint at the base of the thumb is an area prone to early degenerative joint disease. Pain and joint enlargement in this area are quite common. Conservative management usually consists of a CMC joint splint, which supports the area while the patient continues with normal functional activities (Fig. 5). As long as motion in the interphalangeal joint is not painful, this joint can be left free for opposition to the index and long finger. Fitting of this splint is generally easier in men with more soft tissue padding across the dorsum of the hand. Women with thin bony hands sometimes experience discomfort from the pressure over the dorsum of the metacarpals. Care is taken during fabrication to avoid

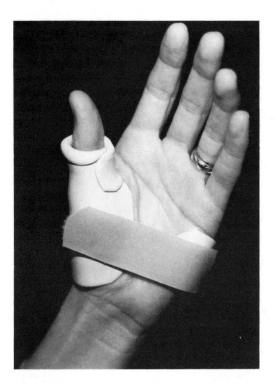

FIGURE 5. Carpometacarpal (CMC) joint splint for control of pain in the first CMC joint.

pressure over the first dorsal interosseous muscle and second metacarpal and to allow the wrist free range of motion.

Occasionally patients with this disorder also have discomfort in the radial aspect of the wrist joint or associated de Quervain's tenosynovitis. These patients do better with a thumb spica splint, although the lack of wrist mobility that this splint entails is somewhat of a nuisance.

Many patients with arthritis in the wrist joint may continue normal activities with light functional splinting. Care is taken not to inhibit full finger flexion or thumb opposition unless there is need to immobilize these joints.

Arthritic patients often benefit from a complete analysis of their normal work and daily activities. Instruction in joint protection principals can help the patient decrease strain of the small joints of the hand and significantly reduce joint pain. General principles include building up tool handles, using larger, more proximal joints to carry loads, and pacing of activities to decrease prolonged stress on involved joints.[20]

THORACIC OUTLET SYNDROME

Thoracic outlet syndrome is a musculoskeletal condition frequently aggravated by work duties. The forward head, rounded shoulder posture is a predisposing factor in the development of thoracic outlet syndrome. Sitting, standing, or repetitious shoulder and scapular motion required to carry out assembly duties or other work can irritate the compromised brachial plexus and bring on symptoms. Therapy directed at control of symptoms and correction of predisposing factors can often be most successful. As with any other condition, the therapist must have a complete understanding of etiology. History and subjective assessment of pain patterns help to determine irritability of the condition. A complete postural exam as well as muscle testing is necessary to establish treatment goals and develop an appropriate treatment plan. Differential testing to exclude cervical, glenohumeral joint, or any other pathology is imperative before initiation of treatment. Because this disorder is complicated and symptoms can mimic other conditions, the therapist must isolate the offending structures and treatment in order to avoid worsening the condition.

Initial treatment may include appropriate modalities to alleviate pain before focusing on posture correction. When symptoms are severe, the patient is taught proper positioning while sitting, standing, and lying. As discomfort subsides, selective stretching of shortened muscles and strengthening of lengthened muscle groups can be initiated in order to restore muscle balance.[5] The patient must be instructed in a home program, because most patients have had poor posture for many, many years, and correction does not happen in a few treatment sessions.

A typical home program includes stretching of the scalene and lateral cervical soft tissues in side-bending and cervical retraction exercises to correct forward-head posture. Shoulder elevation and protraction and retraction are done to increase patient awareness of shoulder position and selectively stretch and strengthen scapular and pectoral musculature. Thoracic extension and brachial plexus stretching exercises are added as they can be tolerated.

Many patients with uncomplicated thoracic outlet syndrome respond quickly, and symptoms are alleviated after only a few sessions of home instructions. Other patients, particularly those with a long history or other associated problems, such as carpal tunnel syndrome or adhesive capsulitis of the glenohumeral joint, can require a lengthy course of treatment.

However, many authors report that a majority of their patients have favorable results with conservative management.[14,19]

REFLEX SYMPATHETIC DYSTROPHY

Reflex sympathetic dystrophy (RSD) is a complication that can follow any type of hand or upper extremity injury and is characterized by pain out of proportion to the extent of the injury. Fortunately, this problem is not seen frequently. RSD is thought to occur in people with a predisposing emotional makeup. At least one study showed significant differences between a test group of RSD patients and a control group in psychological testing results.[13]

Reflex sympathetic dystrophy is characterized by a painful, erythematous, swollen, sweaty extremity and can progress to fibrosis of the joints, soft tissue atrophy, and complete dysfunction of the extremity.[15] Any patient with complaints of pain out of proportion to the injury is an appropriate candidate for therapy. Early intervention can improve the functional outcome of the patient and decrease overall treatment time.

Appropriate treatment can include active exercise as well as heat, contrast baths, and transcutaneous nerve stimulation for control of pain. Recently, Carlson and Watson described a stress loading program to change afferent input to the abnormal central nervous system activity.[6] This program consists of "stress loading" of the affected extremity by using a scrub brush with the shoulder directly over the hand to apply maximum pressure in a back-and-forth motion. A Dystrophile is a commercially made device with a timer and light that may be used in the stress loading program to provide visual cues and encourage patient compliance (Fig. 6). The recommended program starts with approximately 3 minutes of stress loading and gradually progresses to 10-minute sessions three times a day. In addition, the patient carries a weight or weighted bag as tolerated throughout the day while standing or walking. No other form of treatment is recommended until pain and swelling begin to subside. However, use of the hand in activities of daily living is strongly encouraged. The authors describe amazing and almost immediate response with this program.

As pain and swelling subside, attention is given to decreasing stiffness and improving range of motion and strength. Again, it should be

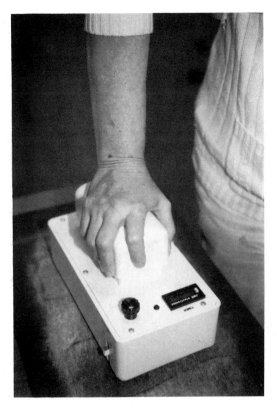

FIGURE 6. The Dystrophile is used by patients with reflex sympathetic dystrophy. Pressure is applied through the shoulder and elbow in a back-and-forth motion for graded "stress loading." (Distributed by North Coast Medical, Inc., Campbell, California.)

noted that if fibrotic changes have occurred, treatment can be lengthy and it can take months to restore good functional use of the extremity. Naturally, a noncompliant patient can lengthen the process even more. In the patient with RSD, painful manipulation of the joints perpetuates the problem and must be avoided.

WORK CAPACITY EVALUATION AND WORK HARDENING

Recently we have been inundated with advertisements and publications on work hardening programs and physical capacity evaluations. It should be pointed out that hand therapy has always included work hardening. The recent development of the capacity evaluation has led to work hardening programs that are significant revenue producers for hospitals and outpatient clinics. Although the sophistication of the examination is a great addition to ther-

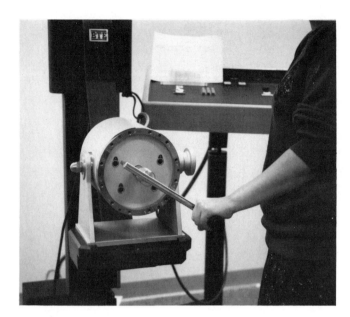

FIGURE 7. The BTE Work Simulator has many attachments that may be positioned to simulate most tasks a patient may be required to perform in his regular job. (Baltimore Therapeutic Equipment, Baltimore, Maryland.)

apy, it should be recognized that work hardening is progressive resistive exercise, which has always been a component of therapy programs.

Individuals lost in the rehabilitation process and destined not to return to their former jobs may well benefit from a work or physical capacity evaluation by a competent therapist. The work capacity evaluation involves a detailed medical history with screening for previous work- and non-work-related injuries, as well as systemic processes that may have made the patient vulnerable to an injury or cumulative trauma disorder. Careful review of previous medical procedures (as well as use of medication, splints, or supports) and previous therapy programs is done.

Physical examination includes observation of the appearance of the involved extremity and measurements of active and passive range of motion. Grip and sensibility testing are done, and edema and atrophy are measured. Subjective reports of pain are reviewed, and subjective and objective findings are correlated.[21]

An analysis of the patient's former job can reveal whether the patient should be expected to return to it. The value of continuing rehabilitation efforts should be considered and appropriate recommendations made.

A work simulation or work hardening program may be recommended on the basis of the outcome of the work capacity evaluation. The BTE Work Simulator has been refined over several years and is now available in many clinics (Fig. 7). This exercise device has numerous attachments that may be applied in various positions to simulate almost any type of work a patient may be called upon to do. The computerized printout gives information on force, distance, and work produced. This can be of great value to the therapist when planning a program for strengthening and work tolerance. Computerized documentation provides positive reinforcement for the well-motivated patient and can assist the therapist in verifying noncompliance in the malingerer.

Job-related tasks such as lifting and carrying may be simulated with simple milk crates and standard clinic weights. Sophisticated equipment is not always necessary.

SUMMARY

Many hand and upper extremity injuries and disorders can be conservatively managed through appropriate splinting, therapeutic exercise, and patient education. A thorough understanding of the anatomy and physiology of upper extremity problems allows the hand therapist to assist the occupational physician in planning a treatment program for the injured worker.

REFERENCES

1. Armstrong TJ: Ergonomics and cumulative trauma disorders. Hand Clin 2:559, 1986.
2. Armstrong TJ, Fine LJ, Goldstein SA, et al: Ergonomic considerations in hand and wrist tendinitis. J Hand Surg 12A:830–837, 1987.
3. Armstrong TJ, Fine LJ, Radwin RG, Silverstein BS: Ergonomics and the effects of vibration in hand-intensive work. Scand J Work Environ Health 13:286–289, 1987.
4. Barber LM: Desensitization of the traumatized hand. In Hunter JM, Schneider LH, Mackin EJ, Callahan AD (eds): Rehabilitation of the Hand: Surgery and Therapy, 3rd ed. St. Louis, C.V. Mosby, 1990, pp 721–730.
5. Barbis J: Therapist's management of thoracic outlet syndrome. In Hunter JM, Schneider LH, Mackin EJ, Callahan AD (eds): Rehabilitation of the Hand: Surgery and Therapy, 3rd ed. St. Louis, C.V. Mosby, 1990, pp 540–562.
6. Carlson LK, Watson HK: Treatment of reflex sympathetic dystrophy using the stress-loading program. J Hand Ther 1:149–154, 1988.
7. Cooney WP: Bursitis and tendinitis in the hand, wrist and elbow. Minn Med 66:491–494, 1983.
8. Curwin S, Stanish WD: Tendinitis: Its Etiology and Treatment. Lexington, MA, Collamore Press, 1984, pp 128–132.
9. Ditmars DM, Houin HP: Carpal tunnel syndrome. Hand Clin 2:525–526, 1986.
10. Evans RB, Hunter JM, Burkhalter WE: Conservative management of the trigger finger: A new approach. J Hand Ther 1:59–68, 1988.
11. Falkenburg SA: Choosing hand splints to aid carpal tunnel syndrome recovery. Occup Health Safety 56:60–64, 1987.
12. Hardy MA: The biology of scar formation. Phys Ther 69:1014–1024, 1989.
13. Hardy MA, Merritt WH: Psychological evaluation and pain assessment in patients with reflex sympathetic dystrophy. J Hand Ther 1:155–163, 1988.
14. Huffman JD: Electrodiagnostic techniques for and conservative treatment of thoracic outlet syndrome. Clin Orthop Rel Res 207:21–23, 1986.
15. Lankford LL: Reflex sympathetic dystrophy. In Hunter JM, Schneider LH, Mackin EJ, Callahan AD (eds): Rehabilitation of the Hand: Surgery and Therapy, 3rd ed. St. Louis, C.V. Mosby, 1990, pp 763–784.
16. Lehmann JF, DeLateur BJ: Diathermy and superficial heat and cold therapy. In Kottke FJ, Stillwell GK, Lehman JF (eds): Krusen's Handbook of Physical Medicine and Rehabilitation, 3rd ed. Philadelphia, W.B. Saunders, 1982, pp 275–280.
17. Lundeberg T, Abrahamsson P, Haker E: A comparative study of continuous ultrasound, placebo ultrasound and rest in epicondylalgia. Scand J Rehab Med 20:99–101, 1988.
18. Madden JW, Peacock EE: Studies on the biology of collagen during wound healing. Ann Surg 174:511–517, 1971.
19. Pang D, Wessel HB: Thoracic outlet syndrome. Neurosurgery 22:105–119, 1988.
20. Phillips CA: The management of patients with rheumatoid arthritis. In Hunter JM, Schneider LH, Mackin EJ, Callahan AD (eds): Rehabilitation of the Hand: Surgery and Therapy, 3rd ed. St. Louis, C.V. Mosby, 1990, pp 763–784.
21. Schultz-Johnson K: Assessment of upper extremity-injured persons' return to work potential. J Hand Surg 12A:950–956, 1987.
22. Taylor Mullins PA: Use of therapeutic modalities in upper extremity rehabilitation. In Hunter JM, Schneider LH, Mackin EJ, Callahan AD (eds): Rehabilitation of the Hand: Surgery and Therapy, 3rd ed. St. Louis, C.V. Mosby, 1990, pp 216–218.
23. Thorson EP, Szabo RM: Tendinitis of the wrist and elbow. Occup Med State Art Rev 4:419–431, 1989.
24. Whipple RR, Unsell RS: Treatment of painful neuromas. Orthop Clin North Am 19:175–185, 1988.

Chapter 34

RETURN-TO-WORK PROGRAMS AFTER HAND INJURIES

Nancy P. McElwain, M.B.A., R.N.

Employees are an employer's greatest asset. In companies of all sizes and types, employees are expected to give 100% effort every day. As industries attempt to compete in a global marketplace, attention to the bottom line demands that the work be carried out efficiently in record time by a minimum number of workers. The very nature of production puts workers at risk for injury. With the proliferation of computers, the number one occupational complaint for 1990 is expected to be "terminal illness" or symptoms stemming from continuous exposure to a video display terminal. As people interact with machines, accidents can result from human carelessness as well as machine breakdown. Furthermore, people, like machines, can suffer the effects of overuse. In spite of national attention to the safety of America's workplaces, the incidence of occupational injuries and illnesses is on the upswing. In 1988, 6.4 million injuries or illnesses were recorded, at a rate of 8.6 per 100 full-time workers.[11] Medical costs grew 14.7% annually from 1980 to 1985.[8] Employers paid $26 million in workers' compensation-related costs in 1987; medical costs, which are physician driven, account for 25–32% of total costs.[5]

With an increased incidence of injury comes a focus on accident prevention. Many employers have active safety programs that serve to educate employees and heighten safety awareness. Employees can receive safety awards, such as cash, plaques, paid time off, and T-shirts, as incentives to reduce accidents. In spite of the focus on prevention, injuries still occur.

Injured employees represent a significant business expense, but one that can be controlled. Workers' compensation laws in all states require the employer to bear the cost (payment of income as well as medical expenses) of an employee injury or illness resulting from work done for the employer. Most employers therefore can gain much from a program that keeps workers at work in a productive capacity.

Return-to-work programs make it possible for employees to return to the workplace as soon as possible after an occupational injury or illness. The ideal situation is for the worker to return to his original job. However, in the event of permanent disabling injuries, the worker may need an altogether new job. Employers can offer vocational training and placement assistance in these circumstances.

More common are the injuries that cause temporary disability, where the worker cannot return to the previous job until healing is complete. Barring unforeseen complications and assuming the treatment regimen is strictly adhered to, the return-to-work date can, in most cases, be predicted by the treating physician. Programs can be designed to return these workers to the workplace earlier, albeit in a different, temporary capacity, to the benefit of the employee, his family, and co-workers, as well as the employer and the insurance carrier. Return-to-work programs create a winning solution for all interested parties.

When an employee is hurt at work and becomes disabled, his daily routine is significantly altered. His activity level is reduced, he

479

becomes somewhat despondent, his image of himself is changed. Without communication from his employer, he may feel alienated from his job and his co-workers.[3,10] The hands are highly visible body parts, and the hand-injured patient may be self-conscious. His self-esteem may be threatened, especially if he is the family breadwinner. Family response can be either sympathetic or apathetic, and loss of economic security is a concern.[1] Workers may blame the company and seek revenge. Prolonged time off the job hampers return to work. Workers may become depressed or angry and often develop a fear of re-injury.[10] All of these factors contribute to prolonged periods of disability.[4] Return-to-work programs counter these negative emotional and financial effects of disability by facilitating timely return to the workplace.

The incidence of disability increases with age. "Disability" here includes illness and disabling conditions such as vision and hearing impairments and cardiac and respiratory disorders. Race and sex have an effect, in that, whereas white males suffer more frequent disabilities than white females, the reverse is true for blacks. Highly educated persons experience fewer disabilities, perhaps because a wider variety of occupational choices are available to them.

ROLE OF THE OCCUPATIONAL PHYSICIAN

As director of the health care team, the physician makes crucial decisions as to the extent of an injury, the employee's capability to return to work, and whether a disability exists. Although the physician's primary responsibility is to the patient, the occupational physician must also balance the needs and concerns of the employee's family, the employer, and the insurance carrier. A conflict of interest need not be a factor here because the employer concerned with protecting employee health and safety demands the highest quality medical care for his employees.

It is not in the company's best interest to coerce the physician into sending the patient back to work too early or in any other way rendering less than appropriate medical care. Short-run costs may be avoided, but long-run expenses can be incurred from, for example, re-injury. Also, employees begin to distrust the employer and to become angry and suspicious of both physician and company.[1] This environment is not conducive to patient recovery and return to work, which is the ultimate goal.

It is to the employee's and employer's advantage to have a dedicated occupational physician. The workplace is a unique setting and the physician should be familiar with all plant operations. Knowledge of this sort aids in making accurate return-to-work decisions.

The plant physician must also be familiar with administrative detail that is of utmost importance to the employer.[6] Special forms may be required to document medical care, work restrictions, and follow-up recommendations. Communication between employer and physician is critically important; the company must be informed of a worker's status. For instance, a physician may be inclined to suggest on Friday that an employee return to work on Monday, not knowing that the employee's next scheduled shift begins on Saturday or Sunday. This may seem a minor point, but it can represent substantial cost to a company.

The employer and physician must work together to ensure that the patient (employee) regains full health and productivity. The employee returns to the job with renewed confidence in the company and better relationships with co-workers; the company benefits from heightened employee morale while avoiding downtime, replacement wages, and significant medical costs; and the physician maintains a positive relationship with both parties with confidence that the patient has received the best possible care.

Pre-employment examinations elicit any history of medical conditions that may predispose employees to injury. The physician must be aware that prospective employees always profess to be healthy and rarely admit to past medical problems, especially if they fear being denied the job.[7] A company should be willing to submit a job description so that the physician can evaluate the worker's ability to perform specific job duties.

ROLE OF THE ERGONOMIST

Accident prevention is important in order to spare the trauma, pain, and expense of disabling injuries. Ideally, a qualified ergonomist should assess the planned work before the workplace is designed to engineer out any activities that unduly stress the human body, such as excessive reaching, bending, and stooping.[9]

If assessment is not done at the outset, costly modifications often are required as medical problems emerge.

Other kinds of suggestions offered by industrial engineers might include[9]:

1. Worker rotation—true rotation means designing tasks so that workers use their hands, wrists, and arms equally.

2. Frequent breaks—ideally, workers should break for 5 minutes each hour, rather than once or twice a shift for 15 minutes.

3. Gradual orientation—in job situations requiring continuous repetitive motions, workers should be allowed to work up gradually to full production speed. This is especially important when quotas are demanded and financial incentives are offered.

4. Room temperature—cold temperatures impair hand and finger dexterity.

5. Appropriate job placement—workers should be assigned to tasks they are physically able to perform.

6. Education/training—Instructing employees in the proper use of tools and other equipment is basic to reducing strain on the hands and wrists. Proper hand positioning should be taught and protective equipment, such as gloves, should be provided. Warm-up exercises to enhance flexibility and strength can also be effective.[7]

ESTABLISHING A RETURN-TO-WORK PROGRAM

Return-to-work programs not only provide the employer with active workers; they also benefit the worker by reinforcing self-esteem and removing the psychological effects of inactivity, ultimately assisting in full medical recovery.[4] A company needs to take three basic steps to establish a return-to-work program.[2,10]

Assessment/Planning

To assess the need for a return-to-work program, a company needs to examine its Occupational Safety and Health Administration (OSHA) record-keeping log for incidents involving lost time that could have been avoided with such a program. If a need is demonstrated, the responsibility for planning the program should be assigned to a specific department, usually the personnel or human resources department or the medical unit. The responsible department head should chair a multidisciplinary committee that includes representatives charged with safety, risk management, and production. Both union and management personnel responsible for production should serve on the committee. Jobs with limited physical requirements should be identified. There may be, for example, one-handed tasks or work that does not require stooping, bending, or lifting. Tasks included should be productive ones, not just busywork, which can be a source of resentment for co-workers.

If the availability of "light-duty" tasks is limited, an alternative is to train returning employees who have been injured on the job to conduct programs on safety awareness, first aid, accident prevention, and health promotion. This keeps employees at the worksite and adds a necessary prevention component to the company's program.

The planning committee should clearly define the process the employee is to follow from the time of injury until return to work. It should communicate to all departments, using a flow chart diagram, the steps to be taken if an injury or illness occurs. All employees should be aware of the company's accident-reporting protocol, especially who to notify at the plant. First aid knowledge is essential for all supervisors, who should also know who is the company physician and where the preferred hospitals are located.

The company physician should be consulted as the plan develops. This person's support and cooperation are important. The committee needs to ensure that the company physician will provide specific functional criteria to assist in placing an injured employee in a job that makes limited physical demands. It is important that the health care provider know that the program is operational and that limited duty is available.

It can make a critical difference in attitude if the injured employee is treated with care and concern by the supervisor and other plant managers. The injured employee should be accompanied to the hospital by a company representative. Visits or telephone calls to the home can be helpful in reassuring the employee that he or she is valued.[7]

Implementation

Once the return-to-work policy is in writing and has been approved, departmental meetings should be held to educate all employees regarding the new program. Each employee should receive a copy and ample time should be set aside for questions and answers. Establish a "start" date to commence only after all employees and health care providers are educated.

Evaluation

A careful tracking system is imperative for measuring the program's success. Indicators to gauge effectiveness are[10]:

1. Decrease in lost time
2. Increase in productivity
3. Decrease in workers' compensation costs (medical and disability payments)
4. Increased employee morale
5. Positive feedback from employees, managers, and health care providers

The committee should meet monthly to discuss modifications of the program, as dictated by feedback. The "limited duty" list of jobs and tasks should be continually updated.

CONCLUSION

Workers' compensation claims in Ohio were studied in the early 1980s to identify workplaces at high risk for cumulative trauma disorders.[12] Reported cases of cumulative trauma disorder increased significantly during the study period, in part because workers' and employers' awareness that such disorders may be related to occupation increased. Effective pre-

vention and control of occupational injuries and illnesses is imperative if workers' compensation costs are to be reduced. It is all too common for companies to react to rising costs by implementing or expanding occupational medicine programs. Prudent employers should be active in establishing programs designed to return the injured employee to the workplace and, in so doing, to prevent short-term disabilities from becoming long-term ones.

REFERENCES

1. Bear-Lehman J: Factors affecting return to work after hand injury. Am J Occup Ther 37:189–194, 1983.
2. Centineo JJ: Return-to-work programs: Cut costs and employee turnover. Risk Management Dec 1986:44–48.
3. Dent GL: Curing the disabling effects of employee injury. Risk Management Jan 1985, pp 30–32.
4. Derebery VJ, Tullis WH: Delayed recovery in the patient with a work compensable injury. J Occup Med 25:829–835, 1983.
5. Dougherty E, Hagin D: Occupational health services gain favor for good reason. Health Care Strategic Management Apr 1989:1–22.
6. Holden JM: Occupational medicine: A job for private MDs. Am Med News, March 3, 1989.
7. Kasdan AS, McElwain NP: Return-to-work programs following occupational hand injuries. Occup Med State Art Rev 4:539–545, 1989.
8. Kirshner E: Medical reviewers take aim at workers comp. Managed Health Care Jan 8, 1990:10–21.
9. Michael B: Firms battle carpal tunnel syndrome costs. Business Insurance Sept 24, 1984:20, 22.
10. Randolph SA, Dalton PC: Limited duty work: An innovative approach to early return to work. AAOHN J 37:446–453, 1989.
11. Survey of occupational injuries and illnesses in 1988. Med Benefits 6(24):1–2, Dec 30, 1989.
12. Tanaka S, Seligman P, et al: Use of workers' compensation claims data for surveillance of cumulative trauma disorders. J Occup Med 30:488–492, 1988.

Chapter 35

UNABLE TO RETURN TO WORK—NOW WHAT?

Terri L. Wolfe, O.T.R./L., Mark S. DiPlacido, M.A., and John D. Lubahn, M.D.

Work-related injuries are a major concern for employers throughout the country. *Accident Facts* reports, "Worker's compensation costs due to hand injuries amount to $1.3 billion annually, including hospital and medical costs plus wage compensation."[1] Pasquale, in the *Monthly Business Report* of the Manufacturers Association of Northwestern Pennsylvania, writes, "The average yearly cost of worker's compensation per employee in Pennsylvania is $248."[9] Economic losses from such injuries obviously affect the employer. Employees may also experience pain, inconvenience, and, in certain cases, permanent disability. Since shortly after 1900, when states began enacting Worker's Compensation Act laws, many different attempts have been made to deal with the problem of work-related injuries. Unfortunately, the lack of uniformity from one state to another has created a complex and sometimes confusing problem for all parties involved. Regardless of the specific workers' compensation system, a team approach involving the patient, employer, physician, nurse, therapist (occupational or physical), and rehabilitation counselor provides the best chance for successful rehabilitation and eventual return to work.

The professionals involved in treatment—physician, nurse, therapist(s), counselor—often need to remember that in addition to suffering a physical injury, the patient may also be experiencing financial difficulty and emotional stress. "Just as important, and often ignored, are the personal costs suffered by the injured employee in terms of feelings of self-worth."[6] The physician, physical or occupational therapist, personnel manager at work, and insurance company claims representative must remember these emotional "costs" when dealing with patients with occupational injuries. Unfortunately, at times, "The illness of work incapacity is experienced in a complex sociopolitical climate so laden with anger, invective, vested interest, bureaucracy, costs and profit taking that it serves the affected unevenly and inefficiently."[2]

TEAM APPROACH

In my experience a team-oriented approach is most effective in returning an injured employee to work. The physician must maintain an open mind in dealing with the employer. If "light duty" or appropriate job modification would allow the patient to return to work without risk, then the physician should ask the employer to comply. Employers should be encouraged to provide light-duty work, with the explanation that the longer the employee is off the job, the harder it will be to return to the workplace.[5] By keeping the worker out of the workplace, there is the risk that the worker may assume the role of "professional patient."[11] Open and accurate communication between the medical personnel caring for the patient and the employer is important to verify that the job description is accurate. "A functional job description delineates the physical requirements of a job in order to evaluate a person's capability of performing the duties of that position whether they are a new employee, an established employee moving into a new position, or an injured employee returning to the job."[4] A videotape of the job may be helpful. The patient, physician, therapist, vocational counselor, and rehabilitation nurse may all view the job and determine whether the worker is physically capable of doing the work or whether, after a period of recuperation or training, the worker will be able to do the work.

To bring the injured worker's physical abilities up to the level required by the former job or a less demanding job, or to introduce a worker to a new job, a work hardening program may be beneficial. For the program to succeed, the worker must follow it faithfully and the worker's progress in endurance and strength must be carefully monitored. "Work hardening programs have developed due to a combination of factors including a rise in the number of industrial injury cases and a lack of adequate comprehensive evaluation intervention services that would facilitate time and cost effectiveness in returning the injured worker to work."[8] Work hardening and rehabilitation have become important as the number of persons in the labor force has declined, mandatory retirement has been eliminated, and the cost of supporting injured workers has become prohibitive. A return to work at a functional level as close as possible to the preinjury status should be the ultimate goal. "There is no single hero in rehabilitation. I have never seen a case of successful rehabilitation in which one person was solely responsible," writes Welch.[12] The following case history illustrates the effectiveness of a team approach.

Case Report. A 54-year-old woman was employed for nearly 20 years as a machine operator when she slipped at work, fell, and injured her right shoulder. Conservative management and therapy were successful in returning her to work for approximately 18 months until she reinjured the same shoulder. An arthrogram revealed a rotator cuff tear, and repair with acromioplasty was performed. The patient complied with her postsurgical treatment program and attended therapy on a regular basis. Steady progress was recorded, and the patient and therapist developed a positive rapport and good working relationship. However, when return to work was suggested, the patient began to experience increased symptoms as well as concern about her ability to return to her former position. The rehabilitation coordinator and therapist visited the employer, who was amenable to modifying the worker's position so that she would use only machines that did not require heavy lifting or movement at or above the shoulder. The worker still expressed doubts about her ability to return to work. Only after a fairly lengthy discussion with the rehabilitation coordinator and therapist did the worker indicate that her main concern was her co-workers' reaction to her limited duty. Although she had an excellent work record for nearly 20 years, she felt that she would be singled out by other employees for not "pulling her own weight."

As this example indicates, "the psychosocial aspects of the work environment have been shown to be of utmost importance for the well-being and health of the employees."[13]

With encouragement from the therapist and after the patient discussed her feelings with the personnel manager at her shop, she agreed to resume work. Although she received some negative comments during the first 3 days of her return, the vast majority of her co-workers were supportive. Within 3 weeks' time, she was performing nearly all of her former duties with no increase in symptoms. After 3 months, she was working at her previous job with no restrictions.

It is important in this case that the patient felt comfortable enough with her therapist to reveal her real concerns about returning to work. The willingness of her employer to modify the job, as well as the encouragement she received from her therapist and physician, resulted in a very successful outcome.

Rehabilitation is also most often successful when the professional members of the team involved with the person who has suffered an occupational injury act primarily as patient advocates. The physician who actively tries to understand the type of work and the atmosphere in which the patient works is able to treat the patient more effectively and to make an accurate decision about the patient's ability to return to work. "The physician should bear in mind that his primary responsibility, as in non-work-related injuries, is to the patient."[5] "Thus, the return-to-work determination is a decision laden with liability, both ethical and legal, impacting significantly on each worker's safety and future."[10] The therapist who understands how and why the injury occurred can design a treatment program that will allow the patient to receive maximum benefit and overall recovery.

The rehabilitation nurse coordinator who more fully understands the patient's expectations, concerns, and goals can best counsel the patient should return to the former position be unavailable. Likewise, the medical professional can provide employers a vast amount of information regarding the injured worker and programs that can reduce the likelihood of future injuries.

JOB DESCRIPTION

Many times a physician or therapist receives a written job description of a patient's work duties from the employer. The purpose of this communication is to provide an accurate description of the position so that the physician can decide whether the patient is capable of performing the job in his or her current physical condition. When the physician discusses the job description with the patient, the patient often indicates that the job description is inaccurate or incomplete. I have found that the actual physical requirements of a position often lie somewhere between the written job analysis provided by the employer and the verbal description given by the patient. In these situations, direct contact with the employer is essential in obtaining an accurate account of the physical requirements of a persons' work.

On-site visits by rehabilitation coordinators, nurses, physical and occupational therapists, and involved physicians is becoming commonplace. These evaluations not only provide insight into the physical demands of a patient's job, but also increase the therapist's credibility because he or she learns how to discuss the requirements of a patient's job in language familiar to the patient. This extra effort by the physician and therapist should increase the patient's confidence without compromising the professional's objectivity. To the patient, the physician should appear to be an advocate. The physician should enhance the patient's self-confidence and self-esteem and thereby increase the likelihood of a successful result. "Successful rehabilitation inevitably involves not only the body but the mind and spirit as well."[6]

PERMANENT DISABILITY

Although many patients eventually resume their original jobs, sometimes a worker suffers a compensible injury so severe that returning to the former position is not possible. Examples are the truck driver who suffers a lower back injury and undergoes surgery but is unable to sit for long periods of time; the typist or data processor who develops bilateral carpal tunnel syndrome or an overuse syndrome such as lateral epicondylitis so severe that symptoms recur when return to the same job is attempted; and the production worker in the meat packaging industry who suffers from an overuse syndrome and can no longer effectively use a trimming knife without increased symptoms. These people face the prospect of intolerance of the demands of their former job. Conservative management, such as medication or therapy, often reduces the symptoms but not to the extent that the patient can return to the former position.

The most appropriate and logical option for the therapist, rehabilitation coordinator, or physician in such cases is to attempt to return the worker to the former employer with work restrictions and guidelines provided by the treating physician. These limitations are usually based on some type of functional capacity evaluation. The costs of failure to achieve this level of rehabilitation are staggering.

Employers throughout the country are quickly realizing that the costs of occupational injuries, both on an emotional and a financial basis, are increasing at a drastic rate. For example, the direct and indirect costs of carpal tunnel surgery can be up to $20,000 per case.[7] As a result, the concept of return-to-work programs is gaining more and more credibility. "These programs are no longer luxuries that only the major industries can afford to provide."[5] They are becoming essential to the survival of businesses, both large and small.

When set up and implemented properly, return-to-work programs can provide numerous benefits to both the employees and the company.

1. The costs of worker's compensation premiums and medical expenses are reduced. Physical and occupational therapy or work hardening is generally not needed if patients perform these activities on the job. Vocational rehabilitation costs are eliminated as well when work the patient can do in his or her present condition is found.

2. Employee morale is improved when necessary, productive work that is within the in-

jured worker's physical capabilities is provided.

3. Would-be abusers of the compensation system are discouraged when it is demonstrated that workers are not allowed to enjoy benefits without being accountable in some way. It is important that such a system actually provide work that is productive rather than simply keep the injured worker off compensation. For injured workers to perform meaningless tasks that are personally degrading only increases their feeling of worthlessness and creates morale problems for both them and uninjured employees. Just as important is the fact that return-to-work programs must fall within a physician's restrictions for the returning worker. Occasionally, an employer who promises light duty actually requires the worker to perform his or her regular tasks a few days after returning. Lastly, it must be understood by both the worker and the employer that the worker will return to the former job as soon as he or she is physically able to do the work.

In the case of the injured worker with a permanent disability that precludes return to the former job, the best option may be to seek another position with the original employer. The therapist or rehabilitation coordinator should learn whether the worker has skills that would allow a transfer to a less strenuous position. In cases like these, difficulties arise when union or company policies do not permit movement to less strenuous positions.

An additional benefit of returning an injured worker to his former employer is mutual familiarity. If a suitable position is available, this may be the best solution for employer and employee.

Case Report. A 52-year-old male machine operator over the last 10 years has been in relatively poor general health. His problems have included hypertension and arteriosclerotic cardiovascular disease. Absenteeism was a problem as was abuse of alcohol and tobacco. While operating a machine with pneumatic controls, the worker developed ulnar artery thrombosis in his dominant right hand. Pain and numbness were severe, and he was unable to perform piecework. Ulnar nerve decompression and arterial resection, along with smoking cessation, were effective in reducing his symptoms, but he could not resume normal duties. His employer eventually placed him in a position that did not require the use of pneumatic tools but was repetitive in nature. Unfortunately, the new work aggravated his

symptoms and his job performance was poor. He was in danger of losing his job.

A discussion with his employer led to an alternative position permitting use of his past experience in inspection and shipping and receiving. Heavy lifting is minimal, and the new job does not require rapid repetitive activity of either upper extremity. Although he at times experiences numbness in the small finger and the ulnar side of the ring finger, he has worked regularly at this job for the last 8 months. Both the worker and the employer are satisfied with this resolution. Cooperation on the part of all involved parties was the only means to this success.

RETRAINING

"In the workplace, vocational rehabilitation specifically focuses on the steps needed to return an employee to work after maximal medical recovery has taken place."[5] When a worker is unable to return to a former position and the employer is unable to change or modify a job permanently, another option is training to enable the injured worker to obtain a position within his or her physical limitations. Such retraining allows return to work with the former employer in another job classification. Once it is established that a worker is unable to return to a former position or employer, the workers' compensation insurance carrier or governmental agency may be willing to provide funding for retraining.

Criteria for retraining include the worker's age, physical capabilities, type of retraining, as well as factors such as the amount of compensation received.

Any retraining program, whether it is to return to work for the former employer or to search for a new position, should follow the following basic guidelines.

1. The training should lead to a readily transferable skill. Programs requiring additional courses or schooling before acquisition of skills that lead to gainful employment are generally considered inappropriate. Programs requiring an extended apprenticeship or on-the-job training without pay should also be avoided.

2. Training should be for a position in which the patient is physically capable of performing required duties.

3. Programs should be of reasonable length. Somewhere in the area of 12–18 months is acceptable. Most insurance carriers do not con-

sider a 4-year college education as reasonable or economically feasible.

4. The training program should be reasonable in price. Depending upon the program and the skills that are being taught, insurance companies often are flexible. However, a commitment from the claims representative or authorized personnel must be obtained before the worker is enrolled in any type of program.

Case Report. A 27-year-old woman who caught both hands in a press at work was retrained for a different position with her employer. She suffered an amputation of her dominant right hand at the wrist with concomitant incomplete amputations of the left index and long fingers. Both digits were nonviable and attached only by flexor digitorum profundus tendons (Figs. 1–3).

The right hand was replanted. The left index finger was amputated, and its nerves, arteries, and veins were used as appropriate graft material for salvaging the left long finger. The patient went through an intense and lengthy physical rehabilitation program of 9 months' duration. She was rated as having approximately 40% of normal

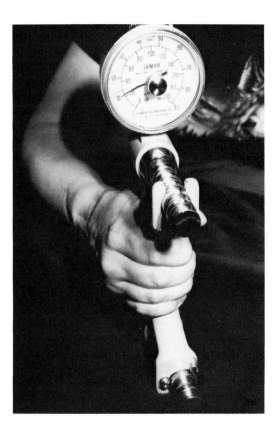

FIGURE 3. Demonstration of strength with a replanted dominant hand.

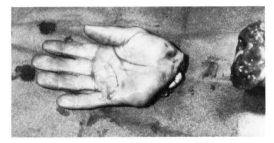

FIGURE 1. Amputated right hand of a 27-year-old worker.

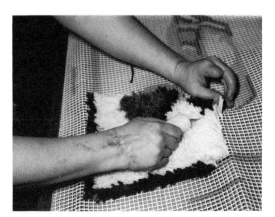

FIGURE 2. The worker in Figure 1 with her right hand replanted and the amputed left index finger used to salvage the left long finger.

function in the right hand and as physically and psychologically incapable of returning to her former job. She entered a 12-month program at a local college and, upon completion of the program, was hired by her former employer to do work using her newly developed skills. She required no further surgery on either hand and has a grip strength of 35 pounds per square inch.

Finally, there is retraining for a transferable skill that is used to locate a position with a different employer. Often, the employee who has suffered an occupational injury experiences significant difficulties in coping with permanent disability. Very often, the insurance carrier or authorized governmental agency allows people to seek counseling in order to assist them through this difficult time. Likewise, before entering a retraining program, the worker may obtain a vocational assessment from an outside agency in order to help assess his or her interests, skills, and aptitudes for areas of retraining. If the physician, physical and occupational therapist, rehabilitation nurse, and rehabilitation coordinator establish a good rapport and working relationship with the employee early on, they can be most helpful in encouraging the worker and providing information regarding alternative career opportunities.

CONCLUSION

The physician and therapist have a special opportunity to support and encourage the worker. They can provide examples of patients who have succeeded from similar situations as theirs and can emphasize the worker's strengths and minimize weaknesses.

These patients are changed physically by the involvement of the physician and therapist, and they come to trust their judgment and skills. Providing an objective and personal perspective of their situation can be a positive influence on their thinking and behavior.

REFERENCES

1. Accident Facts. Chicago, National Safety Council, 1983, p 26.
2. Hadler, NN: Illness in the workplace: The challenge of musculoskeletal symptoms. J Hand Surg 10A:451–456, 1989.
3. Hancock BA, Herrin GD: Monitoring industrial injuries: A case study. J Occup Med 30:43–48, 1988.
4. Isernhagen SJ: Functional job descriptions. Semin Occup Med 2:51–55, 1987.
5. Kasdan AS, McElwain NP: Return-to-work programs following occupational hand injuries. Occup Med State Art Rev 4:539–545, 1989.
6. Kempin LA: Psychological motivation in successful hand therapy. In Hunter JM, Schneider LH, Mackin EJ, Callahan AD (eds): Rehabilitation of the Hand. St. Louis, C.V. Mosby, 1984, p 930.
7. National Institute of Safety & Health Statistics, 1989 (personal correspondence).
8. Ogden-Niemeyer L: Definition and history of work hardening. In Work Hardening: State of the Art. Thorofare, NJ, Charles B. Slack, 1989.
9. Pasquale T: How healthy is workers' comp in Pennsylvania? Manufacturers Association of Northwestern Pennsylvania Monthly Business Rept July 1989:6–12.
10. Schultz-Johnson K: Assessment of upper extremity injured persons' return to work potential. J Hand Surg 12A:950–957, 1989.
11. Schultz-Johnson K: Evaluating the worker's functional capacities for repetitive work. Semin Occup Med 2:31–39, 1987.
12. Welch GT: Why insurance companies are involved in rehabilitation. In Hunter JM, Schneider LH, Mackin EJ, Callahan AD (eds): Rehabilitation of the Hand. St. Louis, C.V. Mosby, 1984, pp 968–970.
13. Wright WL: Psychosocial aspects of the work environment: A group approach. J Occup Med 28:384–393, 1986.

Chapter 36

CUMULATIVE TRAUMA INTERVENTION IN INDUSTRY: A MODEL PROGRAM FOR THE UPPER EXTREMITY

Connie M. Rystrom, B.S, and William W. Eversmann, Jr, M.D.

Prevention of occupational injuries is 1 of 15 prioritized areas identified for improvement by the U.S. Surgeon General. Musculoskeletal disorders resulting from exposure to repetitive motion, vibration, and manual materials handling are listed as the number two research priority by the National Institute for Occupational Safety and Health (NIOSH),[24,32,35,49] the government agency responsible for directing research concerning the nation's occupational disease and injury prevention. Job-related repeated motion disorders of the upper extremity within American service and production industries are becoming more recognized as a potential health epidemic. The U.S. Department of Labor has recently acknowledged a sharp increase in repetitive motion injuries; such disorders as carpal tunnel syndrome and tendinitis account for 48% of all workplace injuries, up from 38% in 1987 and 18% in 1981.[11,22,27] Owing to the insidious nature of cumulative trauma, report of injury by the worker and medical attention given or sought by the employer have heretofore been after the fact. By the time a problem is reported, the condition has often progressed to the point of requiring surgical intervention. Some degree of permanent partial disability and delayed ability or total inability to return to work are not unusual. Delayed problem identification, delayed injury reporting, and delayed

treatment result in higher medical expenses, higher workers' compensation insurance premiums, and increased lost time and productivity to business.

Diagnosis and treatment, important as they are for the restoration of the injured worker to the workplace, cannot, except administratively, address the cause of repetitive motion disorders. Health professionals and employers alike must direct their attention to prevention of repetitive motion disorders to control this upward spiral. The purpose of this chapter is to suggest a multiphase intervention program that has been successfully used in industry to control and reduce repetitive motion disorders.

Traditional approaches to injury reduction in the workplace have focused heavily on ergonomics,[18,19,36] the method of effecting change through manipulation of the physical environment. Work station redesign, tool adaptation, and task modification are the key elements in successful tailoring of a job to the worker performing it. The ergonomic approach validates itself in a growing body of scientific literature and positive outcomes in the work arena. The human-machine interface of ergonomics must be carried from the workplace to the classroom. Worker and management education in ergonomic principles is crucial to any program's success. Education makes ergonomic information more comprehensive. For the worker, it encourages involvement and a responsible attitude toward self and the workplace. For management, it provides the means to independent problem solving and a cornerstone of program perpetuation.

Beyond ergonomics and education, medical consultation broadens the scope of intervention to include active surveillance of the worker population by means of health screens, clinical examinations, and, when indicated, early referral for conservative management. A physician knowledgeable about cumulative trauma disorders and familiar with risks within the workplace is able to treat and rehabilitate injuries optimally for both the worker and the employer.

As part of the medical team, the therapist plays a role that expands beyond the traditional medical model of remediation. Typically therapists deal with people. Their role is to restore health by assisting people to overcome deficiencies and compensate for lost function. Restoration in the workplace involves both tailoring the physical environment to the person and restoring physical capabilities to meet job demands. The occupational therapist, drawing from a specialized background in upper extremity biomechanics, task analysis, and method adaptation is particularly suited to this task.

A reliable medical consultant is often the missing link in intervention efforts. The program presented here encompasses all of these areas—ergonomics, education, and medical consultation—providing a full-circle management approach to cumulative trauma disorders of the upper extremity in the workplace.

PROBLEM IDENTIFICATION

The existence of a problem and the need for intervention are frequently identified by the company. Injury incidence is documented in plant medical records. Incidence may or may not be defined in terms of onset, type of injury, location, worker longevity, and cause. It is not uncommon for an employer to experience an increase in reported injuries after a prolonged period with a stable workforce and little turnover. An increase can also be seen after a period of new employee hiring, institution of a new product line or work operation, or even a change in an established work procedure.

An ideal screening mechanism is capable of identifying all of these parameters. Questionnaires are useful for gathering data. Although questionnaires are probably the most sensitive indicator of the prevalence of cumulative trauma disorders, the literature suggests that screening examinations increase specificity by providing objective confirmation of cumulative trauma.[45] To be most effective, the screening tool should have high sensitivity as well as enable identification of health problems early enough to permit conservative approaches to treatment and control.[13,34,45]

The three-phase surveillance system presented here attempts to offer specificity in terms of population characteristics and exposure, objectivity in physical findings, and sensitivity in identifying early nerve dysfunction.

HEALTH SCREEN

Phase 1—Questionnaire

A medical health questionnaire (see Appendix A) provides the first phase of health screening. The questionnaire enables identification of at-risk workers: those with existing symptoms and those who work in high-risk areas within the plant. Part I obtains identifying information, including name, age, sex, and other items to assist in record-keeping.

Parts II, III, and IV relate to worker exposure. Data from these sections are used in combination with symptoms to target priorities for ergonomic intervention. Questions are designed to gain knowledge of (1) longevity with the company; (2) current work area and responsibilities; (3) work history before and since employment by the company; (4) previous symptoms or treatment; (5) results of treatment; (6) onset, type, duration, and anatomic pattern of current symptoms, if any; (7) precipitating or aggravating activities; (8) lost time and work restrictions; and (9) predisposing medical conditions.

Part V of the questionnaire pertains to symptoms and, in some plants, determines the order in which employees are examined by vibrograms.

While company medical records are a useful indicator of the degree of a problem within the plant, it is erroneous to assume that workers not reporting to the medical department are free of problems. In fact, underreporting is known to occur. Because cumulative trauma disorders develop over time, the onset of symptoms is gradual and not attributable to an accident or specific event. Work-related conditions go unrecognized as such, owing to lack of worker awareness of symptoms and contributing factors. As a result, workers may seek treatment from personal physicians rather than the company medical department. In our experience, a number of workers who report express knowledge of co-workers who experience difficulty and admit to having delayed reporting to avoid surgery. Therefore, screening involves all employees. The plant medical department distributes questionnaires to the entire plant, including production, maintenance, sanitation, shipping, and clerical personnel. Distribution and receipt of questionnaires are logged to ensure that all employees are screened.

Since questions relevant to symptoms are formulated to elicit yes or no responses, break points are easily established. Based on response score, workers are placed in high-, medium-, and low-risk categories with regard to current or potential health problems.

Phase 2—Vibrogram

Because several cumulative trauma syndromes are neuropathic in origin, an objective, noninvasive evaluation of neurological function with a high degree of sensitivity and reproducibility provides an effective surveillance method for workers.[12,34] The digital vibrogram, which measures the amplitude of vibration sensibility at seven frequencies, has proven to be a most sensitive method of evaluating compression neuropathy and a reliable screening technique for use in the workplace. The initial vibrograms are obtained, as questionnaire responses have been, from the entire plant population. In a large facility, the questionnaire has been used to prioritize the order in which vibrograms are obtained, so that employees with the most symptoms are examined first and those with the least symptoms last. After the initial survey, workers at higher risk are re-examined by vibrogram every 3 or 6 months, and the entire plant is re-examined yearly. A pre-employment vibrogram and medical health questionnaire are an important element in determining suitability for work in a repetitive motion job.

The digital vibrogram is evaluated according to the method of Lundborg[29] and graded from 1 to 3, depending on the degree of loss of vibration sensibility at higher frequencies. Using the combined results of the medical health questionnaire and the vibrograms, and subject to the clinical nursing assessment (Phase 3), medical referral for consultation is made as appropriate.

Phase 3—Clinical Examination

Phase 3 of the health screen uses a nursing staff with specific skills in cumulative trauma recognition to clinically examine workers presenting to the plant medical department. The clinical examination supplemented with questionnaire data assists in prioritizing the need for medical referral and alerts the nursing staff to common stresses occurring in a particular area of operation (e.g., a high incidence of lateral epicondylitis among machine operators on a particular work line).

A comprehensive training program for plant nurses by the physician-therapist team precedes inplant examinations. Training requires approximately 5 hours and involves lecture, discussion, demonstration, and practicum evaluation. Course content includes (1) review of upper extremity anatomy and function with respect to joint and ligament structure, peripheral nerves, and muscle tendon function; (2) nerve function with respect to motor and sensory components, common sites of entrapment, stages of neuropathy, and early indicators of dysfunction; (3) typical cumulative trauma disorders in relation to work and leisure activity stresses; (4) conservative management approaches including modalities, splinting, and activity modification; and (5) clinical examination.

The clinical examination is specifically directed at identifying the eight common cumulative trauma disorders (Table 1). The four

TABLE 1. Clinical Examination

Nerve	Tendon
Carpal tunnel syndrome	De Quervain's tenosynovitis of first dorsal compartment
Ulnar tunnel syndrome	Stenosing tenosynovitis of flexor tendon sheath
Cubital tunnel syndrome	Intersection syndrome of second dorsal compartment
Radial tunnel syndrome	Lateral epicondylitis at the elbow

nerve syndromes having in common percussion sensitivity over the nerve also each have a provocative position test such as Phalen's sign, elbow flexion test, or flexor-pronator sign to help confirm the diagnosis.[11] Because each nurse-examiner has a working knowledge of the pertinent upper extremity anatomy, the assessment of the tendon syndromes using localized tenderness over the involved tendon mechanism,[47] crepitus with tendon function, provocative tests such as Finkelstein's test,[14] the intersection syndrome sign or the extensor carpi radialis brevis strength sign can be taught with some assurance that an informed diagnosis may be made.

A vital function in the clinical assessment requires the examiner to correlate the worker's reports of discomfort with his or her work motions so that flexion and extension motions of the wrist can be related to carpal tunnel, ulnar tunnel, and intersection syndromes; elbow flexion and extension to cubital tunnel syndrome; and even ulnar deviation of the wrist to de Quervain's tenosynovitis. These correlations are helpful in making appropriate modifications in work activity to prevent recurrence of problems in the same or other workers.

The importance of trained, reliable plant medical personnel cannot be overemphasized. In our experience, nursing personnel provide a vital link in the coordinated intervention effort. Risk magnitude and demographics (injury type, work location, longevity) frequently surface in medical information. Medical personnel knowledgeable about specific workplace cumulative trauma risks and capable of appropriately evaluating physical complaints in relation to work stresses are able to interpret medical data to assist in targeting ergonomic priorities. Appropriate job assignment to minimize exacerbation of an existing condition or ease re-entry of a recovering injured worker can be advised. Nurses are able to offer counseling regarding potentially hazardous work methods, providing a source of ongoing plant education.

ERGONOMIC INTERVENTION

Health screening data (Fig. 1) facilitate investigation of plant operations by analysis with respect to incidence, frequency, and severity[41,45] of cumulative trauma and are used to target ergonomic priorities. The focus of job intervention based on analysis of population screening should be carefully determined to ensure accurate problem identification and realistic direction for ergonomic efforts.

Ergonomics is a science that seeks to adapt work and the working environment to human capabilities. As such, ergonomics deals with the complex set of interacting human and environmental variables. The ergonomic approach is based largely on the assumption that work activities involving less recognized risk factors are less likely to cause injuries or disorders. Ergonomics seeks to make safe work practices the natural result of tool and workplace design. The goal of ergonomic evaluation is to identify potentially hazardous job elements and reduce risk of injury by tailoring the work to the worker and, conversely, individual capabilities to work demands. In other words, ergonomically designed tools and jobs modify work demands so that a majority of the population can complete the jobs assigned without risk of injury.

The purpose of this section is to cite factors known to contribute to upper extremity cumulative trauma disorders, to present our preferred method of workplace evaluation, and to discuss key considerations for implementing changes in the workplace.

Upper Extremity Risk Factors

Cumulative trauma disorders in soft tissues of the upper extremity are a class of disorders caused, precipitated, or aggravated by tasks requiring repeated or sustained exertions in combination with high forces and nonneutral arm and hand postures.[2,4,47] Specific conditions include tendinitis, tenosynovitis, de Quervain's tenosynovitis, trigger finger, carpal or ulnar tunnel syndrome, cubital tunnel syndrome, and lateral epicondylitis.

Occupational hazards identified by Armstrong and others[5,24,42] include:

1. Repetitive or sustained exertions
2. Forceful exertions
3. Stressful, mechanically inefficient postures including extremes of reach, forearm rotation, wrist flexion, extension, and ulnar deviation
4. Mechanical stresses created by tools held in the hand or soft tissue contact with hard, sharp edges of objects or materials
5. Low temperatures causing physiological stiffness in soft tissue, reduction in circulation, and impaired sensibility

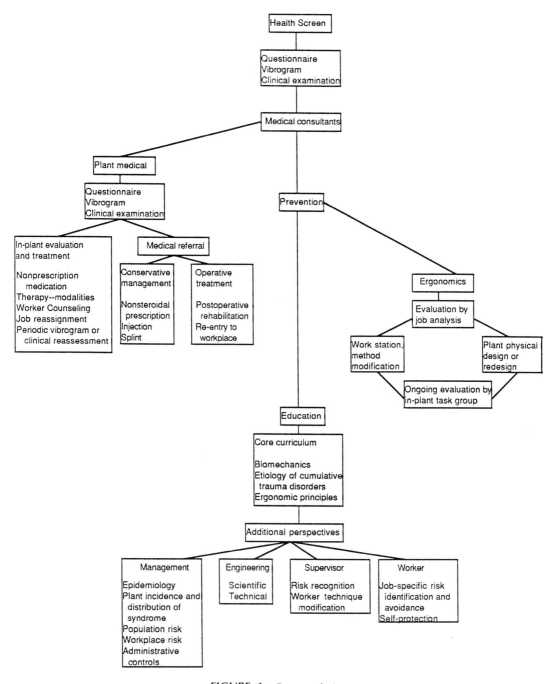

FIGURE 1. Program design.

6. Vibration resulting in soft tissue micro-trauma, scarring, and reduced circulation

7. Poorly designed work stations and methods resulting in potentially injurious work postures requiring a higher degree of work intensity by creating a mechanical disadvantage for the worker

8. Use of gloves

Job Analysis

A variety of evaluation methods are available for job analysis. Important factors need to be considered before a method is selected. From a practical standpoint, the analysis method should be noninvasive, performable in the workplace, and preferably inexpensive. It must be reliable (i.e., yield the same results on repeated application) and lend itself to relevant, practical, and comprehensive interpretations and conclusions.[6]

We prefer a two-stage process of job analysis—task analysis followed by risk identification. Task analysis involves identification of the component parts or series of steps required to perform a job. A "job" may involve a single operation performed by one worker, as in "chain" production line operations, or like tasks performed by several workers simultaneously. Each step is described by the movement involved or the act performed (i.e., reach, grasp box, place box on station, fold flaps, invert box). It is helpful to observe several workers perform the same operation to note individual differences in technique, sequencing, and rate. Frequently, the same job performed by different workers presents varying degrees of risk simply by virtue of work style and technique. Videotaping for later review is helpful to evaluate work technique.

Pertinent force, rate, and distance measurements on each worker or on several workers performing the same job are obtained to gain an impression of risk relative to physical capabilities and individual technique. After work content and requirements have been determined, each task component is analyzed to identify the existence of recognized risk factors; then recommendations are formulated.

Implementation

Recommendations for change must be made with careful consideration. Recommendations must be cost-effective, feasible, and practical. In our experience, often major risk reductions can be obtained through relatively simple, inexpensive adjustments. Many times major stresses are completely eliminated as a result of minor changes.[4] Changes that do not entail major financial implications in terms of time, equipment, and productivity costs are readily accepted and implemented. However, more costly equipment and redesign of tools and physical work stations when they are cost-effective should not be overlooked. In instances where risk factors are combined with a history of repetitive trauma disorders among workers, cost-effectiveness is readily measured.[28,44] Change is relatively inexpensive when compared to the cost of injury. Whatever the change, its cost-effectiveness is borne out in measurable injury reduction.

The most easily implemented changes involve modification of job tasks, worker redistribution, and technique modification, the latter being dependent upon thorough training of workers along with the commitment and cooperation of supervisors.

A number of risk factors can be reduced through appropriately designed task modification. Repetitiveness is often reduced by rate equalization among production line workers, combining or resequencing of job components, task reassignment, worker redistribution, worker rotation among different jobs, increasing the variety of tasks, and expanding available work time (i.e., rate reduction). The employer may initially regard rate reduction, which has obvious productivity implications, with considerable reservation. However in our experience it has been a key intervention, particularly in machine-paced assembly-type operations. Any element of successful job modification in these operations is difficult, if not impossible, without rate reduction.

Because acceptable exposure levels to repetitive risk have yet to be determined,[4,24,41] the ergonomist must rely upon suggestive scientific data when establishing rate recommendations. These include muscle recovery time as a function of holding time, intensity of effort in relation to duration of continuous work, force exertion with respect to physical properties of the object being handled, type of grip, arm and wrist posture, hand span, and whether gloves are used.[6,26,41]

Force and postural stresses are reduced by work station redesign as well as by task modification. Forceful exertions are minimized by tool or object redesign to lessen weights and produce optimal mechanical advantage.[2] Work station redesign controls posture by putting needed items within safe reaching distances and allowing work to be performed with the arm at the side, forearms in neutral rotation, and wrists in neutral deviation. Task modification minimizes force and postural stress by reducing the number of items handled and distributing work loads over large body parts or a combination of joints. Examples include grasping with the entire hand instead of pinching; lifting with two hands rather than one; and bearing the weight of large objects along forearms rather than fingers when carrying.

It should be noted that task modification relies heavily on technique, for which worker compliance is essential. Successful technique modification depends upon worker involvement in the ergonomic correction. *Job-specific* worker education and training are essential.

Worker redistribution is an effective means of dispersing work stresses while using manpower optimally. In many plants, adding workers to dilute stresses is a costly solution. Counseling, combining or eliminating job tasks, and redistributing displaced workers offer alternatives for efficient use of manpower.

Worker rotation is an important intervention. Rotating workers among a variety of tasks reduces stress. Intermittent intense work with short (1–2 minute) breaks alternated with intense efforts is a more efficient work pattern than sustained intense work with longer (15–20 minute) rest periods.[42] Ergonomic evaluation can identify relative work requirements of a specific job or component task. Rotation schedules and patterns can be designed to allow periods of lighter effort interspersed with jobs requiring heavier effort. The feasibility of worker rotation depends on skill levels required for the operations as well as on constraints imposed by union labor grades and job classifications. Worker rotation has been possible in unionized plants, however often with less than the desired latitude.

EDUCATION

Although the success and effectiveness of training programs in reducing musculoskeletal injuries has yet to be clearly substantiated,[25] the NIOSH strategy for reducing musculoskeletal injuries includes training in its suggestions for intervention in jobs where high physical demands pose a risk to the musculoskeletal system.[32,35] The strategy asserts the need to broaden training beyond fundamental issues of safe work practices. It suggests involvement of both management and workers in training designed toward recognition of job hazards and development of the necessary problem-solving skills to participate in hazard control activities.[48]

intervention program concurrent with health screening and ergonomics. The goal of the education phase is to develop in-house ergonomic knowledge at all levels of participation (administration, design, and production) to enable problem recognition and solution. Education provides the foundation for extending the ergonomic effort throughout the plant.

Plant personnel constitute a diverse group. People within the plant have widely varying industrial experience along with varying types and levels of abilities, educational backgrounds, focus, and function relative to position held. Accordingly, education sessions are conducted separately for:

1. Management (plant manager, operations, maintenance, safety and loss control, industrial relations, medical, quality control, marketing, area superintendents)
2. Engineering and design personnel
3. Supervisors (line)
4. Workers

Program content and focus are tailored to each group, and elements pertinent to the interests and function of the participants are emphasized (see Figure 1). Appropriate discussions of anatomy, biomechanics, contributing factors, and ergonomic principles are included in all presentations.

Various training methods are used. Lectures are practical in that large amounts of information can be presented to large groups of people, and content can be structured to accommodate the specific needs of the group. Visual aids such as slides, transparencies, and videotapes enhance lecture material by illustrating concepts and providing examples occurring within the plant. High-speed still photography of work operations is especially helpful; we prefer still pictures to highlight motion risks otherwise obscured in high-rate operations. Anatomical models and props (tools, packaging materials, gloves) can also be demonstrated.

Lectures have been shown to be effective in increasing participants' knowledge of ergonomics, especially when principles are illustrated with anecdotes from personal experience.[38,43,44] It is extremely important to present information in such a way that it can be readily transferred to the workplace. It would be superfluous to instruct the hourly worker about biomechanical force generation in relation to mass and coefficient of friction. A more relevant approach would emphasize use of power grip rather than pinch or selection of gloves that fit properly to reduce hand stress. The former information should be reserved for engineers and those involved in job design.

Management

Education of management includes a broader range of ergonomic issues in comparison to the other groups. Program content includes scope of cumulative trauma disorders in terms of prevalence, incidence, and cost to employers, surveillance approaches for control of injuries within the plant, medical management alternatives for existing injuries, possibilities for re-entry of workers after injury, productivity implications created by change, feasibility of recommendations, labor union issues, and administrative controls such as preselection screening, job placement, job modification, and job rotation.

Input from participants assists in developing a strategy for consultation. Periodic management sessions have been helpful to update on intervention progress and direct or redirect efforts as circumstances dictate.

Engineering and Design Personnel

Industrial and mechanical engineers and design staff are key players in ergonomic change. Workplace design influences body postures during the job, force required for tool use and materials handling, rate, temperature, and vibration. Engineers must be included in ergonomics education to achieve the desired change in existing and new operations. The focus here is to introduce the human element into the existing scientific and technical knowledge base. Topics covered include:[31,36,41]

1. Exertional forces relative to body part being used, direction of movement, size and shape of objects handled
2. Work surface heights in relation to posture
3. Speed pacing in relation to individual performance capabilities
4. Handle designs (curve, length, size, and texture) to maximize strength capability
5. Physiological effect of vibration and thermal conductivity of materials
6. Maximal safe reach and lift parameters
7. Task variety and opportunity for rest
8. Gloves
9. Assistive devices to minimize force and postural stresses

Successful participation in ergonomic redesign requires a sometimes difficult shift in the traditional engineering time-cost-productivity frame of reference.

Supervisors

Education of supervisors emphasizes recognizing and avoiding risks. Program content is focused on developing participants' capability to critique work operations and worker methods. Job-specific examples are used to assist in identifying hazardous motions or postures, excessive forces, and improper gloves. Participation is encouraged for exchange of ideas and group problem solving. When they are able to identify job hazards occurring in their own area, supervisors can facilitate safe work practices on a day-to-day basis. Examples include ensuring proper tool use and choice of gloves, structuring rotation schedules to disperse stresses, controlling material placement, and offering feedback to workers.

Worker training is seen as a primary role of the supervisor. Effective training requires the supervisor's commitment to safety, positive working relationships with employees, and knowledge of learning styles and training methods. The latter often treads new territory in the production industry and has been best addressed by follow-up sessions. The supervisor's role in the intervention effort is a difficult one because this person is in the unenviable position of balancing the often opposing forces of production incentives and accountability for safety.

Workers

Education of workers incorporates three key elements: (1) recognition of the importance of self-protection and responsibility for personal safety, (2) risk recognition and avoidance, and (3) job-specific training.

Resistance to change is inherent in human nature. Among workers, that resistance is heightened when the rationale for change is not clearly defined or when an element of force by superiors is perceived. From this standpoint, worker involvement in the ergonomic effort is crucial.[28,38] The responsibility for worker safety must be shared by both employers and employees. In instances where employer ergonomic intervention affords the opportunity for safe work practices, responsibility for self-protection (through use of recommended work methods or job redesign) shifts largely to the worker. An involved work force is more likely to accept changes and to offer valuable contributions to the overall program. Responsibility for self, at work and away, is a major emphasis of worker education sessions.

Education initially takes place in the classroom. Workers are grouped for sessions according to work area or job operation to allow discussion of job-specific risks and avoidance identified by ergonomic analysis. Focus is on recognition of hazardous motions and activities and work habits to be avoided. Application to home and leisure activities is discussed as well.

The goal of job-specific education is to enhance retention of information and facilitate transfer of learned material into the workplace.[41] In the workplace, education becomes training, and focus shifts from acquisition of knowledge to acquisition of skill.

When ergonomic redesign of tools or work station layout has eliminated risks, little training is required beyond ensuring use consistent with intent. Risk reduction in operations less amenable to physical redesign, on the other hand, requires considerable attention to modifying technique. In addition to overcoming undesirable habits, workers must often learn new methods for accomplishing familiar tasks. Learning new motor skills requires practice. The rate of learning is greater when feedback is given during performance.[41,44] Area supervisors are key figures in training workers in technique. Supervisors must be available to provide immediate positive feedback during on the job learning. In addition, workers must be monitored to ensure practice of learned skills and transfer of skills to new situations. The amount of training necessary for a worker to develop new skills depends on the difficulty of the task, the ability of the trainee, and the ability of the trainer. Supervisor commitment and appropriately focused supervisor education are essential for successful worker training.

TASK FORCE

Ergonomics is a multidisciplinary science requiring effective input from a variety of diverse specialties both inside and outside the organization. At present, ergonomics is not adequately incorporated into the workplace.[28] A common barrier is a management attitude favoring the "quick fix" or "Band-Aid" approach rather than investing the time, manpower, and dollars necessary to implement a full-scale intervention. Communication breakdown among disciplines within the organization, self-interest or noncommitment of a work group, and a general lack of ergonomic and job knowledge

among a portion of the organization important to ergonomic decision making also interfere.

One approach to overcoming these barriers is use of a cross-functional ergonomic task force. Such groups bring together representatives from the various disciplines needed for sound ergonomic design. Research suggests that group decision making is an effective method for effecting technical change.[25,28,38] The ergonomic task force is participative and largely uses in-house expertise. Thorough education to provide ergonomic knowledge is a necessary precursor to group formation. A concerted effort must be made to involve representatives from all levels of the organization: engineering, operations, industrial relations, safety, medical, quality control, marketing, maintenance, production, area supervisors, employee (union), and consultant.

The task force functions to:
1. Identify problems
2. Prioritize areas for intervention
3. Contribute alternative solutions
4. Formulate action plans
5. Charge responsibility for action
6. Review progress and make recommendations
7. Charge responsibility for implementation
8. Conduct follow-up evaluation and make final recommendation
9. Ensure ongoing monitoring of changes

It is important to assign the task force management priority to facilitate consistent attendance at meetings. Poor attendance adversely affects group performance and movement toward goals. Meetings should be scheduled regularly (at least quarterly) and should allot adequate time to cover appointed topics. The group is best structured with an appointed chairperson responsible for scheduling, notification of members, and coordination of meeting agendas.

A well-organized task force with involved participants can address several needs concurrently. Task groups ensure that ergonomics remains a component of the organization's safety program.

CONCLUSION

A well-designed program for cumulative trauma intervention must identify the nature and extent of the problem through health screening and address the problem with an ongoing treatment program of existing disorders. A continuing program managed by the plant medical personnel to evaluate newly identified workers with cumulative trauma symptoms is key to prevention. Our prevention model is based on a detailed program of education founded with a core curriculum for all plant personnel and continued with additional and specific prospectives for management, engineering, line supervisor personnel, and the work force itself. This education program is interfaced with detailed evaluation, by job analysis using ergonomic principles, of individual work stations as well as the plant and its physical design as a whole. The ongoing ergonomic evaluation of the workplace is continued through the formation of an in-plant task group to continue cumulative trauma prevention in the workplace and appropriate changes in the work environment. Through this detailed program a reduction in cumulative trauma cases within the work force, a reduction of surgical treatment needed to resolve those cases, and a reduction of work days lost because of cumulative trauma disorders can be anticipated. An elimination of cumulative trauma from an industrial work force, as we understand it in this country today, is probably not feasible. In clinical experience, however, a meaningful reduction of more than 50% is achievable.

Note

The multiphase program presented here has been instituted within a major U.S. bakery. Various phases of the program have been initiated concurrently since 1987 in six plants across the country. Over a 3-year period one plant alone reported a 64% reduction in medical cases, a 55% reduction in lost work days, and an estimated cost savings of at least $1.5 million.

REFERENCES

1. Armstrong T: An Ergonomics Guide to Carpal Tunnel Syndrome. Akron, Ohio, American Industrial Hygiene Association, 1983.
2. Armstrong TJ: Ergonomics and cumulative trauma disorders, Hand Clin 2:553–565, 1986.
3. Armstrong TJ, Fine LJ, Silverstein BA: Occupational Risk Factors of Cumulative Trauma Disorders of the Hand and Wrist: A Final Report. National Institute for Occupational Safety and Health, contract no. 200-82-2507, Cincinnati, OH, 1985.
4. Armstrong TJ, Foulke J, Joseph B, Goldstein S: An investigation of cumulative trauma disorders in a poultry processing plant. Am Ind Hyg Assoc J 43:103–116, 1932.
5. Armstrong TJ, Radwin RG, Hansen DJ, Kennedy, KW: Repetitive trauma disorders: Job evaluation and design. Hum Factors 28:325–336, 1986.
6. Barnes R: Motion and Time Study: Design and Measurement of Work. New York, John Wiley, 1972.
7. Bleecker ML: Vibration perception thresholds in entrapment and toxic neuropathies. J Occup Med 28:991–994, 1986.
8. Browne CD, Nolan BM, Faithful DK: Occupational repetitive strain injuries: Guidelines for diagnosis and management. Med J Aust 140:329–332, 1984.
9. Chaffin DB, Andersson G: Occupational Biomechanics. New York, Wiley-Interscience, 1984.
10. Dellon AL: Clinical use of vibratory stimuli to evaluate peripheral nerve injury and compression neuropathy. Plast Reconstr Surg 65:466–476, 1980.
11. Eversmann WW Jr: Entrapment and compression neuropathies. In Green DP (ed): Operative Hand Surgery. New York, Churchill Livingstone, 1983.
12. Feldman RG, Goldman R, Keyserling WM: Peripheral nerve entrapment syndromes and ergonomic factors. Am J Ind Med 4:661–681, 1983.
13. Fine L, Silverstein BA, Armstrong TJ, Anderson CA: Detection of cumulative trauma disorders of the upper extremities in the work place. J Occup Med 28:674–678, 1986.
14. Finkelstein H: Stenosing tendovaginitis at the radial styloid process. J Bone Joint Surg 12:509–540, 1930.
15. Forimson A: Tenosynovitis and tennis elbow. In Green DP (ed): Operative Hand Surgery. New York, Churchill Livingstone, 1983.
16. Gelberman R, Szabo R, Williamson R, Dimick M: Sensibility testing in peripheral-nerve compression syndromes. J Bone Joint Surg 62A:632–638, 1983.
17. Goldman R: General occupational health history and examination. J Occup Med 28:966–974, 1986.
18. Grandjean E: Fitting the Task to the Man: An Ergonomic Approach. London, Taylor and Francis, 1980.
19. Hackman JR, Oldham GR: Work Redesign, Reading, MA, Addison Wesley, 1980.
20. Hall DT, Bowen DD, Lewiciki RJ, Hall FS: Experiences in Management and Organizational Behavior, 2nd ed. New York, John Wiley, 1982.
21. Herberts P, Kadefors R, Broman H: Arm positioning in manual tasks: An electromyographic study of localized muscle fatigue. Ergonomics 23:655–665, 1980.
22. Hershenson A: Cumulative trauma: A national problem. J Occup Med 21:674–676, 1979.
23. Hymovich L, Lindholm M: Hand, wrist and forearm injuries—The results of repetitive motions. J Occup Med 8:573–577, 1966.
24. Iserhagen SJ: Work Injury Prevention and Management. Rockville, MD, Aspen, 1988.
25. Joseph BS: Analysis of a Program for Control of Cumulative Trauma Disorders in the Auto Industry. ACGIH Publication, 1987.
26. Kelly JE: Scientific Management, Job Redesign and Work Performance. London, Academic Press, 1982.
27. Kilborn PT: Department of Labor report: Rise in worker injuries is laid to the computer. New York Times, Nov 16, 1989.
28. Liker JK, Joseph BS, Armstrong TJ: From ergonomic theory to practice: organizational factors affecting the utilization of ergonomic knowledge. In Hendrick HW, Brown O Jr (eds): Human Factors in Organizational

Design and Management. Amsterdam, North-Holland, 1984.

29. Lundborg G, Lie-Stenstrom A, Sollerman C, et al: Digital vibrogram: A new diagnostic tool for sensory testing in compression neuropathy. J Hand Surg 11A:693–699, 1986.

30. Luopajarvi T, Kuorinka I, Virolainen V, Holmberg M: Prevalence of tenosynovitis and other injuries of the upper extremities in repetitive work. Scand J Work, Environ Health 5(suppl 3):48–55, 1979.

31. McKenzie F, Storment J, Von Hook P, Armstrong TJ: A program for control of repetitive trauma disorders associated with hand tool operation in a telecommunications manufacturing facility. Am Ind Hyg Assoc J 46:674–678, 1985.

32. Millar JD, Myers MD: Occupational safety and health: Progress toward the 1990 objectives for the nation. Public Health Rep 98:324–336, 1983.

33. Moberg E: Objective methods for determining the functional value of sensibility of the hand. J Bone Joint Surg 40(13):454–476, 1958.

34. Moody L, Arezzo J, Otto D: Screening occupational population for a symptomatic or early peripheral neuropathy. J Occup Med 28:975–986, 1986.

35. National Institute for Occupational Safety and Health: A proposed national strategy for the prevention of musculoskeletal injuries. In Proposed National Strategies for the Prevention of Leading Work-Related Diseases and Injuries, pt 1. Washington DC: Association of Schools of Public Health, 1986, pp 17–34.

36. Nordin M, Frankel VH: Evaluation of the Work Place: An Introduction. Clin Orthop 221:85–88, 1987.

37. Occupational disease surveillance: Carpal tunnel syndrome, JAMA 262:000–000, 1989.

38. Pasmore W, Friedlander F: An action research program for increasing employee involvement in problem solving. Admin Sci Q 27:343–362, 1982.

39. Phalen G: The carpal tunnel syndrome: Clinical evaluation of 598 hands. Clin Orthop 83:29–40, 1972.

40. Punnett L, Robins JM, Wegman DH, Keyserling WM: Soft tissue disorders in the upper limbs of female garment workers. Scand J Work Environ Health 11:417–425, 1985.

41. Rodgers SH: Ergonomic Design for People at Work. New York, Van Nostrand Reinhold, 1986.

42. Rodgers SH: Matching Worker and Worksite—Ergonomic Principles, Work Injury Prevention and Management. Rockville, MD, Aspen, 1988, pp 65–79.

43. Seashore SE, Lawler EE III, Mirvis PH, Cammann C: Assessing Organizational Change, A Guide to Methods, Measures and Practices. New York, John Wiley, 1984.

44. Sell RG: Success and failure in implementing changes in job design. Ergonomics 23:809–816, 1980.

45. Silverson BA: Patterns of Cumulative Trauma Disorders in Industry. Proceedings from 1989 Engineering Summer Conferences, University of Michigan, College of Engineering.

46. Silverstein BA, Fine LJ, Armstrong TJ: Hand and wrist cumulative trauma disorders in industry. Br J Ind Med 43:779–784, 1986.

47. Travers PH: Soft tissue disorders of the upper extremities. In Himmelstein JS, Pransky GS: Worker Fitness and Risk Evaluations. Occup Med State Art Rev 3:271–282, 1988.

48. US Public Health Service: Promoting Health/Preventing Diseases: Objectives for the Nation. US Department of Health, Education and Welfare, 1980.

49. US Public Health Service: Prevention '82. US Department of Health and Human Services, Office of Disease Prevention and Health Promotion, DHHS publication no. 82-51057, 1982.

50. Wells MJ: Industrial incidence of soft tissue syndromes. Phys Ther Rev 41:512–515, 1961.

51. Westgaard RH, Aaras A: The effect of improved work place design on the development of work-related musculoskeletal illnesses. Appl Ergon June 1985, pp 91–97.

52. Wilson R, Wilson S: Tenosynovitis in industry. Practitioner 178:612–625, 1957.

ADDITIONAL READING

1. Accident Facts: Chicago: National Safety Council, 1975.

2. Amis AA, Dowson D, Wright V: Analysis of elbow forces due to high-speed forearm movements. J Biomech 13:825–831, 1980.

3. Armstrong T: Development of biomechanical hand model for study of manual activities. In Easterby R, Kroemer KHE, Chaffin DB (eds): Arthropometry and Biomechanics: Theory and Application. New York, Plenum, 1982, pp 183–192.

4. Armstrong TJ: An ergonomics guide to carpal tunnel syndrome. Am Ind Hyg Assoc J, 1983.

5. Armstrong T, Castelli W, Evans F, et al: Some histological changes in carpal tunnel contents and their biomechanical implications. J Occup Med 26:179–201, 1984.

6. Armstrong TJ, Chaffin DB: An investigation of the relationship between displacements of the finger and wrist joints and the extrinsic finger flexor tendons. J Biomech 11:119–128, 1978.

7. Armstrong T, Chaffin D: Some biomechanical aspects of the carpal tunnel. J Biomech 12:267–570, 1979.

8. Armstrong TJ, Chaffin DB, Foulke JA: A methodology for documenting hand positions and forces during manual work. J Biomech 12:131–133, 1979.

9. Astrand PO, Rodahl K: Textbook of Work: Physiological Basis of Exercise. New York, McGraw-Hill, 1977.

10. Ayoub MA, Ayoub MM, Ramsey JD: A stereometric system for measuring human motion. Hum Factors 12:523–535, 1970.

11. Ayoub M, Presti P: The determination of an optimum size cylindrical handle by use of electromyography. Ergonomics 14:509, 1971.

12. Bjelle A, Hagberg M, Michaelsson G: Clinical and ergonomic factors in prolonged shoulder pain among industrial workers. Scand J Work Environ Health 5:205–210, 1979.

13. Brain WA, Wright A, Wilkinson M: Spontaneous compression of both median nerves in the carpal tunnel. Lancet 1:277–282, 1947.

14. Brammer A, Taylor W: Vibration Effects on the Hand and Arm in Industry. New York, Wiley, 1982.

15. Cannon LJ, Bernacki EJ, Walter SD: Personal and occupational factors associated with carpal tunnel syndrome. J Occup Med 23:255–258, 1981.

16. Chaffin D: Localized muscle fatigue—Definition and measurement. J Occup Med 15:346–354, 1973.

17. Chaffin DB: Ergonomics guide for the assessment of human static strength. Am Ind Hyg Assoc J 35:505–510, 1975.

18. Chaffin DB, Armstrong TJ: Carpal tunnel syndrome and selected personal attributes. J Occup Med 21:481–486, 1979.

19. Chaffin D, Herrin G, Keyserling M: Preemployment strength testing: An updated position. J Occup Med 20:403, 1978.

20. Chaffin DB, Herrin GD, Keyserling WM, Garg A: A method for evaluating the biomechanical stresses resulting from manual materials handling jobs. Am Ind Hyg Assoc J 38:662–675, 1977.

21. Chaffin DB, Lee M, Freivalds F: Muscle strength assessment for EMG analysis. Med Sci Sports Exerc 12:205–211, 1980.

22. Chao E, Opgrande J, Axmear F: Three-dimensional force analysis of finger joints in selected isometric hand functions. J Biomech 9:387–396, 1976.

23. Chapanis A: Research Techniques in Human Engineering. Baltimore, Johns Hopkins University Press, 1959.

24. Clark R: The limiting hand skin temperature for unaffected manual performance in the cold. J Appl Psychol 45:193–194, 1961.

25. Conklin J, White W: Stenosing tenosynovitis and its possible relation to carpal tunnel syndrome. Surg Clin North Am 40:531, 1960.

26. Conn H: Tenosynovitis. Ohio State Med J 27:713–716, 1931.

27. Corlett N, Bishop R: The ergonomics of spot welders. Appl Ergonom 9:23, 1978.

28. Davis PR, Stubbs DA: Safe levels of manual forces for young males. Appl Ergonom 8(pt1): 141–150, 1977a; 8(2):219–228, 1977b; 9(3):33–37, 1978a.

29. de Quervain F: Ueber eine form von chronischer tendovaginitis. Cor Bl Schweiz Aerzte (Basel) 25:389–394, 1895.

30. DeVries H: Method for evaluation of muscle fatigue and endurance from electromyographic fatigue curve. Am J Phys Med 47:125, 1968.

31. Dobyns J, O'Brien E, Linscheid R, et al: Bowler's thumb: Diagnosis and treatment. J Bone Joint Surg 54A:751–755, 1972.

32. Eversmann WW Jr, Ritsick JA: Intraoperative changes in motor nerve conduction latency in carpal tunnel syndrome. J Hand Surg 3:77–81, 1978.

33. Ferguson D: Repetitive injuries in process workers. Med J Aust 2:408–412, 1971.

34. Finkel ML: The effects of repeated mechanical trauma in the meat industry. Am J Ind Med 8:375–379, 1985.

35. Flatt AE: Kinesiology of the hand. American Academy of Orthopaedic Surgeons Instructional Course Lectures, Vol 50. St. Louis, C.V. Mosby, 1961, pp 902–1013.

36. Garrett JW: Clearance and Performance Values for the Bare-Handed and the Pressure-Gloved Operator. AMRL Technical Report 68–24. Wright-Patterson AFB, Ohio: Aeromedical Research Laboratory, 1968, pp 82–93.

37. Gelberman RH, Hergenroeder PT, Hargens AR, et al: The carpal tunnel syndrome. A study of carpal canal pressures. J Bone Joint Surg 63A:380–383, 1981.

38. Goldie I: Epicondylitis lateralis humeri: A pathogenetical study. Acta Chir Scand Suppl 339:119, 1964.

39. Gowitzke BA, Milnar M: Understanding the Scientific Basis of Human Movement, 2nd ed. Baltimore, Williams and Wilkins, 1980.

40. Greenberg L, Chaffin DB: Workers and Their Tools. A Guide to the Ergonomic Design of Hand Tools and Small Presses, Midland, MI, Pendell, 1977.

41. Hadler NM: Industrial rheumatology: Clinical investigations into the influence of the pattern of usage on the pattern of regional musculo-skeletal disease. Arth Rheum 20(4):1019–1025, 1977.

42. Hadler N, Gillings D, Imbus H, et al: Hand structures and function in industrial setting. Arthritis Rheum 21:219, 1978.

43. Hammer A: Tenosynovitis. Med Rec 140:353–355, 1934.

44. Hansen NS: Effects on health of monotonous, forced-pace work in slaughterhouses, J Soc Occup Med 32:180–184, 1982.

45. Harris CM, Tanner E, Goldstein MN, Pettee DS: The surgical treatment of carpal tunnel syndrome correlated with preoperative nerve conduction studies. J Bone Joint Surg 61A, 1979.

46. Hasan J: Biomedical aspects of low-frequency vibration: A selective review. Work Environ Health 6:19–45, 1970.

47. Hazelton FT, Smidt GL, Flatt AE, Stephens RI: The influence of wrist position on the force produced by the finger flexors. J Biomech 8:301–306, 1975.

48. Hempstock TI, O'Connor DE: Assessment of hand transmitted vibration. Ann Occup Hyg 21:57–67, 1978.

49. Hertzberg HTE: Some contributions of applied physical anthropology to human engineering. Ann NY Acad Sci 63:616–629, 1955.

50. Hongell A, Mattsson HS: Neurographic studies before, after and during operation for median nerve compression in the carpal tunnel. Scand J Plast Reconstr Surg 5:103–109, 1971.

51. Hunt JR: Occupational neuritis of the deep palmar branch of the ulnar nerve: A well defined clinical type of professional palsy of the hand. J Nerv Ment Dis 35:673, 1908.

52. Jacobson D, Sperling L: Classification of the hand grip: A preliminary study. J Occup Med 18:396–398, 1976.

53. Jensen R, Klein B, Sanderson L: Motion-related wrist disorders traced to industries, occupational groups. Monthly Labor Review, Sept 1983, pp 13–16.

54. Kelly A, Jacobson H: Hand disability due to tenosynovitis. Ind Med Surg, 57:574, 1964.

55. Kanter RM: The Change Masters. New York, Simon & Schuster, 1983.

56. Kendall D: Etiology, diagnosis and treatment of paresthesia in the hand. Brit Med J 2:1633–1640, 1960.

57. Keyserling WM, Herrin GD, Chaffin DB, et al: Establishing an industrial strength testing program. Am Ind Hyg J 41:730–736, 1980.

58. Kisner W: Thumb neuroma: A hazard of ten pin bowling. Br J Plast Surg 29:225–226, 1976.

59. Kumlin T, Wiikeri M, Sumari P: Radiological changes in carpal and metacarpal bones and phalanges caused by chain saw vibration. Br J Ind Med 30:71–73, 1973.

60. Kurppa K, Waris P, Rokkanen P: Tennis elbow, lateral elbow pain syndrome. Scand J Work Environ Health 5(Suppl 3):15–19, 1979b.

61. Lamphier T, Crooker C, Crooker J: De Quervain's disease. Ind Med Surg 34:849–856, 1965.

62. Landsmeer JMF: Power grip and precision handling. Ann Rheum Dis 21:164–170, 1962.

63. Long C, Conrad P, Hall E, Farler S: Intrinsic-extrinsic muscle control of the hand in power grip and precision handling. J Bone Joint Surg 52:853–867, 1970.

64. Loomis L: Variation of stenosing tenosynovitis at the radial styloid process. J Bone Joint Surg 33A:340–346, 1951.

65. Lord J, Rosati L: Neurovascular compression syndromes of the upper extremity. Ciba Clin Symp 10:35–62, 1958.

66. Lukas E: Lesion of the peripheral nervous system due to vibration. Scand J Work Environ Health 7:67–79, 1970.

67. Lundborg G, Gelberman RH, Minteer-Convery M, et al: Median nerve compression in the carpal tunnel—Functional response to experimentally induced controlled pressure. J Hand Surg 7:252–259, 1982.

68. Mallory M, Bradford H, Freundlich N: An invisible workplace hazard gets harder to ignore. Business Week Jan 30, 1989, pp 92–93.

69. Marie P, Foix C: Atrophie isolée de l'eminence thenar d'origine neuritinque: Rôle du ligament anulaire antérieur du carpe dans la pathogenie de la lesion. Rev Neurol 26:647, 1913.

70. Matthew P: Ganglia of the flexor tendon sheaths in the hand. J Bone Joint Surg 55B:612–617, 1973.

71. Mergler D, Brabant C, Vezina N, Messing K: The weaker sex? Men in women's working conditions report similar health complaints. J Occup Med 29:417–421, 1987.

72. Messing K: Do men and women have different jobs because of their biological differences? Int J Health Serv 12:43–52, 1982.

73. Miller LF: Stenosing tendovaginitis: A survey of findings and treatment in 49 cases. Ind Med Surg 19:465–467, 1950.

74. Mishoe JW, Suggs CW: Hand-arm vibration Part I. Subjective response to single and multi-directional sinusoidal and non-sinusoidal excitation. J Sound Vibrat 35:479–488, 1974.

75. Mishoe JW, Suggs CW: Hand-arm vibration Part II. Vibrational response of the human hand. J Sound Vibrat 53:545–558, 1977.

76. Moberg E: Criticism and study of methods for examining sensibility in the hand. Neurology 12:8–19, 1962.

77. Moberg E: Methods for examining sensibility of the hand. In Flynn SE (ed): Hand Surgery. Baltimore, Williams & Wilkins, 1966, pp 435–449.

78. Muckart R: Stenosing tendovaginitis of abductor pollicis longus and extensor pollicis brevis at the radial styloid. Clin Orthop 33:201–208, 1964.

79. Napier JR: The prehensile movements of the human hand. J Bone Joint Surg 33B:902–913, 1956.

80. Nichols H: Anatomic structures of the thoracic outlet. Clin Orthop 51:17–25, 1967.

81. Niebel B: Motion and Time Study. Homewood, IL, Richard D. Irwin, 1982.

82. Nishiyama K, Watanabe W: Temporary threshold shift of vibratory sensation after clasping a vibrating handle. Int Arch Occup Environ Health 49:21–33, 1981.

83. Partanen TJ, Kumlin T, Karvonen MJ: Subjective symptoms connected with exposure of the upper limbs to vibration. Work Environ Health 7:80–81, 1970.

84. Pelmear PL, Taylor W: The results of long-term vibration exposure with a review of special cases of vibration white finger in industry. In Taylor W, Pelmear PL (eds). London, Academic Press, 1975, pp 83–110.

85. Phalen G: The carpal tunnel syndrome. J Bone Joint Surg 48A:211–228, 1966.

86. Pheasant S, O'Neill D: Performance in gripping and turning—A study in hand/handle effectiveness. Appl Ergonom 6:205–208, 1975.

87. Phillips R: Carpal tunnel syndrome as a manifestation of systemic disease. Ann Rheum Dis 26:59–63, 1967.

88. Poppelsdorf N, Cramer C: An investigation of the effects of gloves on manual and finger dexterity and fatigue. Occupational Health and Safety Engineering Technical Report, Center for Ergonomics, 1205 Beal, Ann Arbor, MI 48109, 1982.

89. Pyykko I, Farkkila M, Toivanen J, et al: Transmission of vibration in the hand–Arm system with special reference to changes in compression force and acceleration. Scand J Work Environ Health 2:87–95, 1976.

90. Quinnell R: Conservative management of trigger finger. Practitioner 224:187–190, 1980.

91. Radwin R, Armstrong TJ: A study of physical stresses associated with pneumatic screwdrivers. Ann Arbor: University of Michigan, College of Engineering and School of Public Health, 1982.

92. Rasmussen G: Human body vibration exposure and its measurement. Technical Review, Bruel & Kjaer 1:3–31, 1982.

93. Reynolds DD, Soedel W: Dynamic response of the hand–Arm system to a sinusoidal input. J Sound Vibrat 21:339–353, 1972.

94. Riley M, Cochran D, Schanbacher C: Force capability differences due to gloves. Ergonomics 28:441–447, 1985.

95. Robbins H: Anatomical study of the median nerve in the carpal tunnel and etiologies of the carpal tunnel syndrome. J Bone Joint Surg 45A:953–966, 1963.

96. Rodgers SH: Job evaluation in worker fitness determination. Occup Med State Art Rev 3:219–239, 1988.

97. Rohmert W: Problems in determining rest allowances. Part I: Use of modern methods to evaluate stress and strain in static muscular work. Appl Ergonom 4:91, 1973.

98. Rothfleisch S, Sherman D: Carpal tunnel syndrome: Biomedical aspects of occupational occurrence and implications regarding surgical management. Orthop Rev 7:107–109, 1978.

99. Schiefer R, Kok R, Lewis M, Meese G: Finger skin temperature and manual dexterity—Some inter-group differences. Appl Ergonom 15:135–141, 1984.

100. Schmidt RT, Toews JV: Grip strength as measured by the Jamar dynamometer. Arch Phys Med Rehab pp 321–327, 1970.

101. Schultz-Johnson K: Evaluating the worker's functional capacities for repetitive work. Sem Occup Med 2(1):31–39, 1987.

102. Seppalainen A: Nerve conduction in the vibration syndrome. Scand J Work Environ Health 7:82–84, 1970.

103. Silverstein BA: Ergonomic Interventions to Prevent Musculoskeletal Injuries in Industry. ACGIH, Lewis Publishers, 1987.

104. Silverstein BA, Fine LJ, Armstrong TJ: Occupational factors and carpal tunnel syndrome. Am J Ind Med 11:343–358, 1987.

105. Smith E, Sonstegard D, Anderson W: Carpal tunnel syndrome: Contribution of flexor tendons. Arch Phys Med Rehab 58:379–385, 1977.

106. Snook SH: The design of manual handling tasks. Ergonomics 21:963–986, 1978.

107. Stone WE: Repetitive strain injuries. Med J Aust 2:616–619, 1983.

108. Streeter H: Effects of localized vibration on the human tactile sense. Am Ind Hyg Assoc J 31:87–91, 1970.

109. Sunderland S: Nerves and Nerve Injuries. Edinburgh, Churchill Livingstone, 1978.

110. Sunderland S: The nerve lesion in the carpal tunnel syndrome. J Neurol Neurosurg Psychiatry 39:615–626, 1976.

111. Tanzer R: The carpal tunnel syndrome. J Bone Joint Surg 41A:626–634, 1959.

112. Taylor N: Carpal tunnel syndrome. Am J Phys Med Rehabil 50:192–213, 1971.

113. Taylor W: Vibration white finger in the work place. J Soc Occup Med 32:159–166, 1982.

114. Thompson A, Plewes L, Shaw E: Peritendinitis crepitans and simple tenosynovitis: A clinical study of 544 cases in industry. Br J Ind Med 8:150–160, 1951.

115. Tichauer ER: Biomechanics sustains occupational safety and health. Ind Engin 8:45–56, 1976.

116. Tichauer ER: Some aspects of stress on forearm and hand in industry. J Occup Med 8:63–71, 1966.

117. Tichauer ER, Gage H: Ergonomic principles basic to hand tool design. Am Ind Hyg Assoc J 38:622–634, 1977.

118. Vihma T, Nurminen M, Mutanen P: Sewing-machine operators' work and musculoskeletal complaints. Ergonomics 25:295–298, 1982.

119. Wasserman E, Taylor W, Behrens V, Samueloff S: Vibration white finger disease in U.S. workers using pneumatic chipping and grinding hand tools I: Epidemiology. U.S. Department of Health and Human Services (NIOSH) Report no. 82–118, 1982.

120. Welch R: The causes of tenosynovitis in industry. Ind Med 41(10):16–19, 1972.

121. Westgaard RH, Aaras A: Postural muscle strain as a causal factor in the development of musculoskeletal illnesses. Appl Ergonom 15:162–174, 1984.

122. Williamson E, Chrenko F, Hamley E: A study of exposure to cold in cold stores. Appl Ergonom 15:25–30, 1984.

123. Woods THE: De Quervain's disease: A plea for early operation. A report on 40 cases. Br J Surg 51:358–359, 1954.

124. Wright I: The neurovascular syndrome produced by hyperabduction of the arms. Am Heart J 29:1–19, 1945.

125. Younghusband O, Black J: De Quervain's disease: Stenosing tenovaginitis at the radial styloid process. Can Med Assoc J 89:508–512, 1963.

APPENDIX A

MEDICAL HEALTH QUESTIONNAIRE

Date _____

Please respond to the following questions as accurately as possible. Your participation will help in identifying health concerns in your workplace. Your answers will be kept confidential and will *not* be used as part of your work record.

I. IDENTIFYING INFORMATION

Name _____ _____ _____ Male   Female
          Last   First   Initial

Social Security Number _____ Employee/Clock No. _____

Birthdate _____ _____ _____ Height _____ Weight _____ Age _____ Date of Hire _____ ___ ___

Do you work in: Production _____   Shipping/Receiving _____   Office/Clerical _____
                   Maintenance _____   Sanitation/Janitorial _____

II. PREVIOUS WORK HISTORY

1. Were you employed prior to Company ABC? (circle one) Yes   No
2. If yes, fill in the job description (or title) and dates of employment beginning with your most recent job first.

Job Description (or title)   Dates Employed (month/year)

_____ from _____ to _____
_____   _____   _____
_____   _____   _____

III. CURRENT WORK HISTORY

1. Do you currently have a part-time job (in addition to ABC)? (circle one) Yes   No
2. If so, what is your part-time position (job title or position)? _____
   How long have you held this position? _____
3. List your work history at ABC.

   Indicate "C" for current   Rate job difficulty from 1 to 10: 1 = easiest
   Indicate "P" for previous

Job		How long on this position (months or years)	Difficulty	Order Worked (1 = current)
_____	Position A	_____	_____	_____
_____	Position B	_____	_____	_____
_____	Position C	_____	_____	_____
_____	Float	_____	_____	_____

4. What shift do you normally work? (circle one)   1st   2nd   3rd   4th   Rotate
5. Do you normally take scheduled breaks and lunches? (circle one) Yes   No
6. When given a choice do you usually work overtime? (circle one) Always   Frequently   Sometimes   Never
7. Approximately how many overtime hours do you work per month? _____

	Yes	No
8. Is there an assigned rotation in your area?	_____	_____
9. If no, do the workers in your area choose to rotate among positions?	_____	_____
10. Do you choose to rotate among positions?	_____	_____
Why? _____		
11. Do you find one (or several) positions more difficult?	_____	_____

If yes, please list _____
_____

12. How long do you work (on the average) at one position before rotating?
    _____

13. Does your current job require any tasks or motion(s) that are repetitious? (circle one)   Yes   No

14. Do any tasks or motion(s) bother you more than others? (Specify)

Task/Motion(s)	(Check all that apply)			
	Shoulder	Elbow	Wrist	Hand
_____	_____	_____	_____	_____
_____	_____	_____	_____	_____
_____	_____	_____	_____	_____

(Use back page if necessary)

15. Do you routinely operate machines or equipment? (circle one)   Yes   No
    If so, specify _____
    Does this operation bother your arms or hands? (circle one)   Yes   No
    How? _____

16. Do you routinely use hand tools? (circle one)   Yes   No
    If so, specify which tools _____
    Do any of the tools bother your arms or hands? (circle one)   Yes   No
    How _____

IV. LEISURE ACTIVITIES

1. Do you participate in any of the following activities?

Gardening	_____	Fishing	_____	Wood working	_____	Painting	_____
Volleyball	_____	Bowling	_____	Needlework	_____	Art	_____
Softball/baseball	_____	Golf	_____	Tennis	_____	Crochet/knit	_____
Weight lifting	_____	Farming	_____	Carpentry	_____		

   Other _____

2. Do any of your leisure activities bother your arms and hands? (circle one)   Yes   No

3. If so, specify _____

V. SUBJECTIVE

	Yes	No
1. Are you right handed?	_____	_____
2. Are you left handed?	_____	_____
3. Do your fingers swell?	_____	_____
4. Do you have pain in the wrist area?	_____	_____
5. When you are having wrist pain, do you have any pain in your forearm or arm?	_____	_____
6. Do you have burning or aching in your wrist or fingers?	_____	_____
7. Have you ever had a fracture of your wrist?	_____	_____
8. Have you ever had any numbness of your fingertips?	_____	_____
9. Are you awakened at night with numbness of your fingers?	_____	_____
10. Have you had any numbness of your fingers during a pregnancy?	_____	_____
11. Do your fingers fall asleep while driving a car?	_____	_____
12. Do you notice any stiffness or clumsiness of your fingers?	_____	_____
13. Did the numbness in your fingers, if you have had any, begin after a fracture of the wrist?	_____	_____
14. When your fingers get numb, do you shake them in order to wake them up?	_____	_____

15. When your fingers are numb, do you let them hang down to wake them up? _____ _____

16. Do you have difficulty picking up small objects such as pins and needles? _____ _____

17. Do you commonly drop objects such as pencils, forks, and spoons? _____ _____

18. Do you drop other objects? _____ _____

19. Is your little finger ever numb? _____ _____

20. Do you have any neurological disorders or nerve disorders (other than nervousness)? _____ _____

21. Does any member of your family have a nerve disorder (other than nervousness)? _____ _____

22. Are you diabetic? _____ _____

23. Is anyone in your family diabetic? _____ _____

24. Have you ever been told that you had a carpal tunnel syndrome? _____ _____

25. Have you ever been told that you have a nerve problem at your elbow? _____ _____

26. If you have had an operation on your wrist, where was it done and by whom?
    Where _____ By whom _____

27. Have you ever missed more than 2 days of work in a row due to an illness/condition? _____ _____

28. In the past year have you stayed off work because of a problem with your arms and/or hands? _____ _____
    What was the problem? _____
    Do you have a problem now? _____ _____

29. When did you first notice the problem? _____
    When did you last notice the problem? _____

30. Does a particular motion or activity bring on or aggravate the problem?
    _____

31. In the past year have you been on restricted duty because of problems with your arm and hands? _____ _____
    What was the restriction? _____

32. Have you requested a change to a different job within the last year? _____ _____

33. Do you have the problem now? _____ _____

Chapter 37

LEGAL CONSIDERATIONS IN OCCUPATIONAL MEDICINE

Susan J. Hauck, J.D.

Occupational medicine physicians who perform services pursuant to a contractual relationship with an employer are a distinct legal entity. They may be subject to different legal standards than "private physicians." Their contractual relationship with the employer may relieve them of some of the malpractice worries of private physicians. On the other hand, they must deal with privacy and discrimination issues that private physicians might never have reason to consider.

This chapter discusses the legal implications of pre-employment physicals, both in terms of malpractice issues and labor and employment law issues. It also discusses strategies for avoiding legal problems before they arise and being prepared in the event of being named in a malpractice lawsuit.

THE LEGAL ASPECTS OF PRE-EMPLOYMENT PHYSICALS

As every occupational physician knows, pre-employment physicals are commonplace. They are also controversial. Everyone is aware of the debate concerning drug and alcohol testing in the workplace. However, x-rays and blood pressure screening have also spurred litigation owing to their possible adverse consequences for black applicants. Height and strength measurements, in some cases, discriminate against female applicants. Then there is the thorny issue of AIDS in the workplace. Federal handicap discrimination laws currently affect all employers receiving federal funds. Proposed legislation may expand handicap discrimination constraints to all employers.

How do these concerns affect the occupational medicine physician? They may involve the physician in litigation, if not as a named defendant, then as an important witness. No one wants to be an unwitting accomplice to illegal employment practices. For these reasons, an understanding of the applicable case law should assist the physician.

The objective of pre-employment examinations is to ensure that employees are physically fit to perform the duties of the job. Employers must be concerned with the safety of the prospective employee, and they must also protect their work force from threats posed by the incapacities of others.

Although pre-employment exams are common and serve legitimate business interests, they have the potential for running afoul of federal and state antidiscrimination statutes and privacy and defamation laws.

Title VII[31] makes it illegal to discriminate against an individual on the basis of race, sex, religion, or national origin. Title VII lawsuits have been brought as a result of employment physicals, with mixed success.

In *Smith v. Olin*,[27] the plaintiff failed to pass an employment physical when an x-ray revealed "bone degeneration with a prognosis of possible aseptic necrosis or further bone degeneration in his spinal region." As a result the plaintiff was disqualified for a position as a manual laborer. The plaintiff claimed his condition was a result of sickle-cell anemia. He charged that if bone degeneration were an automatic disqualification for a job, a higher proportion of black workers would be disqualified.

The court found that employers do not have to justify the exclusion of persons with bad backs from manual labor. It held that this is the case even if such a policy disproportionately affects a class protected by Title VII (i.e., blacks or females).

The legitimate need for x-rays as a part of pre-employment examinations is not disputed. Conditions such as a degenerative back create a risk for the prospective employee, the employer, and the fellow employees. The employer runs the additional risk that his workers' compensation insurance may be taxed for a full disability despite a pre-existing condition.

The Equal Employment Opportunity Commission (EEOC), which enforces Title VII, has generally found physical fitness requirements to be valid, as has the National Labor Relations Board. However, pre-employment examinations may violate Title VII. If the physical requirements are *not* job related and have a disproportionate effect on a protected class, discrimination may be found. If the employer uses the physical examination as a means to further discriminatory hiring practices, a Title VII violation would be found. Also, if the examination itself discriminates against certain persons by disclosing physical conditions that are more prevalent in one protected category of people, and those conditions are the basis for exclusion, there may be liability.[3]

In a case where a pre-employment physical revealed that a black applicant's blood pressure was "too high," the court found that the examination furthered a practice of denying employment to blacks in violation of Title VII.[3]

The EEOC has found it an unlawful employment practice to deny employment to persons who, as a class, tend to fall outside the national norms for weight, if weight requirements are not related to job performance.

The consensus is that as long as physical requirements are necessary for successful performance of the job in question, Title VII laws are not violated by a pre-employment examination requirement. However, when pre-employment physicals tend to disqualify a disproportionate number of people of a certain class, and the physical requirements are not job related, federal laws have been broken. Physi-

cians performing pre-employment physicals should be wary of employers who make physical requirements that bear no relation to the duties of the job. Such practices may land the employer and the physician in the middle of an employment discrimination lawsuit. Physical factors that are considered disqualifications for certain jobs should be analyzed carefully in light of their relation to the actual job duties.

Handicap discrimination laws are an equally important consideration in pre-employment physicals. Employers covered by the Vocational Rehabilitation Act of 1973 and the Vietnam Era Veterans Readjustment Assistance Act of 1974 may not discriminate against otherwise qualified people solely on the basis of handicap. Employers receiving federal financial assistance are covered by these acts.

The statutory definition of "handicapped" is broad, encompassing any person who: (1) has a physical or mental impairment that substantially limits one or more major life activities; (2) has a record of impairment; or (3) is regarded as having such an impairment.[29]

The employer must make "reasonable" accommodations for the known limitations of a handicapped person unless this would cause "undue hardship" to the employer.

These acts receive the most publicity in their relationship to drug and alcohol abuse. They have been interpreted as protecting employees with a history of drug and alcohol abuse.[15] They do not, however, cover current alcohol or drug abuse that prevents a person from performing the duties of the job and poses a direct threat to the property or safety of others.[29]

Although the Rehabilitation Act applies only to "federal employers," many states have their own handicap discrimination statutes. State laws tend to follow the federal legislation. In addition, legislation has been proposed to extend the coverage of the Rehabilitation Act to private employers. If it is enacted, physicians must be very conscious of ensuring that physical prerequisites to employment do not intentionally or unintentionally violate the handicap laws.

Privacy is another important consideration in the context of pre-employment physicals. Two legal concepts are generally referred to as the "right to privacy": the constitutional right to be free from unreasonable "searches and seizures" (the Fourth Amendment) and the common law right to privacy. The taking of blood and urine samples in the workplace is a "search and seizure."

Federal constitutional protections apply only to federal, state, and local governmental action. However, private employers who act in concert with governmental agencies or who function in a quasi-governmental fashion may be subject to constitutional restrictions.[1]

In determining whether searches are unreasonable and prohibited by the Fourth Amendment, the courts balance the need for the particular search against the invasion of personal rights. The scope of the intrusion, the manner in which it is conducted, the justification for initiating it, and the place in which it is conducted are factors in determining the search's legality.

Cases on record appear to state that governmental employees have little expectation of privacy because of the nature of their jobs. Urinalysis has been found to be constitutional in the case of police officers,[28] mass transit workers,[10] state corrections officers,[17] and the racing industry.[26]

Other courts have refused to find that governmental employees have a diminished right to privacy on the grounds that testing in the cases at question, was not based upon "reasonable suspicion." These cases have involved customs employees,[22] school bus attendants,[16] civilian law enforcement personnel,[4] and firefighters.[21]

These decisions involving public employees provide guidance in analyzing cases involving private employers and state constitutions and common law privacy protections.

The common law right to privacy applies to private employers and covers four types of tortious invasion of privacy: (1) the appropriation of another's name or likeness; (2) public disclosure of true, private facts; (3) placing another in a false light in the public eye; and (4) intrusion into another's seclusion.

"Public" dissemination of an employee's or prospective employee's medical condition would constitute a tortious invasion of the employee's privacy. To form the basis of a lawsuit, the dissemination would have to be widespread and made to persons who have no legitimate business interest in the information. For example, where five supervisors were informed about an employee's drinking, the court found that there was no "public disclosure."[14]

However, another court found "tortious invasion of privacy" where an airline's medical examiner disclosed the plaintiff's confidential medical records to her husband and her flight supervisor. The court found that neither person had a "need to know" the confidential information. This case was analyzed as an intrusion into the employee's seclusion.[18]

An invasion of privacy and defamation suit was brought against a company doctor in *Bratt v. IBM*.[9] In this case the physician, who was under contract to IBM, stated in a medical report that Mr. Bratt was "paranoid" and should see a psychiatrist immediately. This information was given to Bratt's supervisors.

The test used for determining whether there was a violation of privacy was whether ". . . the substantiality of the intrusion on the employee's privacy which results from the disclosure outweighs the employer's legitimate business interest in obtaining and publishing the information. The personal nature of the information is one factor. . . [as is] the degree of disclosure."[9]

In the Bratt case an IBM program provided "confidential" counseling to employees with psychological problems. Bratt believed that everything said would be held in confidence. The company doctor neither informed Bratt that she whould report the results of the examination to IBM nor asked him to sign a disclosure form. (It was considered important that Bratt paid the doctor's bill himself and was later reimbursed by his medical insurance and IBM.)

The court recognized the general rule that when an employer retains a physician to examine employees, no physician-patient relationship exists—a rule that is discussed below. However, where the patient reasonably believes that the relationship exists and where the doctor should have known that the patient had such beliefs, the doctor owes a duty of confidentiality to the patient.

Bratt also sued the doctor, IBM, and its medical staff for defamation. Defamation lawsuits are one of the fastest growing areas of litigation, and defamation suits arising out of the workplace are becoming common.

In the context of pre-employment physicals, plaintiffs bring defamation lawsuits when they believe the medical report contained false information and was injurious to their reputation. Truth is a defense; however, the truth of judgmental statements such as "paranoid" or "illegal drug user" may be hard to prove.

Employers and their medical personnel are protected by a "qualified privilege." Communications of matters of common interest to the communicator and the recipient are "privileged," meaning that they cannot form the basis of a defamation action. The "privilege" is conditional and can be exceeded. If the potentially defamatory material is disseminated too widely—i.e., to persons who do not have a "need to know"—the privilege is lost.

If the plaintiff can show "actual malice" on the part of the communicator, the privilege is lost. The definition of "actual malice" differs from state to state. However, the general rule is, if the communicator knew that the statement was false or acted with reckless disregard for the truth or falsity of his statement, there is actual malice.

An occupational medicine physician was sued for defamation when his report of an employment physical stated that the employee was in "very bad shape." The employee claimed that the statement was false and caused him to lose his job.[5] Defamation cases have also arisen where physicians reported alcohol or drug use to the employer.[13]

TO WHOM DO OCCUPATIONAL MEDICINE PHYSICIANS OWE A DUTY?

Employers commonly require pre-employment physicals. They engage physicians to perform these examinations. What is the relationship between the physician and the examinee? What is the relationship between the physician and the employer? Although these questions have no clear-cut answers, some general rules of law apply.

The law imposes on all persons a "duty" to use reasonable care in the performance of their activities. A person who breaches that duty, and thereby causes injury to another, can be sued for negligence.

Physicians are required not only to exercise reasonable care in what they do, but also to possess special knowledge and ability. The general rule is that a physician must have the skill and learning commonly possessed by members of the profession in good standing. Physicians who hold themselves out as "specialists" are held to a higher standard of care. They must use reasonable care in light of their special ability and information and may be negligent where an ordinary physician would not be.[23]

To whom does the occupational medicine physician owe this "duty of care?" A physician owes a duty of care where there is a relationship of doctor and patient as a result of contract, expressed or implied, that the doctor will treat the patient with proper professional skill and the patient will pay for the treatment. The doctor may be sued for malpractice if there has been a breach of professional duty to the patient.[2]

Employers pay the physician for performing pre-employment physicals. The usual doctor-patient relationship does not exist between the prospective employee and the doctor who examines him on behalf of the employer. The purpose of such examinations is to inform the employer of the prospective employee's physical condition, not to treat the patient. For these reasons, the majority of courts have held that for examinations performed by a doctor engaged by a prospective employer, the doctor's duty of care is not the same as that which he owes to his patients.

Doctors have been held not liable for failing to discover a condition of an examinee during an employment physical.[20] The courts have reasoned that there is no usual doctor-patient relationship between the doctor and the prospective employee and that the examination was wholly for the employer's benefit. The doctor's duty to perform the examination in a non-negligent manner is owed only to the employer. The duty the doctor owes the prospective employees is to refrain from injuring them during the examination.

The same is true for a physician performing an examination for the purpose of rating an injury for the employer's workers' compensation carrier. In one recent case[19] an employee noticed numbness in his right thumb and first and second fingers while using a hand scraper at work. Days later he noticed that his right arm was weak and his fingers were tingling. These symptoms persisted and were compounded by pain in the posterior of the neck on the right side. The plaintiff was unable to work after the onset of symptoms. He filed for workers' compensation. The employer's workers' compensation carrier directed the plaintiff to see Dr. Caputi, the defendant. Dr. Caputi found no evidence of intervertebral disc injury or disease or peripheral nerve damage. He concluded that the employee was able to return to work without restrictions or limitations. The plaintiff was later diagnosed as having a brainstem tumor. He sued Dr. Caputi for malpractice.

The court dismissed the complaint against

the physician, holding that at the time of the alleged malpractice there was no doctor-patient relationship. The court found that the doctor examined the patient at the request of the workers' compensation carrier. The examination was not conducted for the purpose of treatment. The plaintiff did not employ the doctor. Accordingly, "where a doctor conducts an examination of an injured employee solely for the purpose of rating the injury for the employer's insurance carrier in a workers' compensation proceeding, neither offers nor intends to treat, care for or otherwise benefit the person examined and has no reason to believe the person examined will rely on his report, the doctor is not liable to the person being examined for failure to properly diagnose a latent brain tumor."[19]

In some instances, doctors have been held liable for malpractice as a result of employment physicals. One of the leading cases is *Hoover v. Williamson*.[12] If the allegations in this case are true, the physician involved acted in a highly unethical manner, but the legal principles involved may impact all occupational medicine physicians.

According to the facts, the defendant, Dr. Williamson, was retained by General Electric. In the course of an annual x-ray examination of the plaintiff's chest, the doctor advised the plaintiff that he had "a little infection on the lungs." The defendant referred the plaintiff to a consultant.

The x-ray examination clearly revealed that the plaintiff had silicosis. The doctor concealed this fact from the patient and also concealed the recommendation of the consultant. As a result, the plaintiff's lung condition became serious and permanent.

The plaintiff sued the doctor for malpractice. The doctor countered that he owed no duty to the plaintiff because there was no doctor-patient relationship. The court disagreed.

When Dr. Williamson undertook to send the plaintiff to a consultant and to advise the plaintiff concerning his condition, he assumed a duty of care to the plaintiff. The general rule of law is that one who assumes to act, even though gratuitously, may thereby become subject to the duty of acting carefully.[25] The court stated: "One who gratuitously undertakes to render services which he should recognize as necessary to another's bodily safety and leads the other in reasonable reliance on the services to refrain from taking other protective steps, or

to enter on a dangerous course of conduct . . . is subject to liability to the other for bodily harm resulting from the actor's failure to exercise reasonable care to carry out his undertaking."

If Dr. Williamson had done nothing more than conduct an x-ray examination of the patient, his only duty would have been to General Electric. By advising the plaintiff concerning his condition, sending the plaintiff to a consultant, and misrepresenting to the plaintiff the seriousness of his condition, he assumed and breached a duty to the plaintiff.

The lesson to be learned is that if, in the course of an employment physical, you undertake to advise or treat the examinee, you assume an obligation of due care to that person.

Physicians have also been successfully sued for malpractice where it was alleged that they injured the examinee during the course of the examination. If a job applicant is burned during the examination, for example, the physician can be held liable.

Liability for injuring a person during the course of an examination seems reasonable; however, the courts have given this rule an interesting application. Some would say that the court in the following case was merely trying to circumvent the no doctor-patient relationship rule and find liability on the part of the doctor. Whatever the motivation of the court, the case shows that liability may be found in circumstances where the physician is acting solely for the benefit of the employer and does not gratuitously undertake to advise the examinee.

In *Armstrong v. Morgan*[5] the plaintiff, upon promotion to the vice presidency of a company, was required to undergo a physical examination by Dr. Morgan, who was retained by the employer. Dr. Morgan examined the plaintiff and reported that Armstrong was "in very bad physical condition." As a result of this report, Armstrong was discharged. He sued Dr. Morgan, contending that the report was false and inaccurate and that the doctor was negligent because he did not exercise reasonable care, attention, observation, and skill in conducting the examination.

The court held that Dr. Morgan owed Armstrong a duty not to injure him during the course of the examination. If Dr. Morgan performed a negligent examination that injured Armstrong by causing his discharge, a lawsuit might be brought.

This case is important. It indicates that an applicant, denied employment as a result of a medical examination, may sue the doctor for malpractice.

Employees who believe they have been injured by a company doctor may also bring a lawsuit against the employer. Under the doctrine of *respondeat superior*, the master is liable for the acts of the servant. Just as an employer is liable for injuries inflicted by his manager or agent, he is also responsible for the acts of a physician whom he employs.

However, the employer may in turn sue the physician for negligence. Company physicians owe a duty to their employer. The case of *Wharton v. Bridges* illustrates the legal principles. The facts of this case are outrageous, but the rule of law applies in less outrageous circumstances as well.

In this case the employer, a trucking company, sent a prospective employee to the defendant doctor for a pre-employment physical. The physician certified the employee as physically fit to drive a truck in interstate commerce. The certification stated that all physical characteristics, including vision, reflexes, and extremities, were normal.

Relying upon this certification, the company hired the applicant as a driver. On his first run, the driver was responsible for a fatal accident. The trucking company was sued and settled out of court for $426,000.

The company then sued the physician for negligence in the performance of the pre-employment physical. The evidence showed that the driver had chorioretinitis in both eyes, resulting in a 95% loss of vision in the left eye and blurred vision in the right eye. He had impaired depth perception, as well as osteoarthritis in his left knee and a 10% loss of flexion and the propensity for the joint to lock, chronic depression, fatigue, and restricted motion.

Pre-employment physicals were a large portion of the physician's industrial medicine practice. He was familiar with the purpose of the pre-employment physicals and their importance to highway safety.

The court held that the doctor owed a duty to the employer to perform the physical in a nonnegligent manner. The trucking company had a right of indemnity against the doctor for breach of his duty to disclose accurately the employee's physical condition.

The court also indicated that the persons involved in the accident could have sued the doctor.

AVOIDING EVEN THE APPEARANCE OF NEGLIGENCE

Although occupational physicians may have limited malpractice exposure, it is still important to be cognizant of the factors that influence a plaintiff's decision to sue and the evidence needed to prevail in a lawsuit. Actual negligence is not necessary for a plaintiff to file a lawsuit. The appearance of negligence suffices.

Many physicians are confident that they maintain such high standards in their practice that they will prevail if they are sued. Unfortunately, being named in a lawsuit is a "loss" in and of itself. Physicians lose time. If a case goes to trial, the amount of the doctor's time involved exceeds 100 hours. This is a disruption of the doctor's practice and personal life.

The defense of a lawsuit is an expensive proposition. Insurance carriers do not necessarily cover all of the expenses. Some insurance carriers require physicians to accept all financial responsibility if they do not accept a settlement offer recommended by the carrier.

Lawyers' time is almost as expensive as doctors' time. Litigation expenses—i.e., filing fees, expert witness fees, and court reporter's fees—can cost thousands of dollars. Not to mention the fees lost while the doctor is absent from the office. The financial tolls can be high.

A malpractice suit also takes an emotional toll. Depression, a loss of confidence, and a loss of nerve may result. The suit may also cause the physician to distrust patients.

For these reasons doctors need to have some understanding of why people sue. What motivates a person to seek out an attorney and sue a doctor? The motivational factor often has more to do with emotions than the quality of medical care received.

A physician who does not pay attention to the common fears of patients or lacks common courtesy may be sued even though he provides excellent medical care. Discourteous receptionists, nurses, and answering services may also contribute to a patient's decision to sue.

A careless, insensitive, or unfeeling remark, coupled with a less than perfect outcome, can spur litigation. An anxious patient with questions who is denied access to the physician may harbor resentment sufficient to motivate litigation. Do not hide behind your receptionist or refuse phone calls. Communication with your patients is essential.

Unfortunately, even the physician who is responsive to both the emotional and the physical needs of patients may be sued. At this point the physician must be prepared to make a defense. The keystone of a solid malpractice defense is good records.[8] The maintenance of neat, complete, and professional medical records is essential for the doctor to prevail.

Attorneys recognize that in the minds of the jury, sloppy, incomplete medical records equal a sloppy, incompetent doctor. Good records equal good medical care. It is estimated that as many as 35–40% of medical malpractice suits are indefensible because of poor medical records, even though the physician was not negligent in his treatment of the patient.[24]

Good medical records should be neat and legible. They should follow a logical sequence and should be contained in neat folders. Your records should contain your thought processes. The reader should be able to understand how you arrived at your diagnosis. Records must establish a probable cause for the patient's problem and outline a treatment plan with enough detail that another physician can understand the problem and continue treatment.

Your treatment plan must be consistent with your diagnosis. If it is not, note the reason for the disparity. You must also document the patient's response to treatment and adjustments to your plan.

Keep careful track of all prescribed medications, noting dosage, method of administration, and refills, if any. Document any changes in dosage, and the patient's response to the medication. A "medication sheet" attached to the file jacket is a good method of recording medications. Your records should also reflect a valid therapeutic indication for the prescription and a dated notation that the patient has been warned of possible side effects.

Good medical records contain documentation of "informed consent," including (1) diagnosis, (2) contemplated tests or treatment, (3) indications, (4) associated risks, complications, or side effects, (5) the goal to be achieved, (6) reasonable available alternatives, (7) result to be expected if nothing is done. Note that these matters were discussed with the patient, that the patient had an opportunity to ask questions, and that the patient understood and agreed to the treatment.[24]

Notations of special circumstances should also be made. Record all emergency calls and instances in which patients are hostile, uncooperative, or intoxicated. It is also a good idea to record all phone calls taken out of the office unless you have total recall of the advice you give out over the phone. This is especially important if you prescribe medications or respond to an emergency situation. Notations should also be made if the patient fails to follow your advice.

Medical records should be retained for a minimum of 7 years in the case of adult patients and 21 years in the case of minors. However, you should retain records indefinitely if possible.

The occupational medicine physician's records should follow all of the above guidelines. They should also clearly reflect on whose behalf the medical services are being provided and the purpose of the medical services.

Knowing what *not* to put in your medical records can be as important as knowing what to include. Never record indiscrete or frivolous remarks such as "fatso" or "crock." In fact, do not include anything in your records that you would not want an unfriendly attorney or jury to read. Judgmental statements about your patients make you sound unprofessional.

Never put notes to your lawyer in the patient's file. These notes may be privileged and should not accidentally fall into the wrong hands.

If you need to make corrections in your records, do not obliterate the original notes. Strike through the originals and then write your correction, explain the need for the correction, and date and initial the correction.

Good record-keeping on the part of the occupational medicine physician is especially important. The odds are that the records of private physicians will never be read by another person. However, the occupational medicine physician's records are disseminated to the employer on whose behalf the services are performed. Complete, professional records are your defense in malpractice and defamation or right to privacy lawsuits that might be brought.

REFERENCES

1. Allen v. City of Marietta, 601 F Supp 482 (1985).
2. 10 ALR 3d 1071: Physician's duties and liabilities to

person evaluated pursuant to physician's contract with such person's prospective or actual employer or insurer.

3. 36 ALR Fed 721: Requirement that employee take and pass physical examination as unlawful employment practice violative of Title VII of the Civil Rights Act of 1964.

4. American Fed. of Governmental Employees v. Weinberger, No. CU 4863531 (S.D. Ga., Dec. 2, 1986).

5. Armstrong v. Morgan, 545 SW2d 45 (1976).

6. Beadling v. Sirotta, 197 A2d 857 (1967).

7. Bell v. Wolfish, 441 U.S. 520 (1979).

8. Belli MM: Belli for Your Malpractice Defense. Oradell, NJ, Medical Economics, 1986, pp 2–93.

9. Bratt v. IBM, 785 F2d 352 (1st Cir. 1986).

10. Division 241, Amalgamated Transit Union v. Suscy, 538 F2d 1264 (7th Cir. 1976).

11. Ferguson v. Wolkin, 499 NYS 2d 640 (1987).

12. Hoover v. Williamson, 203 A.2d 861 (1964).

13. Houston Belt and Terminal Railway Co. v. Wherry, 548 SW2d 743, cert. den. 434 U.S. 962 (1977).

14. Hudson v. S.D. Warren Co., 608 F.Supp. 477 (1985).

15. Johnson v. Smith, 39 FEP 1106 (1985).

16. Jones v. McKenzie, 682 F.Supp. 1500 (1986).

17. King v. McMickens, No. 26086 (NY App. Div. 1986).

18. Levias v. United Airlines, No. 49503 (OH Ct of Apps. 1985).

19. LoDico v. Caputi, 517 NYS 2d 640 (1987).

20. Lotspeich v. Chance Vought Aircraft, 369 SW2d 705 (1963).

21. Lovvorn v. City of Chattanooga, TN., No. 1-86-389 (E.D. TN Nov. 13, 1986).

22. National Treasury Employees Union v. VanRabb, No. 86-3522 (E.D. LA Dec 3, 1986).

23. Prosser WL: The Law of Torts, 4th ed. St. Paul, Minn., West Publishing Co., 1971, pp 161–166.

24. Rasinski DC: Complete medical records are key to liability defense. Info Line V2, Summer 1989.

25. Restatement 2nd, Torts, Sec. 325.

26. Shoemaker v. Handel, 795 F2d 1136 (3rd Cir. 1986).

27. Smith v. Olin Chemical Corp., 555 F2d 1283 (5th Cir. 1977).

28. Turner v. Fraternal Order of Police, 120 LRRM 3294 (1985).

29. 29 USC Sec. 706(7)(B).

30. 29 USC Sec. 794.

31. 42 USC Sec. 2000e et. seq.

32. Wharton Transport Co. v. Bridges, 606 SW2d 521 (1980).

Chapter 38

WORKERS' COMPENSATION—
LEGAL ISSUES

Freeda M. Steinberg, J.D.

Disability—the loss of ability to support one's dependents or oneself—has been a dreaded prospect throughout time. The hazards of the workplace, with its risks that are often unpredictable and beyond the control of the worker, are an age-old cause of injury, illness, and death.

In response to the financial and social needs created by work-related disability and death, laws were enacted in the Middle Ages in England that required employers to compensate injured employees or the dependents of employees who were killed in work-related accidents. With the rise in injuries during the Industrial Revolution, exceptions to employer liability effectively abolished the obligation to compensate in a large majority of cases. Reduced employer liability served the social and economic need to encourage largely unbridled growth of industry and early technological advances, though often at the expense of injured workers, who were reduced to destitution or left to the fickle mercy of the gentry's charity.

In colonial America, workers fared little better. An approach similar to the one that had evolved in England, whereby the injured worker could initiate suit in court against his employer, was adopted. However, recovery was dependent on the worker's (or his survivors') establishing that the injury was the result solely of the employer's "fault" or negligence and that no negligence on the part of either the worker himself or any co-worker had been a factor. Additionally, it had to be established that the work involved did not entail a risk that was known to the worker; that is, that the worker

had not "assumed the risk" (regardless of his lack of power to eliminate or reduce the obvious danger) of the job.

The obvious inequities in this system led individual states beginning in the early 1900s to establish workers' compensation legislation. The essence of such legislation was to establish a largely "no-fault" system, providing compensation for injured employees (or the survivors of employees who were killed) regardless of whose "fault"—the worker's, the employer's, or a co-worker's—had led to the injury. Similarly, the legislation generally provided for compensation even in instances where the employee had "assumed" a known or obvious risk in undertaking to do the work.

Today, all 50 states, the District of Columbia, and the federal government have sets of workers' compensation laws (called acts). Although all the acts share the basic no-fault principles of entitlement to compensation, their many other provisions vary. Federal law covers only federal civilian employees (Federal Employees' Compensation Act) and maritime workers on the United States navigable waters (Longshore and Harbour Workers' Compensation Act). Otherwise, compensation for employee injuries is essentially limited to the recovery provided for under the applicable state act. There is no active movement to enact a federal, or national, uniform workers' compensation law, though the possibility is sometimes discussed.

What follows is a discussion of various issues involved in workers' compensation law. It should be borne in mind that knowledge of the particular provisions of the workers' compensation act in effect in any one state can be gained only by reading that act. Appendix A supplies a list of federal, state, and District of Columbia workers' compensation offices; for a nominal fee, copies of the acts can usually be obtained from these offices. With a general understanding of the theory of workers' compensation law, the reader will be able to understand the specific statutory provisions applicable in one jurisdiction.

COVERAGE OF EMPLOYERS AND EMPLOYEES

Virtually all employers, both private and public (or governmental), are subject to liability under workers' compensation acts. Exceptions typically exempt employers of domestic servants, "casual" employees, or farmworkers, as well as employers with a small number (usually from one to five) of employees.

Generally, employees are automatically covered by the workers' compensation acts in their states. Some states permit an employee to file a waiver, or rejection, of workers' compensation coverage. Such a waiver would be applicable only to injuries that occur after the waiver is filed. The effect of the waiver is to permit the employee to retain his common law right to sue the employer in court for tort damages for negligence in the event of an injury. But by signing the waiver, the employee gives up the statutory right to receive workers' compensation benefits, which would otherwise automatically accrue to him in the event of injury on the job. Thus, an employee who has waived workers' compensation and then is injured at work owing to his or her own negligence cannot claim workers' compensation benefits; and, because contributory negligence (meaning negligence on the part of the person claiming damages for injury) is a complete or partial bar to tort recovery in most states, the worker has no, or very limited, recourse in court against the employer. Further, the worker must prove negligence on the part of the employer in order to recover tort damages in court.

ADMINISTRATION

In all but a few states, the workers' compensation act, or related legislation, provides for a state administrative agency or tribunal that processes and adjudicates workers' compensation claims filed in that state. The agency itself determines all questions of law and issues of fact, such as whether or not the injury is work related, whether the injury has caused any permanent compensable disability, the extent of disability, and whether rehabilitation expenses should be awarded to the employee. The agency, through the particular personnel designated by that state's act, prepares a written decision about these issues, determining whether an award should be made, and if so, the amount of benefits the employee will receive. These agencies have various names in the different states, such as Division of Industrial Accidents, Industrial Board, and Workers' Compensation Board.

In the states that use administrative agencies to decide claims, the court system gets involved only in appeals or enforcement of decisions. In handling appeals, the courts interpret the workers' compensation act or questions of law on issues of evidence. Enforcement petitions arise in instances where the agency has awarded benefits to the employee, the employer then fails to pay the award, and the employee must sue the employer in court to collect the benefits he has been awarded. Through the court enforcement procedure, the employee can obtain a civil judgment that enables him to attach or garnish the employer's assets in order to collect the awarded benefits.

Administrative agencies also decide claims in the District of Columbia and in suits brought under the federal acts mentioned earlier. Appeals from these agencies are brought in the federal, rather than the state, court system.

In Wyoming, Tennessee, New Mexico, Alabama, and Louisiana, workers' compensation claims are administered and decided in the courts rather than by an administrative agency, although in all of these states except Louisiana, a state agency assists the courts in processing, but not in deciding, claims.

LIABILITY-COMPENSATION TRADE-OFF

As noted above, workers' compensation acts provide employees with a right to certain statutorily specified compensation benefits in the event of a work-related injury, *regardless* of fault. In exchange for this protection, the acts provide that the statutory benefits are the employees' *sole* recourse against the employer. Thus, even if the employer was obviously or grossly negligent, the employee cannot sue the employer in court in a common law claim for liability. Tort remedies pursued through court litigation have much broader recovery provisions (such as allowance for pain and suffering) than are available under the workers' compensation acts. The acts, thus, are a trade-off whereby the employer receives immunity from tort liability in exchange for providing more limited workers' compensation benefits to the employee, regardless of fault. The employee is assured of receiving guaranteed, statutorily determined benefits for an injury regardless of fault, in exchange for which he forfeits the right to sue the employer in court for unlimited tort damages in instances where the employer's negligence has caused the injury.

It should be noted that most jurisdictions permit the employee to sue the employer in court for tort damages if the employer intentionally (deliberately) caused the injury or, in some states, if the employer's willful conduct caused the injury. "Willfulness" is a matter of individual state interpretation.

POLICY CONSIDERATIONS

In addition to the trade-off between workers' compensation and tort liability, workers' compensation legislation has other objectives:

1. To increase employer interest and involvement in accident prevention and safety efforts by removing or reducing the employer's motive to conceal or deny fault

2. To reduce the legal expense of and delay in resolving claims that workers would have to litigate in court

3. To assess equitably the cost of workers' injuries to the employer and, ultimately, to the consumer of the goods and services produced through injured workers' efforts

4. To provide rehabilitation and re-employment of the injured worker

SPECIAL FUNDS, SUBSEQUENT INJURY FUNDS, OR SECOND-INJURY FUNDS

A work-related injury or illness occurring to a worker with a previously dormant physical condition may arouse the dormant condition and result in greater permanent disability than the injury or illness otherwise would have caused.

Classically, this situation has arisen in back injuries. A previously dormant degenerative condition in the back is "aroused" or made disabling by a back injury sustained at work. In some cases, no permanent disability would have ensued if the dormant condition had not been present. For example, a diabetic with no previous complications in his extremities may suffer a minimal pinch injury to his foot while at work, and the injury, because of the diabetes, may result in serious ulceration and permanent impairment of the foot.

Most states' workers' compensation acts or related legislation creates a state-administered fund, termed variously a special fund, second-injury fund, or subsequent injury fund. From this fund, workers are paid the proportion of their permanent disability award that is attributable to the pre-existing condition. This provision prevents the unfair assessment against the employer of full liability for disabilities that are, in whole or in part, caused by conditions unrelated to the actual work-related injury or illness. Generally, the monies administered by these funds are collected from amounts assessed against the workers' compensation insurance carriers and self-insured employers that do business in the particular state.

The determination of what portion of the cost of disability should be charged to the actual work event and what part should be charged to the previously dormant condition often is a matter of medical opinion obtained from the various treating or evaluating physicians. A physician must often give an opinion about whether the pre-existing condition was dormant or active before the work-related illness or injury because the employee does not receive compensation, in most instances, for a disability that was active before the work-related injury or illness.

In some jurisdictions, because the difficulty in making apportionments has led to inconsistent decisions, legislation that statutorily determines apportionment for certain medical situations has been passed. For example, Kentucky has recently enacted a law providing that in heart attack and back injury cases, an automatic apportionment of 50% against the employer and 50% against the special fund applies.

FUNDING

The laws of all states require that an employer, in order to do business legally in the state, must qualify under the state's workers' compensation laws by filing a proof either of workers' compensation insurance coverage or of self-insurance. Each state specifies certain requirements an employer must meet in order to operate as a state-insured employer, including a net worth declaration and a deposit of funds or a bond to ensure payment of claims.

In most states, private insurers cover the vast majority of employers' liability for workers' compensation payments.

Provision is made under the state workers' compensation acts for the creation of a state fund that pays the injured employee in the event the employer operates illegally, that is, without workers' compensation insurance or self-insurance, and defaults in paying compensation benefits to the worker. These uninsured employers' funds, like the special fund discussed earlier, are generally funded through assessments made against the self-insured employers and workers' compensation insurance carriers in the state or through state governmental funds, or a combination of both. The existence of these funds enables occupationally injured or ill workers to be paid the benefits they would have been entitled to from their defaulting employers. Administrators of the funds then initiate court action against the uninsured employers to recover the benefits paid. Further, the illegally operating employers are subject to criminal and civil penalties.

TYPES OF BENEFITS

Income Benefits.   Income benefits are cash benefits paid to the worker to partially replace income lost during a period of total inability to work and for any permanent partial disability for which he is entitled to compensation under the particular act.

The initial benefit usually is a temporary total disability benefit for the time the employee is off from work recuperating from the injury or illness. Most states require the employee to be off from work for an elimination period of a specified number of days before temporary total disability benefits are collected. Thus, if the employee is off from work for only 4 days, in a state that has a 7-day elimination period, the loss of income for those 4 days is uncompensated. The amount of a workers' temporary total disability benefit is based on some percentage, usually 50–66⅔%, of his average weekly wage (determined by a statutory formula), subject to a maximum weekly benefit that is determined by his state's average weekly wage.

If an employee becomes totally and permanently disabled, the weekly amount paid for temporary total disability simply continues, either subject to a maximum number of weeks, or, in many states, for the remainder of the employee's life, or until such time as the employer establishes that the employee has regained some ability to return to work. Determination of total disability involves either an objective or a subjective standard, according to the act, similar to the standards discussed hereafter concerning permanent partial disability. In some states, permanent total disability awards are automatically reviewed periodically by the administrative agency or tribunal to determine whether a change in the employee's disability status justifies alteration in the payment of income benefits.

Most states have some statutory provision whereby temporary total disability benefits can be withheld or decreased in the event that the injured worker unreasonably refuses medical treatment. For this reason, physicians should exercise care in discussing possible risks and benefits of treatment and should, at least in a general way, document the information conveyed to the patient. For example, if the suggested treatment has only limited chances of improving the employee's condition or if it has substantial risk of complications or of worsening the employee's condition, the worker's refusal of treatment would not be considered unreasonable.

After the period of entitlement to temporary total disability benefits, which generally ends when the employee has either returned to work or reached "maximum medical improvement" (unless he remains totally disabled, as discussed above), the employee is entitled to compensation for any permanent partial disability sustained from the injury or illness. The employee may also be entitled to a continuation of income benefits under a program of rehabilitation, as is discussed later. Permanent partial disability benefits are usually paid for a number of weeks specified by statute. The amount of the payment is determined by the extent of disability awarded. The provisions in the acts for determination of the extent of permanent partial disability generally fall into one of three theories of compensation:

1. Schedule of Benefits. The majority of states provide a schedule of benefits for certain specific injuries, such as loss of a hand or a finger, that entitle the employee to a stated number of weeks of benefits for the particular injury sustained. These schedules do not take into consideration subjective issues concerning the impact of the injury on the particular employee's ability to work. Thus, a pianist and a factory worker would receive exactly the same benefits for loss of a finger.

2. Functional Impairment. In permanent partial disability awards based on functional impairment, an objective standard, such as the *AMA Guide to the Evaluation of Functional Impairment*, is used to determine disability awards. Awards for injuries not covered by the applicable standard are determined by medical opinions concerning the "whole body" impairment. As with "scheduled" injuries, no consideration is given to subjective criteria.

3. Occupational Impairment. When awards are based on occupational impairment, disability is determined subjectively. Consideration is given to such issues as the particular employee's age, work experience, and education; the work available in the employee's locality; and the extent to which continued work would tend to worsen the employee's condition. Under this type of determination, for example, the loss of an arm may be totally disabling to a 59-year-old laborer with an eighth-grade education, whereas it may be only a partial disability for a younger person with some college education.

Medical Expenses. All workers' compensation acts hold the employer liable for medical expenses reasonably incurred to treat an employee for a work-related injury or illness. There is no cap on benefits, nor does any co-insurance or deductible apply. Medical expenses include, in addition to physician and hospital bills, the cost of prostheses, braces, physical or occupational therapy, home treatment devices, medications, and, in some jurisdictions, the employees' expenses (such as for transportation) in obtaining treatment. Most jurisdictions require medical expenses to be paid within a stated number of days (usually 30–60) after being presented to the employer or its insurer.

Because costs of medical expenses are rising, workers' compensation acts in some jurisdictions have created fee schedules with caps on medical, surgical, and hospital charges for work-related injuries or illnesses. These fee schedules are a matter of significant controversy. At issue is the balance of the need for cost containment against the needs of the injured or ill employees to obtain satisfactory medical treatment. The concern is that physicians will refuse, or limit, treatment of workers' compensation patients in jurisdictions where the fees permitted are viewed as unreasonably low.

Rehabilitation Expenses. Many acts have rehabilitation statutes providing for the employer to bear the cost of rehabilitation therapy, retraining, and job placement if a work-related injury or illness prevents an employee from doing the type of work done in the past. A few jurisdictions also require such employees to be paid income benefits while they are in a retraining or rehabilitation program, although these benefits are generally payable only to people who are permanently and totally disabled.

Death Benefits. All jurisdictions provide for the dependents of employees who die as a result of work-related illnesses or injuries to be paid death benefits to compensate for the lost earning capacity of the deceased worker. Dependency and the amount and duration of benefits paid are determined by statutory provisions in each act. Most acts also provide for the payment of funeral and burial expenses by the employer.

PROCEDURE

Certain procedural elements are common in all jurisdictions. The employee is required to give notice of the work-related injury or illness upon becoming aware of an illness or when an injury is sustained, or as soon thereafter as is reasonably possible. Verbal notice is sufficient in some jurisdictions, whereas others require written notice by the employee. Upon receiving notice, the employer is required to file a written report, often known as a "first report of injury," with the appropriate state board or tribunal.

The employee who is unable to work after the injury or illness receives temporary total disability benefits and payment of medical expenses. During this interval, reports of the treating physicians are often necessary to verify the relationship of the injury or illness to the employee's work and the employee's inability to work. In some jurisdictions, special forms are used for such reports, whereas others rely simply on physicians' narrative reports or personally prepared forms. When no permanent disability is involved, workers' compensation claims end with termination of temporary total disability payments.

If there is permanent disability, either total or partial, several approaches can ensue. The employee can attempt to negotiate a settlement on his own behalf with the employer or its insurance carrier, or he can seek representation by an attorney. The attorney may be able to resolve the permanent partial (or total) disability entitlement of the employee by settlement; if not, a formal workers' compensation claim is filed with the appropriate board or court, depending on the particular jurisdiction. A claim involves preparing and filing various printed forms, often with supporting medical records or reports stating the nature of the injury or illness, its relationship to the work the employee was doing, and the probability of resulting permanent partial or total disability. In jurisdictions that require general reports or records before a claim can be filed, the reports or records are not necessarily considered evidence in the rendering of a decision. The requirements for evidence are determined by each jurisdiction.

The procedure may continue with the taking of depositions from the physicians who have treated the employee, as well as from those who have evaluated the employee at the request of the employer or of the agency. These depositions are submitted as evidence to the agency or court that will decide the claim. All jurisdictions have provisions entitling the employer to have the employee evaluated by an independent physician or physicians of its choice. In some states, in lieu of depositions, physicians' medical reports can be filed with the agency or court as evidence supporting the claimant or the employer or, in instances where it is a party, the subsequent injury fund. For such reports to be accepted as evidence, the physician usually must prepare them on a preprinted form promulgated by the state agency. The reports often obviate physicians' depositions, although the party opposing the party filing the report may take a deposition in order to clarify points raised by the report.

Whether medical evidence is presented by deposition or by report, it generally involves issues of causation, extent of impairment and disability, and pre-existing conditions or disabilities. In jurisdictions that approach disability as an occupational impairment, the physician is also asked to state an opinion about what limitations of activity the injury entails (such as a limitation in grip strength) and what restrictions are medically advisable (such as avoidance of vibratory tools for the employee with carpal tunnel syndrome in order to avoid exacerbating the condition). Additionally, the physician may be called upon to testify about possible or probable side effects from medications necessary for the employee's treatment because these may also limit the choice of jobs (as in situations where medication-induced drowsiness restricts an employee from working with high-powered or dangerous machinery).

At a hearing held by the appropriate board or judge, the employee may testify about the injury or illness, and testimony of lay witnesses, such as co-workers, a foreman, a spouse, or friends who are knowledgeable about the disabling effects of the injury or illness, may be presented. Additionally, the board or judge considers the medical evidence that has been presented by way of deposition or submission of medical reports.

All of this evidence is taken under consideration by the board or judge, and, usually sometime after the hearing, a written opinion is issued, stating whether or not the employee is entitled to benefits and, if so, the extent thereof.

In some cases, by agreement of the parties, all of the evidence is taken by deposition or medical reports, and the case is submitted to the agency or court to decide without a hearing.

After a decision is issued, an unsatisfied party may seek reconsideration of the decision or appeal to the appropriate court.

ISSUES OF ENTITLEMENT

Certain issues determining the entitlement are common to workers' compensation procedure in all jurisdictions.

Existence of Employee-Employer Relationship. Simply put, an injured party can receive workers' compensation benefits only from his or her employer. Occasionally the agency or court handling a claim must decide whether the injured party was employed by the party against whom the claim is made. Usually the matter in dispute is whether the injured person was working as an employee or as an independent contractor, a distinction which turns on the amount of control exerted by the claimed employer over the injured party (such factors as whether the claimed employer set the injured party's hours of work, or whether he set his own hours; whether the worker used his own tools or those of the claimed employer; who directed the specific details of the work; and whether there was a written contract). Occasionally a dispute involves whether the injured party was a partner or joint venturer in the business, as opposed to an employee of the business; owners or partners cannot draw workers' compensation benefits from the business (except in states that, by statute, allow such coverage as an option).

Operation under the Act.   In order to draw workers' compensation benefits, the employee and employer must have been operating, that is, carrying out the employment relationship, under the particular state's act. The employee is automatically working under the act unless he is an exempt worker or has, before the injury, filed a waiver or rejection of workers' compensation benefits. For the employer, operation under the act is mandatory and automatic except for employers of exempt workers. Exempt employees, meaning employees who are, because of the nature of their employment, not eligible to receive workers' compensation benefits, are defined differently under different acts. Categories often included are farmworkers, domestic servants, volunteer workers, temporary or "casual" help, or employees whose employers have fewer than a specified number (usually five or less) of employees. Employers of exempt workers can elect to operate under the act of their state and can thus become liable for payment of workers' compensation benefits.

Work-Relatedness.   The determination of whether an injury or illness is work related generally turns on questions of whether the injury or illness "arose out of and in the course of the employment."

"Arising in the course of the employment" pertains to the time, place, and circumstances of the injury sustained or illness contracted. The standard needs interpretation when the injury occurred while the employee was on break or shortly before or after work began or ended, when it occurred in the parking lot as

opposed to the worksite; or when it occurred while the employee was doing a personal errand during working hours, for example. In recent years, many claims have arisen for cumulative injuries—injuries that develop over time as a result of repetitive trauma (such as carpal tunnel syndrome, back injuries, and chronic strains). Most jurisdictions permit claims that depart from the traditional view of an injury as the result of a single traumatic episode.

"Arising out of employment" pertains to the cause of the injury or illness. In occupational disease cases, for example a communicable disease contracted from a co-worker is not considered an illness "arising out of employment" because the risk was not peculiar to the workplace; whereas pneumoconiosis in a coal miner would "arise out of" the worker's employment. Thus, to "arise out of" the employment, the injury or illness must be a risk occasioned by the employment. A worker who trips on his or her shoelace and sustains injury is probably not entitled to workers' compensation benefits unless he can show that the distraction of the work caused his inattentiveness.

Disability.   Finally, in order to be entitled to benefits, the employee must establish disability—either temporary total disability or permanent total or partial disability under the applicable disability standards discussed earlier.

MISCELLANEOUS PROVISIONS

Thirty-Party Claims.   The injured employee may have a tort claim against a third party other than his employer. For example, a factory worker may have a products liability claim against the manufacturer of an unreasonably dangerous chemical or machine; or, a truck drive for company A may have a personal injury claim against company B, whose forklift operator ran into him as he was unloading delivered goods. In such cases, the employer of the injured worker is still required to pay compensation benefits but may bring a claim directly against the third party or may subrogate against a claim for damages brought by the injured worker in order to recover compensation benefits.

Social Security.   A worker who has become totally disabled by a work-related injury or illness is entitled to both workers' compensation and Social Security disability benefits, providing he meets the Social Security test of having a disability that has lasted, or is expected to last, for at least a year or that is expected to result in death. Where both forms of benefits are received, there is a slight reduction in the amount of benefits received from Social Security.

Reopening. Most jurisdictions allow a workers' compensation claim to be reopened by either party in order to request an increase or reduction of the agreed-upon or awarded benefits. In some jurisdictions reopening can be done only upon showing that the physical condition of the worker has changed. Others allow reopening upon showing change of occupational disability, as where the employer proves that a worker drawing total disability benefits has been working, or where a worker with a hand injury was initially allowed to return to work by the employer but has now been terminated and is unable, because of a hand injury, to find a job. In the latter case, the worker who was initially awarded no or minimal permanent disability benefits may be entitled to reopen the claim and obtain an award or an increase in the amount previously awarded.

Statutes of Limitation. All acts provide a deadline, or statute of limitation, for filing a claim. (Where a claim is settled by agreement, without a formal claim, the required filing of agreement papers with the agency or court constitutes the filing of a claim for the purpose of preserving the right of the claimant to reopen the claim.) If a claim is not filed by the injured or ill employee within the time provided, compensation benefits cannot be claimed for income, medical expense, or rehabilitation, and the claim cannot be reopened.

Penalties. All acts provide for civil and criminal penalties to be assessed against persons making false claims or employers failing to comply with statutory record-keeping requirements, to provide insurance or self-insurance, or to pay benefits.

Some jurisdictions also permit employees to bring civil suits against their employers for certain conduct, such as firing the employee in retaliation for a workers' compensation claim.

CONCLUSION

The foregoing overview of workers' compensation law and procedure should benefit those who become involved in such claims, whether as physicians, adjusters, company representatives, claimants, or employers.

APPENDIX A

Workers' Compensation Administrative Offices

U.S. Department of Labor

Employment Standards Administration
200 Constitution Ave., N.W.
Washington, DC 20210
202-523-6191
Workers' Compensation Programs
Office of State Liaison and Legislative Analysis
200 Constitution Ave., N.W., Rm. N-4414
Washington, DC 20210
202-523-9575

State Laws

Alabama
Department of Industrial Relations
Workmen's Compensation Office
Montgomery, AL 36130
205-261-2868

Alaska
Workers' Compensation Division
Department of Labor
P.O. Box 1149
Juneau, AK 99802
907-465-2790

Arizona
Industrial Commission
1601 West Jefferson
P.O. Box 19070
Phoenix, AZ 85005
602-255-4411

Arkansas
Workers' Compensation Commission
Justice Building
State Capitol Grounds
Little Rock, AR 72201
501-372-3930

California
Division of Industrial Accidents
525 Golden Gate Avenue, Room 617
San Francisco, CA 94101
415-557-3542

Colorado
Division of Labor
1313 Sherman Street, Room 314
Denver, CO 80203
303-866-2861

Connecticut
Workers' Compensation Commission
1890 Dixwell Ave.
Hamden, CN 06514
203-789-7783

Delaware
Industrial Accident Board
State Office Building, 6th Floor
820 North French Street
Wilmington, DE 19801
302-571-2884

District of Columbia
D.C. Department of Employment Services
1200 Upshur Street, N.W.
Washington, DC 20011
202-576-6265, 7088

Florida
Division of Workers' Compensation
2590 Executive Center Circle E
Tallahassee, FL 32301
904-488-2514

Georgia
Board of Workers' Compensation
10th Floor
1000 South Omni International
Atlanta, GA 30335
404-656-3875

Hawaii
Disability Compensation Division
Department of Labor and Industrial Relations
830 Punchbowl Street
Honolulu, HI 96812
808-548-4180

Idaho
Industrial Commission
317 Main Street
Boise, ID 83720
208-334-3250

Illinois
Industrial Commission
160 North LaSalle Street
Chicago, IL 60601
312-793-6500

Indiana
Industrial Board
601 State Office Building
100 N. Senate Avenue
Indianapolis, IN 46204
317-232-3808

Iowa
Industrial Commission
507 10th Street
Des Moines, IA 50319
515-281-5934

Kansas
Division of Workers' Compensation
217 S.E. Fourth St.
Topeka, KS 66603
913-296-3441

Kentucky
Workers' Compensation Board
U.S. 127 South, 127 Building
Frankford, KY 40601
502-564-5550

Louisiana
Office of Workers' Compensation
P.O. Box 94094
910 N. Bon Marche Drive
Baton Rouge, LA 70804
504-925-7211

Maine
Workers' Compensation Commission
Station 27, Deering Building
August, ME 04333
207-289-3751

Maryland
Workmen's Compensation Commission
6 N. Liberty St.
Baltimore, MD 21201
301-659-4700

Massachusetts
Industrial Accident Board
Leverett Saltonstall Office Building
100 Cambridge Street, 17th Floor
Boston, MA 02202
617-727-3400

Michigan
Workers' Disability Compensation Office
Department of Labor
P.O. Box 30015
Lansing, MI 48909
517-373-3480

Minnesota
Department of Labor and Industry
444 Lafayette Road
St. Paul, MN 55101
612-296-2432

Mississippi
Workers' Compensation Commission
P.O. Box 5300
Jackson, MS 39216
601-987-4200

Missouri
Division of Workers' Compensation
Department of Labor & Industrial Relations
P.O. Box 58, 722 Jefferson St.
Jefferson City, MO 65102
314-751-4231

Montana
Division of Workers' Compensation
5 S. Last Chance Gulch
Helena, MT 59601
406-444-6500

Nebraska
Workmen's Compensation Court
State House
Lincoln, NE 68509
402-471-2568

Nevada
State Industrial Insurance System
515 E. Musser Street
Carson City, NV 89714
702-885-5284

New Hampshire
Department of Labor
19 Pillsbury Street
Concord, NH 03301
603-271-3172

New Jersey
Division of Workers' Compensation
Department of Labor
John Fitch Plaza, CN 110
Trenton, NJ 08625
609-292-2414

New Mexico
Labor and Industrial Commission
1596 Pacheco St.
Santa Fe, NM 87501
505-827-9876

New York
Workers' Compensation Board
180 Livingston Street
Brooklyn, NY 11248
718-802-4903

North Carolina
Industrial Commission
Dobbs Building
430 N. Salisbury Street
Raleigh, NC 27611
919-733-4820

North Dakota
Workmens' Compensation Bureau
Russel Building—Highway 83 N.
Bismarck, ND 58501
701-224-2700

Ohio
Bureau of Workers' Compensation
246 N. High Street
Columbus, Ohio 43215
614-466-1238

Oklahoma
Workers' Compensation Court
Jim Thorpe Building
2101 N. Lincoln
Oklahoma City, OK 73105
405-521-8025

Oregon
Workers' Compensation Department
Labor and Industries Building
Salem, OR 97310
503-378-3304

Pennsylvania
Bureau of Workers' Compensation
Labor and Industry Building
Harrisburg, PA 17120
717-783-5421

Rhode Island
Division of Workers' Compensation
220 Elmwood Avenue
Providence, RI 02907
401-277-2722

South Carolina
Workers' Compensation Fund
800 Dutch Square Blvd.
Ste. 160
Columbia, SC 29210
803-758-6290

South Dakota
Department of Labor
Division on Labor and Management
700 N. Illinois Street
Pierre, SD 57501
605-773-3681

Tennessee
Division of Workers' Compensation
Department of Labor
501 Union Building, 2nd Floor
Nashville, TN 37219
615-741-2395

Texas
Industrial Accident Board
200 East Riverside Drive
Austin, TX 78704
512-448-7900

Utah
Industrial Commission
160 East 300 South
Salt Lake City, UT 84145-0580
801-530-6800

Vermont
Department of Labor and Industry
State Office Building
120 State St.
Montpelier, VT 05602
802-828-2286

Virginia
Industrial Commission
Worker's Compensation Division
1000 DMV Drive
Richmond, VA 23220
804-257-8600

Washington
Department of Labor and Industries
General Administration Building, HC-101
Olympia, WA 98504
206-753-6376

West Virginia
Workers' Compensation Fund
Department of Labor
601 Morris Square
Box 3151
Charleston, WV 25332
304-348-2580

Wisconsin
Workers' Compensation Division
P.O. Box 7901
Madison, WI 53707
608-266-6841

Wyoming
Workers' Compensation Division
122 West 25th St.
Cheyenne, WY 82002-0700
307-777-7441

Chapter 39

ERGONOMIC DESIGN OF HANDHELD TOOLS TO PREVENT TRAUMA TO THE HAND AND UPPER EXTREMITY*

Susan L. Johnson, O.T.R., C.V.E.

The Industrial Revolution took the worker from the farm to the factory and assembly-line production. Over time, this interaction between man and workplace has compromised optimum performance in terms of efficiency, health, and human wellness. In any man/machine system there are tasks that are better performed by man than by machine and vice versa. Man excels in adaptability, not repetitiveness. If man is asked to perform repeatedly and beyond his forced capabilities, breakdown will occur. Cumulative effects of physical stress are insidious and can suddenly result in injury. Frequently it is the tool handle, linking the worker to his work, that is the source of the undue stress.

Silverstein, in 1985, suggested that hand and wrist symptoms increased by 37% with high force/high repetition job tasks.[1] The results supported the findings of the National Institute of Occupational Safety and Health (NIOSH) and the U.S. Surgeons General's Office with regard to cumulative trauma disorders (CTD): "When job demands . . . repeatedly exceed the biomechanical capacity of the worker, the activities become gradually trauma-inducing."[2] Therefore, biomechanical analysis and human anatomy must be considered in the design of tool handles to prevent injury to the human body. The costly consequences of CTD have given way to ergonomics: the relationship between man and his workplace to achieve op-

timum performance and reduced trauma. When tool design is inappropriate, the hand and upper extremity become vulnerable to injury.

For example, in 1986 the state of Colorado identified claims totalling \$34,789.009.[3] In the United States there were over 500,000 workers' compensation injuries in 1987, resulting in 20 billion dollars in lost time, medical care, retraining of personnel, and the processing of claims.

Armstrong cites the most common risk factors of CTD as repetitiveness, force, mechanical stress, posture, vibration, and temperature.[4,5] Meager identifies the most important elements of tool design with regard to the human factor as size, shape, texture, ease of operation, shock absorption, and weight.[6,7]

Cumulative trauma disorders that may occur secondary to poor hand tool design are trigger finger, synovitis, nerve compression, arterial compression, chronic strain, muscle strain, aggravation of arthritis, epicondylitis, vibratory trauma, carpal tunnel syndrome, de Quervain's disease, tenosynovitis, and tendinitis (Table 1).

HANDLE SIZE AND SHAPE

Tool handle size is an essential consideration in tool design to maximize grip strength, reduce stress on digital flexor tendons, and avoid stress to the first carpometacarpal (CMC) collateral ligament.[8] Considering anthropomet-

* Adapted from Johnson SL, Journal of Hand Therapy, 3:86–93, 1990, with permission.

TABLE 1. Cumulative Trauma Disorders*

Cumulative Trauma Disorder	Associated Risk Factors and Postures
1. Lateral epicondylitis	Radial deviation of the wrist with pronation
2. Tenosynovitis of the digital extensors	Ulnar deviation of the wrist with supination
3. Tenosynovitis of the digital flexors	Forceful wrist flexion Repeated digital flexion
4. Tendonitis of the extensor compartments	Repetitive wrist flexion/extension Repeated radial deviation of the wrist combined with forceful exertions of the thumb Repeated ulnar deviation of the wrist in combination with forceful exertions of the thumb Manipulations of more than 2,000 per hour Direct blunt trauma Any repetitive motion that is forceful and fast
5. Nerve compression: Radial tunnel syndrome	Resistive supination with the elbow extended
Superficial radial nerve	Direct pressure or repetitive blows
Pronator syndrome	Repeated and resistive forearm pronation with the elbow in flexion
Carpal tunnel syndrome	Repeated wrist flexion or extension; sustained wrist flexion Repeated forces at the base of the palm and wrist
Cubital tunnel syndrome	Sustained elbow flexion
Ulnar tunnel syndrome	Sustained wrist flexion Direct trauma
Digital neuritis	Contact over the neurovascular bundles on the side of the fingers
6. Ganglion cysts	Repeated manipulations with extended wrist Repeated twisting of the wrist
7. Trigger finger	Direct pressure from hard objects to the flexor tendon at the level of the metacarpal head

*Adapted from Armstrong T, et al: An investigation of cumulative trauma disorders in a poultry processing plant. Am Ind Hyg Assoc J 43:103–116, 1982.

rics, the male and female hands are often different sizes. One size does not fit everyone. The smaller female hand with its smaller muscle mass will not tolerate inadequately levered tool handles or inadequate shock absorption.[9] When a handle diameter is too large and the forces are applied at the distal phalanx of the fingers (Fig. 1A), the tendon forces can be 2–

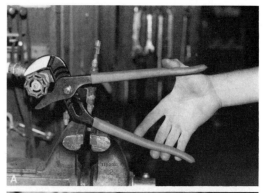
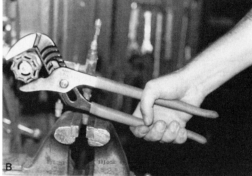
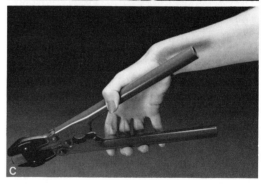

FIGURE 1. *A*, A handle diameter that is too large results in tendon forces 2–3 times greater than when force is applied at the middle phalanx (*B*), especially when the wrist is flexed (*C*).

3 times greater than when the force is applied at the middle phalanx (Fig. 1B). Conversely, with a small handle, the fingers cannot effectively apply force because of the mechanically disadvantaged, shortened position of the extrinsic finger flexors. Small handles can also result in intrinsic muscle overcompensation and strain. This compromised position and its adverse effects are compounded when the wrist is flexed (Fig. 1C).

Therefore, when applying maximal crimping force, the wrist should be held in approximately 30° of extension with small hand joints slightly flexed, thus allowing the extrinsic flexor muscles to work in a mechanically efficient position and in synergy with the intrinsic muscles. Milner has shown that a partially stretched muscle will contract more forcefully than an unstretched muscle at the time of firing.[10] Greenberg and Chaffin state that grip span for crimping tools should be restricted to approximately 5–8 cm for maximal strength.[11] A maximum grip strength is usually achieved at a span of 7.5 to 8.0 cm,[10] which is measured from the center of the hand, at the base of the third metacarpal to the long finger middle phalanx.

Crimping tools should have a spring opening. The spring handle should open the tool no more than 11.5 cm in width.[11] Should the handle spring open further, the thumb CMC joint may be subjected to stresses, leading to partial joint dislocation, joint capsule injury, or aggravation of arthritis. In addition, all volar finger joint capsules are vulnerable to injury from tool handles that are too large in diameter, because the fat pad is nonexistent at the digital skin crease over the volar joint.

In cylindrically shaped tools, such as pneumatic tools, the optimal grip span would be smaller. Grip strengths on round objects were determined by Ayoub and LePresti.[12] They found that maximum grip strengths were recorded when the diameter was 4 cm.[12]

The specific diameters are important, as the small muscles of the hand are susceptible to undue stress. They stabilize the hand during forceful use and balance the long flexor and extensor tendons during prehension and fine manipulation. The tool handle diameter can easily stress these muscles, as an overstretched or understretched muscle does not contract efficiently.[11] The intrinsic muscles fatigue quickly if the diameter of the handle is too large or too small and require unnecessary energy for tool retention.

Inappropriate handle size can also stress the flexor tendons in the finger, where they are held close to the phalanges by a pulley and sheath system. This system prevents bowstringing during flexion. An area of frequent injury is the proximal opening of the tendon sheath in the area of the first and second annular ligaments. This pulley can be traumatized by narrow tool handles or constant pressure. Inflammation and swelling of the tendon in this area may result in compression of the tendon, causing a nodule to form, resulting in trigger finger.

HANDLE LENGTH

The length of the handle should be designed to minimize pressure to the median or ulnar nerve at the distal palm or wrist. The force of the handle should be disturbed over the thenar and hypothenar eminences and digits two through five. The median nerve arteries, and synovium of the flexor tendons are quite superficial and thus susceptible to any downward pressure, as may occur with handheld staplers or short-handled pliers. It is recommended that handles be at least 9 cm long to distribute forces evenly.[13] Incorrect size of the handle can cause pressure to underlying tendons, sheaths, and nerves, resulting in CTDs such as trigger finger, tenosynovitis, digital neuritis, joint capsulor injury, carpal tunnel syndrome, and Guyon canal syndrome.

TOOL CONTOUR

Handles should have a small contour to coincide with the curve of the transverse palmar arch and allow for even application of force. On the digital side, the handle should follow the natural palmar curve of the fingers as they flex toward the palm in order to distribute muscle loading evenly to the digits.[7] A "reverse curvature"[8] has been adapted by Bob Brown, Hewlett and Packard Business computer group. This curve is contoured to accommodate the natural curve of the thenar eminence. Short handles do not permit this accommodation and should be avoided or used only when light force is applied.

Profiling of handles using digit separators is an example of poorly designed contour from a biomechanical standpoint. Profiling restricts the range of the hand, impairing comfortable grasp of the tool. The prominences on the handle can cause joint capsule injury, trigger finger, neurovascular injury, or intrinsic strain (since the digits are held in abduction while they are trying to flex fully).[15] Because the neurovascular bundles are superficial on each side of the finger just lateral to the palmar fat pads, they lack protection and are susceptible to direct trauma. The edges of the finger separators on profiled handles can easily compress these structures (Fig. 2).

Finger rings on handles should be avoided for the same reason. If ill-fitting, improperly contoured, used forcefully, or held constantly,

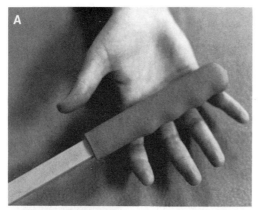

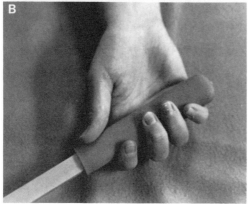

FIGURE 2. Profiling of handles can cause neurovascular injury to the fingers as a result of compression by the finger separators.

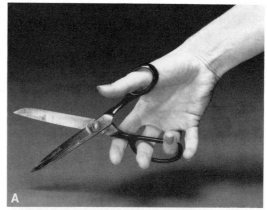

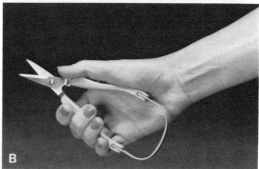

FIGURE 3. *A*, Scissors can cause compression of digital neurovascular structures. *B*, Loop-design scissors help to distribute the pressure more evenly.

these rings may cause intrinsic strain or neurovascular compression.

Compression of the digital arteries and nerves can be produced by other tools, such as scissors, that apply pressure to the sides of the fingers during use (Fig. 3A). For this problem, loop-design scissors with a built-in spring opening alleviates the stresses to these digital neurovascular structures and applies pressures more evenly (Fig. 3B).

UPPER EXTREMITY POSTURE DURING TOOL USE

It is important to assume a correct posture when using tools to prevent shoulder strain, carpal tunnel syndrome, tenosynovitis, de Quervain's disease, or epicondylitis. Tools should be designed so that use does not entail greater than 20° of abduction of the shoulder in the vertical position. Normally this shoulder position will not create an excessive load; how-

ever, abduction greater than 20° increases the amount of shoulder strain.

A heavy hand-tool markedly compounds the moment requirement of arm abduction. Chaffin[16] found that if shoulder abduction was approximately 30°, muscle fatigue occurred after a period of time 3 times longer than when abducted 60°, and 6 times longer than when abducted 90°. Stick drawing and templates, developed by Drillis, can be used to determine the best working height for a person to avoid shoulder abduction or wrist ulnar deviation (Fig. 4).[17] The height that is ideal for tall workers may require short workers to turn their wrists or abduct their shoulders.

Holding a tool with the wrist in prolonged ulnar deviation may cause carpal tunnel syndrome. It may also promote tenosynovitis, de Quervain's disease, and epicondylitis.[18] In 1978, Tichauer compared two groups of trainees in electronic assemblies.[15] When the wrist was maintained in ulnar deviation, creating ulnar drift of the tendons and tendon sheaths, there was gradual increase in tenosynovitis, epicon-

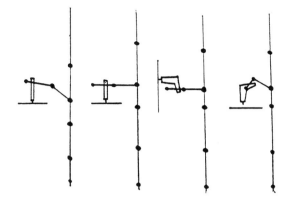

FIGURE 4. Stick drawing and templates can be used to determine the best working height for a person to avoid shoulder abduction or wrist ulnar deviation. (Adapted from Drillis R, Contini R, 1966.[17])

dylitis, and carpal tunnel syndrome,[15] owing to the altered position of the flexor tendons.

It is important to design the job and the handle so that the wrist is maintained in a neutral position, with the radius aligned with the second metacarpal. Figure 5A demonstrates a pneumatic torque driver being used improperly. By adjusting the posture and type of tool, and instructing the employee to keep the wrist straight, malalignment of the wrist is corrected (Fig. 5B). If the posture cannot be adapted because of restrictions in design, the tool must be adapted. Job-site evaluations are sometimes needed to evaluate whether a cylindrical driver or a pistol-shaped driver is more appropriate for the job to be performed with the wrist in a neutral position. The orientation of the work space and location of work pieces relative to the worker's arm are decisive factors (Fig. 5C).

The use of pliers often results in positioning the wrist in ulnar deviation (Fig. 6A). This is corrected by bending the handles of the pliers with respect to the work station. John F. Bennet has developed a 19° double-ellipse bend to reduce hand fatigue and to provide the grip strength required to hold the tool (Fig. 6B). This design keeps the wrist straight and is thus incorporated in many hand tools. Future research may show that angulations of greater than 19° are even more efficient (Fig. 6C).

Armstrong performed biomechanical job evaluations and found that poultry processing operations with a common, straight-handled knife required extreme wrist flexion and ulnar deviation (Fig. 7A).[19] The cumulative trauma incidence rate for hand and wrist injuries in these industries was approximately 17% each year, occurring in boning, cutting, and filleting operations,[19,20] The knife commonly used in these jobs was adapted to have a pistol-grip and wrap-around handle (Fig. 7B).[19] EMG studies supported the implementation of this adaptation by showing that muscle fatigue was reduced when the wrap-around handle was used.[19] Additionally, relaxing the hand be-

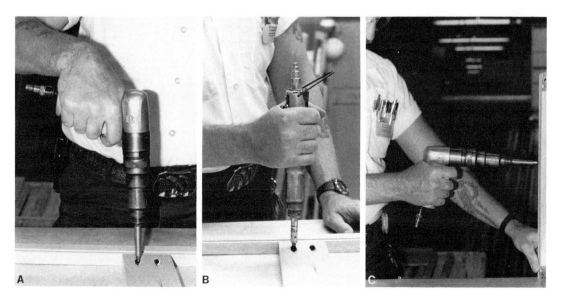

FIGURE 5. A, Improper use of pneumatic torque driver. B, Correction of malalignment of the wrist. C, Configuration of the work space and location of work pieces relative to the worker's arm are important.

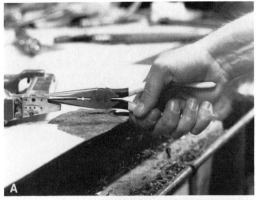

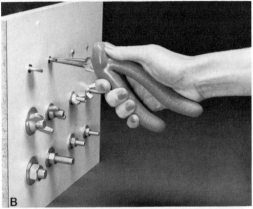

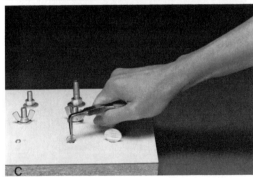

FIGURE 6. *A*, The use of pliers often results in positioning the wrist in ulnar deviation. *B*, A 19° double-ellipse bend reduces hand fatigue. *C*, Angulation of greater than 19°.

tween cuts and performing the task with the wrist in a neutral position were effective in reducing injuries.

Stirex or Intercodev, Inc. has adapted other tools to maintain good wrist alignment and reduce hand fatigue. Pain rollers, paint brushes, files, trowels, rakes, and hoes have all been revised with pistol-shaped handles (Fig. 8).

Excessive radial deviation in tool use can lead to lateral epicondylitis, particularly with

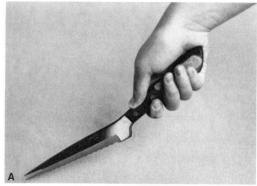

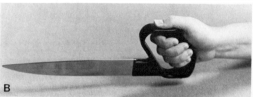

FIGURE 7. *A*, Common, straight-handled knife requires extreme wrist flexion and ulnar deviation. *B*, Adaptation of same knife with pistol-grip and wrap-around handle.

wrist extension and full pronation. Wire brushes or polishing tools may have to be held in this poor posture.

TEXTURE OF HAND TOOLS

Texture of the tool handle is an important design consideration. Comaish and Bottoms provided a basis in their study for including texture as one of the most important elements of tool design.[21] They found that a handle with a slippery finish or a dry hand requires added strength to retain the tool. If the texture is too coarse, skin irritation and reduced efficiency occur. A correctly textured tool allows for tool retention with minimal energy expenditure. Cross-cut patterns and resilient rubber are good textures.

Tools must be designed to avoid transmission of shock or vibration to the hand and upper extremities. Such transmission has been documented to contribute to vibration white finger syndrome (VWF), osseous injury, carpal tunnel syndrome, vasoconstriction, and Raynaud's syndrome. Tool vibration may adversely affect the digital arteries, causing permanent injury to the arterial walls.

Handheld tools generate random vibrations from a wide range of 2–2,000 Hz. Low-fre-

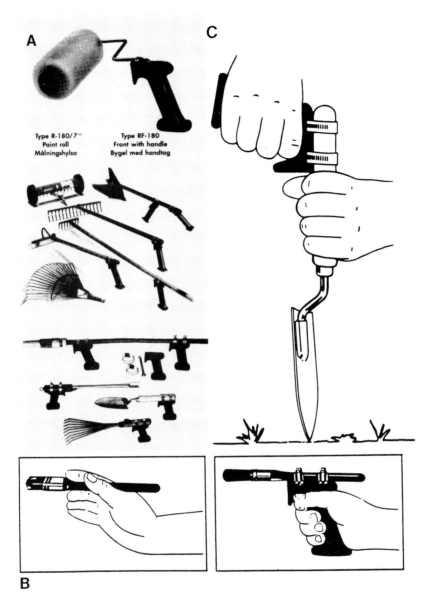

FIGURE 8. *A*, Pistol-shaped handles on various tools. *B*, The wrist is held in ulnar deviation when using a normal paint brush. When a pistol handle is added, the grasp is changed to maintain correct wrist alignment during use. *C*, The same principle is demonstrated with use of a trowel with a pistol handle. (Reproduced with permission from Intercodev, Inc., Holbrook, NY.)

quency (20–25 Hz) vibrations are usually most damaging to the joints. Higher frequency vibrations are largely absorbed by superficial tissue where actual cell damage can occur; this may happen with a frequency as low as 100 Hz. Frequencies of 50–200 Hz cause vasoconstriction and 30–50 are mostly associated with CTS.

Standards and guidelines for dose relationship have been developed but should still be regarded as recommendations rather than firm design specifications. The University of Michigan proposes no more than 30 minutes ex-

posure to vibration. Some experts recommend use of antivibration gloves to reduce the transmission of vibration.

It is necessary to select work gloves carefully for proper fit and to reduce the tendency for irritants to be embedded in the gloves. Wearing gloves tends to make gripping the tool more difficult. The worker wearing gloves grasps the tool more tightly, resulting in fatigue. Hertzberg showed that pilots wearing gloves reduced their strength by 30%.[22] Gloves that are too thick separate the fingers and require over-

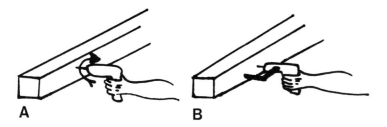

FIGURE 9. Torque bars help to decrease rotational forces. (Adapted from Armstrong T, 1983.[5])

tight gripping; intrinsic strain and functioning can occur, as the glove acts as digital separators. In some situations it may be better to design an energy-absorbing tool that does not require the worker to wear gloves.

Torque bars are beneficial in decreasing rotational forces (Fig. 9). The driving torque of the tool creates a tendency for the tool to rotate in the worker's hand unless it is gripped firmly. If the wrist is forced into a deviated posture, there is an increased risk of CTD. Tichauer found that the maximum amount of torque absorbed in the hand from a straight driver should not exceed 12 inch pounds.[20,23] VanBergeijk set specifications at Ford Industry for *straight tools*, not to exceed 28 inch pounds of rotational torque, and for *pistol-grip and right-angled tools*, not to exceed 60 inch pounds.[24]

The tools should be aligned with the axis of rotation of the wrist, and the tool center of gravity weighted at the middle of the palm in order to reduce rotatory forces. External cords or ground wires should be avoided to reduce rotation and may need to be counterbalanced overhead (Fig. 10). The tool or the arm may be supported during use. The hand should be held in a relaxed neutral position, neither over-supinating nor overpronating.

Impact vibration must be considered with repetitive use of hammers. Repetitive hammering may contribute to percussion injuries to tissues and "hypothenar hammer syndrome" (injuries to the vessels of the hypothenar eminence).[25] This can cause temporary spasm of the muscles in the blood vessels with the potential for clot formation. Attention should be given to types of handles that absorb shock. Resin is strong but heavy and transmits shock. The excess weight in the grip impairs its balance and causes overgripping. Hickory wood is the best shock absorber in hammer handles.

Dead-blow hammers have shot in hollow heads. As the partially filled head strikes the work, the shot follows through to sustain the blow, stop the rebound, and control the hammer, allowing more accuracy.

TOOL WEIGHT

Tool weight is as important as handle design. Light tools for light tasks is a good rule. Heavier tools can cause intrinsic strain, muscle spasm,

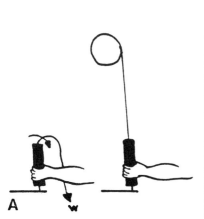
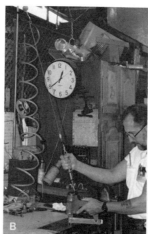
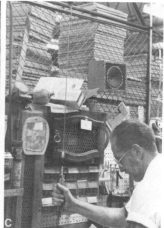

FIGURE 10. External cords or ground wires on tools should be avoided to reduce rotation, and may need to be counterbalanced overhead. (Adapted from Armstrong T, 1983.[5])

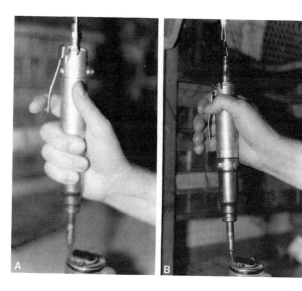

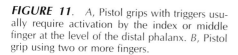

FIGURE 11. *A*, Pistol grips with triggers usually require activation by the index or middle finger at the level of the distal phalanx. *B*, Pistol grip using two or more fingers.

tendinitis, and epicondylitis, but also possess adequate inertia to prevent transmission of excessive vibration. An overhead counterbalance, padded arm supports, or both should be considered to reduce the load moment on the shoulder. Tool balancers work by counterbalancing the weight of the tool with a long spring suspended over the work area (Fig. 10C). These are effective if the work area is limited in size to below the tool balance and the tool is used in one general orientation (vertical or horizontal) but not both.

The lesser strength of the female hand can lead to cumulative trauma when women on utility line work must use tools designed for male strength.[9] The use of excessively heavy tools can contribute to epicondylitis and should be counterbalanced. The tool must be balanced so that the center of gravity of the tool is aligned with the center of the grasping hand.

Reaching overhead for a tool repetitively should be avoided to reduce the risk of thoracic outlet syndrome. Suspended or counterbalanced tools should be close to shoulder height.

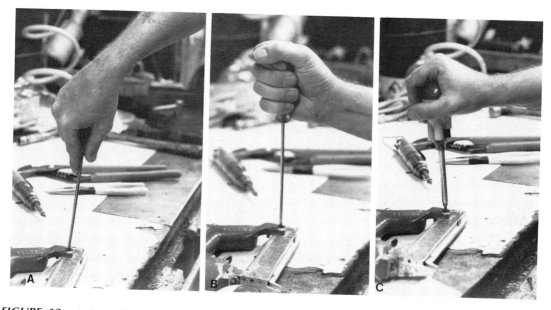

FIGURE 12. *A*, Screwdrivers requiring downward force position the wrist in ulnar deviation. *B*, Phalange handle encourages the operator to hold the screwdriver like a dagger. *C*, Rachet design eliminates the need for repeated forearm supination and pronation.

ACTIVATION DEVICES ON HAND TOOLS

Pistol grips equipped with triggers usually require activation by the index or middle finger at the level of the distal phalanx (Fig. 11A). Triggers should permit flexion of the middle phalanx of the index before flexing of the distal phalanx. If the distal phalanx flexes first, a nodule on the tendon may develop that will not allow the nodule to move within the tendon sheath or pulley. An adaptation for this situation is the use of two finger triggers instead of one for frequent work (Fig. 11B).[26] A four-finger operation to activate the tool's trigger distributes the force and further reduces risk for tenosynovitis.[26]

In some tools, the triggers are often situated too high on the pistol grip, requiring the wrist to hyperextend when activating the trigger and imposing an extra load on the thumb. This can result in pressure on the median nerve, as in carpal tunnel or deQuervain's syndrome. With cylinder pneumatic drills, the thumb is often required to maintain an extended position to activate the trigger. In this type situation, a digital trigger using all four fingers is preferred.

Screwdrivers requiring downward force position the wrist in ulnar deviation (Fig. 12A). A phalange handle encourages the operator to hold the screwdriver like a dagger. Thus, the wrist is kept in a neutral position and sustained ulnar deviation is avoided (Fig. 12B). A ratchet design eliminates the need for repeated forearm supination and pronation (Fig. 12C). A thumb stop can also be used to provide forward thrust through the thumb musculature instead of the palm.

CONCLUSION

Using ergonomic design and appropriate selection of hand tools for the prevention of cumulative trauma disorders is paramount. The principles and designs presented should help to reduce the biomechanical stresses on the worker's hands, arms, and shoulders. Proper tool design and use can improve productivity and promote human wellness. In addition, the employer is able to reduce the costs of worker compensation premiums by reducing injury within the industry. Frequently it is the rising number of workers' compensation claims that becomes the impetus for changes.

Acknowledgments

The author would like to gratefully recognize her father and mother and to thank her children, Anna and Erica; the Colorado Department of Labor; Chris Warren; Jim Burnett; Riviera Cabinets; Intercodev; Corona Industries; Ken Boyer and Heidi Graff for their assistance in the illustrations; and Hazel Jackson, Debbie Bohne, Tracy Pierce for their technical assistance in preparing the manuscript.

REFERENCES

1. Silverstein BA: The prevalence of upper extremity cumulative trauma disorders in industry. The University of Michigan, Occupational Health and Safety Engineering, 1985.
2. Proposed Strategies for the Prevention of Leading Work-Related Diseases and Injuries. Associated Schools of Public Health under a cooperative agreement with the National Institute for Occupational Safety and Health, 1986, p 19.
3. Lewis JH: Final Report of the Independent Study of the Colorado Workers' Compensation System.
4. Armstrong TJ. Ergonomics and cumulative trauma disorders. Hand Clinics, Vol 2, No 3, August 1986: 553–565.
5. Armstrong T: An ergonomics guide to carpal tunnel syndrome. Akron, Ohio, AIHAJ Ergonomic Guide Series, 1983.
6. Meagher SW: Human factors engineering. Contemp Orthop 8:73–80, 1987.
7. Meagher SW: Tool design for prevention of hand and wrist injuries. Hand Surg 12A:855–857, 1987.
8. Chaffin DB, Andersson GBJ: Occupational Biomechanics. New York, John Wiley & Sons, 1984, p 362.
9. Meagher SW: Design of hand tools for control of cumulative trauma disorders: An ergonomic interventions to prevent musculoskeletal injuries in industry. America Conference of Government Industrial Hygienists. Chelsea, MI, Lewis Publishers, 1987, pp 111–115.
10. Meagher SW: Hand tools: Cumulative trauma disorders caused by improper use of design elements. Trends in ergonomics. Human Factors 3:581–587, 1986.
11. Gowitzke BA, Milnar A: Understanding the Scientific Basis of Human Movement, 2nd ed. Baltimore, Williams and Wilkins, 1980, p 95.
12. Greenberg L, et al: Workers and Their Tools: A Guide to the Ergonomic Design of Hand Tools and Small Presses. Midland, MI, Pendell Publishing Company, 1977.
13. Ayoub MM, LoPresti P: The determination of an optimum size cylindrical handle by use of electrobiography. Ergonomics 4:503–518, 1971.
14. Webb Associates: Anthropometric Source Book, Vol II. Washington, DC, NASA Reference 1024, 1978, pp 43–47.
15. Tichauer ER: The biomechanical basis of ergonomics. New York, Wiley Interscience, 1978, pp 41–43, 69–70.
16. Chaffin DB: Localized muscle fatigue—definition in measurement. J Occup Med 15:346–354, 1973.

17. Drillis R, Contini R: Body Segment Parameters. Department of Health, Ed., and Welfare, New York, New York, University School of Engineering, 1966.
18. Chaffin DB, Andersson G: Hand tool design guidelines. In Chaffin DB, Andersson G: Occupational Biomechanics. New York, John Wiley, 1984, pp 355–368.
19. Armstrong T, Foulke J, Joseph B, et al: An investigation of cumulative trauma disorders in a poultry processing plant. Am Ind Hyg Assoc J 43:103–116, 1982.
20. Wilkes B, et al: Job demands and work health in machine-paced poultry inspection. Scand Work Environ Health 7:12–19,
21. Comiash S, Bottoms E: The skin and friction: Deviations from Amton's laws and effects of hydration and lubrication. Br J Dermatol 84:37–43, 1971.
22. Hertzberg T: Some contributions of applied physical anthropometry. Ann NY Acad Sci 63:616–629, 1955.
23. Tichauer ER: Some aspects of stress of forearm and hand in industry. J Occup Med 2:63, 1966.
24. Van Bergeijk E: Selection of power tools and mechanical assist for control of occupational hand and wrist injuries. Handout presented at 1985 Ergonomic Conference at the University of Michigan, Ann Arbor, Michigan.
25. Benedict K, et al: The hypothenar hammer syndrome. Radiology 111:57–60, 1974.
26. Lindquist B: How to Design Tool Handles and Triggers for Low Physical Load, Ergonomic Tools of Our Time. Stockholm, T.R. Tryck, 1986, pp 24–31.
27. Tichauer ER: Ergonomic Principles to Hand Tool Design. Ergonomics Guide. New York, New York University Dept. of Industrial Engineering, 1977.
28. National Safety Council: Ergonomics: A Practical Guide. Chicago, National Safety Council, 1988.
29. Eastman Kodak Company: Ergonomics Groups: Ergonomic Design for People at Work, Vol II. New York, van Nostrand Reinhold, 1986.
30. Putz-Anderson V: Cumulative Trauma Disorders: A Manual for Musculoskeletal Diseases of the Upper Limbs. NIOSH, New York, Taylor and Francis, 1988.
31. Ayoub M, Ashton NA: Guide for Preventing Upper Extremity Disorders. Lubbock, TX, Texas Tech University, Institute for Biotechnology, February 1984.
32. Brammer AJ: Vibration Effects on the Hand and Arm in Industry. New York, John Wiley and Sons, 1981.
33. Grand Geane E: Fitting the Task to the Man. London, Taylor and Francis, 1981.
34. Rogers S: Recovery time needs for repetitive work. Semin Occup Med 2:19–24, 1985.

Chapter 40

ERGONOMIC CONSIDERATIONS AND JOB DESIGN

Bradley S. Joseph, Ph.D. and Donald S. Bloswick, P.E., Ph.D

Upper extremity cumulative trauma disorders (UECTDs) are a major problem in industry. These chronic injuries are associated with jobs that place excessive physical demands on the operator. Extensive research in ergonomics and related fields has produced ample evidence for the specific kinds of stresses, (or risk factors) that can cause a variety of painful and sometimes disabling injuries to the human musculoskeletal, nervous, and circulatory systems. Intervention strategies have been developed to address these problems, consisting primarily of techniques for job design that reduce or eliminate known stresses. Although ergonomic hazards have been recognized as an occupational problem for several years, until recently the analysis and correction of many stressful jobs have been possible only for highly trained experts. This chapter describes a simplified, "factor-floor" approach to this difficult problem.

The chapter covers three topics:
1. The outcomes of poor job design—a review of what can happen to the employee and to the organization as a result of poor job design.
2. Identification and definition of risk factors associated with occupational UECTDs.
3. A road map for use of ergonomic information in job design and analysis.

We would like to thank the UAW/Ford National Joint Committee on Health and Safety for their contributions to this manuscript.

OUTCOMES OF POOR JOB DESIGN

The outcomes or indicators of poor job design can be separated into two types: health effects and operational effects. Health effects are physical disorders and injuries resulting from exposure to stressful working conditions. In the case of the upper extremity, most of these health effects belong to the category of cumulative trauma disorders. Operational effects include both the effects on personnel (absenteeism, turnover) and the decrements in quality and productivity that result from impaired job performance associated with work that causes pain, discomfort, and inconvenience.

Health Effects

Cumulative trauma disorders (CTDs) are defined as disorders of the nerves, muscles, tendons, and bones that are caused, precipitated, or aggravated by repeated exertions or movements of the body. Injuries of the upper extremity are classified as acute or chronic. Acute injuries usually occur suddenly during a single event or accident. Chronic injuries develop over a long period of time, and usually result from repeated exposures to physical stresses. Cumulative trauma disorders of the upper extremity such as the fingers, hands, arms, shoulders, and neck are chronic injuries of special interest.

Industrial case studies of the incidence and prevalance of CTDs suggest that UECTDs occur in epidemic proportions in some industries (Table 1). For example, in a study conducted at a poultry processing plant, Armstrong et al.[4] showed UECTD incidence rates on some jobs as high as 129.6 cases per 100 workers per year, and a plant-wide rate of 12.8%. One medium-sized poultry plant, with 700 workers, reported an incidence rate of 38.6 injuries per 100 full-time workers. Similar rates have been reported for other industries, including manufacturing, assembly, and service (see Table 1). For example, Silverstein[23] found prevalence rates of 11.9% for hand and wrist tendinitis and 8.1% for carpal tunnel syndrome in a variety of industries.

Operational Effects

Although there is a considerable body of data on ergonomics-related injuries and illnesses, there is little documentation to date on the *operational* effects of poor job design in industry. Longmate and Hayes[18] note a 10–12% increase in productivity, along with a decrease in medical problems, when ergonomic modifications were implemented in a Johnson & Johnson facility. Wick[28] noted a 100% increase in productivity and significant decreases in poor posture and poor biomechanical conditions when a packaging line was redesigned to reduce ergonomic problems. Much of this data is anecdotal, however, and better data need to be collected. One can speculate, however, that jobs which are poorly designed will require more effort to perform and lead to increased fatigue and frustration in operators. It is likely that the attendant discomfort and distractions are responsible for reduced quality, increased error and scrap rates, and a greater chance of on-the-job accidents.

Research has associated a variety of occupations and activities with increased incidence of UECTDs. Table 2 presents some of those most frequently mentioned. This very diverse list of occupations shares one common element: the repeated use of the hands.

The problem with UECTDs is so alarming that industry is undertaking many efforts to resolve it. Many of these efforts are in the form of joint union and company programs. Ergonomics committees, with membership from a variety of job functions, are being formed to review jobs for sources of stress and to develop solutions. However, these joint efforts are not without problems. These groups must be trained in techniques for recognizing job stresses and for developing and implementing effective solutions. Therefore, a layman's methodology for job analysis is essential. This chapter outlines a generic approach. It should be noted that, while more sophisticated analysis techniques are available to the layman, they often are not needed. However, it is assumed that when more sophisticated analyses are required, the reader will seek the proper help in the identification of job stresses.

IDENTIFICATION AND DEFINITION OF RISK FACTORS

Associated Risk Factors for Occupational UECTDs

Three primary risk factors (or generic characteristics) of work have been associated with chronic occupational disorders affecting all parts of the body:

1. The repetitiveness of the task
2. The force requirements of the task
3. The postural requirements of the task.

TABLE 1.   Examples of Studies Reporting the Magnitude of CTDs in Industry

Study	Industry	Incidence/Problems	Prevalence
Wherle, 1976	Automotive trim production	Carpal tunnel	2.0/200,000 man-hours plant wide & 25.6/ 200,000 in selected dept.
Armstrong, Foulke, Joseph, & Goldstein, 1982	Poultry trim operations	Cumulative trauma disorders	Range from 7.1 to 129.6/ 200,000 man-hours
Silverstein, 1985	High repetitiveness & high force	Hand and wrist tendinitis and carpal tunnel syndrome	Overall prevalence was 11.9/100. Risk was up to 31.7 times greater in jobs with high force and repetitiveness

TABLE 2. Occupations and Activities Associated with Increased Frequency of Cumulative Trauma Disorders*

Aircraft assembly	Waiting tables
Automobile assembly	Inspecting
Buffing machine operator	Musicians
Core making	Packaging
Electronics assembly	Postal workers
Fabric cutters/sewers	Textile workers
Fruit packers	Tire & rubber
Gardening	Typing/VDT operation
Hay making	Meat processing
Housekeeping	

* From Armstrong T, et al: Analysis of Cumulative Trauma Disorders and Work Methods. Cincinnati, OH, National Institute for Occupational Safety and Health, 1981.[2]

TABLE 3. Reported Risk Factors of Cumulative Trauma Disorders

1. High hand and finger forces, especially with pinch grip
2. Posture:
   a. Shoulder: Elbow above mid-torso; reaching down and behind
   b. Forearm: Inward or outward rotation with bent wrist
   c. Wrist: Palmar flexion or full extension
   d. Hand: Pinch forces
3. Repetitive exertions
4. Mechanical stress concentrations/contact trauma:
   a. Over the base of the palm
   b. On the palmer surface of the fingers
   c. On the sides of the fingers
5. Vibration
6. Environment, cold, gloves

Mechanical stress concentrations, vibration, and environmental conditions are also recognized as hazard factors. Table 3* summarizes some of the more commonly cited risk factors for occupational CTDs of the upper extremity. In addition to force, frequency, and posture, Table 3 includes other risk factors more nearly unique to the upper extemity—mechanical stress, temperature extremes, glove use, and the use of vibrating and nonvibrating tools. Because these factors normally occur in combination, and because of their diversity and possible interaction with one another, it is difficult to determine the distinct contribution of any single factor to the development of CTDs. Accordingly, studies that aim to quantify the contribution of each factor to disease are currently being done. Silverstein[23] reports one such study that shows a relationship between high levels

of repetitiveness and force, and the prevalence of UECTDs. Jobs with high force and repetitiveness requirements had a predicted risk for tendinitis 32 times greater than that of jobs with low force and repetitiveness requirements. The predicted risk of carpal tunnel syndrome in the study jobs was 19 times higher than in the control jobs.

The Risk Factors—Definition and Measurement

The previous section summarized the several risk factors associated with CTDs. When designing or redesigning jobs to control UECTDs, one must evaluate these risk factors for two reasons:

1. In order to pinpoint the features of a job that need modification.
2. Once corrections have been made, in order to determine their effectiveness in reducing the degree of risk.

Since research to date is inconclusive about which risk factors or interaction of factors contributes most to the development of disease, the most reliable way to assess the risk of injury is to measure all the risk factors. Below is an overview of the techniques used to measure and to evaluate their effects on the upper extremity. Many of these measurement techniques are not practical for the industrial environment. Instead, these techniques are useful for research to develop exposure models. This overview is intended only to familiarize the reader with risk factor assessment. The actual method of using this information will be explained later.

Repetitiveness. The concept and measurement of repetitiveness have their origin in modern time study. Frederick W. Taylor introduced modern time study in 1895 when he developed a system based on the concept of a task: a day's work.[19] In his system, management planned each day's work and provided the worker with a written task description every day. To define a task, Taylor proposed breaking the work assignment into smaller units called elements.[25] Elements were individually timed, and a day's work was based on the total time necessary to complete the elements in a task description.

Gilbreth furthered the notion of time study by developing modern motion study. Motion study investigates the body motions used in

*A more complete listing of this Table with references can be seen in Armstrong, 1986[6].

performing an operation "with thought toward improving the operation by eliminating and simplifying unnecessary motions, and then establishing the most favorable motion sequence for maximum efficiency."[19] The elements in Gilbreth's system (called "Therbligs") can be grouped in a series, defined as the cycle of a job. Table 4 lists the Therblig elements and information pertaining to movement and force. Barnes[7] defines a cycle as "a series of elements that occur in regular order and make possible an operation. These elements repeat themselves as the operation is repeated." He defines elements as "a division of work that can be measured with stop-watch equipment and that has readily identified terminal points." Armstrong[6] simplifies the concept, describing elements as the "fundamental movements or acts required to perform a job." Thus, elemental analysis, often the first step to identifying the job requirements, provides a consistent way to familiarize oneself with the essential components of the study job.

The traditional way to measure repetitiveness is simply to count the number of cycles occurring during a shift. On the basis of this definition, jobs with short cycle times are more repetitive than jobs with longer cycle times because they require the operator to repeat the sequence more often. A study conducted by Armstrong et al.[5] considered cycle times shorter than 30 seconds (jobs with 1000 or more cycles per shift) to be highly repetitive.

Often, jobs with cycle times longer than 30 seconds require the operator to repeat many similar motions within a single cycle. In such cases, measuring the number of cycles per shift may not be an adequate way to determine job repetitiveness. Consequently, the concept of fundamental cycles was developed. Fundamental cycles are defined as a repeated set of motions or elements within a cycle. Jobs with at least 50% of the cycle time spent performing the same fundamental cycles are considered as repetitive as jobs with a cycle time less than 30 seconds.[5]

Cycles and fundamental cycles together constitute one classification system for repetitiveness. But this system considers only the speed at which the operator is performing the job, not the actual movements. Repetitiveness can also be measured in terms of the number of movements or posture changes per shift. Several studies have associated movements with the prevalence of UECTDs. Hammer[14] found that jobs requiring greater than 2000 hand manipulations per hour were associated with the development of tendinitis. This high number of repetitions is not in conjunction with the finger forces and awkward postures often found in industrial tasks, so it should not be considered as an upper, acceptable level. Repeated wrist flexion and extension have been correlated with carpal tunnel syndrome.[2,9,22,24]

Posture. Part of Table 3 lists, by joint, some of the stressful postures associated with UECTDs. Appendix I (adapted from Armstrong, 1984[5]) illustrates some of these stressful postures. Observers can determine if a certain posture occurs during a cycle either by observing the job directly or by reviewing a videotape of the job. Postural problems can also be identified directly by a trained observer, although this method is not as accurate as recording the number of postures from a videotape. A person trained to recognize the potentially stressful posture(s) can review a job and write a detailed description of the task in which the stressful posture(s) occur. An estimate is then made of the number of times the stressful posture(s) occurs in the cycle. This type of analysis usually results in a checklist to record the problems for future reference. Often, videotape is made to supplement the analyst's records.

Other, more accurate research methods for posture recording are available. One system, developed by Armstrong[4] and based on the work of Corlett et al.,[11] divides the upper ex-

TABLE 4.   Therblig Work Elements for Documentation of Manual Work Activities*

Element	Movement	Force
Search	Yes	No
Select	Maybe	No
Grasp	Maybe	Yes
Reach	Yes	No
Move	Yes	Yes
Hold	No	Yes
Release	Maybe	No
Position	No	Yes
Preposition	No	Yes
Inspect	Maybe	Maybe
Assemble	Yes	Yes
Disassemble	Yes	Yes
Use	Maybe	Maybe
Unavoidable delay	No	No
Avoidable delay	No	No
Plan	No	No
Rest to overcome fatigue	No	No

* Elements requiring movement and force are indicated.

tremity into its individual joints and defines their position in space with reference to the body. The positions of the joints are analyzed for each plane and degree of freedom of movement, including three degrees of freedom for the shoulder and two for the elbow and wrist. Because it is impossible to analyze the angles of each joint to the nearest degree, zones or ranges of angles are used to estimate the position within a specific range. This analysis allows the categorization of postures into zones of stressfulness. In this system, hand postures, for example, are described by categorizing the dominant grip type and noting which fingers are involved. The job analysis is recorded on videotape so that the data can later be played back and stopped at specific intervals (usually 3 Hz). The output for the system is a series of data points indicating both the location of a particular joint in space in reference to the body and the work element in which it occurs. Data reduction is done by combining certain postures into indices of stressfulness, and determining the percentage of time spent in a particular posture and the frequency with which the posture occurs.

Drury and Wick[13] described another posture recording system for use in ergonomic applications in a shoe factory. Their system requires an analyst to review videotape and to record those elements with "damaging" postures. Such elements are identified by looking for specific stressful postures and checking the appropriate boxes on the job analysis form. The output from the system is a count of stressful postures used during a shift.

It should be noted that the analysis system developed by Armstrong and Wick requires both a certain baseline level of equipment and analyst expertise. Consequently, these sytems are often not practical for in-plant use if many jobs require analysis or if simpler job analysis techniques will suffice.

Force. Force can be measured in a variety of ways. In most cases, force estimates can be done by looking at the grip posture, the weight of the objects, the duration of the action, and the location of the loads. But depending on these and other factors, force may change. Consequently, this method does not give an accurate indication of the actual force required to hold the object in the hand. If an accurate measurement of force is required, then another more sophisticated approach should be chosen. One such system incorporates the use of elec-

tromyography (EMG) to measure muscle activity in the finger flexor muscles of the forearm. Electromyography essentially measures the motor unit potential of twitching muscle fibers.[10] Because muscle tension increases with EMG activity,[8,12,17] it is possible to make a reasonable estimate of muscle force, in this case grip force, by measuring EMG activity.

Another relatively new method of force measurment involves the use of thin, pressure-sensitive, force measurement devices that are attached to the hands or fingers or mounted in gloves. These devices allow the direct measurement of the forces on the hands or fingers. Care must be taken to minimize the effect of this type of device on the tactile sensitivity of the hand. If tactile sensitivity is decreased, the hand force may be higher than actually required to perform the task.

It should be noted that the methods described above require a certain level of equipment and expertise and are often not practical for in-plant use if many jobs require analysis and if routine job analysis will suffice.

Tools, Vibration, Gloves, and Mechanical Stress. Measuring these factors of job stressfulness is usually done through observation. Observers must document the factors' existence and relative severity. In the case of hand tools, tool shape, size, and type—whether power-operated or not—may all contribute to the stressfulness of a job. In addition, it is often important to measure the frequency and power of vibration.

In many industrial facilities, gloves are worn to protect the hands from abrasion, harmful chemicals, or other forms of exposure. However, since gloves are often available in limited sizes and types, operators may have to wear gloves that are either too big and bulky or too small. When gloves fit improperly, the hand force required by the job can be increased, causing additional stress on the operator. The glove may also decrease the coefficient of friction between the "hand" and the tool or work piece, or desensitize the receptors in the hands and cause the worker to grip the tool harder than necessary.

Mechanical stress concentrations on the sensitive tissues of the palm, sides, and backs of fingers, forearm, elbow, and armpit can be caused by contact with the hard, sharp edges of tool handles, work surfaces, containers, work pieces, and other elements of the workstation. Prolonged or repeated stress concentrations have been associated with a variety of upper extremity disorders.[16,26] Occurrences of mechanical stress should be noted and their sources identified during job analysis.

ERGONOMIC ROAD MAP

As with any aspect of occupational health and safety science, the main goal of occupational ergonomics is to help create a workplace free from recognized hazards. Applying the principles of ergonomics into job design can help accomplish this goal.

In traditional problem-solving, there are essentially three main steps: (1) identification of the problem, (2) evaluation of the problem and determination of potential solutions, and (3) implementation of solutions and follow-up (Fig. 1). Using ergonomic information in job design can be thought of as a problem-solving loop or cycle.

When using ergonomic information, the first step is to identify jobs that exhibit *indicators* that an ergonomic stressor exists. Often this involves the collection and statistical analysis of data from the plant health and safety records (e.g., OSHA 200 logs, first accident visits, first aid log, etc.).

Second, the jobs are analyzed for potential ergonomic factors and several recommendations are made to prevent or resolve problems. This involves traditional methods of job analysis and the use of anthropometric data.

Third, solutions are implemented and followed up to determine their effectiveness. This involves data acquisition to determine if the solution has solved the problems it set out to solve. Many of the statistical techniques used in the charting of quality control (e.g., statistical process control, etc.) can be used at this stage.

Finally, once job changes are implemented and validated, the process cycles to the beginning and starts over again.

The following sections describe the road map

and provide an example, through a case study, of how it can be used.

Step I: Identification of Priority Jobs

There are two types of jobs that are a priority for ergonomic analysis: existing jobs and new jobs. Existing jobs are those that have been involved in production for a period of time. Often, these jobs have a great deal of historical data that enable one to monitor the operational effectiveness of the job—quality, productivity (the number of parts produced), through-put (the number of good parts being produced), absenteeism, employee turnover—and to monitor the employee health—injury and illness data. Typically, these data exhibit some "normal" level or trend that indicates the process is in control (not exhibiting abnormal indicators). Because of this historical data, existing jobs are easy to monitor for indicators of poor job design.

New jobs are jobs that have not been active in production and are either on the drawing board or are ready to be started up. These jobs do not have historical data and are more difficult to monitor. However, records from other jobs in the facility or in the company that have similar operations or processes can be used to identify potential problems.

There are three ways to identify a job for ergonomic analysis:

1. Statistical analysis of the data—often this analysis is done on existing jobs with adequate sources of data.
2. Informal reports—through informal plant organizations and structures, jobs exhibiting problems are reported directly to the appropriate people. This can be done on either existing or new jobs.
3. Proactive analysis—before any problem is demonstrated, jobs may be reviewed for potential issues.

A discussion of each method and how it can be used to identify jobs for analysis follows:

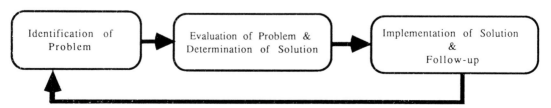

FIGURE 1. Ergonomic problem solving cycle.

Statistical Analysis. The use of statistical analysis is probably the most common method to identify jobs for analysis. Typically, many different records are kept on jobs in plants. These records vary by type but are all used for a common purpose—to monitor trends and to identify variations in those trends. Some of the most common records kept in industrial plants are statistical process control charts (SPC charts) to monitor critical factors in quality control, productivity charts that note through-put on the line and line rates, and health and safety charts to record the incidence and severity of injury and illness in the plants. As stated in the introduction, all three issues can be useful in identifying potential ergonomic problems in industry.

The most useful indicators of an ergonomic problem are injury and illness data. Jobs that exceed human limitations are more likely to result in an injury.* In the case of ergonomics, some injuries are classified as CTDs. In most injury and accident reporting systems, this injury type can occur under a variety of titles. The most typical is strain and sprain. However, present medical recording systems often make the task of identifying problem jobs very difficult. This is primarily because medical systems were not designed to identify specific jobs. Instead they were designed to accommodate federal or state reporting requirements for worker compensation, regulatory agencies, etc.

When an employee develops a medical condition, a typical procedure to manage and monitor that employee works as follows:

Step 1. Employee may **report a medical problem** in four different ways:

a. Reports to foreman and gets permission to go to medical.

b. Goes straight to Emergency Room of affiliated hospital.

c. Reports to main hospital the next day before shift.

d. Reports problem to family doctor. If the doctor judges it to be work-related, then the employee will usually report the problem to plant medical within a few working days.

Step 2. **Plant hospital case history or equivalent.** Once the employee reports the

problem to the medical department, a case history report or equivalent is filled out. Typically, this form contains information that identifies the employee by his/her name, social security/employee number, home address, telephone number, sex, age, shift, plant department number, date/time of injury, date/time injury reported, cause of accident/injury, the job classification at time of injury, and

Step 3. Depending on the severity of the case, an **accident investigation** may be done. The purpose of this report is to determine exactly how the incident occurred and what corrective actions are being taken to prevent further occurrences. If the case results in lost or restricted work days, then the number of days will be recorded.

Step 4. **Application for compensation and lost time.** If the injury is sufficiently severe to require medical attention beyond initial treatment at the medical office, or if the injury prevents the employee from performing normal work duties, then the employee can apply for workers' compensation. Depending on the state and the rules, compensation for specific types of injuries may be available. Often workers' compensation records only the most severe cases and does not provide an accurate picture of the true incidence of illness or injury in a plant.

This medical recording system is often called **passive surveillance**. It has a number of weaknesses for use as a basis for identifying jobs for ergonomic stress.

First, the system is not designed to associate a specific injury with a specific job. Instead, it provides a picture of "global" trends of injury for large areas of the plant. This picture makes it possible to evaluate the overall effectiveness of health and safety efforts, and to pinpoint large "hot spots" where further attention is needed. But because one cannot use the data to relate the incidence of injuries to specific jobs, their value in identifying specific jobs is limited.

The data may be used to identify departments or "zones" in the plants. If careful follow-up of this data is done, it may be possible to identify the specific job or jobs that are causing the problems.

Second, passive surveillance systems alone, or analysis of existing medical records, may not indicate the actual prevalence of UECTDs. Cumulative trauma disorders and related mus-

---

*Medically we may consider CTDs as injuries. However, the Bureau of Labor Statistics recordkeeping requirements for the workplace classifies most CTDs as illnesses. For more information refer to the Recordkeeping Guidelines for Occupational Injuries and Illnesses, U.S. Department of Labor, September 1986, OMB #1220-0029.

culoskeletal disorders often have nonspecific symptoms that occur after-hours and on weekends. Employees often do not relate these symptoms to the job and do not seek medical attention until after the symptoms have progressed enough to hamper their work efforts. Often these late-stage cases indicate only the tip of the iceberg of job effects.

For every compensable case, there are many more cases of employees with subclinical complaints. Consequently, OSHA logs and workers' compensation data often identify late-stage (tip-of-iceberg) disorders and complaints, reflecting only a subset of the population afflicted by these disorders. However, the plant medical case reports may be useful as an early indicator of medical incidents. Because these reports are filled out for all cases other than simple first aid, they can give a more accurate indication of the number of work-related injuries and illnesses in the plant. Still, the accuracy of these records depends on many uncontrollable factors.

Third, the period elapsing from the time when the operator notices the initial symptoms of the injury and when he/she seeks medical attention often is lengthy, and the employee may have moved to a new department or job or jobs. Consequently, it is hard to pinpoint the job that caused the injury or to correlate the job type with specific injury type.

Fourth, passive surveillance systems depend on the employee to report the injury to the plant medical department. If employees are not knowledgeable about the symptoms and do not associate them with their work activity, or if employees do not have a good relationship with the plant medical department, they may neglect to report the injury. This can result in an under-estimation of the numbers of work-related injuries in the plant.

An alternative method for determining the extent of work-related injuries is active surveillance. Active surveillance can be done in a number of ways, of which two are discussed.

One method involves noninvasive diagnostic examinations by trained medical professionals. The examinations are designed to detect symptoms of CTDs and other ergonomics-related injuries. Although relatively accurate, this method is expensive and inconvenient. The employee must be off the job for the period of the examination. Furthermore, it requires the services of trained medical specialists.

Another passive surveillance method uses self-administered questionnaires. The main advantage of this method is that it is relatively inexpensive. The employee can fill out the questionnaire during work breaks or on his/her own time. While no special personnel are required to administer the questionnaire, some expert assistance may be required in its development or interpretation. However, the questionnaires are probably not as reliable as the examinations in producing data about subclinical cases. Furthermore, the success of the program depends on the timeliness and accuracy with which the questionnaires are completed and returned. The OSHA Red Meat Packing Guidelines for Ergonomic Programs[20] suggest this method of active surveillance.

A word of warning: Employee expectations for correcting ergonomic problems must be carefully monitored. Passing out questionnaires without an adequate support structure to correct problems can lead to false expectations and poor employee relations. Therefore, it is recommended that whenever active surveillance is used, the industrial facility has a well-developed system in place to correct areas that are identified as having problems.

The best strategy is to combine these two methods. For example, one approach is to administer the questionnaire to all employees, and then, based on their responses, to select a subset of employees who have a high probability of disease. These employees are then examined by medical specialists in order to confirm the diagnosis.

Medical visits should be analyzed to determine if they relate to particular jobs or job classifications and to monitor the costs associated with particular types of medical cases (UECTDs for example):

1. *Job identification system.* Most plants have a structure for dividing up responsibilities on the production floor. Typically, this structure has at least three levels: superintendent, general supervisor, and supervisor. The superintendent has responsibility for all the general supervisors in a particular area, who are defined by various factors such as similarity of products or operations. A general supervisor controls several supervisors, each of whom oversees from 20–30 operators. Therefore, a method should be developed to match a particular employee to a specific supervisor so that a medical incident can be tied to 1 of 20 jobs.

It should be noted that a mechanism already exists in most plants to help identify specific jobs—namely, the job-process sheets completed by the plant engineers. These sheets are typically developed and maintained by industrial and process engineering. They outline the specific tasks the operator must go through to complete the job. All jobs have a unique sheet.

2. *Medical cost system*. There are several costs associated with a medical incident, whether it involves a single medical visit or a lost-time compensation. The cost of a medical visit includes the time away from the job, the time for the doctor or nurse to make an examination, treatment time, and materials associated with treatment.* These costs should be recorded, on existing medical record forms, along with the major costs associated with the workers' compensation, days restricted, or days lost from work.

In many industrial facilities formal record-keeping chores are becoming computerized. This should facilitate in identifying problem jobs. Company "systems people" or consultants can help provide the necessary resources to automate these procedures.

It should be noted that other indicators of ergonomic problems can be monitored in the same way as medical indicators. In fact, often plant information systems are already developed and in place to monitor these operational indicators.

Informal Reports.   Many ergonomic problems are identified through informal "networks" within the plant environment. These reporting systems are an important source of information. One of the most common is the network that occurs between the operator and his/her labor representative and the production department supervisors. In unionized facilities, this labor representative may be the department representative (committeeman), the health and safety representative, or other plant union representatives. Often, an operator experiencing problems on a job will report the problems to the supervisor and to the labor representative. If the issue(s) cannot be resolved immediately, then a variety of mechanisms through the collective bargaining agreement can then be used to get action. Facilities that have established health and safety programs and ergonomic programs usually deal with these issues directly.

Proactive Analysis.   New manufacturing and assembly systems and their associated jobs are a prime candidate for ergonomic analysis. Early in the process lifecycle, many changes can be made that normally would not be possible if the job were producing at or near capacity. Therefore, it is to the benefit of the facility to review these incoming jobs as early as possible in their development.

Step II: Job Analysis and Solution Development

Job analysis for occupational risk factors can be considered complete only when all the components that make up the work environment are analyzed for potential risk. Jobs exhibiting the indicators of poor design must be analyzed to determine the causes. After causes are identified, corrective measures can then be taken to reduce or eliminate the stresses. In order to perform a complete job analysis, a thorough understanding of what makes up the work environment must be made.

There are five basic components or *work parameters* that together form the work environment. These *parameters* are the basic building blocks of any job. When job stresses are identified, they can usually be traced to one or more of these parameters. Correcting the problems identified in job analysis usually involves changing one or more parameter. The parameters are as follows:

1. Workstation
2. Hand tools and equipment used to perform the job
3. Parts and materials involved in the work
4. Work methods
5. Environmental conditions.

The **workstation** is the work space occupied by a worker. It includes all the furniture and machinery in the work space, such as the work table or bench, stools or chairs, platforms, controls and displays, conveyor systems, etc.

Hand tools and equipment include both manual and power hand tools that are used to perform the job tasks, material handling devices, personal protective equipment, jigs to hold parts, etc.

The **parts and materials** include the work pieces and hardware, the components of assembly that are installed or processed, subassemblies, containers, etc. This also includes

---

* In fact, some plants studies estimate that medical visit costs may average 50 dollars.

the shape, specifications, and tolerances of the parts.

The **work methods** are the postures and movements used by each particular operator.

The **environment** is the atmosphere surrounding the worker. Environmental conditions to note include noise levels, air quality, temperature, lighting, etc.

In general, there are three steps to an ergonomic analysis—(1) the job summary, (2) determining job stresses, and (3) matching the stresses to the responsible work parameters. The job summary is designed to determine what is involved in doing the job. Determining job stresses involves investigating and discovering what risk factors are caused by the job. Matching the stresses to the work parameters involves looking at each stress and determining what parameter of the job is the most likely cause of the stress.

This analysis system is not unlike what a physician does in treating a patient. A patient who is experiencing symptoms enters a physician's office. The physician asks the patient a series of questions to get a background about him or her and what he or she does—the job summary. This portion of the examination is very important because it gives the physician a useful history on which to build a diagnosis.

The next step is for the physician to determine the symptoms experienced from the illness. These symptoms can be in the form of aches and pains, etc. From the symptoms and the history, the physician can usually begin to form a diagnosis—determining job stresses.

The last step is to match the stresses to the information in the history and determine possible work-related causes (or non–work-related causes) and what has to be changed to eliminate the "illness"—matching stresses to work parameters.

Figure 2 illustrates a form that can be used to facilitate job analysis. The form contains at two main sections—a summary section and an analysis section. The analysis section contains four columns with the following labels: Task Description, Job Stress, Work Parameter: Corrective Actions/Comments. Individuals who correctly complete both the summary sections and the four columns of the analysis section will have performed an ergonomic job analysis.

Ergonomic Analysis: Job Summary. The job summary is the first and probably most important step in ergonomic analysis. Another name for the job summary is "getting the facts." It involves collecting data that will be used in understanding how the operator does the job and in matching ergonomic stress to job work-parameters.

There are two sources available for collecting this information—direct observation and consultation. In most cases, both methods should be used when collecting the necessary data. During direct observation, the analyst goes to the job site and closely observes the operation while it is performed by the employee. If a video tape system is available, it should be used to record the operation. It is recommended that several complete cycles of the job be videotaped for future reference. Appendix II is a form sometimes used to assist in this video tape procedure.

Although direct observation is a useful method of data collection, the best source of information about a job is from the person or persons associated with the job on a daily basis. Consultation involves getting this information through interviewing these people. During consultation, either the industrial engineer assigned to the area, the supervisor or equivalent management person responsible for coordination of the area, or the worker should be interviewed formally or informally. Typically, these interviews are done at the job site so that specific job stresses can be identified and reviewed while the operation is running.

The amount of information that must be collected depends on a number of factors specific to the facility. It depends on the type of operation, the age of the plant, the make-up of the work force, and many other factors too numerous to list here. At a minimum, the following information should be collected:

The Job Title/Job Location. The job title is important for documentation. Typically, only a few words are necessary; however, the terms used to describe the job should coincide with terminology used by the plant. In most cases, the supervisor can be helpful in getting this information. It is helpful if the job title used in the job summary in some way correlates with the job title listed in the Medical Department (see "Identification of Priority Jobs: Statistical Analysis").

An example of a Job Title/Job Location is as follows:

Job Number 10005—installing master cylinder onto vehicle

Job Title: Job Location: Cycle Time (seconds):	Job Indicators	**Ergonomic Job Analysis Form**
Parts & Materials	Workstation Layout	
Handtools & Equipment		
Environmental Conditions		

Task Description	Job Stress	Work Parameter	Corrective Action/ Comments

FIGURE 2.   Ergonomic job analysis form.

Job Location—Final line

Job Indicator.   Recall that there are two types of effects or indicators of poor job design—health and operational. In ergonomic analysis, it is important to understand the way a particular job was identified to help direct and focus the type of analysis. Often, one indicator (e.g., health indicator—carpal tunnel syndrome) will be accompanied by the other indicator (e.g., operational indicator—poor quality). A typical set of indicators that identify a particular job may be:

Medical Department reports:
  3 cases of carpal tunnel syndrome
  2 cases of shoulder tendinitis
Engineering reports: poor quality

Summary of the Main Tasks.   Recall from the discussion of repetition that jobs are made up of a series of steps called tasks. In general, complicated or "enriched" jobs usually require more tasks than simple and repetitive jobs. Analyst should identify each major task and sequentially record them. In the example above, installing the part onto a vehicle may have the following task list:

Job Number 1005—installing master cylinder onto vehicle

Task #1. Operator gets two parts and places them into jig on work bench

Task #2. Operator subassembles parts

Task #3. Operator installs part onto the fire wall in vehicle

Persons familiar with traditional industrial engineering practices can be helpful in gathering this data.

Individual Task Descriptions. After the task list is developed, the next step is to describe how the operator completes each task. Typically, a sentence or two is all that is necessary. However, the level of detail depends on a number of factors, including how complicated the tasks are, the time between the tasks, the level of analysis needed to adequately identify the risk factors from the job, etc.

Below is an example of a task description from the vehicle installation example;

Task 2. Operator subassembles parts. First the operator places both parts into a jig. Second, the operator gets four screws from a parts bin and hand starts each screw into the parts. Finally, the operator gets a power tool and tightens each screw onto the part.

The Time to Complete a Cycle. A set of tasks that repeat themselves is called a cycle. Cycle time, measured in seconds, is the elapsed time between two cycles. This information is important because the data can be useful in estimating how repetitive a job is. In the master cylinder install example, a typical time for one complete cycle would be 60 seconds.

Layout. A simple sketch of the workplace should be drawn from two views, top view and side view (Fig. 3). The top view is useful in determining where the main components of the workstation are placed (e.g., worktable or bench, stools or chairs, platforms, controls and displays, conveyor systems, etc.) and where the operator is placed within the workstation.

Hand Tools and Equipment Used During the Operation. A list of hand tools and equipment should be made. Often, specialized equipment is used that can contribute to poor

job design. For the master cylinder job, a list of hand tools and equipment may be as follows:

Right-angle, air-powered nut runner

In-line, air-power nut runner

Jig to hold parts

Parts bin

Work bench.

Parts and Materials Used. Parts and materials should be documented. Often, the quality of the parts at the time of assembly, the weight of parts, the method for delivery to the production line—all can contribute to poor job design. In the example, a parts and materials list would include the following:

Master cylinder

Reservoir

4 bolts and nuts

4 screws

Environmental Conditions. To reiterate, ergonomics is the study of the relationship between the worker and the work environment. Most of the time, ergonomics looks only at the worker/machine interface. However, poor environmental conditions can contribute to poor job design. For example, an excessively hot or noisy environment can require an increased effort on the part of the operator. Often, if this increased effort is combined with known risk factors, the job may be more likely to lead to health and/or operational effects.

Operator Input. Again, the best source of information is the operator who performs the job. Before completing the job summary, all data should be checked and verified with the operator. In addition, ask the operator to point out data that were missed and/or went unrecorded.

Summary information and the task descriptions should be placed in the form as soon as possible after collection. It is helpful if these data are collected on the factory floor near the vicinity of the job. Often the supervisor or the industrial engineer (or equivalent) can be useful in collecting this data. Many times, these data are available on "process sheets" or allocation sheets that contain specific information about the job. Figure 4 shows an example of the form filled out with the summary information for the master cylinder job.

Ergonomic Analysis: Determining Job Stresses. The risk factors associated with poor job design have already been outlined. The next step is to use this knowledge in isolating those risk factors in order to identify stressful job tasks. Recall that a cycle consists of a series

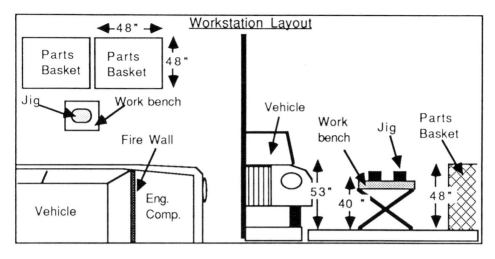

FIGURE 3. Workplace layout—*master cylinder installation.*

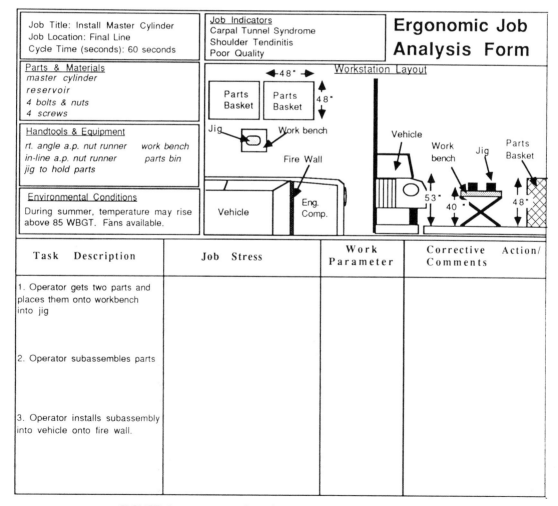

FIGURE 4. Ergonomic Job Analysis Form—with summary information.

of tasks. It is the job of the analyst to determine, first, if the risk factors exist, second, if the risk factors are significantly contributing to overall job stress and leading to or associated with the indicators of ergonomic problems, and third if the risk factors are associated with a particular task or with many tasks within the cycle. In this way, risk factors that are shown to be contributing to injuries or operational effects can later be corrected. This is accomplished by gathering data from the same two sources as in the job summary—direct observation and consultation.

Recall that direct observation involves looking at the job and pinpointing areas of risk. When determining job stresses, direct observation is most useful when the identified risk factors are easily seen by the analyst. Typically, these risk factors are postural problems. However, because the harmful effects of postural problems are often through combinations of force and repetitiveness, all three factors should be considered in the analysis.

In many cases, the best way to observe the job is through the use of videotape. Videotaping allows the analyst to slow the sequences of tasks down and closely observe the job for postural risk factors. If one is identified and if other risk factors are present, the analyst is often required to consult with either the operator, the supervisor, or the engineer. Again, asking a person or persons familiar with the job is helpful in getting a clear picture of the other risk factors and their contribution to poor job design.

Often, when performing this part of the job analysis, it is helpful to have a list of identified risk factors to check against. The postural factors from Table 3 (described above) can be used to develop such a list. As risk factors are identified, they can be documented by the task number(s) they occurred with, the relative frequency of occurrence during a task or cycle, and the force requirement when doing the task.

Figure 5 outlines the jobs stresses for the master cylinder job on the Job Analysis Form. It must be emphasized that completion of the job stress column of the form can be done in a variety of ways. For example, ergonomic stress to the lower back can be objectively measured by a variety of tools that assess strength data and compressive force on the critical regions of the spine. These measures are based on "models" developed and tested over many years at major universities and hospitals throughout the world. However, for the upper extremity, very little or no "objective" system of measurement exists. Data are being collected, but a true exposure model is not yet available. Therefore, the most common way to measure exposure on the upper extremity is through direct observation of the job.

Direct observation is effective in assessing the exposure as long as the analyst constantly reviews the job indicators. For example, if the indicator for a job were a large incidence of carpal tunnel syndrome, then concentrating on risk factors associated with the lower back may be a waste of time and resources. However, as scientists working in ergonomics develop new data on exposure, better exposure assessment tools can be used. Often, these exposure tools are in the form of a checklist, simple mathematical formulae, or graphical information. Appendix III is a checklist sometimes used to assist in the analysis of UECTDs.

When exposure models are available, they can and should be used to verify job stress exposure data collected through direct observation. This verification will not change the form or the contents of the form. Instead, the job stresses listed in the job stress column should be denoted by the method of analysis or the analytical tool used to verify the exposure (Fig. 6).

Ergonomic Analysis: Matching Job Stresses to Work Parameters. The final step in ergonomic job analysis is to match the job stresses to responsible work parameters. Recall that the work parameters are defined as those factors that together form the entire work environment. Specifically work parameters are the workstation, the hand tools and equipment, the parts and materials, and the environmental conditions. In this last step of job analysis, the analyst reviews each risk factor and determines in which task it was found and which parameter(s) is causing it to exist. In other words, this part of the analysis involves matching the risk factor to a parameter in order to determine the "root cause" of the job stress. Figure 7 shows the responsible work parameters for the example job.

Solution Development.   Recall that the primary risk factors for ergonomic stress are force, frequency, and posture. Alone or in some combination, these risk factors can contribute to ergonomic stress and may lead to ergonomic indicators. When developing solutions, it is best to eliminate first the obvious and most visual

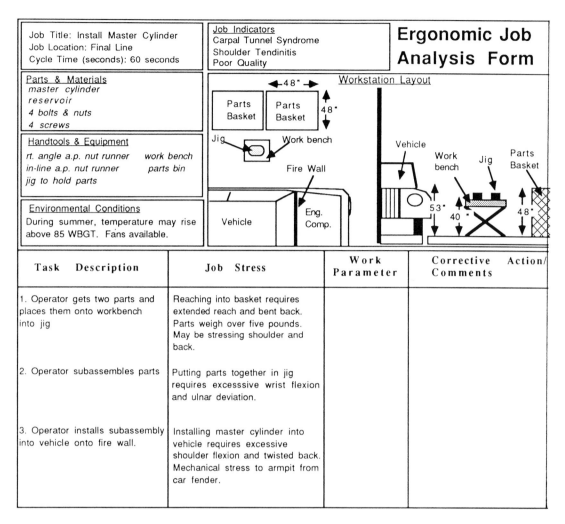

FIGURE 5. Ergonomic Job Analysis Form—with job stress information.

factors that directly correlate to an indicator or potential indicator. When these factors are related to repeated and/or forceful awkward postures, an effective strategy for developing solutions is systematically to eliminate situations that lead to the awkward postures. If this cannot be done, then reducing the force or number of times the posture is repeated should be attempted.

Data from the exposure models used to identify stress can be useful to identify ways to eliminate the stress. Once the job stress and the root cause (responsible work parameter) are identified, then the best and most efficient method to remove them can be developed.

Removing ergonomic stress cannot be done in a vacuum. The analyst must be acutely aware of job requirements, the constraints of the workstation and tooling, the product, and the

operator before any job change can be attempted. Often, these are referred to as the 3 Ps of the job—people, process, and product. In most cases, the plant engineering department has a very good understanding of the process and the product; however, they do not consider, nor understand, the person. It is important that they be made aware of human limitations before attempting to correct a job.

There are two types of solutions that can be used to reduce risk factors: engineering solutions, or controls, and administrative solutions. Engineering controls involve the redesign of the workstation, tools and equipment, parts and materials, work methods, and environment. Administrative solutions involve little or no change to the *physical* workplace layout. Instead, they involve training, worker selection, exercise and conditioning, job rotation,

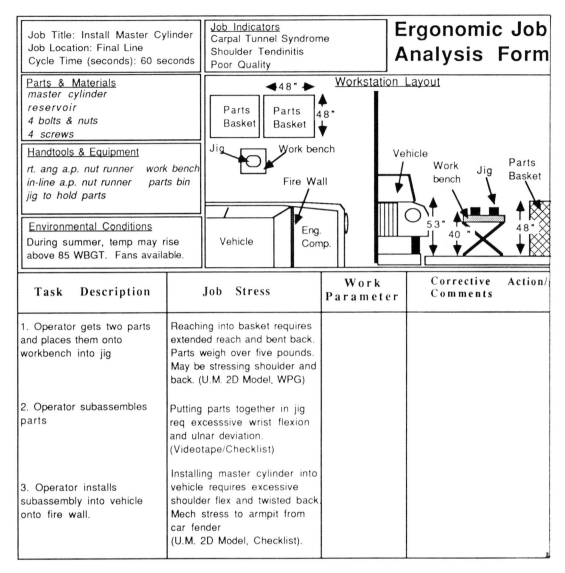

FIGURE 6. Ergonomic Job Analysis Form—with job stress information and verification from ergonomic analysis tools.

and job enlargement. Two of the common administrative solutions are job rotation (systematically changing the person from one job to another) and work enlargement (adding more work content to the job to reduce the frequency of a particular stress). Caution must be exercised when using administrative solutions. First, if rotation or enrichment is used, the added work elements must be analyzed to insure the operator is not getting more exposure to the same risk factors. Second, plant work rules negotiated with labor may make it difficult to use administrative controls. A general summary of controls related to UECTD is noted in Table 5.

Control methodologies also may be thought of as those that decrease the exposure *level* of the CTD hazard and those that decrease the *exposure duration* of the worker or work population to the hazard. This type of grouping is presented in Table 6 along with a notation as to the general control methodology category (**E**ngineering or **A**dministrative) which might be best associated with each item.

As can be seen from Table 6, the decrease of exposure level requires both engineering and administrative efforts, whereas the decrease of exposure *duration* requires solely administrative efforts. The activities in Step III, "Implementation of Solution and Follow-up," are di-

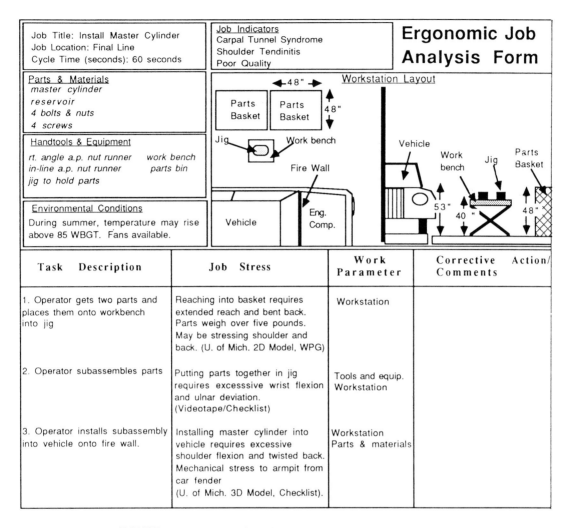

Task Description	Job Stress	Work Parameter	Corrective Action/ Comments
1. Operator gets two parts and places them onto workbench into jig	Reaching into basket requires extended reach and bent back. Parts weigh over five pounds. May be stressing shoulder and back. (U. of Mich. 2D Model, WPG)	Workstation	
2. Operator subassembles parts	Putting parts together in jig requires excesssive wrist flexion and ulnar deviation. (Videotape/Checklist)	Tools and equip. Workstation	
3. Operator installs subassembly into vehicle onto fire wall.	Installing master cylinder into vehicle requires excessive shoulder flexion and twisted back. Mechanical stress to armpit from car fender (U. of Mich. 3D Model, Checklist).	Workstation Parts & materials	

FIGURE 7. Ergonomic Job Analysis Form—matching work parameters.

rected to decrease the exposure level and exposure duration by dealing with the factors noted above.

Probably the most effective way to remove stress from a workstation is to design the physical layout to fit human measurements. This is a type of engineering control. One of the most effective tools to achieve this is the use of anthropometric data. Anthropometry is the study of human body sizes. It has been used by many consumer industries for years to insure that their products will meet the widest possible range of consumers. For example, interior design engineers in the auto industry use anthropometry extensively in product design. If one considers the "cockpit" of an automobile to be a workstation, then the same principles can be used in the industrial setting. In gen-

eral, it is desirable to accommodate at least 90% of the population when designing jobs. To achieve this goal there are three basic rules in using anthropometry:

1. **Don't** design for the average. Designing for the average may not accommodate larger and smaller people.

2. Design for the extremes. Try to accommodate large and small people in the design.

3. Design for adjustability or a range. Adjustable workstations can be used by a variety of people for a variety of jobs.

There are many anthropometric data sources available in a variety of texts that can be used.[15, 21] The key is to insure that the data being applied to the redesign best depict the population performing the job.

Typically, the final decision on any solution

TABLE 5.   Summary of Control Methodologies for Upper Extremity Cumulative Trauma Disorder Hazards

Force:	Tool design—decrease hand force
	Use power grip as opposed to pinch grip
	Improve mechanical advantage
	Improve friction characteristics
	Automate, use power tools
	Use appropriate grip span (not very large or very small)
Posture:	Workplace design/work orientation—keep hands in front of body below mid-torso, minimize reaches and arm rotation
	Tool design—minimize wrist deviation
	Work methods—use fixtures to properly orient parts
	Provide adjustable, ergonomic chairs
Frequency:	Increased cycle time
	Worker rotation
	Alternate hands
	More rest breaks
	Automation
	Job enlargement, decrease specialization
	Discourage piecework, incentive programs
Contact trauma:	Padding on tools, benches
	Spread force among several fingers
	Alternate hands
	Tool and workplace redesign
Vibration:	Minimize exposure by tool selection/modification, vibration damping, padding, worker rotation
Adverse Env:	Minimize exposure, use appropriate gloves

TABLE 6.   Control Methodologies for Upper Extremity Cumulative Trauma Disorder Hazards

1. Decrease exposure level (incompatibility between the worker and the work)
   a. Decrease stressors associated with the parameters that form the work environment
      Workstation (E)
      Hand tools and equipment (E)
      Parts and materials (E)
      Work methods (E)
      Environmental conditions (E)
      Training (A)
   b. Increase worker capacity
      Selection (A)
      Exercise and conditioning (A)
2. Decrease exposure duration
   a. Job rotation (A)
   b. Work enlargement (A)

E = engineering; A = administrative.

is based on an understanding of the process, on feasibility, and on intuition and common sense. Often, communicating with same group of people that were consulted with during the job summary and the risk factor identification steps will yield positive results. In any case, several alternative solutions should always be listed before any final decision can be made.

Figure 8 depicts some specific solutions that may be useful for this job redesign. Note the solutions are worded in such a way to allow several alternative engineering solutions to be attempted.

Step III: Implementation of Solution and Follow-up

In Step II, "Job Analysis and Solution development," the basic parameters that form the work environment were presented as:
1. Workstation.
2. Hand tools and equipment.
3. Parts and methods.
4. Work methods.
5. Environmental conditions.
In addition, the two general types of "solutions" to reduce risk factors were discussed. These were **engineering controls**, such as designing the work station/process to fit the human operator, thereby reducing the *level* of the hazard for a worker or population of workers, and **administrative solutions**, such as job rotation or work enlargement, which reduce the worker's *exposure* to the hazard.

In this section, some guidelines will be presented to assist in the implementation of the ergonomic "process," including administrative and engineering controls, to affect the work parameters in a way to reduce the risk of UECTDs. Information on procedures for the documentation and follow-up of ergonomic intervention efforts will be discussed. The importance of an appropriate medical management program for CTDs in an ergonomic intervention effort will also be noted.

Ergonomics Program/Process Implementation.   Once Step I, "Identification of Priority Jobs," and Step II, "Job Analysis and Solution Development," have been completed, an ergonomics program/process must be implemented. An ergonomics *program* may be interpreted by some to mean a single event that will solve all ergonomics problems. The concept of an ergonomics, *process* is sometimes preferred, because it suggests a systematic, closed-loop effort, including periodic evaluation and feedback relating to ergonomics intervention.

The purpose of the ergonomics process is to

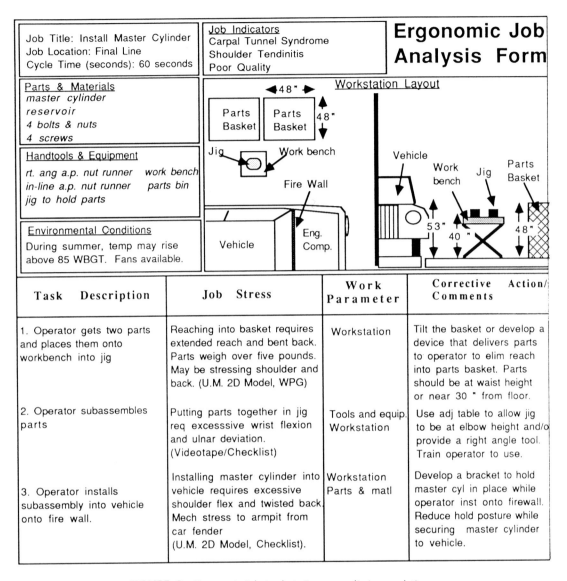

FIGURE 8. Ergonomic Job Analysis Form—preliminary solutions.

reduce the level and duration of hazard exposure for workers in jobs identified in Step I by applying the principles of job analysis discussed in Step II. Two important factors in ergonomics process implementation are: (1) the **determination of the order** in which the jobs identified in Step I as hazardous are to be "attacked" and (2) a recognition of the **human environment** within which the process takes place.

The order in which jobs are "attacked" (and sometimes the order of specific corrective actions for a particular job) depends on criteria established by the organization. If data are available on the frequency or costs of injuries and illnesses related to UECTDs, it is possible to establish criteria based on these issues. The frequency and costs of UECTDs for jobs identified as hazardous may be available from the passive or active surveillance analysis techniques discussed in Step I. If data relating to injury frequency or cost are not available, the order may be based on the number of people exposed to UECTDs.

The number exposed is the number of employees who perform operations in the area identified as containing the particular UECTD. This number may be difficult to determine exactly in cases where employees rotate through jobs that have been identified as hazardous.

A third criteria considers the **cost of implementation**. This should include the costs of (1) external consultants, (2) internal design, engineering, tooling, and materials, (3) down time during modification, and (4) operator and maintenance training. When possible, these costs can be compared to potential benefits of the ergonomic redesign to establish a cost-benefit ratio. Potential benefits may include (1) reduction in UECTDs, (2) reduction in accidents, (3) reduction in turnover and absenteeism, and (4) improved production efficiency. The cost-benefit ratio will assist in the ranking of ergonomic redesign possibilities and may also assist in the justification of the ergonomic redesign project to management and budget personnel.

A fourth criteria is based on the **regulatory environment**. Federal and state OSHA programs have placed increasing emphasis on ergonomic hazards during site inspections. Ergonomic hazards are cited according to Section 5.a.1. of the OSHA Act, or the "General Duty Clause," which notes that employers must provide " . . . employment and a place of employment which are free from recognized hazards that are causing or are likely to cause death or serious physical harm. . . ." When hazards are detected in the work place by a OSHA Compliance Officer, it is generally assumed that a competent industrial safety or health person should have "recognized" the same hazard. Since UECTDs are also generally considered to be "serious," they are therefore cited under the general duty clause. An additional factor not included in the OSHA Act is that there must be feasible and useful abatement. The term *feasible* is not well defined but generally is meant to include technological and economic factors. When an OSHA citation is issued, the employer must either comply with the abatement recommendations or contest the citation. In some cases a criminal action may be initiated. The compliance with OSHA citations may therefore take precedence over the previous three criteria.

The **human environment** within which the process takes place consists of workers, supervisors, managers, and engineers. For the ergonomics process to be successful, all of these groups must be considered. Workers must have a feeling of "ownership" and understanding of the ergonomic redesign for it to be successful. They must have the desire to make the ergonomic redesign work and enough understanding of the basics of ergonomics so that they perform the job correctly from an ergonomic standpoint. Supervisors must recognize the benefits of the ergonomics process and realize that it will assist them in meeting their performance goals. They must support and assist workers to perform the job correctly from an ergonomics standpoint. Managers must understand that the ergonomics process will likely improve overall performance and profitability. They must be receptive to ergonomics projects and understand the cost/benefit ratio and regulatory environment as noted above, so that these projects can compete successfully with other funding requests. Engineers must understand and incorporate the principles of ergonomics into all phases of the design and redesign process so that ergonomic hazards can be avoided and not just corrected after process implementation.

It is important that the ergonomics process include all of the above groups to be successful in the long run. One way to facilitate this cooperation is through the implementation of working committees that include, as a minimum, workers, supervisors, managers, engineers, and safety/health care representatives. These committees may exist at several levels within a corporation (work area, plant, operating division), with cooperation between different levels.

In order for workers, supervisors, managers, and engineers to contribute to the ergonomics process, it is necessary that they be given appropriate ergonomics training. Workers and supervisors must be taught the basics of ergonomics so that they perform the job correctly. Managers must be given a general awareness of the principles and cost effectiveness of ergonomics. Engineers must be given a more in-depth understanding of ergonomics and be provided with the analytical tools to incorporate ergonomic considerations into the design (or redesign) process.

Documentation and Follow-up. The data contained on the Ergonomic Job Analysis Forms shown on the previous figures indicate the information necessary to reduce the ergonomic hazards associated with a particular job. In addition to this, it is important to establish a procedure to track the progress of the corrective actions.

Whatever technique is developed to track this progress, it should include the following (based on the UAW-Ford Ergonomics Process, 1989)[27]:

1. *Project Date:* Date when tracking form initiated.

2. *Project Name/Number:* Short name or number to identify the project.

3. *Job Description:* Name of the job, department, etc. and responsible personnel in this area.

4. *Baseline Data:* Data relating to ergonomic incidence, absenteeism and turnovers, and production problems.

5. *Proposed Ergonomic Modifications:* "Corrective Action" from Ergonomic Job Analysis Form.

6. *Planned Completion Date:* Self-explanatory.

7. *People Responsible:* Personnel responsible for the proposed ergonomic modifications noted in Item 5 above.

8. *Status:* Record and date of all actions taken.

After the ergonomic intervention is complete, it is necessary to evaluate how well the ergonomics process has reduced the ergonomic hazards associated with a particular job. This is actually a two-phase effort.

Initially the job is analyzed to determine and record how the corrective actions implemented during the ergonomics process have reduced the job stressors noted on the Ergonomic Job Analysis Form presented in Step II," Job Analysis and solution Development." Since the job priority and the corrective actions noted on the Ergonomic Job Analysis Form are evaluated against the organizational criteria discussed earlier in this section, all jobs may not be redesigned and all corrective actions may not be implemented completely.

In addition, the passive or active surveillance techniques discussed in Step I are monitored to determine if the corrective actions have been effective in reducing the frequency and/or costs of UECTDs. It should be noted that there may be an initial increase in the reported incidence of UECTDs after the implementation of an ergonomics process due to the emphasis on early reporting of these disorders. Hopefully this will actually result in a long-term decrease in related costs due to early diagnosis and conservative management of these incidents. It is also advisable to determine, to the maximum extent possible, the actual benefits of the project in terms of (1) reduction in the number and/or cost of UECTDs, (2) reduction in accidents, (3) reduction in turnover

and absenteeism, and (4) improved production efficiency.

If, during this follow-up, it is determined that an ergonomic problem still exists, the process moves again to Step II, in which the job is analyzed and solutions proposed. In Step III the job is re-evaluated and prioritized against other jobs requiring modification.

Medical Management. A medical management program is necessary in addition to the implementation, documentation, and follow-up of ergonomic solutions noted earlier in this section. A successful medical management program requires the efforts of a physician or occupational health nurse with training in ergonomics. This person may be a full-time employee assigned to the plant or work area, a part-time employee, or a contract employee. It is the primary responsibility of this person to:

1. Assure that employees with UECTDs are properly identified and diagnosed. The identification might involve assistance with passive or active surveillance methods. Employees should be encouraged to report early symptoms of UECTDs.

2. Assure that employees with UECTDs are properly treated and rehabilitated. This should include a systematic approach that recognizes the utility of conservative treatment in the overall program.

3. Screen employees. This may involve the establishment of a baseline against which changes in health status can be evaluated and to establish work capabilities.

4. Develop or monitor a worker conditioning program, if appropriate.

The medical management program might also include assistance with the: (1) identification of UECTD hazards in the workplace, (2) identification of light duty jobs, and (3) an overall ergonomics training program.

SUMMARY

This chapter outlined some of the outcomes of poor job design, identified and defined risk factors associated with poor job design, and gave a brief overview of a layman's approach to job analysis. With this information, persons interested in fixing jobs that have ergonomically poor designs can begin to develop a working understanding of the problem, what caused it, and some consideration in its solution.

APPENDIX I
(From Armstrong, 1984)

STRESSFUL POSTURES ASSOCIATED WITH UPPER EXTREMITY CUMULATIVE TRAUMA DISORDERS

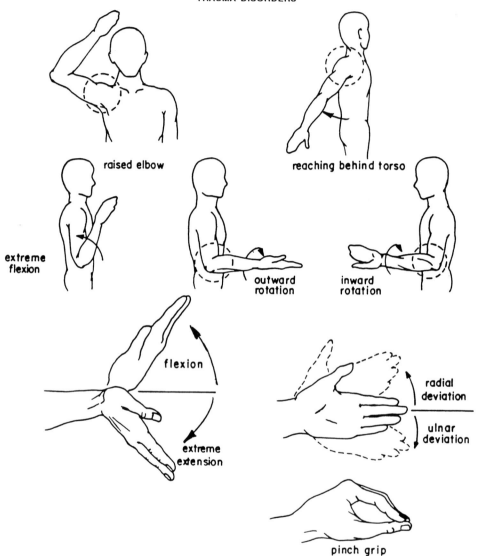

APPENDIX II

GUIDELINES FOR PREPARING VIDEO TAPE

UPPER EXTREMITY CUMULATIVE TRAUMA DISORDER

NOTE: This is not intended to be a complete Upper Extremity Cumulative Trauma Disorder (UECTD) checklist. It is meant to assist in the preparation of a video tape and provision of task information that will allow the review of this video tape by internal or external ergonomic experts.

Equipment Required:

1. Video camera, blank tapes
2. Tripod
3. Batteries for camera (at least 2)
4. Battery charger if taping projected to be longer than 1 hour
5. Clip board and paper
6. Tape measure
7. Device to weigh objects
8. Writing utensils (pens, large markers for signs that must be visible on tape, etc.)
9. UECTD checklists

1. Record the following information at the beginning of the video tape and at the top of the narrative diary of the tape:

   a. Name and location of facility
   b. Date and time of day
   c. Name of person using camera.

2. It is important that the tape reviwer be easily able to follow the tape and the tape narrative diary. Key the narrative diary to the sequential numbers printed on the video tape. If you are using a camera without the capability to "print" the numbers on the tape, you may video tape a piece of paper with a number and the name of the task written on it immediately before the task is taped and then use that name/number in the narrative diary and task description. If possible also note the name of the task on the audio portion of the tape at the beginning of each task.

3. **Taping Procedure:**

   a. Tape each job or task long enough to observe all aspects of task. Tape 5–10 minutes for all jobs, including approximately 10 cycles. Generally a cycle is considered to be a set of repeated motions during which one part or assembly is processed. Sometimes, however, jobs have relatively long cycle times (in excess of 30–60 seconds or so) during which many similar motions (sometimes called "fundamental cycles") are repeated. In these cases fewer than 10 complete cycles may be taped if all aspects of the job are recorded at least 3–4 times. Hold the camera still. Use a tripod if available. Don't walk with the camera unless absolutely necessary to record the task. When you must change locations move slowly and minimize recorded camera movement.
   b. Begin taping each task with a whole-body shot of the worker. Include the seat/chair and the surface on which the worker is standing. Hold this for 2–3 cycles, then zoom in on the arms/hands.
   c. It is best to tape several workers to determine the hazard level for workers with different anthropometry. If possible, try to tape one "worst case" situation (where the worker appears to be mismatched to the task), a "best case" (where the worker and job are appropriately matched), and an "average" case that seems to represent the "normal" situation. The worst case situation is often indicated by symptoms/complaints of CTD.
   d. Tape from an angle that will allow determination of wrist flexion, arm posture, etc. Tape

from both sides and front if possible. A view from the top is helpful (but often not possible). The total cycles included in the views from both sides, front, and top are included in the 10 minute/10 cycle (or 10/10) procedure noted above. While you should include the entire upper body, be sure to focus on the following task aspects for these particular suspected problems:

Wrist problems/complaints	Hands, wrist, forearms
Elbow problems/complaints	Arms, elbows
Shoulder problems/complaints	Arms, shoulders

    e. Tape one or two cycles of the task immediately preceding and following the task in question.

    f. Be sure the tape is light enough. If the camera has a high-speed shutter, turn the high-speed shutter off. It requires too much light for most industrial tasks. If you are taping a worker with dark clothes on a light background, activate the "back lit" capability on the camera.

4. For each taped task, determine the following parameters (to the maximum extent possible):

    a. Task or cycle frequency per shift. (This information may be available from the worker, supervisor, or production records.)

    b. Note if the task is continuous or sporadic. Does the worker perform the task for the entire shift or does he/she rotate tasks with other workers? If rotation exists, briefly tape these tasks also.

    c. Approximate dimensions of workspace. For example:
Work-bench height
Maximum reaches required to part bins and finished item bin
Chair height (or note if adjustable)
Note if (and how) the worker's movement is restricted due to a confined workspace.

    d. Determine the types of hand tools:
Size (span of grips when maximum force is applied)
Weight
Type of grips (size, shape, texture)
Do the tool handles cause stress concentrations on the base of the palm, or back or sides of fingers?
For powered tools note the following
    Weight of tool (if a counterbalance is installed, is it properly adjusted?)
    Vibration of tools during operation
    Vibration of tools when the clutch slips at pre-set torque
    Air exhaust onto workers hand

    e. Type of handwear
Is the handwear material slippery?
Do the gloves fit properly?

    f. Are any of the items/parts cold or is the work performed in a cold environment? Which hand is affected?

    g. Weight of part if significant (over 2–3 lbs). If possible, an estimate of grip or pinch forces on parts or on tools should be made and recorded.

If several different tasks are performed during the cycle, an estimate should be made for each. If the worker is required to maintain a static force application for more than 10 seconds, note the force level.

5. For each taped worker, determine the following information and parameters to the maximum extent possible:

    a. Name
    b. Height and weight
    c. Age
    d. History of: cumulative trauma disorders

            acute trauma (wrist fracture)
            ganglionic cyst

e. History of: arthritis
            gout
            hypertension
            diabetes
            kidney disorders
            thyroid disease
            pregnancy
            use of oral contraceptives

  f. Time on the job being taped
  g. Other jobs performed
  h. Time on previous jobs that may relate to any complaint of UECTD
  i. Do nonoccupational activity factors exist (hobbies such as golf, tennis, weightlifting, knitting, etc).?

6. Make any other notes that you feel would assist the reviewer of the tape in determining the UECTD hazard of the workplace.

APPENDIX III

CHECKLIST FOR UPPER EXTREMITY CUMULATIVE TRAUMA DISORDER

NOTE: This Upper Extremity Cumulative Trauma Disorder (UECTD) checklist is meant to assist with the determination of the hazard associated with a particular task. The user should also attempt to determine the incidence (history) of UECTD through a review of available epidemiological data (OSHA 200s, workers' compensation records, insurance records, etc.) and prevalence (existence) of UECTD through on-site discussions with management, union representatives, and workers. It is expected that personnel using this checklist will have some familiarity with the causes and preventions of UECTD.

Date _____ Time _____

Name of inspector _____

Home Office _____

_____

Facility/plant inspected _____

Address _____

_____

_____

Department _____

Job name _____

Job description _____

_____

_____

_____

Number of employees who perform job _____

1. GENERAL TASK PARAMETERS:

Task or cycle frequency per shift._____.
This information may be available from the worker, supervisor, or production records. Generally this reflects the number of items produced or complete cycles performed. When a job cycle is relatively long (one minute or so), many similar motions (sometimes called fundamental cycles) are performed. When this is the case, note below the types of movements that are repeated frequently.

_____

_____

_____

Note if the task is continuous or sporadic. Does the worker perform the task for the entire shift or does he/she rotate tasks with other workers? _____

_____

_____

2. WORK SPACE PARAMETERS:

Work bench height: _____

Does workbench have sharp edges? _____

Maximum reaches required to part bins and finished item bin (note length and direction):

_____

_____

Chair height: _____

Is chair height fixed? _____

If chair is adjustable, how is adjustment performed? _____

_____

Is the neck or torso bend over the work? _____

Is "sit-stand" seating available? _____

Note if (and how) the worker's movement is restricted due to a confined workspace: _____
_____
_____

Worker standing surface: _____

Worker standing surface slippery? _____

3. HANDTOOL/EQUIPMENT PARAMETERS:

Name of tool: _____

Size (span of grips when maximum force is applied): _____

Weight: _____

Type of grips (size, shape, texture, frictional characteristics): _____
_____

Do the tool handles (or parts) cause stress concentrations on base of the palm, back, or sides of fingers? _____

For powered tools note the following:

    Weight of tool (if a counterbalance is installed is it properly adjusted?): _____

    Vibration of tools during operation: _____

    Vibration of tools when the clutch slips at pre-set torque: _____

    Air exhaust onto workers hand: _____

4. PARTS/MATERIAL:

Weight of part: _____

(If possible, an estimate of grip or pinch forces on parts or on tools during assembly operations should be made and recorded.) _____

Do parts have sharp edges that contact the hands or arms? _____
_____

5. WORK METHODS:

Is a pinch grip required? _____

Are elbows above mid-torso? _____

Do arms reach down and behind? _____

Is there wrist deviation? _____
_____

Is there arm rotation, in particular with bent wrist? _____
_____

6. ENVIRONMENTAL PARAMETERS:

Are any of the items/parts cold or is the work performed in a cold environment? _____

Which hand is affected? _____

Is the handwear material slippery? _____

Are the gloves bulky? _____

Are the gloves too large or too small? _____

Do the gloves require excessive force to manipulate? _____

If several different tasks are performed during the cycle an estimate should be made for each. If the worker is required to maintain a static force application for more than 10 seconds, estimate the force level.

7. WORKER PARAMETERS

For each worker of interest, determine the following information and parameters (to the maximum extent possible):

a. Name _____

b. Height and weight: H _____ W _____

c. Age _____

d. Symptoms/complaints of UECTD (soreness, tingling, numbness, abnormal sensation, or pain in the shoulder, arm, hand, or wrist during work or nonwork activities): _____
_____

    Symptoms occur (day, night, etc.): _____

    Date of first symptoms: _____

    Activities that exacerbate or alleviate complaint: _____

    Medical treatment: _____

    Task modification: _____

e. History of: cumulative trauma disorders _____

              acute trauma (wrist fracture) _____

              ganglionic cyst _____

f. History of: arthritis _____

              gout _____

              hypertension _____

              diabetes _____

              kidney disorders _____

              thyroid disease _____

              pregnancy _____

              use of oral contraceptives _____

g. Time on job(s) in which symptoms first appeared or became aggravated: _____

h. Other jobs performed: _____

i. Time on previous jobs that may relate to any complaint of UECTD: _____
_____

j. Do nonoccupational activity factors exist (hobbies such as golf, tennis, weightlifting, knitting, etc.)? _____
_____

Make any other notes that you feel would assist in determining the UECTD hazard of the workplace.

_____
_____
_____
_____
_____

REFERENCES

1. Armstrong T: University of Michigan Course Notes, 1984.

2. Armstrong T, Chaffin D: Carpal tunnel syndrome and selected personal attributes. J Occup Med 21:481–486, 1979.

3. Armstrong T, Foulke J, Goldstein S, Joseph B: Analysis of Cumulative Trauma Disorders and Work Methods. Report to National Institute for Occupational Safety and Health. Cincinnati, Ohio, Robert A. Taft Center, January 1981.

4. Armstrong T, Foulke J, Joseph B, Goldstein S: Analysis of cumulative trauma disorders in a poultry processing plant. Am Ind Hyg Assoc J 43:103–116, 1982.

5. Armstrong T, Joseph B, Woolley C: Analysis of Jobs for Control of Upper Extremity Cumulative Trauma Disorders. Proceedings of the 1984 International Conference on Occupational Ergonomics, 1984.

6. Armstrong T, Radwin R, Hansen, D, Kennedy K: Repetitive trauma disorders: job evaluation and design. Hum Factors, 1986.

7. Barnes R: Motion and Time Study, Design, and Measurement of Work. New York, John Wiley & Sons, 1972.

8. Bouisset S: EMG and muscle force in normal motor activities. In Desmedt JE (ed): New Developments in Electromyography and Clinical Neurophysiology. Basel, Karger, 1973, pp 547–583.

9. Brain, Wright, Wilkinson: Spontaneous compression of both median nerves in carpal tunnel. Lancet i:277–282, 1947.

10. Chaffin D, Andersson G: Occupational Biomechanics. New York, John Wiley & Sons, 1984.

11. Corlett E, Medeley S, Manenica I: Posture targetting: A technique for recording working postures. Ergonomics 22:357–366, 1979.

12. DeVries H: Efficiency of electrical activity as a phys-

iological measure of a functional state of muscle tissue. Am J Physiological Med 47:10–22, 1968.

13. Drury C, Wick J: Ergonomic Applications in the Shoe Industry. Proceedings of the 1984 International Conference on Occupational Ergonomics. Toronto, May 7–9, 1984, pp 489–493.

14. Hammer AW: Tenosynovitis. Medical Record, October 3, 1935, 353–355.

15. Grandjean E: Fitting the Task to the Man: A Textbook of Occupational Ergonomics. New York, Taylor & Francis, 1988.

16. Kendall D: Aetiology, Diagnosis, and Treatment of Paraesthesiae in Hands. Br Med J 2:1633–1640, 1960.

17. Lippold O: The relation between integrated action potentials in a human muscle and its isometric tension. J Physiol 117:492–499, 1952.

18. Longmate A, Hayes T: Making a difference at Johnson & Johnson: Some ergonomic intervention case studies. IM March/April 1990, 27–30.

19. Niebel BW: Motion and Time Study. Homewood, Ill, Richard D. Irwin, 1967.

20. OSHA: Ergonomic Program Management Guidelines for Meat Packing Plants, 1990.

21. Pheasant S: Bodyspace, Anthropometry, Ergonomics and Design. New York, Taylor & Francis, 1986.

22. Phalen G: The carpal tunnel syndrome. J Bone Joint Surg 48A:211–228, 1966.

23. Silverstein B: The Prevalence of Upper Extremity Cumulative Trauma Disorders in Industry. Ph.D. Dissertation. Ann Arbor, MI, University of Michigan, Department of Epidemiology, 1985.

24. Tanzer R: The carpal tunnel syndrome. J Bone Joint Surg 41A:626–634, 1959.

25. Taylor FW: Shop management. Transactions of the ASME 28:1337–1480, 1903.

26. Tichauer E: Biomechanics sustains occupational safety and health. Industrial Engineering 46–56, 1976.

27. UAW-Ford: The UAW-Ford Ergonomics Process, 1989.

28. Wick JL: Productivity and ergonomic improvement of a packaging line: A case study. Trends in Ergonomics/Human Factors IV 97–102, 1987.

INDEX

Entries in boldface type indicate complete chapters.

Abrasions, first aid for, 138
Abscesses, digital, 427, 428
Accident prevention programs, essentials of, 47
Accidents, causes of, 48–49
  cost of, 48
Acid injuries, first aid for, 140–141
Acromioclavicular joint separation, 91–96
Acro-osteolysis, x-ray of, 111–112
Adhesive capsulitis, 288
  imaging of, 95
Adson's test, 281–282, 335, 361
Alkaline caustics, burns from, 59
Alkyl mercuric agents, burns from, 266
Allen's test, 133, 332
  for carpal tunnel syndrome, 377
Allergens, industrial, 447
Allergic contact dermatitis, 446, 448–450
Allergic reactions, to anesthetic agents, 145–147
Allodynia, definition of, 124
American National Standards Institute (ANSI), 49
Ames distorted room, 23, 24–25
Ammonia, burns from, 266
Amputation(s), care of part from, 222, 223
  fingertip, 161–162, 163–166, 168
  first aid for, 138–139, 222–223
  level of, and functional outcome, 216–219
  long-term sequelae of, 229–230
  microsurgical instruments for, 223
  of surgeons' hands, 4–5
  postoperative management of, 229
  power presses and, 49
  preoperative care for, 156
  prostheses for, 229
  recovery and, 10
  replantations and, **215–231**
  surgical procedure for, 229
  vs. replantation, 219
Anesthesia, for infection, 426
  for upper extremity, **143–157**
Anesthetic agents, local
  administration of, 143–144, 147–151
  anxiety reaction to, 145, 146
  choice of, 147
  effectiveness of, 144

Anesthetic agents, local, (*Continued*)
  malignant hyperthermia and, 145–146
  maximum dosage of, 145
  pharmacology of, 144–145
  toxic reaction to, 145–147
    prevention of, 146
    treatment of, 146–147
Anesthetic injections, diagnostic, for shoulder pain,
    283–284
Aneurysm, 330–333
  of upper extremity, 322–324
  in crushing injuries, 241
Anterior interosseous nerve, 370, 372
  anatomy of, 70
Anterior interosseous nerve syndrome, 373–374
  etiologic factors in, 374
  palsy in, 374
Antidepressants, chronic pain and, 40–41
Arc injuries, 252, 264
Arcade of Frohse, 122, 389–390
Arteries, injuries and diseases of, **319–339**
Arthritis, **455–468**
  definition of, 455
  differential diagnosis of, 455–457
  degenerative, of elbow, 293
    of wrist, 305
  diagnostic studies of, 459–460
  medical history and, 457–458
  physical examination of, 458–459
  post-traumatic, shoulder pain and, 286
  rehabilitative therapy for, 473–474
  signs and symptoms of, 455–459
Arthritis profile, 467
Arthrodesis, wrist, 303, 305–307
Arthrogram, of elbow, 100
  of shoulder, 94, 285
  of wrist, 105–107, 302–303
Asphalt, burns from, 266
Assessment, pain, methods of, 81–87
  psychological, 76–79
Atypical mycobacterium infections, 430
Avulsion amputations, definition of, 216
  safety ring, 50
Axial instability, of wrist, 308

Axillary block, 149, 151, 152
  pain after, 442
Axillary nerve, 364
  anatomy of, 121–122
Axonotmesis, 272–273
  nerve compression and, 369

Bands of Fontana, 369
Bankart fracture, imaging of, 93
Bayonet position, 315
Beck Depression Inventory, 81–82
Beham's wheel, 19
Behavior therapy, 35
Benefits, of workers' compensation, 518–519
Bennett's fracture, 193, 194, 316
Biceps tendon, ruptured, 292
Bicipital tenosynovitis, 408
Bier block, 149
Biobrane gloves, 260–261
Blade-of-the-hoe position, 423
Bleeding, See Hemorrhage
Blocks, local and regional, **143–157**
Blood-nerve barrier, 118
Bone, crushed, 246–247
Bone biopsy, 460
Bone scan, 90
  for arthritis, 460
Boss, CMC, 317–318
Bouchard's nodes, 464
Boutonnière deformity, 67, 174–175
  in rheumatoid arthritis, 461
  in thermal burns, 263
  x-ray of, 111
Boxer's fracture, 198
Brachial artery, anatomy of, 71
Brachial plexitis, 123
Brachial plexus, anatomy of, 119–120, 122–123, 362
  occupational injuries to, 364–366
Brachial plexus neuropathy, 362–366
Brain, environment and, 25–27
  hemispheres of, 32–33
Brewerton view, 109, 184, 198
Brown-Séquard syndrome, 117
BTE Work Simulator, 476
Buddy taping, 472
Bupivacaine, 147
Burn, preoperative care for, 156
Burns, 58–59, **259–269**, See also Electrical injuries
  chemical, 58–59
  degrees of, 259
  electrical, 59
  emergency management of, **259–269**
    chemical, 265–268
    electrical, 264–265
    thermal, 259–264
  first aid for, 140
  thermal,
    infections in, 263
    boutonnière deformity in, 263
    contractures in, 263–264
    surgical therapy for, 261–263
Bursitis, elbow, 292
  olecranon, 58, 99, 292–293
  subacromial, 285

Calcific tendinitis, 409
Calcium hydroxide, burns from, 266
Cantharide, burns from 266

Carpal instability, 297–300
  algorithm for, 302
Carpal instability–combined (CIC), 300, 305
Carpal instability–dissociative (CID), 299
Carpal instability–nondissociative (CIND), 300, 308
Carpal tunnel, anatomy of, 62, 375
  plain film view of, 104, 106
Carpal tunnel syndrome, 55, **341–352**, 374–379
  acute, 344
  anatomy of, 342
  chronic, 344–345
  conditions predisposing to, 379
  conservative treatment of, 348–349
  cost of, 485
  diagnosis of, 345, 376
  dynamic, 347
  ergonomics and, 379
  evaluation of, 124
  fluid imbalance and, 343–344
  neuroanatomy and, 70
  occupational causes of, 376–379
  pathogenesis of, 342–344
  postoperative course of, 350
  presentation of, 341
  prevalence of, 341–342
  rehabilitative therapy for, 469–471
  repetitive motion and, 344
  shoulder pain and, 282
  splinting for, 469–471
  steroid injection for, 348–349
  surgical management of, 349–350
  testing for, 376, 377, 378
  traumatic, 244, 246
  treatment of, 379–380
  vibration syndrome and, 325–326
  vs. pronator teres syndrome, 372
Carpal tunnel view, 184, 192
  plain film of, 104, 106
Cartilage, destruction of, 456
Casts, complications of, 441–442
  for replantation, 225, 226
  hand, safe position for, 203
  splitting of, 437
  surveillance case definition of, 54
  thumb spica, 191
Causalgia, definition of, 115, 124
Celery, contact dermatitis and, 448
Cell proliferation, in healing, 240
Cement, burns from, 266
Cervical spondylosis, 356–359
  treatment of, 358–359
Cervicobrachial occupational diseases, 354–362
Change, medical categories of, 34–35
  problems and opportunities for, 32–37
  readiness for, 41
Cheiralgia paresthetica, 122
Chemicals, vascular disease and, 333–334
Cherry pitter's thumb, 380
Chromates, contact dermatitis and, 449
Chronic acid, burns from 266
Chronic pain, injured worker and, **13–45**
  predisposition toward, 26
Chronic pain disorder, features of, 39
Chronic pain patient, clinical depression and, 38
  identification of, 37–39
  inner perspective of, 22–24
  "pain game" and, 17–18
  rehabilitation contract and, 41
Chuck pinch, 167, 168

Citrus fruits, contact dermatitis and, 448–449
Clawed hand, ulnar nerve lesion and, 384
Cleland's ligaments, 71
Clenched fist syndrome, 76–77
Clinical Analysis Questionnaire, 82
Clinical electrophysiology test, for carpal tunnel syndrome, 347–348
Clinical neurophysiologic testing, 125–129
  report of, 128–129
Clostridium tetanus, 132
Codman exercises, 285
Cognitive therapy, 35–37
Communication, in the rehabilitation process, 5, 7–8
Compartments, dorsal, of wrist, 412–416
Compartment syndrome, complications of, 437
  in crushing injuries, 242
Compensation neurosis, 78
Complete anterior interosseous nerve palsy, 374
Complete posterior interosseous nerve palsy, 390
Complications, of surgery, 435–436
Compression neuropathies, 55, **353–402**
  vibration syndrome and, 325–326
Computed tomography, *See* anatomical part
Confidentiality, 509
Connective tissue disease, Raynaud's phenomenon and, 466
Contact dermatitis, **443–454**
  criteria for evaluating occupational causation of, 452–453
  definition of, 444
  irritant, 444, 448–450
  of hand, 58
  prevention of, 450–451
  substances causing, 447–448
Contact urticaria, 447, 448
Contraction, wound, 240–241, 242
Contractures, in thermal burns, 263–264
Conversion disorders, 78
Conveyors, safety rules for, 51
Cords, formation of, 363
Cost system, medical, 547
Costoclavicular maneuver, 361
Cozen's test, 411
Creams, barrier, for contact dermatitis, 451–452
Creosol/creosote, burns from, 266
CREST syndrome, 466
Crush amputations, definition of, 216
Crush injuries, **239–247**
  blood vessel injuries in, 241–242
  bone injuries in, 246–247
  muscle injuries in, 242–243
  nerve injuries in, 243–246
  phalangeal, 208, 209
  skin and subcutaneous tissue in, 240–241
  tendon injuries in, 243
Cubital tunnel, anatomy of, 380, 381
Cubital tunnel syndrome, 55, 381–383
  differential diagnosis of, 383
  elbow pain and, 294–295
  electrodiagnostic tests for, 383
  signs and symptoms of, 382–383, 384
  treatment for, 383
Cumulative trauma disorders, 53, 54–55, **353–402**
  control methodologies for, 556
  ergonomics and, **539–567**
  force and, 543
  in garment workers, 56
  in musicians, 55–56

Cumulative trauma disorders, (*Continued*)
  in VDT keyboard operators, 56
  interventions for, **489–505**
    education and, 495–497
    program of, 493
  occupations/activities associated with, 541
  outline of, 354
  postures associated with, 542–543
  prevalence of, 54–55, 540
  risk factors for, 492–493, 527, 528, 540–544
  upper extremity, checklist for, 564–566

Data processors, injuries in, 55–56
Days lost from work, 47–48
Death benefits, from workers' compensation, 519
Degenerative osteoarthritis, of shoulder, imaging of, 94–95
Dependency, dealing with, 8–9
De Quervain's disease, 57, 392, 403, 413–414
  treatment of, 414
Dermatitis, contact, 58, **443–454**
  types of, 443–450
Diaphysics, 181
Dichromate salts, burns from, 266
Digital artery, comparative diameter of, 221
Digital nerve block, 148
Digits, ligament injuries of, 314–315, 316–318
  replantation of, 218–219
Dinner fork deformity, 137
Disabling work injuries, cost of, 47
  numbers of, 47
Disability, 480
  compensation for, vs. rehabilitation, 6–7
  definition of, 17
  insurance for, 29–30
  permanent, 485–486
  workers' compensation benefits and, 518–519
  workers' compensation procedures and, 519–520
Dislocations, compound, of PIP joint, 136
  elbow, imaging of, 98
  hand, **181–213**
  illustration of, 183
  MCP joint, 201, 202
  PIP joint, 203, 205–207
  thumb, 314
  thumb MCP joint, 314
Disk-Criminator test, 378
Doctor-patient relationship, 510–512
Dominance, hand, 32–33
Donor sites, postoperative care of, 435
Doppler mapping, of hand, 321
Dorsiflexion intercalated segment instability (DISI), 298, 299, 308
Double crush syndrome, 342, 393
Dressing, splitting of, 436–437
Drug dependence, 9
Drugs, anesthetic, 144–145
  chronic pain and, 40–41
Drummer boy's palsy, 415
Duty of care, 510
Dystrophile, 475

Edema, complications of, 436
  in crushing injuries, 242
Education, for ergonomic change, 495–497
  engineering and design personnel, 496
  management, 495–496

Education, for ergonomic changes, (*Continued*)
  supervisors, 496
  workers, 496–497
Effort thrombosis, 336
E. I. du Pont de Nemours, safety record of, 47
Eikenella corrodens infections, 429
Elbow
  anatomy of, 289
  arthritis of, 293
  bone scan of, 101
  disorders, history and physical examination of, 289–290
  golf, 403, 410
  imaging of, 97–102
    arthrogram of, 100
    displaced fat pads and, 99
    plain films, 97–98
    magnetic resonance imaging, 102
  inflammatory conditions of, 100
  injuries of, 57–58
  loose bodies in, imaging of, 99–100
  myositis ossificans in, imaging of, 99
  occupational disorders of, **289–296**
  osteoarthritis of, 101
  pain, differential diagnosis of, 411–412
    neurologic causes of, 293–294
  posture of, in cubital tunnel syndrome, 381–382
  radial tubercle of, 101
  radiographic anatomy of, 97
  soft tissue abnormalities of, 98–99
  tendinitis of, 290, 410–412
  tennis, 57, 100–101, 290–292, 410
  vascular conditions of, 101
Electrical injuries, **249–257**
  evaluation of, 251–253
  first aid for, 141
  management of, 251–256
  pathophysiology of, 250–251
  resuscitation from, 251–253
  wound management in, 253–256
    debridement, 255
    fasciotomy, 253
Electrical properties of tissues, 250
Electricity, physics of, 244–250
Electrodiagnostic studies, for carpal tunnel syndrome, 347–348, 378
Electromyography, 125–126
  in neurogenic thoracic outlet syndrome, 360
Elevation, for infection, 426
  in postoperative care, 434–435
Emotional reaction, cognitive theory of, 34
Employability, 40
Employers, communication with, 9
Employment physical examination, legal aspects of, 507–510
Enthesopathy, 456
Entitlement, for workers' compensation, 520–521
Entrapment neuropathies, definition of, 368
Epicondylitis, 410
  lateral, 57, 100
  medial, 57
Epiphysis, 181
Epithelialization, 240
Equal Employment Opportunity Commission, 508
Erb's palsy, 122
Erb's point, 128
Ergonomic intervention,
  for cumulative trauma, 492–495

Ergonomic intervention, (*Continued*)
  implementation of, 494–495
  task force for, 497
Ergonomic job analysis, job identification and, 544–547
  job stresses and, 550, 552
  solution development from, 552–556
  solution implementation following, 556–559
    cost of, 558
  statistics in, 545–547
  steps of, 548
Ergonomic job analysis form, 548, 549
  with job stress information, 553
    with ergonomic verification, 554
  with matching of work parameters, 555
  with preliminary solutions, 557
  with summary information, 551
Ergonomic solutions,
  documentation of, 558–559
  follow-up of, 558–559
  human environment and, 558
  implementation of, 556–558
    cost of, 558
  medical management of, 559
  regulatory environment and, 558
Ergonomics, cumulative trauma interventions and, 489–500
  definition of, 353–354
  in anterior interosseous nerve syndrome, 374
  in carpal tunnel syndrome, 379, 380
  in cervical spondylosis, 359
  in cubital tunnel syndrome, 383
  in myofascial pain syndrome, 356
  in posterior interosseous nerve syndrome, 391
  in pronator teres syndrome, 372–373
  in Wartenberg's syndrome, 393
  injury prevention and, 480–481
  job design and, **539–567**
  problem-solving cycle of, 544–559
  tool design and, 527–537
Etiologies, of upper extremity injury, **53–60**
Examination, for cumulative trauma, 491–492
Exercise, in postoperative care, 435
  for tennis elbow, 291
Extensor muscles, of upper extremity, 65–68
Extensor tendinitis, 412–413
Extensor tendon injuries, 171–176
  Zone I, 172–173
  Zone II, 173–176
  Zone III, 176
  Zone IV and V, 176
Extrapyramidal system, 116
Extrinsic muscles, of upper extremity, 65–68

Factitious disorders, 77
False aneurysm, 322
Fasciotomy, in electrical injuries, 253–265
Felon, 427, 428
Fibro-osseous pulley system, 68
Fingernails, anatomy of, 73
Fingertip, anatomy of, 160
Fingertip, injuries of, **159–169**
  first aid for, 138–139
  prevention of, 159–160
  treatment of, 162–166, 169
Finkelstein's test, 392, 414
Fish fancier's digit, 405
First aid, for amputation, 222–223
  for hand injuries, **131–142**

Flaps, 167, 168, 240
  volar advancement, 167
Flexor tendon injuries, 135, 176–178
  Zone I, 177
  Zone II (no-man's-land), 177–178
  Zone III, 178
  Zone IV and V, 178
Flexor tendinitis, 416–419
Flexor tenosynovitis, 416–417, 417–419
Floral workers, contact dermatitis and, 450
Food handlers, contact dermatitis and, 448–449
Force, measurement of, in cumulative trauma
      disorders, 543
Forearm, imaging of, 102
Foreign bodies, first aid for, 141
Formic acid, burns from 266
Fracture-dislocation, digital, 317
  Monteggia, 102
  PIP joint, 203, 205–207
  thumb, 316
Fractures, Bankart, 93
  Bennett's, 193–194, 316
  boxer's, 186, 198
  distal phalanx, 161, 163, 164
  elbow, imaging of, 98
  examination of, 136–137
  first aid for, 139–140
  Galeazzi, 102
  hand, **181–213**
    treatment of, 187–210
      capitate, 191
      hamate, 191–192
      lunate, 192–193
      metacarpals, 198–203
      PIP joint, 203–207
      phalanx, 207–210
      scaphoid, 187, 189–190
      summary of, 188–189
      thumb, 193–198
      trapezium, 190
      triquetrum and pisiform, 193
  healing of, principles and assessment, 186–187
  Hill-Sachs, 93, 284
  history of, 183–184
  internal fixation of, 186
  mallet, 182–173
  malrotation of, 199
  phalangeal, 110, 198–210
    baseball, 209
    internal fixation for, 203
    mallet, 209
  physical examination of, 183–184
  postoperative care of, 434
  radiographic examination of, 184–185
  rehabilitation of, 212
  reverse Bennett's, 200
  Rolando's, 193, 194, 195
  rotational malalignment of, 182, 183
  sesamoid, 109–110
  terminology of, 181–183
  treatment of, general principles, 185–186
Freon, burns from, 266–267
Frostbite injury, 59
Frozen shoulder, idiopathic, 286
  imaging of, 95
Full interface pattern, 126
Functional impairment, workers' compensation and, 519
Fungus infections, 430
F-wave, 127

Galeazzi fracture, 102
Gamekeeper's thumb, 312
Garment workers, injuries in, 55–56
Gasoline, burns from, 267
Germinal matrix, 73
Gloves, Biobrane, 260–261
  cumulative trauma disorders and, 543
  hairdressers and, 449
  hand-held tools and, 533–534
  horticulturists and, 450
  prevention of contact dermatitis and, 451
  surgical, for thermal burn, 261
  tendinitis with, 404–405
Goals of recovery, 6–7, 8
Golf elbow, 403, 410
Graft(s), free nail, 165, 167
  full-thickness skin, 168
  nerve, 275
  postoperative care and, 435
Grayson's ligaments, 71
Grinding injury, 131, 134
Grip, weakness of, 77
Guarding devices, 49
Guillotine amputations, definition of, 216
Guyon's canal, anatomy of, 385
Guyon's canal compression syndrome, 385

Hairdressers, contact dermatitis and, 449–450
Hand-arm vibration syndrome, 324–330, *See also* Vibration and Vibration syndrome
  classification of, 324–330, 326–327
  clinical features of, 325–326
  diagnosis of, 328
  pathogenesis of, 326–328
  prevention of, 329
  treatment of, 329
Hand, anatomy of, **61–73**
  imaging of, 109–113
    foreign bodies and, 111
    fractures, 110, 111
    MRI, 112
    plain films, 109
  immobilization of, safe position for, 203, 211
  infections of, **423–431**
    factors affecting, 425
    management of, 426
    organisms responsible for, 424–425
  injuries of, first aid for, **131–142**
    history of, 132–133
    physical examination for, 133–137
    prevention of, **47–52**
  ligament injuries of, **311–318**
  radiographic anatomy, 109–110
  role of motivation in recovery of, **1–11**
Hand pain, psychological evaluation of, **75–88**
Hand splinting, for first aid, 137–138
Hand therapy, **469–477**
Hand tools, *See* Tools
Handicap, definition of, 17, 508
Handlebar palsy, 121
Handles, tool, 527–529, 533
Hardiness, 80–81
Healing, process of, 239–240
Heberden's nodes, 464
Hematoma, complications of, 438–439
  of nail bed, 161, 162–163
  under nail plate, 138
Hemispheres, brain, 32–33
Hemorrhage, complications of, 436, 437–438

Hemorrhage, complications of, (*Continued*)
  partial arterial injury and, 437–438
Herpes simplex infection, 429
High-compression injection injuries, 59
High-pressure injection injuries, **233–237**
  case studies of, 234
  examination of, 235
  pathophysiology of, 233–235
  radiographic evaluation of, 236
  treatment of, 236
Hill-Sachs fracture, imaging of, 93, 284
HLA-B27, 456, 463
Horner's syndrome, 362
Honeymoon paralysis, 371
Horseshoe infection, 429
Horticulturists, contact dermatitis and, 450
H-reflex, 127
Hydrocarbons, burns from, 267
Hydrochloric acid, burns from, 267
Hydrofluoric acid, burns from, 58–59, 267
Hyperabduction syndrome, 334
Hyperesthesia, definition of, 124
Hyperextension injury, to PIP joint, 173, 205–207
  to thumb MCP joint, 313–314
Hyperpathia, definition of, 124
Hypochondriasis, 78
Hypothenar hammer syndrome, 56, 330, 385
Hysterical neuroses, 78

Idealism, reality vs., 30–32
Imaging, of upper extremity, **89–113**
Immobilization, hand, safe position for, 203–211
Impairment, definition of, 17
Impingement syndrome, 280, 286, 406–408
  Neer's stages of, 407
Incomplete anterior interosseous nerve syndrome, 374
Industrial irritants, 446
Infection(s), complications of, 440–441
  treatment of, 441
  first aid for, 141
  joint, 456–457, 459
  of hand, **423–431**
    factors affecting, 425
    management of, 426
    organisms responsible for, 424–425
  postoperative, 440–441
    treatment of, 441
Inflammation, 239
  in arthritis, 455–457
Infraclavicular plexus, 363
Injection injuries, high-pressure, **233–237**
Injuries, disabling, summary of, 48
Innervation density tests, 345–346
Instruments, microsurgical, for replantation, 223
Intersection syndrome, 414–415
  treatment of, 415
Intravenous regional blockade, 149
Intrinsic-plus position, 203, 211
Ischemia, complications of, 436, 439–440

Jersey finger, 177
Job, physical requirements of, law and, 508
Job analysis, 493–494
Job description, return-to-work program and, 485
Job design, ergonomics and, **539–567**
  poor, outcomes of, 539–540
    health effects, 539–540
    operational effects, 540

Job identification system, 546–547
Job summary, ergonomic analysis and, 548–552
Joint(s), *See also* Arthritis
  digital, tendon injuries and, **171–179**
  digital CMC, injuries to, 316–318
  digital MCP, ligaments of, 314–315
  infection of, 456–457, 459
  MCP, dislocations of, 201, 202
    injuries to, 174–176
    puncture wounds of, 175–176
  PIP, dislocations of, 203, 205–207
    flexion deformity of, 173–176
    injuries to, rehabilitative therapy for, 471–472
  thumb CMC, injuries to, 315–316
  thumb MCP, fractures of, 195–196
    ligaments of, 311–315
  trapeziometacarpal, fractures of, 195–196
Joint disease, musculoskeletal disorders and, 455–457
Joule's law, 250

Kanavel, Allen, 423–424, 428
Key pinch, 160
Kienböck's disease, 192–193, 305

Laboratory tests, preoperative, 156
Laceration injuries, 59
  simple, first aid for, 137
Landburg's syndrome, 417
Lateral cord, 363
Lateral epicondylitis, 290–292, 410–411
Legal considerations, in occupational medicine, **507–514**
Liability, for workers' compensation, 516
  of the physician, **507–514**
Liberty wrist support, 470
Lidocaine, 147
  administration of, 148
Ligament of Struthers, 121
Ligaments, digital MCP collateral, injuries to, 314–315
  of hand, injuries to, **311–318**
  of wrist, injuries to, **297–309**
  thumb radial collateral, injuries to, 313
  thumb ulnar collateral, injuries to, 311–313
Ligamentotaxis, 195
Lightning injuries, 265
Lindburg's sign, 417
Lister's tubercle, 415
Lithium, burns from, 267
Litigation, influence of, in recovery, 7
  settlement of, 9–10
Local anesthesia, **143–157**
  administration of, 147–151
Local sepsis, 441
Lumbrical plus, 178
Lye, burns from, 267

Machines, inspection of, 51
Macro EMG, 126
Magnetic resonance imaging (MRI), 90
  See also anatomical parts
  for arthritis, 460
Malingering, 7, 29–30, 77–78, 486
Mallet finger, 67, 111, 172, 173
  first aid, 139–140
  x-ray of, 110
Malpractice, employment physicals and, 511
Management, education of, for ergonomic change,
  495–496

Medial cord, 363
Medial epicondylitis, 292, 411
Median nerve compression test, 347
Median nerve, 364
  anatomy of, 69–70, 120–121
    at the wrist, 375–376
  compression of, 370–380
    sites of, 371
  injuries to, in palm and digits, 380
Median palmar digital neuropathy, 380
Medical cost system, 547
Medical expenses, workers' compensation and, 519
Medical health questionnaire, 503–505
Medical records, law suits and, 513
Mesotenon, 404
Metastatic disease, of shoulder, imaging of, 96
Metaphysis, 181
Millon Behavioral Health Inventory, 82
Millon Clinical Multiaxial Inventory, 82
Minnesota Multiphasic Personality Inventory, 82
Motivation
  definition of, 2–3
  examples of, 4–5
  latent, cultivation of, 8–9
  role of, in recovery of hand, **1–11**
  spectrum of, 3–5
  use of, in rehabilitation, 7–10
Motor dysfunction, 116
Motor testing, for carpal tunnel syndrome, 346–347
Motor unit, 125, 126
Motor unit potential, 126
Mucous cyst, 427
Multiple crush syndromes, 393
Munchausen syndrome, 77
Muriatic acid, burns from, 267
Muscle, crushed, 242–243
Musicians, injuries in, 55–56
  tendinitis in, 404
Myelin degeneration, focal, in acute nerve
    compression, 368
Myelin sheath, 366
Myoelectric prostheses, 229
Myofascial pain syndrome, 355–356
  treatment of, 356, 358
Myopathy, joint disease and, 457
Myositis ossificans, of the elbow, 99

Naffziger syndrome, 281
Nail, infections of, conditions that mimic, 427
  missing, stent for, 163
Nail bed injuries, 136, **159–169**
  prevention of, 159–160
  treatment of, 162–166, 169
Nail-gun injury, 134
Nail plate avulsions, 161, 162
Narcotics, chronic pain and, 40–41
National Institute for Occupational Safety and Health
    (NIOSH), 47
Neer decompressions, 286
Negligence, 510–513
  avoiding, 512–513
Nerve, See also specific nerve
  anterior interosseous, 370, 372
  cross section of, 118
  crushed, 243–246
  lateral cutaneous, 364, 365–366
  localization of, 123–124
  long thoracic, 364

Nerve, See also specific nerve, (Continued)
  median, compression of, 370–380
  musculocutaneous, 364, 365, 366
  peripheral, anatomy of, 366–368
    injuries to, **271–277**
    pressure on, 367–368
    stretching of, 367
  suprascapular, 364
Nerve blocks, **143–157**
Nerve compression, acute, 368
  chronic, 369–370
  neural response to, 368
  syndromes of, 362–397
Nerve conduction studies, 127
Nerve conduction velocity, 127
  test for, in carpal tunnel syndrome, 347–348
Nerve entrapment, 55
  of upper extremity, summary of, 394–396
  pathologic response to, 369–370
Nerve graft, 275
Nerve supply, upper extremity, 69–71
Nervous system, environment and, 25–27
  parts of, 115–116
Neural lesions, classification of, 272
Neurologic evaluation, of upper extremity, **115–130**
Neurolysis, for carpal tunnel syndrome, 349–350
Neuromas, 275–276
  therapy for, 472–473
Neurapraxia, 272–273
  nerve compression and, 369
Neurorrhaphy, 274–275
Neurotmesis, 272–273
  definition of, 369
Neurovascular system, of upper extremity, 71–72
Nitric acid, burns from, 268
Nociception, 79
"No-man's-land" (flexor tendon, Zone II), 177–178
  anesthesia and, 148–149
Nonsteroidal anti-inflammatory drugs, 466–468
Norgaard projection, 109, 191
NSAIDs, 466–468
Numbness, postoperative, 442

Objective, definition of, 18
Occlusive diseases, occupational, 330–333
Occupational hand therapy, **469–477**
Occupational impairment, workers' compensation and,
    519
Occupational injury, pain and, **13–45**
Occupational occlusive disease, 330–333
  treatment of, 332–333
Occupational physician, duty of, 510–512
  legal considerations of, **507–514**
  return-to-work decision and, 480
Occupational Safety and Health Administration
    (OSHA), 47
Ocular dominance columns, 25–26
Ohm's law, 250
Olecranon bursitis, 292–293
  imaging of, 99
Operant conditioning, 35
Operating microscope, 223, 224
Orf, 429
Organization, living, 20–21
Osteoarthritis, 464–465
  lost time from work and, 464
Overuse injuries, prevalence of, 53
Overuse syndrome, 54

Overuse syndrome, (*Continued*)
  See also Cumulative trauma disorders *and* Repetitive
     motion injuries
Oxygen, for toxic reactions to anesthesia, 146–147

Pain, acute vs. chronic, 14–15, 40
  categories of, 15–16
  concept of, 79
  chronic, **13–45**, *See also* Chronic pain patient
    change and, 34
    drugs and, 40–41
    evaluation of, 39–40
    failed surgery and, 35
    language and, 27–29
    predisposition toward, 26
    readiness for change and, 41
    recognition of, 37–38
    states of, 17
    therapeutic programs for, 32–37
    treatment of, 37–42
  definition of, 14–17
  dimensions of, 14
  duration of, 15–16
  elbow, 411–412
    imaging of, 101–102
    neurologic causes of, 293–294
  financial loss and, 13
  "good" vs. "bad," 435
  hand, psychological evaluation of, **75–88**
  in combat vs. hospital, 80
  learned behaviors and, 26
  motivation in dealing with, 9
  past experiences and, 24–27
  phantom, 26–27
  postoperative, 441–442
  psychogenic, 78–79
  returning to work with, 80
  shoulder, 408–409
  wrist, algorithm for, 103
Pain assessment, methods of, 81–87
Pain behavior, 79, 80
"Pain game," 17–18
Pain-prone disorder, clinical features of, 38
Pain stimulus, location of, 15–16
Painful arc syndrome, 283
Painful shoulder, causes of, 280, 281–282
  diagnosis of, 282–285
  treatment of, 285–286
Palm, replantation and, 221–222
Palmar spaces, 430
  infections of, 428–429
Palsy, median, 70
Pancoast's tumor, 282
Parkinson's disease, 116
Paronychia, acute, 426–427
  chronic, 427
Pasteurella multocida infection, 429
Patient education, 7–8
Patient, chronic illness and, 39
  chronic pain, *See* Chronic pain patient
  goals of, in recovery, 6–7, 8
Perception, nature of, 18–21
  objective vs. subjective, 19
Peripheral nerve, injuries to, **271–277**
  classification of, 272
  complications of, 275–276
  compression, 55
  pathophysiology of, 272

Peripheral nerve, injuries to, (*Continued*)
  rehabilitation of, 275
  treatment of, 273–275
    penetrating injuries, 273–275
Peripheral nervous system, anatomy of, 366–368
  examination of, 135
  parts of, 117
  physiology of, 366–368
Peripheral neuroanatomy, 271–272
Peritendinitis calcarea, imaging of, 94
Permanent disability, 485–486
Phalen's test, for carpal tunnel syndrome, 347, 377
Phantom pain, 26–27
Phenol, burns from, 268
Phosphorus, burns from, 268
Physical examination, employment, legal aspects of,
    507–510
  for hand injuries, 133–137
Physician's duty, 510–512
Pillar pain, 350
Pinch, pulp-to-pulp, 274
Pinning, percutaneous, of proximal phalanx, 202
Pins, postoperative care of, 434
Pliers, ulnar deviation when using, 531–532
Pollicization, 227
Position of function, 423
Positron emission tomography, 36
Posterior cord, 363
Posterior fat pad sign, 99
Posterior interosseous nerve, anatomy of, 69
Posterior interosseous nerve syndrome, 391
Postoperative care, **433–442**
Post-traumatic stress disorder, 77
Postures, cumulative trauma disorders and, 542–543
  stressful, 560
Potassium, burns from, 268
Potassium hydroxide, burns from, 268
Potassium permanganate, burns from, 268
Poultry processing, tool design and, 531–532
Povidone-iodine, burns from, 268
Power press injuries, 49–50
  during maintenance and repair, 49–50
Pre-employment physical examination, legal aspects of,
    507–510
Preoperative care, **155–157**
Presses, power injuries and, 49
Pressure sores, 442
Prevention, of cumulative trauma, **489–505**
  of hand injuries, **47–52**
Prilocaine, 149
Privacy, right to, 508–509
Pronator syndrome, elbow pain and, 295
  vs. carpal tunnel syndrome, 295
Pronator teres syndrome, 371–373
  treatment of, 372
  vs. carpal tunnel syndrome, 372
Propane, burns from, 268
Prostheses, for amputations, 229
  recovery and, 10
Protective clothing, for contact dermatitis, 451
Psoriatic arthritis, 462–463
Psychogenic patient, 39
Psychological assessment, clinical case examples of,
    83–87
  of hand pain, **75–88**
Psychological Pain Inventory, 81
Psychological symptoms, 76–79
Pulp space infection, 427
Pulse volume recording, 321, 332

Pyarthrosis, 141
Pyogenic granuloma, 429, 430
Pyramidal system, 116
Pyroxidine deficiency, in carpal tunnel syndrome, 348

Radial artery, anatomy of, 71
Radial nerve, 121–122, 364
    anatomy of, 69, 388–389
    entrapment of, at the brachium, 389
Radial nerve compression neuropathies, 388–393
Radial nerve palsy, high, 389–390
    occupational cause of, 389
Radial nerve wrist block, 150, 151
Radial sensory nerve, 392–393
Radial sensory nerve entrapment, 391–393
    treatment of, 393
    vs. de Quervain's disease, 392
Radial tunnel syndrome, 55, 390–391
    differential diagnosis of, 391
    elbow pain and, 293–294
    test for, 390
    treatment of, 391
    vs. lateral epicondylitis, 411
Radiographic evaluation, **89–113**
    See also anatomical part
    of joints, 459–460
    of shoulder, 91–96
    of upper extremity, **89–113**
        technical principles of, 89
Radionuclide imaging, 90
    See also anatomical part
Ramazzini, Bernardo, 354
Rapid reversible physiological block, in acute nerve
        compression, 368
Raynaud's disease, 56–57, 465–466
Raynaud's phenomenon, 56–57, 321–322, 323, 334,
        465–466
    occlusive diseases and, 330–333
    vs. secondary Raynaud's phenomenon, 321–322
Reactive arthritis, 463
Real, definition of, 18
Reciprocal determinism, theory of, 34
Recovery, litigation and, 7
    motivation and, **1–11**
Reflex sympathetic dystrophy, 276
    rehabilitative therapy for, 475
Reflexes, of upper extremity, 125
Reflex sympathetic dystrophy, 123
    psychological aspects of, 77
Regional blockade, intravenous, 1
Rehabilitation, hand, **469–477**
    motivation and, **1–11**
Rehabilitation benefits, from workers' compensation, 519
Rehabilitation program, discipline of, 9
Rehabilitation team, education of, 8
Reiter's syndrome, 463–464
Renaut bodies, 118, 369–370
Repetitive motion injuries, See also Cumulative trauma
        disorders
    interventions for, **489–505**
        program of, 492
    prevalence of, 53
Repetitive strain syndrome, 54
Repetitive trauma, of elbow, 290
    occlusive disease and, 330–333
Repetitiveness, definition and measurement of, 541–542
Replantation, affected parts and, 220–221
    anatomical considerations for, 221–222

Replantation, affected parts and, (Continued)
    contraindications for, 219–221
    dressing for, 225
    failure of, 226
    functional outcome of, 216–219
        age and, 219
        amputation level and, 216–219
        criteria for, 218
    indications for, 219–221
    intravenous fluid for, 225
    ischemic time and, 219–220
    long-term sequelae of, 228–229
    major, definition of, 216
    minor, definition of, 216
    patient considerations and, 221
    post-discharge, management of, 226
        physical therapy for, 226–227
    postoperative management of, 225
        medications for, 226
        monitoring for, 226
    re-exploration of, 226
    retraining and, 487
    secondary surgery for, 227
    survival of, 216
    technique of, 222–225
        order of repair for, 223–225
        surgical procedures, 223–225
    upper extremity, **215–231**
    vs. amputation, 219
Respondeat superior, doctrine of, 512
Retraining, for return to work, 486–488
Return to work, 156
    failure to, **483–488**
Return-to-work programs, 6, **479–482**
    ergonomist and, 480–481
    establishment of, 481–482
    evaluation of, 482
    job description and, 485
    occupational physician and, 480
    team approach to, 483–485
Revascularization, definition of, 215
Reverse Bennett's fracture, 200
Reverse Phalen's test, for carpal tunnel syndrome, 377
Rheumatoid arthritis, 460–462
    tenosynovitis in, 405
Ring, safety, 50
Ring injuries, 50
    avulsion, 134
Risk factors, for cumulative trauma, 492–493
    identification of, 540–544
    measurement of, 541–544
    solutions to, 552–556
Robert's view, 184, 194, 196, 198
Rolando's fracture, 193, 194, 195
Rotator cuff tear, 286
    imaging of, 93–94
Rucksack compression injury, 364–365
Runaround, 426

Safe position, 236, 423, 424
Safety features, of machines, 49–51
Saturday night palsy, 121–122
Scalenus-anticus syndrome, 281
Scapholunate advanced collapse (SLAC), 30
Scaphocapitate syndrome, 191
Scaphoid view, 187, 190
Scapula, winging of, 362, 363
Scar formation, 240

Scars, therapy for, 472–473
Schedule of Recent Experience, 82
SCL-90-R, 82
Scleroderma, 466
Screening, for cumulative trauma, 490–492
   clinical examination in, 491–492
   program of, 493
   questionnaire, 490–491
   vibrogram, 491
Secondary gain, 7, 24, 486
Self-employment, recovery and, 4
Semmes-Weinstein monofilaments, 345
   test, for carpal tunnel syndrome, 376, 378
Sensibility, tests of, for carpal tunnel syndrome, 345–
      346
Sensory impairment, 116
Sensory testing, for carpal tunnel syndrome, 376, 378
   of upper extremity, 125
Sentinel Event Notification System for Occupational
      Risks (SENSOR), 55
Sepsis, rapidly spreading, 440–441
Shock, from hemorrhage, 438
Shoulder, anatomy of, 279–280, 407
   function of, 281
   imaging of, 91–96
      dislocations, 92, 93
      fractures, 92, 93
   injuries of, 58
   occupational disorders of, **279–287**
   radiographic anatomy of, 91
   radiographic evaluation of, 91–96
      algorithm for, 91
   tendinitis of, 406–410
      treatment of, 409–410
Shoulder-hand syndrome, 282
Shoulder impingement, imaging of, 95–96
Shoulder pain, 96
   causes of, 280, 281–282
   diagnosis of, 282–285
   differential diagnosis of, 408–409
   history and physical examination of, 282–283
   radiographic evaluation of, 284
   range of motion testing in, 283
   treatment of, 285–286
Sickness Impact Profile, 36
Silvadene, for thermal burns, 261
Single fiber EMG, 126
Skeleton, upper extremity, 61–64
Skier's thumb, 312
Skin, in crushing injuries, 240–241
   of hand, anatomy of, 72–73
      examination of, 133
Skin diseases, 58, **443–454**
   hazardous occupations for, 447
Skin graft, 240
Snuffbox, anatomic, 190
Social Security disability benefits, 521–522
Sodium, burns from, 268
Sodium hydroxide, burns from, 268
Sodium hypochlorite, burns from, 268
Somatization disorder, 78–79
Somatizer, 76
Somatoform disorders, 78
Somatosensory evoked potentials, 128
   dermatomal, 128
Speed's test, 408
Spinal segmental anatomy, 118–120
Splinting, for infection, 426

Splint, aluminum-foam, 209–210
   CMC joint, 474
   complications of, 441–442
   cylinder, 175
   for hand fractures, 210–212
   for thermal burns, 260
   hairpin, 172–173
   hand, safe position for, 203, 211
   hand-based, for thumb MCP joint, 313
   materials for, 211
   palmar, for trigger finger, 473
   splitting of, 436–437
   stack finger, 210
   temporary, 184
Spondyloarthropathy, 456
Stability, vs. change, 34
Stamping machine injuries, 49–50
State-Trait Anxiety Inventory, 81–82
Stenosing tenosynovitis, rehabilitative therapy for, 472
Sterile matrix, 73
Steroid injection, for carpal tunnel syndrome, 349
   for tennis elbow, 291
Stockinette, use of, in postoperative care, 434–435
Streptococcus, postoperative infection with, 440–441
Stress, response to, 80–81
Stress x-ray, 185
Styloidectomy, 303, 305
Subluxation, 181, 182
Suffering, definition of, 79
Suits, law, reasons for, 512–513
Sulfuric acid, burns from 268
Supraspinatus tendon, 407–408, 409
Surveillance, for cumulative trauma, 490–492
   passive, 545–546
Swan-neck deformity, 173
   in rheumatoid arthritis, 461
Swelling, complications of, 436
Symptom exaggeration, learned, 30
Synovial biopsy, 460
Synovial fluid analysis, 459
Synovial osteochondromatosis, imaging of, 96
Synovitis, chronic, 456
   crystal-induced, 456
   postinjection flare, 410
Syringomyelia, 116, 117
Systemic lupus erythematosus, 466

Tachistoscope, 32
Tajima suture, 224
Tar, burns from, 266
Task analysis, 494
Task modification, 494–495
Taylor-Pelmear classification, 326
Team, rehabilitation, education of, 8
Technetium-99m bone scan, for fractures, 185
Tendinitis, 55, **403–421**
   bicipital, 285–286
   calcific, 409
   diagnosis of, 405–406
   epidemiology of, 404
   etiology of, 404–405
   in dorsal compartments of wrist, 412–416
   of elbow, 290, 410–412
      treatment of, 412
   of shoulder, 406–410
      treatment of, 409–410
   of wrist and hand, 412–419

Tendinitis, (*Continued*)
  rehabilitative therapy for, 471
  repetitions and, 542
  terminology of, 403
  treatment of, 405–406
Tendon(s), anatomy of, 403–404
  biceps, rupture of, 292
  crush injuries to, 243
  examination of, 135–136
  flexor digitorum profundus, injuries to, 177–178
  hand, injuries to, **171–179**
Tendon sheath infection, 427–428, 429
Tendons,
Tennis elbow, 100–101, 290–292, 410
Tenosynovitis, 55
  atypical *Mycobacterium* infection and, 405
  carpal tunnel syndrome and, 343
  definition of, 403
  digital flexor, of the wrist, 417–418
  flexor, of the digits, 418–419
  flexor carpi radialis, 417
  flexor carpi ulnaris, 417
  in dorsal compartments of wrist, 412–416
  in rheumatoid arthritis, 405
  in spondyloarthropathies, 405
Tests, *See also* specific tests
  for carpal tunnel syndrome, 345–348
  sensibility, 345–346
Tetanus, prophylaxis for, 138, 426
  wounds prone to develop, 137
Textile machine injury, 132
Thalamic syndrome, 116
Thenar infections, 428–429
Therblig work elements, 542
Third parties, influence of, in recovery, 10
Third-party claims, workers' compensation and, 521
Thoracic outlet compression, 334–336
  treatment of, 335–336
Thoracic outlet syndrome, 55, 123, 334–336, 359–362
  categories of, 359–360
  criteria for, 359
  evaluation of, 361–362
  neurological, 360
  rehabilitative therapy for, 474–475
  shoulder pain and, 281–282
  treatment of, 362
  vascular, 360–361
Threshold tests, 345–346
Thrombosis, 330–333
  in crushing injuries, 241
  of hand, 324
Throwing arm injury, 293
Thumb, arterial anatomy of, 222
  CMC joints of, injuries to, 315–316
  fractures and dislocations of, 193–198
  ligament injuries of, 311–314, 315–316
  MCP joint of, 311–314
  neural entrapments in, 380
  reconstruction of, 227–228
  replantation of, 218
Time and motion study, 541–542
Tinel's test, for carpal tunnel syndrome, 347
Title VII, 507–508
Tomography, *See also* anatomical part
  for fractures, 185
Tools, hand, contour of, 529–530
  posture during use of, 530–532
  texture of, 532–534

Tools, hand, contour of, (*Continued*)
  work parameters and, 547–548
  hand held, ergonomic design of, 527–537
   handles of, 527–529, 533
   hand-held activation devices and, 536
   in cumulative trauma disorders, 543–544
   weight of, 534–535
Tourniquet, complications of, 441–442
  for hemorrhage, 438
Tourniquet test, 347
Transcutaneous electrical nerve stimulation (TENS), 406
Transfer, emergency, procedure for, 155
Trapezius myalgia, 409
Triangular fibrocartilage complex, 63
Trichloroacetic acid, burns from, 268
Trigger finger, therapy for, 472
Trigger points, characteristics of, 355–356, 357
Triggers, on hand held tools, 536
Tumor, of shoulder, imaging of, 96
Two-hand devices, 49
Two-point discrimination test, 160, 274
  for carpal tunnel syndrome, 345

Ulnar carpal abutment syndrome, 306
Ulnar collateral ligament, of the thumb, 64
Ulnar nerve, 364
  anatomy of, 70, 121, 380–381
   in the forearm, 385
   in Guyon's canal, 385–386
   sensory distribution of, 382
Ulnar nerve compression, 380–388
  in the forearm, 383–385
Ulnar neuropathies, at the wrist, classification of, 386–387
  occupational causes of, 387
  management of, 387–388
Ulnar nerve wrist block, 150, 151
Ulnar palsy, neuroanatomy and, 70–71
Ulnar snuff box, 301
Ultrasound, of shoulder, 94
Upper extremity, **1–567**, *See also* Hand
  amputations of, **215–231**
  anatomy of, **61–73**
  anesthesia for, **143–157**
  cost of work-related accidents to, 48, 53
  motor examination of, 124–125
  nerve root innervation of, 119
  neurologic evaluation of, **115–130**
   examination and, 124–129
  occupational injuries to, etiologies and prevalence of, **53–60**
  postoperative care of, 434
  radiography of, **89–113**
  reflexes of, 125
  replantations of, **215–231**
  sensory dermatomes of, 119
  sensory testing of, 125
  venous drainage of, 71–72
Upper extremity injuries, costs of, 53
  etiologies of, **53–60**
  prevalence of, **53–60**
Urticaria, contact, 447–448
U.S. Department of Labor, 522

Vasa nervorum, 118
Vascular injuries and diseases, upper extremity, **319–339**

Vascular injuries and diseases, (*Continued*)
  assessment of, 319–321
  chemically induced, 333–334
  neurological symptoms of, 324
  presentation of, 319
  tests for, 320–321
Vascular supply, to hand, examination of, 133–134
Vascular system, of upper extremity, 71–72
Vasoconstriction, from vibration, 326–327
Venous claudication, 336
Venous occlusion, 336
Vibration, exposure to, clinical manifestations of, 325
  exposure standards of, 328–329
  in cumulative trauma disorders, 543–544
  measurement of, 326
  tool design and, 534
Vibration injuries, prevalence of, 53
Vibration syndromes, 324–330
  diagnosis of, 328
  pathogenesis of, 326–328
  prevention of, 329
  treatment of, 329
Vibration testing, in acute nerve compression, 368
Vibration white finger disease, 56–57, 324–330
Vibrogram, 491
Video display terminal, cumulative trauma syndrome
    and, 56
Video display terminals, 479
Videotape, in job analysis, 552
  of upper extremity cumulative trauma disorders,
    guidelines for preparing, 561–563
Vinyl chloride disease, 333–334
Visual analog scale, 36
Vitamin B$_6$, for carpal tunnel syndrome, 348, 379
Vocational rehabilitation, 486–488
Vocational Rehabilitation Act of 1973, 508
Volar flexion intercalated segment instability (VISI), 298,
    299, 308
Volar plate, injuries to, 313–314, 315
  rupture of, 313–314
Von Frey pressure test, 345

Wallerian degeneration, 126
  in acute nerve compression, 368
Wartenberg's syndrome, 391–393
Weber two-point discrimination test, 345–346
West Point view, 92, 284, 285
White finger disease, 56–57, 324–330
Woodworking injuries, 50
Work accidents, classification of, 47
Work capacity evaluation, 475–476
Work hardening, 475–476

Workers' compensation, administration of, 516
  offices for, 522–525
  benefits of, 518–519
  coverage of, 516
    liability trade-off of, 516–517
    objectives of, 517
  entitlement to, 520–521
  funding of, 518
  goals of the patient and, 7
  legal issues of, **515–525**
  physician's duty and, 510–512
  procedures of, 519–520
  Social Security benefits and, 521–522
  special funds of, 517
  third-party claims and, 521
Workers' compensation claims, from contact dermatitis,
    452
  penalties related to, 522
  preexisting conditions and, 453
  reopening of, 522
  statutes of limitations of, 522
Workers' compensation insurance, 29–30
Work parameters, 547
Workplace, unsafe acts in, 48–49
Workplace layout, 551
Work-relatedness, workers' compensation and, 521
Workstation, 547
Wright's hyperabduction test, 361
Wrist, anatomy of, 62–63
  arthrography of, 105–107
  carpal instability of, 297–300
  computed tomography of, 107
  conjunct rotation of, 297, 298
  diagnostic evaluation of, 301–303
  dorsal compartments of, 412–416
  function of, 297
  imaging of, 103–108
  injuries to, 57
  instability of, 297–300
  ligament injuries of, **297–309**
    treatment of, 303–308
  MRI of, 107–108
  plain films of, 104
  radiographic anatomy of, 103–104
  radiographic evaluation of, 301–303
  radiocuclide imaging of, 104–105, 106
  tomography of, 104
Wrist block, 148, 150

X-ray evaluation, *See* Radiographic evaluation

Yergason's test, 408